Football Traumatology

Piero Volpi
Editor

Football Traumatology

New Trends

Second Edition

Springer

Editor
Piero Volpi
Knee Orthopedics and
Sport Traumatology Unit
Humanitas Clinical Institute IRCCS
Milan
Italy

Head of Medical Staff FC
Internazionale Milan
Milan
Italy

ISBN 978-3-319-18244-5 ISBN 978-3-319-18245-2 (eBook)
DOI 10.1007/978-3-319-18245-2

Library of Congress Control Number: 2015944540

Springer Cham Heidelberg New York Dordrecht London

Printed on acid-free paper

Springer International Publishing AG Switzerland is part of Springer Science+Business Media (www.springer.com)

Foreword I

Football is not only a fantastic and unique sport with benefits in terms of cultural diversity, social and ethnic mix, and education; it also has numerous positive effects on well-being and health. Many conditions, such as obesity and drug addiction, can be combated through the promotion of football activities. This has recently been recognized by FIFA's original and promising program "FIFA for Health." The prevention of disease is a key aspect of participation in football, and on a related note, some famous players have been involved in promoting vaccinations and other actions.

On the other hand, it is self-evident that participation in the sport can be halted at any moment by a serious injury. For many years, medical doctors, physios, coaches, and players have therefore been keen to identify effective treatments that will enable return to full sporting activity within the shortest possible time. This book identifies those treatments that are most appropriate in different circumstances, providing state-of-the-art descriptions of surgical and medical treatment options relating to, for example, particular joints or specific types of injury. It also addresses two other crucial aspects: prevention of injuries and long-term outcomes. When speaking of the "health" of the footballer, it is necessary to consider not only the period during which the sport is played but the entire lifetime of the player.

Taking into account the fact that football is played everywhere in the world by males and females and by amateurs and professionals, there is no doubt that the management of traumatic injuries, from prevention to treatment and return to the pitch, must be performed by educated and informed professionals. This book, written by recognized experts and coordinated by an outstanding staff, offers a unique contribution to the current knowledge of sports traumatology in football and will be of great practical value.

Philippe Neyret
Académie Médicale du Football de Lyon,
ISAKOS President,
Lyon, France

Foreword II

As a past professional footballer and current President of the Italian Footballers' Association, I am naturally interested in all aspects of injuries to players, including prevention, treatment, and rehabilitation. During my footballing career I had personal experience of injuries, both minor and very serious, including one major injury suffered when I was 30. That injury did, however, have one positive outcome in that it enabled me to understand the consequences of serious injury for the player, including the psychological impact, in a way that otherwise would not have been possible. I recovered and returned to play with even more energy (if that was possible!) than previously, but I did so with a particular sensitivity to the disruption that a traumatic event can cause to a successful professional career.

Within football, injuries are unfortunately a constant and recurring event. As an executive and a former professional player, I have observed that the limited time devoted to injury prevention is playing an important role in the increase in muscle injuries and trauma. Regrettably, sport activity planning too rarely takes account of the player as an athlete, being oriented instead to the footballer as a showman. Thus the player has more games, including more luxury friendly matches, and spends more time touring while devoting less time to training, preparation, and recovery – and recovery has been the subject of our recent conservations with players. In this context, last season we produced a short but very informative video on overmedication. Our goal has been, and continues to be, to persuade athletes, who are often very young and focused on other matters, to take care of their bodies. Each athlete has to work with his or her own body, and looking after it properly is the first rule that must be followed in order to become a true professional.

Excessively hasty return to playing following an injury and the use of drugs and therapies to accelerate a return or to enhance the capacity for training and exercise may have serious repercussions after a professional career is over. It is essential both to allow the correct recovery time after a traumatic event and to realize the potential long-term impacts of heavy use of drugs and "invasive" therapies.

This is a hot issue since playing at all costs often appears to be in everybody's interest: the player's, the coach's, the doctor's, the supporter's, and the president's. It is difficult but necessary work to gain a sufficiently deep knowledge of the risks and benefits of different therapies and approaches, and of their contraindications, as a sound basis for decision making.

The Italian Footballers' Association has always been attentive to the issue of the health of players, and we are most grateful to Dr. Volpi for his valuable work in this field. This publication bears witness to his extremely high levels of competence and professionalism. The in-depth analysis in this book, which brings together expertise from several countries, is most welcome and should significantly raise awareness of issues surrounding the prevention of injuries, as well as their evaluation, treatment, and rehabilitation.

Finally, I would like to offer a bitter reflection that may nevertheless also offer hope for the future. If we are unable to take care of footballers' bodies through appropriate preventive and rehabilitative strategies, the high number of absences of "showmen" players will continue unabated. Perhaps even the cynical business interests in the sport will come to realize that impacts are to be felt not only on the health of the athlete but also on the quality and profitability of events.

Damiano Tommasi,
President, Italian Footballers' Association,
Vicenza, Italy

Preface

Over recent decades, much has been done in football to promote health protection, particularly in the context of sports trauma prevention. Significant progress has been made in sports medicine as applied to football, with the introduction of innovative diagnostic tests and therapeutic methods. Furthermore, the knowledge of the medical staff of football teams with respect to trauma prevention and management has improved significantly.

The desire to decrease the incidence of trauma in professional and amateur sportspeople reflects the primary need to preserve their physical integrity and health, even after the end of their sporting careers. With regard to football, recent data show a constant increase in the frequency and severity of trauma during both matches and training. This is particularly true for athletes of high-level professional teams due to the pressures of additional national and international matches. The high number of matches restricts the opportunity for rest between matches and hinders regular and effective training. However, similar problems are also reported by footballers who play on a weekly basis. Moreover, modern football differs in many respects from football in the past: the game is more intense, the players' movements are faster and more explosive, and their physical structure is more powerful.

On the regulatory front, there have been several interesting proposals, for instance, to increase the number of substitutions permitted during a match. At the same time, early season preparation tends to be too short, with too many official engagements. Furthermore, many athletes would prefer a longer winter break in order to ensure a proper recovery for the second part of the season.

Football needs not only competence and professionalism but also passion. Only those who love this sport, experience its fascination, rejoice in victory, and suffer the inevitable setbacks can express their feelings on the field and help football to mature further. Passion will be essential in order to innovate and to maintain and defend the values that are the essence of this marvellous sport.

Piero Volpi
Knee Orthopedics and Sport Traumatology Unit,
Humanitas Clinical Institute IRCCS,
Milan, Italy

Head of Medical Staff FC Internazionale Milan,
Milan, Italy

About the Editor

Piero Volpi is an Orthopedic Surgeon and Sports Medicine Specialist and Director of the Knee Surgery and Sport Traumatology Unit at Humanitas Clinical Institute IRCCS, Milan. He played professional football from the beginning of the 1970s until 1985 while maintaining his medical studies. He is now Head of Medical Staff FC Internazionale Milan, Italy, and is also Responsible Physician of the Italian Association of Football Players (AIC). He has also recently been appointed as member of U.E.F.A. Medical Committee. Dr. Volpi is Teaching Professor at the Specialty School of Orthopedics and Traumatology at the University of Milan. He is also Vice-President of Italian Arthroscopy Society (SIA) and member of several national and international scientific societies: SIOT, SIGASCOT, FMSI, ISAKOS, ESSKA, AND EKA. He is the author of more than 300 publications and over 600 contributions, including book chapters, articles, and presentations to scientific national and international meetings. He is Editor in Chief of the *Journal of Sports Traumatology* and Member of Editorial Board of *Medicina dello Sport Journal.*

Contents

Part I

General Concepts

1 Epidemiology in Professional Footballers

Cristiano Eirale

Epidemiology is the science that studies the patterns, causes and effects of health and disease conditions in defined populations.

The study of professional footballers' injury epidemiology has recently gained importance due to the high number of players involved and the economic interests linked to professional football. Injures have a considerable economic impact in a club: if we consider that, on average, 10–15 % of the team is always unavailable due to injuries, it becomes clear how we can speculate that this percentage of the players' wages is wasted.

Moreover, it has been shown that injuries have a direct impact on the results [1, 2], therefore again an indirect influence on the economy of the club.

The way to reduce injury incidence is called prevention. Conducting an injury surveillance study is the fundamental first step in order to implement an adequate programme of prevention.

For these reasons, professional clubs and national and international associations have implemented epidemiological researches in professional footballers. FIFA (Fédération Internationale de Football Association) has implemented surveys during its competitions [3–6], while UEFA (Union of European Football Associations) has started a prospective study on its most important competition at club level, the UEFA Champions League [7, 8]. Some national federations have implemented epidemiological researches as well [9, 10].

1.1 Methodology

Unfortunately, the results of different researches are often incomparable due to the different methodology utilized.

The main debatable concept to be considered is the injury definition.

In early studies, reports from emergency departments and insurance claims have been utilized. It is clear that these definitions have many limitations; the most important is that, counting only injuries which are referred to a specific hospital or for which an insurance claim to a definite company has been performed, only serious injuries are usually recorded, while minor complains are lost. Moreover, the lack of exposure time doesn't allow a calculation of the incidence [11].

The "medical attention" definition focuses on those injuries for which the footballers seek the help of a clinician. This may help to collect a high number of injuries, also the lesions that doesn't oblige the player to stop his activity but may have an impact of further injuries or at least on his performance. If this definition provides a wide picture of the impact of the injuries on the athletes, it also relies on factors like the

C. Eirale
Aspetar – Qatar Orthopedic and Sport Medicine Hospital, Doha, Qatar
e-mail: Cristiano.eirale@aspetar.com

P. Volpi (ed.), *Football Traumatology: New Trends*, DOI 10.1007/978-3-319-18245-2_1

availability of medical staff and the players' pain threshold.

The time-loss injury definition indicates that the injury forces the athlete to miss at least a future training session or a match [12]. This definition is often utilized in the prospective cohort studies on football [13, 14], especially at club level [7, 9, 15–17], and therefore it has the advantage that allows the comparison of the results. Moreover, this definition allows a good identification of the injuries impacting the footballer's activity; however, its main limitation is that all the injuries, despite which the player continues his football activity, are not recorded and therefore missed. Since footballers often compete with minor injuries [18], especially overuse in aetiology [19], this definition may not offer a correct picture of the injury epidemiology in football.

In addition to the different definitions, also other major methodological dissimilarities were present in early epidemiological researches, such as the exposure and injury data collection modalities.

For this reasons, a meeting among experts has taken place in 2006 during which guidelines on football epidemiological studies were established [12].

1.2 Main Challenges

An important factor is the reliability of data. Football epidemiological studies often require the involvement of multiple clubs and therefore clinicians with different backgrounds may be involved. This can be a source of bias. First, it has to be verified that all participants utilize the same medical approach in diagnosis and prognosis. In this view, it is better that all clinicians involved in the data collection are part of the same professional category, for example, sport medicine physicians, orthopaedic surgeons or physiotherapists. Sometimes, this is not enough because they may be part of different medical schools; some studies involve teams from all over the world [20] with an undeniable different approach to sport medicine.

Another important matter is not only the quality of the data but also their completeness. Prospective studies may last an entire season or even more. A continuous supervision is fundamental in order to ensure complete collection. New technologies such as mobile phones, table PC and specific softwares have been implemented with this aim. In addition, recent literature shows the need for a revision of the best definition of injury to be utilized, in order to capture at the best kinds of injuries and complaints [19].

1.3 Epidemiological Researches in Professional Football

The highest expression of club-level football in the world is arguably represented by the UEFA Champions League. Since 2001, UEFA has implemented an injury analysis among some clubs participating to this competition, with the aim of reducing injuries which, at this level, have a high economic impact. Actually, this study involves more than 20 European top-level football clubs from different countries. Each day, injury data, together with information on the football activity exposure of each player, are collected by the medical staff of these clubs [21]. The results of this survey have been extensively published in the scientific literature [7, 22–25] and helped to identify the most common injuries and their characteristics. This may favour the implementation of prevention programmes at club level.

Similarly, FIFA is also conducting surveys in all its main competitions at male, female and youth level [3, 4, 6, 20, 26]. Many national associations [9, 10, 27, 28] have implemented injury registries and numerous clubs have developed independent injury data for their teams [29].

1.4 Injury Incidence

It has been estimated that its overall risk of injury in football is about 1,000 times higher than for typical industrial occupations generally regarded as high risk [30].

Luckily, while in the last three decades the training and match volume has increased, the risk of injury has not augmented. This is perhaps due to the improvement of athlete healthcare and to the implementation of prevention programmes. According to the UEFA Champions League injury study, a professional football team can expect about 50 time-loss injuries per season, and on average, 12 % of the squad is unavailable due to injury at any moment of the season [31]. Anyway, on average every player can expect at least one injury every season. In terms of incidence, the rate in football is included between 10 and 35/1,000 match hours, increasing with the level of play, especially during matches [32].

The injury rate increases during tournaments, compared with the course of the season. This is certainly due to the higher match exposure but possibly also to other factors like psychological pressure and fatigue. These risk factors, however, have still to be confirmed by the scientific evidence.

At club level, it has been reported a higher incidence of injuries, especially overuse in aetiology, at the beginning of the season. This may be due to the fact that players may not have reached optimal physical and physiological states at that time [27].

The debate about possible differences in injury rates between positions in the field is still open. It seems that strikers have a higher injury rate than midfielder and defenders [33]. However, other researches showed a higher rate in defenders [34] and midfielders [35]. Most of the studies show a lower incidence in goalkeepers, compared with field players [36].

1.5 Match and Training Injury Rates

Most injuries occur during matches, where there is five times higher risk of injury compared with training. This is possibly due to the high intensity of the match play and to the higher amount and energy of duels and impacts. Other factors like the pressure of the results, fair play and psychological and environmental factors should be taken into consideration. It has to be also considered how there is no possibility, during matches, of seeking medical care if not for a few minutes, while during training injuries may be evaluated more carefully by the medical staff and preventive player changes can be performed. In particular, the last 15 min of each half is the period in which players are most vulnerable to injuries and fatigue plays probably a major role in this.

1.6 Reinjuries

In general, a reinjury is defined as an injury at the same side and location of a previous lesion. When it occurs within 2 months from the return to play, it is usually defined as early reinjury and is often seen as a failure of the treatment.

Therefore, reinjury rate is sometimes considered as a medical staff performance indicator. In effect, while injury frequency may be mostly affected by technical and performance activities, reinjuries, as determined by an early return to play and incomplete rehabilitation, are often associated with medical staff performance. In more recent football studies, a reinjury rate between 12 % and 30 % has been reported [7, 13, 14, 27, 28]. Frequently, reinjuries are generally associated with higher severity (return to play time) compared with first injuries. This, together with the relatively high incidence, underlines the importance of the utilization of correct guidelines in the return-to-play decision. There is a need for new football-specific medical and physical tests to assess athletes before they return to play. Objective data could help the clinician avoid an attitude that is too aggressive (which could increase the risk of reinjury) or too conservative (which would have a negative impact on the lay-off time of the athletes).

1.7 Types and Locations of Injury

In epidemiological studies based on a time-loss definition of injuries, the most common injury location is the thigh, followed by the knee, groin and ankle, while the most common type of injury is strain, followed by contusion and sprain [31]. When considering medical attention injuries, contusions are the most common type of injuries. However, a contusion seldom obliges a player to stop his sport activity; therefore they are less recorded in studies utilizing a time-loss definition. This example highlights the importance of choosing an appropriate injury definition in according with the sport and the environment. Also, it is fundamental to interpret the results of any epidemiological study in according with the chosen definition.

Hamstring strains are the most common subtype of injuries and a typical 25-player team can expect about seven hamstring strains per season [23, 31]. It is therefore evident how, like in many other sports, many efforts are focused on the prevention and treatment of this injury.

Despite their relative low incidence (<1 % of all injuries), anterior cruciate ligament (ACL) ruptures are the most attention-drawing pathology in football due to the long absence from sport activity that they imply. Nowadays, in football, ACL lesions are generally treated surgically and the average time to return to play is between 6 and 7 months. While some decades ago it was a career-ending injury, progress in sport surgery and rehabilitation has led to a return-to-football outcome at the same level as before the injury in 90 % of the patients. However, on return to play there is an increased risk of new knee pathologies, especially overuse in aetiology [37]. This may indicate knee abuse due to the absolute necessity of professional footballers of returning to play [38].

The hip and the groin are normally the third-fourth most common injury location in prospective epidemiological studies based on a time-loss injury definition [9, 31]. It seems that the real magnitude of the problem has been underestimated so far, due to the relatively difficult diagnosis of the pathologies located in that region, not always allowing their clear identification and classification. Moreover, groin injuries are often overuse in aetiology and may be underestimated in researches based on a time-loss injury definition [19]. In the UEFA Champions League study, an average of seven groin injuries per team per season has been estimated [39], but, for the above-mentioned reasons, this may be only the tip of the iceberg. In fact, it is well known among clinicians that the groin pain syndrome is often a difficult pathology to be treated, frequently requiring long treatments and an appropriate management of training and match loading, in other words, an impacting lesion in football, no matter what statistics may show.

The ankle is the most common injury location in many sports [40]. While first football epidemiological researches performed in the eighties were reporting that the ankle was the most common location of injury (around 30 % of total number of injuries), more recent researches show a much inferior incidence rate [8]. This decreasing trend can be the result prevention strategies (e.g. neuromuscular training, bracing, taping), which have proved to be effective in reducing the incidence of ankle sprain, or this may be due to changes of the rules of the game which have been applied, such as a red card for a tackle from behind. In any case, this finding has to be taken into account as an example of the possibility of reducing injuries in football.

1.8 Overuse and Traumatic Injuries

In according with their aetiology, injuries are classified in overuse and traumatic. For overuse injuries a specific moment in which the injury occurred cannot be identified [41]. There is evidence that overuse football injuries have a higher incidence during the preseason. This is probably due to the increased workload. For what concern other periods of the season, different trends of seasonality are linked to different regions and their specific environmental conditions.

1.9 Injury Trends

If the injury rate has decreased for ligament injuries, overall training, match injury rates and the rates of muscle injury and severe injury have not been reduced [8]. It is difficult to understand the reasons of this; theoretically the increasing number of evidence-based prevention programmes should be a crucial tool in the hands of the clinicians. This may be due to the increasing demands on footballers (higher numbers of season games, higher intensity) or possibly to the difficulties in implementing such programmes at elite level.

1.10 Women Football

Women's football has gained more and more prominence in the last years. The number of participants has quickly increased together with the discipline's professionalism. While males have a general higher risk of injury compared with female players, the risk of sustaining a moderate to severe injury (>1 week absence) does not vary between men and women. Injury patterns are also basically comparable but women have relatively more knee injuries while men more groin pathologies [42]. Female players are particularly more vulnerable for ACL injuries. It has been estimated that the risk is two to three times higher than their male counterparts. Females also tend to sustain their ACL injury at a younger age and have a higher risk of injury especially during match play, while no significant gender-related variation has been described during training sessions [42]. These data have provided the basis for an extensive scientific research on the prevention for ACL injury in female footballers [42, 43].

1.11 Youth Football

Young footballers' injuries are more overuse in aetiology compared with adults. Of vital importance seems to be a strict training load monitoring. The huge differences in growth between subjects and the unpreparedness to too intense training loads may be a serious risk factor [44–47]. Female players tend to suffer more knee-related injuries, while males are more prone to ankle injuries. Common pathologies are Sever and Osgood-Schlatter diseases.

1.12 Influence of the Medical Staff on Injuries

Epidemiological data highlight the importance of the medical staff, whose role in many clubs and federations is still undervalued. The impact on prevention of injuries and reinjuries may be notable.

Often, investments on medical personnel and equipment are still overlooked, even in professional football, and there is debate on the methods of medical staff recruitment and its effective impact on the economy of the clubs [48]. It has been already stated at the beginning of the chapter that injury rates are correlated with the results of the clubs [1, 2]: this should lead professional football managers to carefully evaluate the possibility of providing their athletes with the best medical care, not only to preserve their health but also with the ultimate purpose of influencing the team performance.

References

1. Eirale C, Tol JL, Farooq A, Smiley F, Chalabi H (2013) Low injury rate strongly correlates with team success in Qatari professional football. Br J Sports Med 47(12):807–8
2. Hägglund M, Waldén M, Magnusson H, Kristenson K, Bengtsson H, Ekstrand J (2013) Injuries affect team performance negatively in professional football: an 11-year follow-up of the UEFA Champions League injury study. Br J Sports Med 47(12):738–42
3. Dvorak J, Junge A, Derman W, Schwellnus M (2011) Injuries and illnesses of football players during the 2010 FIFA world cup. Br J Sports Med 45(8):626–630
4. Dvorak J, Junge A, Grimm K, Kirkendall D (2007) Medical report from the 2006 FIFA world cup Germany. Br J Sports Med 41(9):578–581, discussion 581
5. Junge A, Dvorak J (2013) Injury surveillance in the World Football Tournaments 1998-2012. Br J Sports Med 47(12):782–8
6. Junge A, Dvorak J, Graf-Baumann T (2004) Football injuries during the world cup 2002. Am J Sports Med 32(1 Suppl):23S–27S
7. Walden M, Hagglund M, Ekstrand J (2005) UEFA Champions League study: a prospective study of injuries in professional football during the 2001–2002 season. Br J Sports Med 39(8):542–546
8. Ekstrand J, Hagglund M, Kristenson K, Magnusson H, Walden M (2013) Fewer ligament injuries but no preventive effect on muscle injuries and severe injuries: an 11-year follow-up of the UEFA Champions League injury study. Br J Sports Med 47(12):732–737
9. Eirale C, Farooq A, Smiley FA, Tol JL, Chalabi H (2013) Epidemiology of football injuries in Asia: a prospective study in Qatar. J Sci Med Sport 16(2): 113–117
10. Bjorneboe J, Bahr R, Andersen TE (2010) Risk of injury on third-generation artificial turf in Norwegian professional football. Br J Sports Med 44(11): 794–798
11. Junge A, Dvorak J (2000) Influence of definition and data collection on the incidence of injuries in football. Am J Sports Med 28(5 Suppl):S40–S46

12. Fuller CW, Ekstrand J, Junge A et al (2006) Consensus statement on injury definitions and data collection procedures in studies of football (soccer) injuries. Clin J Sport Med 16(2):97–106
13. Eirale C, Hamilton B, Bisciotti G, Grantham J, Chalabi H (2012) Injury epidemiology in a national football team of the Middle East. Scand J Med Sci Sports 22(3):323–329
14. Ekstrand J, Walden M, Hagglund M (2004) Risk for injury when playing in a national football team. Scand J Med Sci Sports 14(1):34–38
15. Hassabi MM, Mortazavi SM, Giti MR, Mansournia M, Shapouran S (2010) Injury profile of an Iranian professional soccer team, in the Premier League. Asian J Sports Med 4:201–208
16. Morgan BE, Oberlander MA (2001) An examination of injuries in major league soccer. The inaugural season. Am J Sports Med 29(4):426–430
17. Hagglund M, Walden M, Ekstrand J (2003) Exposure and injury risk in Swedish elite football: a comparison between seasons 1982 and 2001. Scand J Med Sci Sports 13(6):364–370
18. Hammond LE, Lilley JM, Pope GD, Ribbans WJ (2014) The impact of playing in matches while injured on injury surveillance findings in professional football. Scand J Med Sci Sports 24(3):e195–200
19. Bahr R (2009) No injuries, but plenty of pain? On the methodology for recording overuse symptoms in sports. Br J Sports Med 43(13):966–972
20. Junge A, Dvorak J, Graf-Baumann T, Peterson L (2004) Football injuries during FIFA tournaments and the olympic games, 1998–2001: development and implementation of an injury-reporting system. Am J Sports Med 32(1 Suppl):80S–89S
21. Hagglund M, Walden M, Bahr R, Ekstrand J (2005) Methods for epidemiological study of injuries to professional football players: developing the UEFA model. Br J Sports Med 39(6):340–346
22. Hagglund M, Zwerver J, Ekstrand J (2011) Epidemiology of patellar tendinopathy in elite male soccer players. Am J Sports Med 39(9):1906–1911
23. Ekstrand J, Hagglund M, Walden M (2011) Epidemiology of muscle injuries in professional football (soccer). Am J Sports Med 39(6):1226–1232
24. Nilsson M, Hägglund M, Ekstrand J, Waldén M (2013) Head and neck injuries in professional soccer. Clin J Sport Med 23(4):255–60
25. Lundblad M, Waldén M, Magnusson H, Karlsson J, Ekstrand J (2013) The UEFA injury study: 11-year data concerning 346 MCL injuries and time to return to play. Br J Sports Med 47(12):759–62
26. Junge A, Dvorak J (2007) Injuries in female football players in top-level international tournaments. Br J Sports Med 41(Suppl 1):i3–i7
27. Hagglund M, Walden M, Ekstrand J (2005) Injury incidence and distribution in elite football–a prospective study of the Danish and the Swedish top divisions. Scand J Med Sci Sports 15(1):21–28
28. Hagglund M, Walden M, Ekstrand J (2006) Previous injury as a risk factor for injury in elite football: a prospective study over two consecutive seasons. Br J Sports Med 40(9):767–772
29. Hassabi M, Mohammad-Javad Mortazavi S, Giti MR, Mansournia MA, Shapouran S (2010) Injury profile of a professional soccer team in the premier league of iran. Asian J Sports Med 1(4):201–208
30. Fuller CW, Junge A, Dvorak J (2012) Risk management: FIFA's approach for protecting the health of football players. Br J Sports Med 46(1):11–17
31. Ekstrand J, Hagglund M, Walden M (2011) Injury incidence and injury patterns in professional football: the UEFA injury study. Br J Sports Med 45(7): 553–558
32. Dvorak J, Junge A (2000) Football injuries and physical symptoms. A review of the literature. Am J Sports Med 28(5 Suppl):S3–S9
33. Carling C, Orhant E, LeGall F (2010) Match injuries in professional soccer: inter-seasonal variation and effects of competition type, match congestion and positional role. Int J Sports Med 31(4):271–276
34. Peterson L, Junge A, Chomiak J, Graf-Baumann T, Dvorak J (2000) Incidence of football injuries and complaints in different age groups and skill-level groups. Am J Sports Med 28(5 Suppl):S51–S57
35. Arnason A, Sigurdsson SB, Gudmundsson A, Holme I, Engebretsen L, Bahr R (2004) Risk factors for injuries in football. Am J Sports Med 32(1 Suppl):5S–16S
36. Eirale C, Tol JL, Whiteley R, Chalabi H, Hölmich P (2014) Different injury pattern in goalkeepers compared to field players: a three-year epidemiological study of professional football. J Sci Med Sport 17(1):34–8
37. Walden M, Hagglund M, Ekstrand J (2006) High risk of new knee injury in elite footballers with previous anterior cruciate ligament injury. Br J Sports Med 40(2):158–162, discussion 158–162
38. Ekstrand J (2011) A 94% return to elite level football after ACL surgery: a proof of possibilities with optimal caretaking or a sign of knee abuse? Knee Surg Sports Traumatol Arthrosc 19(1):1–2
39. Werner J, Hagglund M, Walden M, Ekstrand J (2009) UEFA injury study: a prospective study of hip and groin injuries in professional football over seven consecutive seasons. Br J Sports Med 43(13):1036–1040
40. Fong DT, Hong Y, Chan LK, Yung PS, Chan KM (2007) A systematic review on ankle injury and ankle sprain in sports. Sports Med 37(1):73–94
41. Orava S (1980) Exertion injuries due to sports and physical exercise. A clinical and statistical study of nontraumatic overuse injuries of the musculoskeletal system of athletes and keep-fit athletes. University of Oulu, Oulu
42. Walden M, Hagglund M, Werner J, Ekstrand J (2011) The epidemiology of anterior cruciate ligament injury in football (soccer): a review of the literature from a gender-related perspective. Knee Surg Sports Traumatol Arthrosc 19(1):3–10
43. Moses B, Orchard J (2012) Systematic review: annual incidence of ACL injury and surgery in various populations. Res Sports Med 20(3-4):157–179

44. Backous DD, Friedl KE, Smith NJ, Parr TJ, Carpine WD Jr (1988) Soccer injuries and their relation to physical maturity. Am J Dis Child 142(8):839–842
45. Bergeron MF, McKeag DB, Casa DJ et al (2005) Youth football: heat stress and injury risk. Med Sci Sports Exerc 37(8):1421–1430
46. Brito J, Rebelo A, Soares JM, Seabra A, Krustrup P, Malina RM (2011) Injuries in youth soccer during the preseason. Clin J Sport Med 21(3): 259–260
47. Carter CW, Micheli LJ (2011) Training the child athlete: physical fitness, health and injury. Br J Sports Med 45(11):880–885
48. Orchard JW (2009) On the value of team medical staff: can the "Moneyball" approach be applied to injuries in professional football? Br J Sports Med 43(13):963–965

2 Epidemiology in Young Football Players

Oliver Faude and Roland Rössler

2.1 Introduction

Football is the most popular sport worldwide [1]. There is growing evidence that playing football is beneficial for cardiovascular and neuromuscular fitness and health during the whole lifespan [2–4]. Thus, playing football has a great potential to support a healthy lifestyle and to contribute to public health. Football is a high-intensity sport with many changes in movement direction and velocity and many situations of direct contact between players. Thus, there is a high risk to sustain an injury. These harmful side effects have to be considered when the health benefits of playing football were assessed. Efforts have to be made to reduce the risk of injury [5].

Fifty-eight percent (22 out of 38 million) of all officially registered football players worldwide are under the age of 18 years [1]. Thus, effective prevention of injuries in youth football results in a relevant direct benefit for a large number of young players. Furthermore, injuries in young athletes can lead to a reduction in current and future sports participation [6, 7]. Injuries as well as insufficient physical activity are associated with a large economic burden and the utilization of medical, financial, and human resources [7, 8]. Therefore, successful injury prevention starting early in life is also relevant from a long-term public health perspective.

The first step in sports injury prevention is to establish the extent of the injury problem [9, 10]. Epidemiological data on football injuries are the basis to developing successful injury prevention programs. A large amount of research has been done on injury epidemiology in adult and high-level football [11–14]. In addition, injury prevention programs have been developed and evaluated in adolescent and adult players of both sexes and particularly in adolescent female players targeting severe knee injuries [11, 15–18].

The present overview is based on a previous systematic review on football injuries in children and adolescent players [19]. The objectives of this review were to describe the current scientific data on football injuries in players younger than 19 years of age. We analyzed prospective cohort studies on injuries in youth players and additionally population-based descriptive surveys from emergency departments. These data may build a basis to develop promising injury prevention programs in children's and youth football.

2.2 Injury Incidence and Prevalence

Most available data are related to players aged between 13 and 19 years. Studies reporting data for younger age groups are rare. Overall injury

O. Faude (✉) • R. Rössler
Department of Sport, Exercise and Health, University of Basel, Basel, Switzerland
e-mail: oliver.faude@unibas.ch; roland.roessler@unibas.ch

P. Volpi (ed.), *Football Traumatology: New Trends*, DOI 10.1007/978-3-319-18245-2_2

incidence was between 2 and 7 injuries per 1,000 h of exposure. Whereas incidence in training was usually low between 1 and 5 injuries per 1,000 h, match incidence was higher by a factor of 3–6 and tended to increase with age. In the oldest players match incidence reached values which are similar to adult football. Only few studies analyzed injuries in youth players of the highest level of play [20–23]. Reported injury incidences in high-level players were within the upper range of those observed in players of sub-elite level. Sex differences in injury incidence were not obvious. Similarly, data on possible differences between playing football outdoors and indoors are rare, and no conclusive statement is possible at the moment.

This summary is based on average values from a large number of studies. Few single investigations reported considerably higher (51.7 injuries per 1,000 match hours [24]) or lower (1.5 injuries per 1,000 match hours [25]) incidences. Such large discrepancies are probably due to methodological differences between studies, for instance, regarding injury definition, data collection strategies, or observation period. Although there exists a consensus on methodological issues in studies on football injuries [26], its application in children and adolescents is to some extent limited as standardized injury surveillance, particularly for minor injuries, as well as documentation of football exposure is complicated [19].

Having a closer look on data from population-based approaches which analyzed injuries from a large number of emergency room visits in North America [27–29] may result in a broader perspective of the injury problem associated with playing football. Although minor injuries which are usually the most frequent ones are missed in such analyses, this approach allows for a broad overview of severe injuries and their exact diagnosis. The majority of football injuries (about 60 %) presented to emergency departments resulted from unorganized football [27]. Injury rates were reported to be on average between 1.5 and 2.5 injuries per 1,000 children per year [28, 29] or between 6 and 7.6 annual injuries per 1,000 children participating in football [29].

2.3 Injury Characteristics

Information on the characteristics of injuries is also important from an injury prevention perspective (for summary, see Table 2.1). As children and adolescents are not miniature adults and growth spurts and maturation may relevantly affect injury events, it is of particular importance to obtain valid data on injury characteristics for all age groups in youth football.

2.3.1 Mechanisms of Injury

About half of all injuries in youth football are contact injuries, i.e., players had contact with an opponent or with an object (e.g., ball, ground, or posts). Whereas contact injuries occur mostly during match play, the incidence of noncontact injuries is higher during practice sessions. An interesting observation is that injuries resulting from player-to-player contact increase with age, whereas contact with an object becomes less relevant in older youth players [27].

About three quarters of all injuries are caused by a single traumatic event, whereas the remaining injuries resulted from repetitive microtrauma (overuse injuries). Traumatic injuries tend to be more frequent during matches [30, 31]. Recurrence rates are reported to be between 3 % and 19 % of all injuries. These numbers are very similar to those observed in adult football players.

2.3.2 Location of Injury

As well as in adult players, injuries in youth players also occur most often at the lower extremities (nearly 80 % of all injuries) with the ankle, knee, and thigh being mostly affected. Half of the remaining injuries are located at the trunk (including back complaints). Injuries to the upper extremities as well as to the head/face are less frequent. Although not very frequent, head injuries may have serious consequences for an individual, particularly regarding the long-term development of central nervous system structure

Table 2.1 Summary of findings on injury characteristics in children's and youth football.

Injury mechanism [%]	Contact			Overuse			Trauma			Recurrent	
	51 (35–68)			24 (10–43)			77 (57–90)			4 (3–19)	
Body part affected [%]	Lower extremities	Thigh/upper leg	Ankle	Knee	Lower leg	Foot/toe	Hip/groin	Upper body	Trunk/ spine	Upper extremities	Head/face
	79.5 (58–89)	16.5 (6–30)	23 (15–38)	17 (8–36)	8 (5–16)	9.5 (0.3–19)	7.5 (2–10)	20 (11–42)	10 (5–17)	6.5 (3–12)	3.5 (0.3–12)
Type of injury [%]	Strain		Sprain			Contusion		Fracture		Concussion	
	10 (9–25)		22 (20–32)			33 (29–47)		6 (4–9)		2 (1–7)	
Injury severity [%]	Mild (<7–8 days)			Moderate (7–8 to 28–30 days) [%]					Severe (>28–30 days) [%]		
	52 (27–67)			32 (20–52)					14 (10–37)		

Based on data from Faude et al. [19]. Data are presented as median (min–max) from available prospective cohort studies and functioning (see also Sect. 2.4.4). An interesting and important observation is that upper body injuries are more frequent during match play (nearly one third of all match injuries) [19]. Particularly, the number of injuries to the upper limbs (nearly 15 %) as well as to the head (up to 17 % of all injuries [32]) can be increased during games.

An interesting observation in youth players is that the proportion of upper body injuries decreases with increasing age. Studies analyzing players younger than 15 years [22, 33, 34] revealed that 20–29 % of all injuries were located to the upper body, whereas this proportion was between 11 % and 21 % in players older than 14 years [21, 23, 35–37]. This is mainly due to a difference in injuries to the upper limbs and, particularly, to fractures of the arm, wrist, or hand. A decrease in the proportion of fractures with increasing age has also been reported in other studies [27, 28, 38]. It might be hypothesized that less developed coordination skills and less playing experience increase the likelihood of falls. In conjunction with skeletal immaturity, this may result in an increased frequency of fractures to the upper limbs [27].

2.3.3 Type of Injury

As in adult football the most common injury types in youth football are contusions, joint–ligament injuries (sprains), and muscle–tendon injuries (strains). When looking particularly on those studies which analyzed boys and girls separately, it seems that sprains were comparably frequent to strains in boys (each 15–30 %) [22, 33, 36, 39, 40], whereas girls suffered from a higher proportion of sprains (about 35 % vs. 20 % strains) [21, 35, 37, 41]. There is evidence that the proportion of sprains and strains increases with age [27, 38, 39, 42]. One study showed that the proportion of sprains increased with age in girls, whereas the proportion of strains increased particularly in boys [42].

Fractures and concussions are less frequent, but such injuries may have serious consequences. There is evidence that the risk of sustaining a fracture or a concussion is higher during match play [43, 44]. The severity of these injury types is underlined by data from American emergency departments. Fractures and dislocations contributed to 23–31 % of all injuries resulting in presentation to an emergency room [45]. Fractures and sprains were the most frequent injuries leading to layoff times of more than 3 weeks [45]. Interestingly, there was also a sex difference with boys incurring more fractures (42 vs. 22 %) and fewer sprains (24 vs. 46 %) than girls, and the proportion of knee injuries in girls was twice as high as in boys (50 vs. 23 %) [45].

A particular problem in youth football is growth-related conditions, such as osteochondral disorders with Osgood–Schlatter and Sever's disease being the most prominent ones [20, 22, 46] (see also Sect. 2.4.3). A French study group found that Osgood–Schlatter disease was together with fractures the most common major injury in elite youth players [20, 22].

2.3.4 Severity of Injury and Return to Play

The severity of injuries is usually assessed by the number of days players are not able to fully take part in training and/or match play [26]. In youth football, match and training schedules are often not as tight and consistent as in adult football, and thus, particularly the proportion of mild injuries with short layoff times might be underestimated when this approach is applied. Nevertheless, figures on injury severity are very similar as compared to adult players. About half of all time-loss injuries lead to an absence between 1 day and 1 week, one third is of moderate severity (absence between 1 week and 1 month), and 10–15 % of all injuries are severe (layoff more than 1 month). The average layoff time per injury is about 15 days [19].

From those injuries which are presented to emergency departments, up to 5 % result in hospitalization and/or surgery [27–29, 44] with a higher risk for hospitalization and/or surgery in boys as compared to girls [27, 29] and for match injuries than for training injuries [27, 44]. Most of those injuries concerned the head/face, the neck, or the trunk [27]. The number of fatal accidents while playing football has been estimated being about 5 per 100,000 accidents presented to emergency rooms [29].

2.4 Injury Types of Particular Relevance in Youth Football

Some types of injury need to be particularly considered as they are very frequent and/or have severe consequences for an individual pediatric athlete either in the short (long layoff times) or the long term (adverse effects on physical or cognitive development). The following chapters summarize the major issues with regard to these types of injuries.

2.4.1 Strains and Sprains

In adolescent players strains and sprains are similarly frequent as it is known from adult football. Ligament injuries usually occur at the knees and ankles, whereas muscle injuries most often concern the thigh and, particularly, hamstring muscles. Ligament ruptures and muscle tears often result in long layoff times. It has been repeatedly observed in adult players that, for instance, previous ankle or knee ligament injuries as well as muscle injuries are among the most important predictors of future injuries of the same type. To avoid a cascade of recurrent sprains and/or strains, injury prevention should begin at an early age. To date, there is convincing evidence from studies in adolescents and adults that sprains and strains can be prevented by appropriate intervention programs [47].

The most important and serious ligament injury in football is a rupture of the anterior cruciate ligament (ACL). ACL injuries are particularly frequent in adolescent girls and typically lead to layoff times of about half a year and may potentially result in serious long-term consequences, for instance, pain and functional impairments due to early osteoarthritis. Therefore, it is of particular importance to early prevent ACL injuries. This issue was a major topic of scientific research during the last two decades. The majority of ACL injuries result from noncontact situations [14]. Several studies have dealt with possible prevention programs. Most of them have proven beneficial. A recent meta-analysis showed that about 70 % of all knee injuries (most studies focusing on ligament and ACL sprains) can be prevented by appropriate neuromuscular training in young female players [47].

2.4.2 Fractures

In young athletes fractures are more frequent as compared to adolescents or adults. Fractures are among the most frequent severe injuries in youth football. Children are particularly vulnerable to shearing injuries at the growth plates at the epiphyseal–metaphyseal junction [48]. Such physeal injuries might have considerable long-term consequences for children and, thus, prevention of these injuries is of particular importance. For instance, growth plate injuries can result in disturbed physeal growth and, in consequence, in limb length discrepancies, angular deformity, or altered joint mechanics. Also, osteoarthritis may be caused by growth plate injuries [48]. As particularly goalkeepers are prone to fractures of the upper limbs (own unpublished data in 7–12-year-old children), prevention should also focus on this playing position. Preventive programs may include the learning of fall techniques as it is established in martial arts. There is evidence that teaching specific landing skills can potentially reduce fall-related injuries in junior Australian rules football [49].

2.4.3 Overuse Complaints Related to Growth and Maturation

Osteochondral disorders are overuse injuries which are common among growing children [50, 51]. Usually, such complaints occur with a gradual onset and worsen with exercise, particularly while running, jumping, and/or kneeling. Therefore, these injuries are common in high-impact sports like football. Complaints are usually relieved during rest periods. It is speculated that recurrent shear stress at the bone–growth plate interfaces results in multiple small avulsion fractures at tendon–bone junctions. In child and adolescent athletes, this occurs frequently at the calcaneal (Sever's disease) or tibial apophysis (Osgood–Schlatter syndrome). These osteochondral disorders are more common among boys as compared to girls. Whereas Sever's disease usually occurs at the beginning of puberty in the under-11 age group, Osgood–Schlatter peaks during later stages of puberty (about 12 years in girls, up to an age of 15 years in boys).

Such complaints are usually self-limiting and have a good prognosis. Commonly, pain is present for 2–3 months, but it can last up to 2 years. Severe long-term consequences are very seldom; however, a relevant problem might develop as the layoff times are usually associated with sports reduction or complete cessation. Cessation is only necessary in case of severe exercise-induced pain. A graded reduction of training duration, frequency, and intensity may allow for a recovery of the complaints in most instances. In high-impact sports like football, it might be advisable to change some running or jumping exercises by non-weight-bearing alternatives. This procedure can be assisted by the application of ice/cryotherapy for pain management and physical therapy including stretching and strengthening exercises to reduce muscle imbalances [50, 51].

2.4.4 Head Injuries and Concussions

Head injuries and, particularly, concussions are serious and potentially catastrophic. Pediatric concussions are generally considered a public health concern [48]. In youth football, the frequency of head/face injuries is greatest during match play. The frequency of concussion varies between 1 % and 7 % [19]. Harmon et al. estimated that 3.8 million sports-related concussions occur in the USA every year with a large amount of unreported concussions [52]. In gender-comparable sports the concussion rate was reported to be about 70 % higher in girls as compared to boys [53].

Typical symptoms of concussions are headache, nausea, dizziness, concentration and memory difficulties, sleep disturbances and/or confusion, and emotional lability [48, 54]. Symptoms and management of concussions in adolescents down to the age of 13 years are similar to those of adults. In children younger than 13 years, symptoms may be more subtle and are reported differently from children than from adults (e.g., abdominal pain or behavioral changes) [48, 54]. Symptoms typically last 7–10 days, but may be present for weeks to months. Sim et al. observed that high school athletes showed longer memory dysfunction after a concussion as compared to college students [55]. In general, recovery from concussion in children and adolescents usually takes longer and injury management and return to play should be handled more cautiously [54].

Direct impacts to the head or to the body which transmit forces to the brain can potentially cause concussions. Most concussions result from player-to-player contact or from contact with the playing surface [56]. In addition, there might be danger that brain injuries can result from heading. O'Kane et al. observed in 11–14-year-old female football players that nearly one third of the reported concussions resulted from heading [56]. It has to be emphasized that nearly 60 % of those girls continued playing with symptoms. In addition, Janda et al. evaluated the effect of repetitive head impacts due to heading on cognitive function in a cohort of 11.5-year-old football players and observed that the number of ball impacts was inversely related to verbal learning [57].

2.5 Conclusions and Potential for Injury Prevention

Injury incidence in youth football increases with age, reaching values known from adult football in the oldest age categories. Injury characteristics in adolescent players are comparable to adults. Thus, it seems reasonable that prevention programs proven beneficial in adults are also efficacious in youth football players. A recent meta-analysis showed that exercise-based injury prevention programs have the potential to reduce overall injury rate in organized youth sports by an average of 46 % [47]. When a prevention program focuses on a particular type of injury (e.g., knee sprains), the preventive effect tends to be even greater. Poor compliance seems to be a major factor compromising the efficacy of prevention programs [58, 59].

Although injury incidence is lower in younger players, injury prevention in these age groups seems of particular importance as most youth players are younger than 15 years of age. Injury characteristics in (pre)pubescent players seem to differ from adolescent and adult footballers. Younger players have more fractures but fewer strains and sprains. The upper body and, particularly, the upper limbs are more frequently affected. Growth-related conditions as well as skeletal and coordinative complaints associated with maturation are age-specific injury characteristics during pubertal stages. Data on injury in prepubertal children is nearly completely missing. Injury prevention programs particularly tailored for children before and during puberty based on the specific needs and characteristics in these age groups need to be developed and evaluated.

Acknowledgment The Ph.D. studies of Roland Rössler on the "Epidemiology of Football Injuries in Youth Players" were financially supported by FIFA.

References

1. FIFA Communications Division (2007) FIFA big count 2006: 270 million people active in football. Zurich
2. Krustrup P, Christensen JF, Randers MB, Pedersen H, Sundstrup E et al (2010) Muscle adaptations and performance enhancements of soccer training for untrained men. Eur J Appl Physiol 108:1247–1258
3. Krustrup P, Hansen PR, Andersen LJ, Jakobsen MD, Sundstrup E et al (2010) Long-term musculoskeletal and cardiac health effects of recreational football and running for premenopausal women. Scand J Med Sci Sports 20(Suppl 1):58–71
4. Faude O, Kerper O, Multhaupt M, Winter C, Beziel K et al (2010) Football to tackle overweight in children. Scand J Med Sci Sports 20(Suppl 1):103–110
5. Verhagen E, Bolling C, Finch CF (2015) Caution this drug may cause serious harm! Why we must report adverse effects of physical activity promotion. Br J Sports Med 49:1–2
6. Maffulli N, Longo UG, Gougoulias N, Loppini M, Denaro V (2010) Long-term health outcomes of youth sports injuries. Br J Sports Med 44:21–25
7. Maffulli N, Longo UG, Gougoulias N, Caine D, Denaro V (2011) Sport injuries: a review of outcomes. Br Med Bull 97:47–80
8. Collard DC, Verhagen EA, van Mechelen W, Heymans MW, Chinapaw MJ (2011) Economic burden of physical activity-related injuries in Dutch children aged 10–12. Br J Sports Med 45:1058–1063
9. Bahr R, Krosshaug T (2005) Understanding injury mechanisms: a key component of preventing injuries in sport. Br J Sports Med 39:324–329
10. van Mechelen W, Hlobil H, Kemper HC (1992) Incidence, severity, aetiology and prevention of sports injuries. A review of concepts. Sports Med 14:82–99
11. Junge A, Dvorak J (2004) Soccer injuries: a review on incidence and prevention. Sports Med 34:929–938
12. Junge A, Dvorak J, Graf-Baumann T, Peterson L (2004) Football injuries during FIFA tournaments and the Olympic Games, 1998–2001: development and implementation of an injury-reporting system. Am J Sports Med 32:80S–89S
13. Ekstrand J, Hagglund M, Walden M (2011) Injury incidence and injury patterns in professional football: the UEFA injury study. Br J Sports Med 45:553–558
14. Faude O, Junge A, Kindermann W, Dvorak J (2005) Injuries in female soccer players: a prospective study in the German national league. Am J Sports Med 33:1694–1700
15. Junge A, Lamprecht M, Stamm H, Hasler H, Bizzini M et al (2011) Countrywide campaign to prevent soccer injuries in Swiss amateur players. Am J Sports Med 39:57–63
16. Steffen K, Emery CA, Romiti M, Kang J, Bizzini M et al (2013) High adherence to a neuromuscular injury prevention programme (FIFA 11+) improves functional balance and reduces injury risk in Canadian youth female football players: a cluster randomised trial. Br J Sports Med 47:794–802
17. Mandelbaum BR, Silvers HJ, Watanabe DS, Knarr JF, Thomas SD et al (2005) Effectiveness of a neuromuscular and proprioceptive training program in preventing anterior cruciate ligament injuries in female athletes: 2-year follow-up. Am J Sports Med 33:1003–1010
18. Walden M, Atroshi I, Magnusson H, Wagner P, Hagglund M (2012) Prevention of acute knee injuries in adolescent female football players: cluster randomised controlled trial. BMJ 344:e3042
19. Faude O, Rössler R, Junge A (2013) Football injuries in children and adolescent players: are there clues for prevention? Sports Med 43:819–837
20. Le Gall F, Carling C, Reilly T (2007) Biological maturity and injury in elite youth football. Scand J Med Sci Sports 17:564–572
21. Le Gall F, Carling C, Reilly T (2008) Injuries in young elite female soccer players: an 8-season prospective study. Am J Sports Med 36:276–284
22. Le Gall F, Carling C, Reilly T, Vandewalle H, Church J et al (2006) Incidence of injuries in elite French

youth soccer players: a 10-season study. Am J Sports Med 34:928–938

23. Müller-Rath R, Schmidt C, Mumme T, Andereya S, Miltner O (2006) The injury pattern following the introduction of the junior premier league in Germany compared to professional senior football (soccer). Sportverletz Sportschaden 20:192–195
24. McNoe BM, Chalmers DJ (2010) Injury in community-level soccer: development of an injury surveillance system. Am J Sports Med 38:2542–2551
25. Emery CA, Meeuwisse WH, Hartmann SE (2005) Evaluation of risk factors for injury in adolescent soccer: implementation and validation of an injury surveillance system. Am J Sports Med 33:1882–1891
26. Fuller CW, Ekstrand J, Junge A, Andersen TE, Bahr R et al (2006) Consensus statement on injury definitions and data collection procedures in studies of football (soccer) injuries. Br J Sports Med 40:193–201
27. Giannotti M, Al-Sahab B, McFaull S, Tamim H (2011) Epidemiology of acute soccer injuries in Canadian children and youth. Pediatr Emerg Care 27:81–85
28. Adams AL, Schiff MA (2006) Childhood soccer injuries treated in U.S. emergency departments. Acad Emerg Med 13:571–574
29. Leininger RE, Knox CL, Comstock RD (2007) Epidemiology of 1.6 million pediatric soccer-related injuries presenting to US emergency departments from 1990 to 2003. Am J Sports Med 35:288–293
30. Schmidt-Olsen S, Bunemann LK, Lade V, Brassoe JO (1985) Soccer injuries of youth. Br J Sports Med 19:161–164
31. Rosenbaum DA, Silvis ML, Williams JE, Davis SW (2009) Variation in injury risk over the course of a two-day youth club soccer tournament. Inj Prev 15:266–269
32. Maehlum S, Dahl E, Daljord O (1986) Frequency of injuries in a youth soccer tournament. Phys Sportsmed 14:73–79
33. Kakavelakis KN, Vlazakis S, Vlahakis I, Charissis G (2003) Soccer injuries in childhood. Scand J Med Sci Sports 13:175–178
34. Schiff MA (2007) Soccer injuries in female youth players. J Adolesc Health 40:369–371
35. Steffen K, Andersen TE, Bahr R (2007) Risk of injury on artificial turf and natural grass in young female football players. Br J Sports Med 41(Suppl 1):i33–i37
36. Junge A, Cheung K, Edwards T, Dvorak J (2004) Injuries in youth amateur soccer and rugby players–comparison of incidence and characteristics. Br J Sports Med 38:168–172
37. Söderman K, Adolphson J, Lorentzon R, Alfredson H (2001) Injuries in adolescent female players in European football: a prospective study over one outdoor soccer season. Scand J Med Sci Sports 11:299–304
38. Berger-Vachon C, Gabard G, Moyen B (1986) Soccer accidents in the French Rhone-Alpes soccer association. Sports Med 3:69–77
39. Brito J, Malina RM, Seabra A, Massada JL, Soares JM et al (2012) Injuries in Portuguese youth soccer players during training and match play. J Athl Train 47:191–197
40. Inklaar H, Bol E, Schmikli SL, Mosterd WL (1996) Injuries in male soccer players: team risk analysis. Int J Sports Med 17:229–234
41. Soligard T, Myklebust G, Steffen K, Holme I, Silvers H et al (2008) Comprehensive warm-up programme to prevent injuries in young female footballers: cluster randomised controlled trial. BMJ 337:a2469
42. Froholdt A, Olsen OE, Bahr R (2009) Low risk of injuries among children playing organized soccer: a prospective cohort study. Am J Sports Med 37: 1155–1160
43. Yard EE, Schroeder MJ, Fields SK, Collins CL, Comstock RD (2008) The epidemiology of United States high school soccer injuries, 2005–2007. Am J Sports Med 36:1930–1937
44. Rechel JA, Yard EE, Comstock RD (2008) An epidemiologic comparison of high school sports injuries sustained in practice and competition. J Athl Train 43:197–204
45. Darrow CJ, Collins CL, Yard EE, Comstock RD (2009) Epidemiology of severe injuries among United States high school athletes: 2005–2007. Am J Sports Med 37:1798–1805
46. Price RJ, Hawkins RD, Hulse MA, Hodson A (2004) The football association medical research programme: an audit of injuries in academy youth football. Br J Sports Med 38:466–471
47. Rössler R, Donath L, Verhagen E, Junge A, Schweizer T et al (2014) Exercise-based injury prevention in child and adolescent sport: a systematic review and meta-analysis. Sports Med 44:1733–1748
48. Caine D, Purcell L, Maffulli N (2014) The child and adolescent athlete: a review of three potentially serious injuries. BMC Sports Sci Med Rehabil 6:22
49. Scase E, Cook J, Makdissi M, Gabbe B, Shuck L (2006) Teaching landing skills in elite junior Australian football: evaluation of an injury prevention strategy. Br J Sports Med 40:834–838, discussion 838
50. Gholve PA, Scher DM, Khakharia S, Widmann RF, Green DW (2007) Osgood schlatter syndrome. Curr Opin Pediatr 19:44–50
51. Hendrix CL (2005) Calcaneal apophysitis (Sever disease). Clin Podiatr Med Surg 22:55–62, vi
52. Harmon KG, Drezner JA, Gammons M, Guskiewicz KM, Halstead M et al (2013) American medical society for sports medicine position statement: concussion in sport. Br J Sports Med 47:15–26
53. Marar M, McIlvain NM, Fields SK, Comstock RD (2012) Epidemiology of concussions among United States high school athletes in 20 sports. Am J Sports Med 40:747–755
54. McCrory P, Meeuwisse WH, Aubry M, Cantu B, Dvorak J et al (2013) Consensus statement on concussion in sport: the 4th international conference on concussion in sport held in Zurich, November 2012. Br J Sports Med 47:250–258

55. Sim A, Terryberry-Spohr L, Wilson KR (2008) Prolonged recovery of memory functioning after mild traumatic brain injury in adolescent athletes. J Neurosurg 108:511–516
56. O'Kane JW, Spieker A, Levy MR, Neradilek M, Polissar NL et al (2014) Concussion among female middle-school soccer players. JAMA Pediatr 168:258–264
57. Janda DH, Bir CA, Cheney AL (2002) An evaluation of the cumulative concussive effect of soccer heading in the youth population. Inj Control Saf Promot 9:25–31
58. Steffen K, Myklebust G, Olsen OE, Holme I, Bahr R (2008) Preventing injuries in female youth football–a cluster-randomized controlled trial. Scand J Med Sci Sports 18:605–614
59. Pfeiffer RP, Shea KG, Roberts D, Grandstrand S, Bond L (2006) Lack of effect of a knee ligament injury prevention program on the incidence of non-contact anterior cruciate ligament injury. J Bone Joint Surg Am 88:1769–1774

Epidemiology in Female Football Players

3

Astrid Junge

3.1 Introduction

It was estimated that about 10 % of all football players worldwide are female, which is about 29 million [1]. Due to the growing popularity of women's football, the number of female players increased between 2000 and 2006 by 50 %. A survey in 2006 by the Federation International de Football Association (FIFA) reported that there were over seven million female football players in the USA, 1.8 million in Germany, one million in Mexico and 794 000 in Canada [1]. In the Confederation of North, Central American and Caribbean Association Football (CONCACAF), 23 % of all football players were women (USA: 40 %; Canada: 33 %) [1].

The first women's football World Cup was held in China in 1991, and since 1994 a women's football tournament is part of the Olympic Games. In 2002, FIFA organised the first U-19 Women's World Championship, which was changed in 2006 to the U-20 Women's World Cup. The FIFA U-17 Women's World Cup was introduced in 2008. All six continental football federations organise at least one tournament for women and two (U-16/17 and U-19/20) for junior female players. In many countries a national league is played; however, the level of professionalism (training and playing conditions) of these leagues still varies greatly between countries.

The scientific literature on female football players has grown in recent years. Several authors have reported epidemiological data on injuries in female football players [2–17], and additional information is available from injury prevention projects [e.g. 18, 19]. However, most studies focus on adolescent players (for details see Chap. 2).

Twelve prospective epidemiological studies were found on exposure-related injury rates of adult female football players during the season [2–13] and three during top-level international tournaments [14–16]. All studies on injuries during the season were conducted in Scandinavia, Germany or the USA; information from other countries/continents could not be found. All studies (except the two on college and university teams) were conducted in top-level teams. Exposure-related injury data of recreational female players are extremely rare. Data from a nationwide injury prevention programme in Switzerland [19] indicate that the average incidence of training and match injuries of recreational players might be within the range of the prospective epidemiological studies reported in Table 3.1. However, it should be kept in mind that the information described below is based on a small and highly selected subgroup and thus might not be representative for all female football players around the world.

A. Junge
FIFA Medical Assessment and Research Centre (F-MARC), Zurich, Switzerland

Medical School Hamburg (MSH), Hamburg, Germany
e-mail: Astrid.Junge@F-MARC.com

P. Volpi (ed.), *Football Traumatology: New Trends*, DOI 10.1007/978-3-319-18245-2_3

Table 3.1 Prospective studies on incidence of injury in adult female football players during a year or season

Author/year	Country	No. of players	Skill level	Age (years)	Study period	Injuries per 1,000 h	
						Match	Training
Engström et al. 1991	Sweden	41	Premier, 2nd division	16–28	1 year prior 1991	24	7
Östenberg and Ross 2000	Sweden	123	Senior players, different skill levels	14–39	1 season 1996	14.3	3.7
Giza et al. 2005	USA	202	Women's United Soccer Association		2 years 2001/02	12.6	1.2
Faude et al. 2005	Germany	165	First national league	22.4 ± 5.0	1 season 2003/04	23.3	2.8
Fuller et al. 2007a, b	USA	64/72 teams	College and university teams		2 seasons 2005–6	21.8/19.2	2.6/2.8
Dick et al. 2007	USA	19,871	College teams	>= 18	1988–2003	(16.4) (athletes exposure)	(5.23) (athletes exposure)
Jacobson and Tegner 2007	Sweden	195	Premier league (12 teams)	23 ± 4.0	1 season 04–10/2000	13.9	2.7
Tegnander et al. 2008	Norway	181	Elite (10 teams)	17–34	2001	23.6	3.1
Hägglund et al. 2009	Sweden	228	(12 clubs)		Season 2005	16.1	3.8
Gaulrapp et al. 2010	Germany	254	Premier league (12 teams)	16–35	1 year	18.5	1.4
Ekstrand et al. 2011	Sweden		First division (5 teams)	23 ± 4 15 − 38	2003–2008	14.9 12.5	2.9 2.8

Table 3.2 Prospective studies on incidence of time-loss injury in female football players during tournaments

Author/year	Type of tournament	No. of tournaments	Year of the tournament (s)	No. of matches	Injuries per match (95%CI)
Walden et al. 2007	UEFA Women's EURO	1	2005	15	1.0
Hagglund et al. 2009	UEFA Women's U-19 Championship	3	2006–2008	45	0.7
Junge and Dvorak 2013	FIFA Women's World Cup™	3	2003–2011	96	1.0 (0.8–1.2)
Junge and Dvorak 2013	FIFA Women's U-19/U-20 World Cup	6	2002–2012	180	1.0 (0.9–1.2)
Junge and Dvorak 2013	FIFA Women's U-17 World Cup	3	2008–2012	96	0.7 (0.5–0.9)
Junge and Dvorak 2013	Women's Olympic Football Tournament	4	2000–2012	88	1.0 (0.8–1.2)

3.2 Injury Rate

For adult female football players, the incidence of time-loss injuries during the season varied between 12.5 and 23.6 per 1,000 exposure hours for match injuries and between 1.2 and 3.8 (7) per 1,000 exposure hours for training injuries (see Table 3.1).

During tournaments the incidence is approximately one time-loss injuries per match, equivalent to 30.3 per 1,000 match hours (see Table 3.2). The average incidence of time-loss injuries was similar in FIFA Women's World Cups™, FIFA U-19/20 Women's World Cups, UEFA Women's EURO and the Olympic Football Tournaments and lower in FIFA U-17 Women's World Cups and UEFA Women's Under 19 Championships [14, 16].

While an increase of the injury rate was observed in the FIFA Women's World Cups from 2003 to 2007, the FIFA U-17 Women's World Cups 2008–2012 and the Olympic Football Tournaments 2000–2008, a decrease was observed in the UEFA Women's Under 19 Championships from 2006 to 2008 [14, 16]. Changes in the incidence of injuries in top-level tournaments may be influenced by the playing style, refereeing, quantity and intensity of match play.

3.3 Type and Location of Injury

The majority of injuries affect the lower extremity (see Table 3.3). Most frequently injured body parts are the knee (12–34 % of all injuries) and ankle (9–35 %) followed by the thigh (11–27 %). The proportion of injuries to the trunk ranged between 1.9 % and 13.2 %; upper extremity injuries represent less than 10 %. The proportion of head injuries during the season ranges between 4 % and 14 %. For tournaments the results were similar, except a higher proportion of head injuries which is most probably due to the injury definition (not restricted to time loss) used by FIFA. From the NCAA data [6–8], it seems that head and knee injuries are more frequent in matches and thigh injuries in training.

Most injuries affected either joints/ligaments (19–57 %) or muscles (11–42 %). Contusions are frequent. The percentage of fractures ranged between 1 % and 11.6 %. Concussions represent up to 8.6 % of match injuries (Table 3.4).

Injuries of the anterior cruciate ligament (ACL) are a special concern in women's football due to their severity and long-term consequences (see below). The incidence of an ACL injury is three to seven times higher in female athletes compared to their male counterparts [20–23]. Female football players also incur ACL at a younger age than men [20–22]. Further a previous ACL injury is a risk factor for a subsequent one [24]. Thus, prevention of ACL injuries is of great importance. It has been shown that exercise-based prevention programmes can substantially reduce the rate of ACL injuries in female football players [18, 25] (for details see Chap. 6).

Also a higher incidence of concussion in female compared to male players has been reported [16, 26]. It is unclear whether the female brain is more sensitive to impacts or the discrepancy is influenced by differences between the genders in the reporting of symptom. Diagnosis, treatment and return to play after head injury are outlined in the Consensus Statements of the Concussion in Sports Group [27–30].

3.4 Long-Term Health Consequences

Only very few studies concern the long-time health consequences of playing (professional) football, and most related to osteoarthritis (OA). Almost all studies focus on male players or gender is not mentioned; only one focussed on female players [31]. In Sweden, all 106 female football players who sustained an ACL tear during football play 12 years earlier were contacted and asked to complete questionnaires and have radiographic examinations of their knees. Of the 103 former players (aged 26–40 years) investigated, 82 % had radiographic changes in their index knee, and 51 % fulfilled the radiographic criterion for knee OA [31].

Neuropsychological and/or cognitive impairment as consequence of heading and concussion in football has been discussed in the literature [e.g. 32–35]. However, none of these studies regard long-term sequela in former elite female football players. A study on 22 female university-level football players after a first concussion suggests that cognitive functions related to cognitive processing speed are most vulnerable to concussion and are still impaired 6 months after injury [36].

Table 3.3 Total number of time-loss injuries and percentage of different body parts

	Total	Head/face	Trunk/spine	Upper extremities	Hip/groin	Thigh/upper leg	Knee	Lower leg	Ankle	Foot/toe
Author, year	*N*	%	%	%	%	%	%	%	%	%
Östenberg and Ross 2000	**52**	–	1.9	3.8	1.9	26.9	15.4	5.8	34.6	9.6
Giza et al. 2005	**173**	10.4					33.8		9.3	9.3
Faude et al. 2005	**241**	6.7	7.4	5.4	5.9	18.2	18.7	8.3	17.8	11.2
Fuller et al. 2007 (training)	**774**	8.2	12.6	4.4	8	16.5	15.3	14	14.7	6.5
Fuller et al. 2007 (match)	**946**	13.9	8.6	7.2	4.5	11	22.9	7.6	16.8	7.6
Dick et al. 2007 (training)	**5,836**	3.9	13.2	4.2	7.6	21.3	12.1	5.8	16.7	
Dick et al. 2007 (match)	**5,373**	13.8	8.4	6.3	3.2	10.7	19.3	5.9	19.4	2.7
Jacobson and Tegner 2007	**237**	6	3	2	7	19	25	11	13	7
Tegnander et al. 2008	**189**	7.4	6.9	4.8	9	17.5	16.4	7.4	23.8	6.9
Hägglund et al. 2009	**299**	4	9	2	11	23	22	7	16	5
Gaulrapp et al. 2010	**246**	7.1			1.7	12.9	31	9.4	22.1	4.6
Ekstrand et al. 2011	**222**	7.7	3.2	4.1	7.2	24.8	19.8	6.3	21.6	5.4
Walden et al. 2007	**31**	5.6		5.6		16.7	22.2	22.2	16.7	11.1
Junge and Dvorak 2013	**419**	17.4[a]	9.1[a]	8.1[a]	2.5[a]	9.6[a]	12.6[a]	14.7[a]	20.3[a]	5.7[a]

[a]Percentages relate to all injuries ($n = 1,116$)

Table 3.4 Total number of injury and percentage of different injury types

Author, year	Total N	Fracture %	Joint/Ligament injury %	Muscle injuries/strain %	Concussion %	Contusion %
Östenberg and Ross 2000	**52**	3.8	57	29		11.5
Giza et al. 2005	**173**	11.6	19	30.7	2.9	16.2
Faude et al. 2005	**241**	4.7	29	15.2		20.7
Fuller et al. 2007 (training)	**774**	5	32.7	41.6		9.5
Fuller et al. 2007 (match)	**946**	5.6	41	16.6		23.6
Dick et al. 2007 (training)	**5,836**	1.2	18.1	32.7	2.2	1.2
Dick et al. 2007 (match)	**5,373**	1.1	19.3	11.8	8.6	13.8
Jacobson and Tegner 2007	**237**	1	25	29	4	8
Tegnander et al. 2008	**189**	5.3	31	36	(3.7)	7.4
Hägglund et al. 2009	**299**	3	23	28	2	11
Gaulrapp et al. 2010	**246**	5.8	35	10.8	5.3	15.8
Ekstrand et al. 2011	**222**	4.1	38	31.5	5	17.6
Walden et al. 2007	**31**	11.1		16.6	5.6	44.5
Junge and Dvorak 2013	**419**	2.1[a]		7.8[a]	3[a]	51.3[a]

[a]Percentages relate to all injuries (n = 1,116)

Conclusion

Epidemiological information on injuries of adult female football players is very limited. The 15 prospective epidemiological studies found in the literature were all conducted in one of four countries (which were winner or second in the FIFA Women's World Cup™) or during the FIFA or UEFA tournaments. Studies on recreational female players and female players from other continents are lacking. Future epidemiological studies should also analyse injury mechanism and risk factors to make specific recommendations for injury prevention for adult female football players. Exercise-based prevention programmes proved to be effective in adolescent female players; similar studies should be performed also in adult female players.

References

1. FIFA communications division (2007) FIFA big count 2006: 270 million people active in football. Zurich
2. Engstrom B, Johansson C, Tornkvist H (1991) Soccer injuries among elite female players. Am J Sports Med 19(4):372–375
3. Ostenberg A, Roos H (2000) Injury risk factors in female European football. A prospective study of 123 players during one season. Scand J Med Sci Sports 10(5):279–285

4. Giza E, Mithöfer K, Farrell L, Zarins B, Gill T (2005) Injuries in women's professional soccer. Br J Sports Med 39(4):212–216
5. Faude O, Junge A, Kindermann W, Dvorak J (2005) Injuries in female soccer players: a prospective study in the German national league. Am J Sports Med 33(11):1694–1700
6. Fuller CW, Dick RW, Corlette J, Schmalz R (2007) Comparison of the incidence, nature and cause of injuries sustained on grass and new generation artificial turf by male and female football players. Part 2: training injuries. Br J Sports Med 41(Suppl 1):i27–i32
7. Fuller CW, Dick RW, Corlette J, Schmalz R (2007) Comparison of the incidence, nature and cause of injuries sustained on grass and new generation artificial turf by male and female football players. Part 1: match injuries. Br J Sports Med 41(Suppl 1):i20–i26
8. Dick R, Putukian M, Agel J, Evans TA, Marshall SW (2007) Descriptive epidemiology of collegiate women's soccer injuries: national collegiate athletic association injury surveillance system, 1988–1989 through 2002–2003. J Athl Train 42(2):278–285
9. Jacobson I, Tegner Y (2007) Injuries among Swedish female elite football players: a prospective population study. Scand J Med Sci Sports 17(1):84–91
10. Tegnander A, Olsen OE, Moholdt TT, Engebretsen L, Bahr R (2008) Injuries in Norwegian female elite soccer: a prospective one-season cohort study. Knee Surg Sports Traumatol Arthrosc 16(2):194–198
11. Hägglund M, Waldén M, Ekstrand J (2009) Injuries among male and female elite football players. Scand J Med Sci Sports 19(6):819–827
12. Gaulrapp H, Becker A, Walther M, Hess H (2010) Injuries in women's soccer: a 1-year all players prospective field study of the women's Bundesliga (German premier league). Clin J Sport Med 20(4):264–271
13. Ekstrand J, Hägglund M, Fuller CW (2011) Comparison of injuries sustained on artificial turf and grass by male and female elite football players. Scand J Med Sci Sports 21(6):824–832
14. Waldén M, Hägglund M, Ekstrand J (2007) Football injuries during European Championships 2004–2005. Knee Surg Sports Traumatol Arthrosc 15(9):1155–1162
15. Hägglund M, Waldén M, Ekstrand J (2009) UEFA injury study–an injury audit of European Championships 2006–2008. Br J Sports Med 43(7):483–489
16. Junge A, Dvořák J (2013) Injury surveillance in world football tournaments 1998–2012. Br J Sports Med 47:782–788
17. Faude O, Rössler R, Junge A (2013) Football injuries in children and adolescent players: are there clues for prevention? Sports Med 43(9):819–837
18. Rössler R, Donath L, Verhagen E, Junge A, Schweizer T, Faude O (2014) Exercise-based injury prevention in child and adolescent sport: a meta-analytic review. Sport Medicine 44(12):1733–1748
19. Junge A, Lamprecht M, Stamm H, Hasler H, Bizzini M, Tschopp M, Reuter H, Wyss H, Chilvers C, Dvorak J (2011) Country-wide campaign to prevent football injuries in Swiss amateur players. Am J Sports Med 39(1):57–63
20. Arendt E, Dick R (1995) Knee injury patterns among men and women in collegiate basketball and soccer. NCAA data and review of literature. Am J Sports Med 23:694–701
21. Roos H, Ornell M, Gardsell P, Lohmander LS, Lindstrand A (1995) Soccer after anterior cruciate ligament injury: an incompatible combination? A national survey of incidence and risk factors and a 7-year follow-up of 310 players. Acta Orthop Scand 66:107–112
22. Bjordal JM, Arnly F, Hannestad B, Strand T (1997) Epidemiology of anterior cruciate ligament injuries in soccer. Am J Sports Med 25:341–345
23. Prodromos CC, Han Y, Rogowski J, Joyce B, Shi K (2007) A meta-analysis of the incidence of anterior cruciate ligament tears as a function of gender, sport, and a knee injury-reduction regimen. Arthroscopy 23:1320–1325
24. Smith HC, Vacek P, Johnson RJ, Slauterbeck JR, Hashemi J, Shultz S, Beynnon BD (2012) Risk factors for anterior cruciate ligament injury: a review of the literature—Part 2: hormonal, genetic, cognitive function, previous injury, and extrinsic risk factors. Sports Health 4(2):155–161
25. Alentorn-Geli E, Myer GD, Silvers HJ, Samitier G, Romero D, Lázaro-Haro C, Cugat R (2009) Prevention of non-contact anterior cruciate ligament injuries in soccer players. Part 2: a review of prevention programs aimed to modify risk factors and to reduce injury rates. Knee Surg Sports Traumatol Arthrosc 17(8):859–879
26. Dick RW (2009) Is there a gender difference in concussion incidence and outcomes? Br J Sports Med 43(Suppl 1):i46–i50
27. Aubry M, Cantu R, Dvořák J, Graf-Baumann T, Johnston K, Kelly J, Lovell M, McCrory P, Meeuwisse W, Schamasch P (2002) Concussion in sport group. Summary and agreement statement of the first international conference on concussion in sport, Vienna 2001. Recommendations for the improvement of safety and health of athletes who may suffer concussive injuries. Br J Sports Med 36(1):6–10
28. McCrory P, Johnston K, Meeuwisse W, Aubry M, Cantu R, Dvořák J, Graf-Baumann T, Kelly J, Lovell M, Schamasch P (2005) Summary and agreement statement of the 2nd international conference on concussion in sport, Prague 2004. Br J Sports Med 39(4):196–204
29. McCrory P, Meeuwisse W, Johnston K, Dvořák J, Aubry M, Molloy M, Cantu R (2009) Consensus statement on concussion in sport: the 3rd international conference on concussion in sport held in Zurich, November 2008. Br J Sports Med 43(1 Suppl):i76–i90
30. McCrory M, Meeuwisse WH, Aubry M, Cantu B, Dvořák J, Echemendia RJ, Engebretsen L, Johnston K, Kutcher JF, Raftery M, Sills A, Benson BW, Davis GA, Ellenbogen RG, Guskiewicz K, Herring SA, Iverson GL, Jordan BD, Kissick J, McCrea M, McIntosh AS, Maddocks D, Makdissi M, Purcell L, Putukian M, Schneider K, Tator CH, Turner M (2013) Consensus statement on concussion in sport: the 4th international conference on concussion in sport held

in Zurich, November 2012. Br J Sports Med 47: 250–258
31. Lohmander LS, Ostenberg A, Englund M, Roos H (2004) High prevalence of knee osteoarthritis, pain, and functional limitations in female soccer players twelve years after anterior cruciate ligament injury. Arthritis Rheum 50(10):3145–3152
32. Matser EJ, Kessels AG, Lezak MD, Jordan BD, Troost J (1999) Neuropsychological impairment in amateur soccer players. JAMA 282(10):971–973
33. Matser JT, Kessels AG, Jordan BD, Lezak MD, Troost J (1998) Chronic traumatic brain injury in professional soccer players. Neurology 51(3):791–796
34. Rutherford A, Stephens R, Potter D (2003) The neuropsychology of heading and head trauma in association football (soccer): a review. Neuropsychol Rev 13(3): 153–179
35. Vann Jones SA, Breakey RW, Evans PJ (2014) Heading in football, long-term cognitive decline and dementia: evidence from screening retired professional footballers. Br J Sports Med 48(2): 159–161
36. Ellemberg D, Leclerc S, Couture S, Daigle C (2007) Prolonged neuropsychological impairments following a first concussion in female university soccer athletes. Clin J Sport Med 17(5):369–374

Risk Factors

4

Piero Volpi and Cristiano Eirale

4.1 Risk Factors

In epidemiology, a risk factor is a variable associated with an increased risk of disease. Sometimes, when a variable may be associated with either increased or decreased risk, the term determinant is utilised as well.

Risk factors or determinants are correlated with the risk of injury or disease, but they are not necessarily causal, because correlation does not demonstrate causation. In order to assess the strength of an association and to provide causal evidence, specific statistical methods have to be utilised.

In football, injury risk is multifactorial [1]. Determining the individual risk factors for each type of injury is an imperative step for the consequent development of prevention programmes. Once the injury profile has been determined, the risk factors and injury mechanisms have to be identified [2].

Both intrinsic and extrinsic risk factors have to be taken into consideration. They can either be modifiable or non-modifiable.

P. Volpi
Knee Orthopedics and Sport Traumatology Unit, Humanitas Clinical Institute IRCCS, Milan, Italy

Head of Medical Staff FC Internazionale Milan, Milan, Italy

C. Eirale (✉)
Aspetar – Qatar Orthopedic and Sport, Medicine Hospital, 29222 Doha, Qatar
e-mail: Cristiano.eirale@aspetar.com

Intrinsic risk factors can be categorised as physical or psychological [3]. Examples of intrinsic risk factors are weight, eight, age, gender, ethnicity, previous injury history, muscle strength, imbalance and tightness, aerobic fitness, ligamentous laxity, central motor control and psychological and psychosocial factors. Among the main extrinsic risk factors, we can mention the climatic conditions, the playing surface and its conditions, the intensity of the performance during matches and training, the player exposure during training and matches, the composition of the training, the playing position, the equipment, the rules of the game and the social and lifestyle factors.

4.2 Intrinsic Risk Factors

Among the intrinsic risk factors, age, career duration and previous injuries have been shown having a negative effect on the athlete injury risk. Players with positive injury history have been shown to be two to three times more likely to suffer an identical injury in the subsequent season [4]. Though some studies have shown no relation [5] between previous injury and injury risk, most researches have shown a correlation. In particular, studies that utilised a multivariate analysis, a method that is certainly more appropriate in the risk factor analysis, confirmed these findings [4, 6]. Inadequate rehabilitation has also been identified as a possible risk factor for football injuries [3]. There is evidence that

P. Volpi (ed.), *Football Traumatology: New Trends*, DOI 10.1007/978-3-319-18245-2_4

the professional players are nowadays heavier and taller than some decades ago [7]. It can be hypothesised that these parameters may increase the energy of the contacts and therefore the injury risk. However, this thesis has not been confirmed by scientific data, so far. Several researches showed also a greater muscle strength in the lower limbs of the current professional player [8, 9]. Also in this case, it can be speculated that this may have increased the injury risk; on the other hand, however, this can be also considered a protective factor.

Mechanical instability in ankles or knees, joint laxity or functional instability also seems to predispose players to injuries, in particular of the hamstrings, groin and knee [8, 10–13]. Other potential intrinsic risk factors, like ethnicity and mental characteristics, may play a role, but the scientific literature is still inconclusive and further research is warranted.

Some researches have investigated the relationship between sports injuries in general [14] and psychological factors, and some of them have explored this in relation to football, finding a positive correlation [15, 16].

The analysis of intrinsic risk factor may allow clinicians to prepare individual programmes of prevention.

4.3 Extrinsic Risk Factors

The influence of extrinsic risk factors needs to be analysed as well.

Physical and psychosocial stress appears to increase the injury risk. However, the role of testing the level of stress of the footballers is still generally underestimated. In order to prevent injuries, it seems at least necessary a close training load monitoring.

As stated initially by Ekstrand [17] and confirmed by successive researchers [6, 7, 18, 19], a high training/match ratio is a protective factor in football. This is probably due to the fact that physically well-trained and mentally prepared players can bear the physical stress during the game with a reduced risk of injury.

Also, the relative shortness of the period of physiological preseason preparation can be considered a potential contributing factor to the occurrence of accidents [7].

The "economic value" of the game is today definitely higher than the previous. Also, the constant pressure of the media is contributing to increase the stress on footballers and therefore may put them at further risk. In addition to this, also the increased performance during the game, the different training methodologies and technical and tactical innovations are aspects to consider in modern football. Indeed, the widespread use in tactical solutions, such as the pressing, the offside trap and the double marking, made at maximum intensity, is a potential risk factor for injury.

Moreover, modern football involves tactical situation in which many players are present in a limited area of the field, increasing the possibility of contacts. In addition to this, the exasperated physical preparation may predispose the players to high force contacts which can results in acute (ligament injuries of the knee, in particular ACL lesions, tendon ruptures, etc.) and chronic (tendonitis, enthesitis, chondropathies, etc.) pathologies.

As previously discussed, a congested calendar and relative limited time for training, recovery and preseason preparation are potential contributing factors to the occurrence of accidents. However, if it seems that a period of 3 days between matches and a correct rotation of the players may help to avoid an increasing of the injury risk [20–23], not all the teams have the possibility to rotate players due to the limited numbers of players at their disposal. There is certainly an advantage for richer teams that may dispose of a higher number of good level players and therefore can apply this rotation. Teams with lower financial possibilities may not be able to adequately apply player turnover, missing the opportunity of this prevention strategy. This is a classic example of a possible intervention on the rules of the game, for preventive purposes. It may be hypothesised, in fact, that more changes during a game (e.g. 5 instead of 3) may allow a more adequate in-game turnover. This further turnover possibility may possibly impact the risk of injuries, perhaps also reducing the gap between teams. Of course, this has to be confirmed by epidemiological studies, but it is certainly a good example of applying science to football for impacting the health of the players and therefore for increasing the level of the game.

Despite there are no studies confirming this, also the pressure of the media is contributing to increase the pressure on footballers, especially of elite level, and may affect the injury risk.

The association between the playing position and injury risk is still undefined. While the majorities of the studies showed no relation [24–27], there is some evidence of a higher incidence of injuries in defenders [28], halfbacks [29] and midfielders [1, 30]. As a confounder factor, modern football requires defending actions in forwards and attaching phases of the game in defenders. Moreover, players may change role during the season or even during a game. These may be reasons of an indeterminate link between injury risk and playing position.

Football pitches have certainly to be taken into consideration as a potential extrinsic risk factor. Despite that the results of the scientific research are still controversial [31–33], it seems that there is not an increased risk of injury associated with playing on last-generation artificial turfs. However, ankle sprain incidence is increased, while quadriceps strains decreased on this surface [32, 34, 35]. This may suggest the use of specific preventive measures for teams playing or training regularly on this surface.

Moreover, weather and pitch conditions seem to affect injuries, creating regional differences in match injury incidence. Teams from northern Europe have a higher general risk of injury than the teams from southern Europe, possibly due to poorer climate and surface conditions. Conversely, there is a trend towards an increased risk of ACL injury in Mediterranean countries, where it has been hypothesised that the pitches, with higher rotational and traction forces, may be the most important risk factor [36]. These data seems to be confirmed by some researches on Australian football [37, 38] and underline the importance of developing regional epidemiological studies in order to define and characterise the particular injuries for each country.

In this view, attention must be also paid on the choice of footwear and cleats, in order to avoid excessive ground-shoe rotational forces that may increase the number of injuries, in particular located to the knee.

With the 2012 Olympic Games and the 2014 FIFA World Cup both being organised during the period of Ramadan (Islamic holy month of fasting), there was a debate about the possible effects of fasting on physical performance and injury.

A study of injury epidemiology in Qatari footballers [39] has allowed the investigation of the influence of Ramadan on football injury incidence and patterns. In a population with a majority of Muslim footballers competing in a Muslim country, no significant difference of injury incidence, characteristics and patterns has been shown during Ramadan compared to the rest of the football season. On the contrary, there is some evidence that non-Muslim footballers competing in a Muslim country suffer more during this time as they struggle to cope with the changes in social and sports life during this period such as training time modifications.

In modern football, despite this has never been explored in scientific researches, the frequent changes of coaches and technical staff can be considered a possible risk factor. Another aspect to take onto account is the high number of players for each professional team: if this may ensure an appropriate turnover allowing a better recovery of tired and injured players and therefore can be seen as a protective factor, on the other hand, the pressure and the competitiveness between the players may increase, leading to a higher risk of injury during training.

While some of these risk factors are not easy to be corrected, the player lifestyle represents a central risk factor that can be quickly modified or corrected. For example, smoking is an element of absolute toxicity and alcohol and, even when taken occasionally, can be contra-productive for the performance [7].

Also an excessive use of drugs in order to continue sports activity despite an injury or to speed up the recovery time should be considered as an important risk factor to the footballers' health [7].

On top of these considerations, fair play among players, coaches and managers and the central role of the referee in the protection of the players are key risk factors that national and international federation should continuously take into consideration, in order to perform the adapted adjustments. Football scientists should continuously monitor the impact of the fair play, of the referees' activity and of the rules of the game on the injury risk [40, 41].

In this sense, there is evidence in the literature that football medicine has contributed decreasing the injury rates by changing the rules of the game. It has in fact been shown that injury rates were reduced by the introduction of the red card for a tackle from behind [42] and for the use of the elbow to hit an opponent during a duel [42].

References

1. Fuller CW, Junge A, Dvorak J (2012) Risk management: FIFA's approach for protecting the health of football players. Br J Sports Med 46:11–17
2. van Mechelen W, Hlobil H, Kemper HC (1992) Incidence, severity, aetiology and prevention of sports injuries. A review of concepts. Sports Med 14:82–99
3. Dvorak J, Junge A, Chomiak J et al (2000) Risk factor analysis for injuries in football players. Possibilities for a prevention program. Am J Sports Med 28:S69–S74
4. Hagglund M, Walden M, Ekstrand J (2006) Previous injury as a risk factor for injury in elite football: a prospective study over two consecutive seasons. Br J Sports Med 40:767–772
5. Trojian TH, McKeag DB (2006) Single leg balance test to identify risk of ankle sprains. Br J Sports Med 40:610–613, discussion 613
6. Arnason A, Sigurdsson SB, Gudmundsson A et al (2004) Risk factors for injuries in football. Am J Sports Med 32:5S–16S
7. Volpi P, Taioli E (2012) The health profile of professional soccer players: future opportunities for injury prevention. J Strength Cond Res 26:3473–3479
8. Fousekis K, Tsepis E, Poulmedis P et al (2011) Intrinsic risk factors of non-contact quadriceps and hamstring strains in soccer: a prospective study of 100 professional players. Br J Sports Med 45:709–714
9. Requena B, Gonzalez-Badillo JJ, de Villareal ES et al (2009) Functional performance, maximal strength, and power characteristics in isometric and dynamic actions of lower extremities in soccer players. J Strength Cond Res 23:1391–1401
10. Hagglund M, Walden M, Ekstrand J (2013) Risk factors for lower extremity muscle injury in professional soccer: the UEFA Injury Study. Am J Sports Med 41:327–335
11. Engebretsen AH, Myklebust G, Holme I et al (2011) Intrinsic risk factors for acute knee injuries among male football players: a prospective cohort study. Scand J Med Sci Sports 21:645–652
12. Engebretsen AH, Myklebust G, Holme I et al (2010) Intrinsic risk factors for groin injuries among male soccer players: a prospective cohort study. Am J Sports Med 38:2051–2057
13. Witvrouw E, Danneels L, Asselman P et al (2003) Muscle flexibility as a risk factor for developing muscle injuries in male professional soccer players. A prospective study. Am J Sports Med 31:41–46
14. Junge A, Dvorak J, Rosch D et al (2000) Psychological and sport-specific characteristics of football players. Am J Sports Med 28:S22–S28
15. Taimela S, Osterman L, Kujala U et al (1990) Motor ability and personality with reference to soccer injuries. J Sports Med Phys Fitness 30:194–201
16. Chomiak J, Junge A, Peterson L, Dvorak J (2000) Severe injuries in football players. Influencing factors. Am J Sports Med 28:S58–S68
17. Ekstrand J, Gillquist J, Moller M et al (1983) Incidence of soccer injuries and their relation to training and team success. Am J Sports Med 11:63–67
18. Ostenberg A, Roos H (2000) Injury risk factors in female European football. A prospective study of 123 players during one season. Scand J Med Sci Sports 10:279–285
19. Hagglund M, Walden M, Ekstrand J (2003) Exposure and injury risk in Swedish elite football: a comparison between seasons 1982 and 2001. Scand J Med Sci Sports 13:364–370
20. Carling C, Le Gall F, Dupont G (2012) Are physical performance and injury risk in a professional soccer team in match-play affected over a prolonged period of fixture congestion? Int J Sports Med 33:36–42
21. Dellal A, Lago-Penas C, Rey E et al (2013) The effects of a congested fixture period on physical performance, technical activity and injury rate during matches in a professional soccer team. Br J Sports Med
22. Dupont G, Nedelec M, McCall A et al (2010) Effect of 2 soccer matches in a week on physical performance and injury rate. Am J Sports Med 38:1752–1758
23. Ekstrand J, Walden M, Hagglund M (2004) A congested football calendar and the wellbeing of players: correlation between match exposure of European footballers before the World Cup 2002 and their injuries and performances during that World Cup. Br J Sports Med 38:493–497
24. Engstrom B, Forssblad M, Johansson C, Tornkvist H (1990) Does a major knee injury definitely sideline an elite soccer player? Am J Sports Med 18:101–105
25. Hawkins RD, Fuller CW (1999) A prospective epidemiological study of injuries in four English professional football clubs. Br J Sports Med 33:196–203

26. Ekstrand J, Gillquist J (1983) Soccer injuries and their mechanisms: a prospective study. Med Sci Sports Exerc 15:267–270
27. Ekstrand J, Gillquist J, Liljedahl SO (1983) Prevention of soccer injuries. Supervision by doctor and physiotherapist. Am J Sports Med 11:116–120
28. Peterson L, Junge A, Chomiak J et al (2000) Incidence of football injuries and complaints in different age groups and skill-level groups. Am J Sports Med 28:S51–S57
29. McGregor JC, Rae A (1995) A review of injuries to professional footballers in a premier football team (1990–93). Scott Med J 40:16–18
30. Arnason A, Sigurdsson SB, Gudmundsson A et al (2004) Physical fitness, injuries, and team performance in soccer. Med Sci Sports Exerc 36:278–285
31. Kristenson K, Bjorneboe J, Walden M et al (2013) The Nordic football injury audit: higher injury rates for professional football clubs with third-generation artificial turf at their home venue. Br J Sports Med 47:775–781
32. Sousa P, Rebelo A, Brito J (2012) Injuries in amateur soccer players on artificial turf: a one-season prospective study. Phys Ther Sport
33. Soligard T, Bahr R, Andersen TE (2012) Injury risk on artificial turf and grass in youth tournament football. Scand J Med Sci Sports 22:356–361
34. Ekstrand J, Hagglund M, Fuller CW (2011) Comparison of injuries sustained on artificial turf and grass by male and female elite football players. Scand J Med Sci Sports 21:824–832
35. Bjorneboe J, Bahr R, Andersen TE (2010) Risk of injury on third-generation artificial turf in Norwegian professional football. Br J Sports Med 44:794–798
36. Walden M, Hagglund M, Orchard J et al (2011) Regional differences in injury incidence in European professional football. Scand J Med Sci Sports. doi:10.1111/j.1600-0838.2011.01409.x
37. Orchard J, Rodas G, Til L et al (2008) A hypothesis: could portable natural grass be a risk factor for knee injuries? J Sports Sci Med 7:184–190
38. Orchard J, Seward H, McGivern J, Hood S (1999) Rainfall, evaporation and the risk of non-contact anterior cruciate ligament injury in the Australian football league. Med J Aust 170: 304–306
39. Eirale C, Tol JL, Smiley F et al (2013) Does Ramadan affect the risk of injury in professional football? Clin J Sport Med 23:261–266
40. Andersen TE, Engebretsen L, Bahr R (2004) Rule violations as a cause of injuries in male norwegian professional football: are the referees doing their job? Am J Sports Med 32:62S–68S
41. Fuller CW, Smith GL, Junge A, Dvorak J (2004) The influence of tackle parameters on the propensity for injury in international football. Am J Sports Med 32:43S–53S
42. Junge A, Dvorak J (2013) Injury surveillance in the world football tournaments 1998–2012. Br J Sports Med 47:782–788

5 Football Injury Prevention

Mario Bizzini and Jiri Dvorak

5.1 Introduction

With about 300 million people playing the game, football (soccer) is the most popular sport worldwide [1]. Playing football requires various skills and abilities, including endurance, agility, speed and a technical and tactical understanding of the game. Playing football has many health benefits, but it is also associated with a certain risk of injury.

Injury prevention within the game is one important task of the Medical Committee of the Fédération Internationale de Football Association (FIFA). In 1994 FIFA established its Medical Assessment and Research Centre (F-MARC) with the aim "to prevent football injuries and to promote football as a health-enhancing leisure activity, improving social behaviour" [2].

There is extensive literature on the frequency and characteristics of football injuries, and several scientific studies on injury prevention programmes in amateur football players have been published. However, the implementation of injury prevention programmes in the real world of sports represents a major challenge [3].

5.2 Why Is Injury Prevention Important?

Besides the slogan "prevention is better than cure", there are clear arguments in favour of injury prevention research and implementation.

From a medical perspective, every single injury increases the risk for a subsequent injury (especially if there has been insufficient rehabilitation and retraining), and severe injuries (such as ACL or cartilage) may increase the risk of osteoarthritis in the long term [4].

From a coach and players' perspective, staying injury free is the only way to perform to one's potential and to enable a team to have all the players at disposal. It has been shown that elite teams with less injured players are more successful in terms of better results and championship ranking [5]. An additional benefit is that injury prevention programmes may play a role in enhancing performance, which can further improve the compliance of coaches and players [6].

From a socio-economic perspective, the burden of injuries causes a significant impact on the health-related costs (medical treatment, rehabilitation, etc.). For example, in Switzerland (with 7.9 million inhabitants) the healthcare costs for injuries in amateur football were nearly 170 million US dollars in 2010 [7].

M. Bizzini (✉) • J. Dvorak
Schulthess Klinik, FIFA-Medical Assessment and Research Centre (F-MARC),
Lengghalde 2, Zürich, ZH 8008, Switzerland
e-mail: mario.bizzini@f-marc.com; jiri.dvorak@f-marc.com

P. Volpi (ed.), *Football Traumatology: New Trends*, DOI 10.1007/978-3-319-18245-2_5

5.3 Injury Prevention Research

The development and implementation of measures for injury prevention should follow the four-step sequence proposed by van Mechelen et al. [8]. After having established the extent of the injury problem (step 1) and analysed the aetiology and mechanisms of injuries (step 2), possible preventive measures should be introduced (step 3). Finally (step 4) the effectiveness of the preventive interventions should be assessed by repeating step 1. Ideally, randomised controlled trials (RCTs) should be performed to scientifically investigate the preventive interventions [9, 10].

The epidemiology of football injuries, injury mechanisms and risk factors have been presented in the previous chapters and will not be addressed here. However, it should be acknowledged that there is a lack of research in children (younger than 14 years of age) at all levels.

Football injuries mainly affect the lower extremity. The most frequent locations are the ankle, knee and thigh. Sprains, strains and contusions are the most common types of injury. Specifically, ankle and knee ligament injuries (with the ACL more prevalent in women) and hamstring muscle lesions (more prevalent in men) are the most often documented injuries in football players. About two thirds of traumatic injuries are caused by the action of another player (contact injuries), and 12–28 % of all injuries are caused by foul play [11]. The percentage of noncontact injuries (e.g. during running, twisting, cutting, landing from a jump) varies from 26 % to 59 % [11]. Overuse injuries (e.g. tendinopathy, low back pain) account for 9–34 % of all injuries, and perhaps this figure could be even higher considering the methodological problems with the injury definitions used in many studies [12].

Another figure of major concern is that about a quarter of injuries (mostly noncontact) are reinjuries of the same type and location.

The types of injury have direct implications in terms of preventive strategies. Although the contact injuries may only be tackled with a severe application of the laws of the game (and the promotion of fair play), it is possible that the noncontact injuries may be targeted with specific exercises or programmes.

5.4 Prevention of Injuries: Scientific Evidence

The first RCT study investigating the effectiveness of injury prevention measures in football players was performed by Ekstrand et al. in 1983 [13]. It was then almost another 20 years before Junge et al. (2002) [14] published a controlled trial on injury prevention in football. Both authors showed that a multimodal intervention programme (comprising adapted equipment, warm-up routine, prophylactic ankle taping, controlled rehabilitation, specific stabilisation and coordination exercises for the trunk, ankle and knee joints) was effective in reducing the overall incidence of injuries by 75 % in male senior [13] and by 21 % in male youth teams [14]. Currently as many as 30 scientific studies exist on injury prevention measures in football players. For example, Heidt et al. found that a preseason neuromuscular training programme (cardiovascular conditioning, plyometrics, strength, flexibility) was found to reduce the number of overall injuries in female youth players [15], and Lehnhard et al. reported a reduction of 47 % for overall injuries when a 1-year progressive strength training programme was performed in a male college football team [16]. Emery et al. [17] reported the positive preventive effects of a neuromuscular programme for injuries in general and the acute onset injury in youth male and female players. FIFA's "The 11", which is a simple injury prevention programme, was implemented in a 4-year nationwide campaign in Switzerland and showed a 12–25 % reduction of injuries in male and female amateur players of different age and level of play [18]. With its consequent impact on the healthcare costs, this study demonstrated how injury prevention in football may have a significant socio-economic impact. The FIFA 11+ was also found to reduce the incidence of injuries by 30–50 % in youth female football players after performing this "complete warm-up" at least twice a week [19]. The importance of compliance, a crucial aspect for the effectiveness of the prevention programme, was also evaluated in the aforementioned study [20]. The results showed that players with high compliance had a significant lower risk of injury and that positive coach attitudes towards prevention were correlated with high compliance and lower injury risk [20].

While these studies aimed at reducing the injury incidence in football, other studies have focused on specific types of injuries. Most studies have addressed ankle sprains [21]. Balance training (on unstable surfaces) and the use of semirigid ankle orthoses have been effective in reducing (approximately 80 %) the recurrence of ankle sprains in previously injured male and female players, but not in healthy players [22–25].

Specific hamstring eccentric strengthening exercises were found to be effective in reducing hamstring strains (by approximately 30 %) in male elite and amateur football players [26–28], and Croisier et al. [29] described how the restoration of normal strength decreased the incidence of hamstring injuries in professional male players. Further support for these findings was provided by a study by Holmich et al. [30] which found a trend (not significant) for less groin injuries in amateur players performing a specific strengthening and core stability programme.

Prevention measures for ACL and severe knee injuries have been addressed in different studies. Caraffa et al. [31] showed a significant reduction in ACL injuries in male professional and amateur players with balance board proprioceptive training, while Sodermann et al. [32] found no preventive effects with the same intervention on the incidence of acute knee injuries in female adult players. Neuromuscular programmes including plyometrics, strength and stabilisation training were specially developed to target the high incidence of noncontact ACL injuries in female football players [33]. Hewett et al. [34] published the first paper in this field and reported a trend towards reduction in knee injuries in young female players performing such programmes. The PEP (Prevent and Enhance Performance) was evaluated in two studies [35, 36] and showed its effectiveness in reducing noncontact ACL tears in youth female college players. Similar findings were demonstrated in a large RCT in adolescent female players with a 15 min neuromuscular warm-up programme [37], and by implementing an adapted programme (warm-up, balance, strength and core stability), Kiani et al. [38] documented an impressive reduction of acute knee injuries and noncontact knee injuries in youth female players. Hägglund et al. [39] showed how a 10-step progressive rehabilitation programme for injured players was able to reduce (66–75 %) recurrent injuries in those same players following this programme.

Interestingly, Fredberg et al. [40] did not find any preventive effect with specific eccentric exercises in the prevalence of Achilles and patellar tendinopathy in male professional players. A study by Johnson et al. [41] reported a lower injury frequency with training in mental skills (cognitive-behavioural training) among high-risk elite male and female players, whereas no effects on acute injuries was found with an educational video-based injury awareness programme .

Back in 2006 and following F-MARC research [42–46], the International Football Association Board (IFAB) decided that any incident of elbow to the head should be sanctioned with a red card (as IFAB did for the tackles from behind and the two-footed tackles from the side). The consequent application of these decisions helped in reducing the number of head (including concussions) and ankle injuries caused by elbowing and dangerous tackles. Data from previous male FIFA World Cups (2006, 2010) proved that the reinforcement of the laws of the game and the subsequent stricter refereeing during the competitions were crucial in protecting the health of the players [2, 47, 48] (Fig. 5.1).

To summarise the published studies, it seems that between 20 % and 50 % of all noncontact football injuries can be prevented with exercise-based prevention programmes [14, 17, 19, 35–37]. The best available evidence is for female adolescent players, whereas the impact of such programmes in male players has been demonstrated only recently [49]. Based on the current evidence, the key elements of effective injury prevention programmes are core stability/strength, neuromuscular control and balance, eccentric training of the hamstrings, plyometric and agility (Table 5.1).

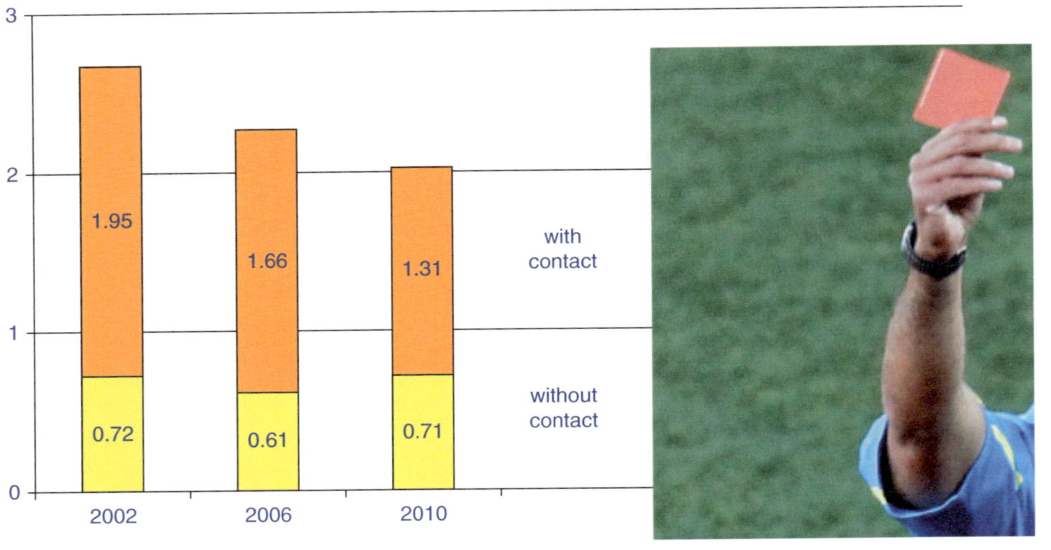

Fig. 5.1 Role of refereeing in preventing contact injuries at the FIFA World Cups 2002–2010 (number of injuries per match; 64 matches per World Cup) (Courtesy of F-MARC)

Table 5.1 Injury prevention programs in football/soccer

Year	Authors	Design	Nr. subjects	Gender	Age (range)	Sports	Prev. program	Effect
2005	Mandelbaum	CCT	1,041	f	14–18	Soccer	PEP	+
2006	Pfeiffer	CCT	1,439	f	14–18	Soccer, basket, volley	–	–
2007	Emery	RCT	920	m/f	12–18	Basket	–	+
2008	Gilchrist	RCT	1,435	f	Av.19	Soccer	PEP	+
2008	Steffen	RCT	2,020	f	13–17	Soccer	The 11	–
2008	Pasanen	RCT	457	f	Av. 24	Floorball	–	+
2008	Soligard	RCT	1,982	f	13–17	Soccer	11+°	+
2010	Kiani	RCT	1,506	f	13–19	Soccer	HarmoKnee	+
2010	Emery	RCT	744	m/f	13–18	Soccer	–	+
2011	LaBella	RCT	1,558	f	Av.16	Soccer, Basket	KIPP	+
2012	Longo	RCT	121	m	13–15	Basket	11+°	+
2012	Beijsterveldt	RCT	456	m	18–40	Soccer	The 11	–
2012	Walden	RCT	4,564	f	12–17	Soccer	Knäkontroll	+
2014	Owoeye	RCT	414	m	14–19	Soccer	FIFA 11+	+
[a]	Silvers	RCT	1,769	m	18–23	Soccer	FIFA 11+	+

CT cohort trial, *RCT* randomized controlled trail, *f* female, *m* male, *PEP* prevent and enhance performance
[a]Not yet published, 11 + ° = FIFA 11+; –/+: negative versus positive injury prevention effect of the programme

5.5 Development and Research Around FIFA 11+

F-MARC conducted an initial study on the prevention of football injuries, with results showing 21 % fewer injuries in the intervention compared to the control group [14]. The interventions were focused on improving the structure and content of the training by educating and supervising the coaches and players. The programme included preventive interventions such as improvement of warm-up, regular cooldown, taping of unstable ankles, adequate rehabilitation, promotion of the spirit of fair play and ten sets of exercises designed to improve coordination, stability of the ankle and knee and flexibility and strength of the trunk, hip and leg muscles. Based on the experiences with this pilot study and in cooperation with international experts, F-MARC developed a basic injury prevention programme for amateur football players called "The 11".

"The 11" comprises of 10 evidence-based or best-practice exercises (core stability, balance, dynamic stabilisation and eccentric hamstring strength) and the promotion of fair play. The programme was designed to reduce the most common football injuries (ankle and knee sprains, hamstring and groin strains). It can be completed in 10–15 min and requires no equipment other than a ball. "The 11" was implemented in two nationwide campaigns (Switzerland and New Zealand) in cooperation with the national accident insurance company and the national football association [18, 50].

In Switzerland, the implementation of "The 11" and its effect on the injury rate were carefully evaluated by an independent research company [18]. Four years after the launch of the programme, teams that included "The 11" as a part of their warm-up had 11.5 % fewer match injuries and 25.3 % fewer training injuries than teams that warmed-up as usual. In New Zealand, the implementation of "The 11" resulted in a 2.4 dollar return of investment for the national accident insurance company after 2 years [51]. In other RCTs, the compliance of the intervention group (with "The 11") was too poor for a statistically significant effect of the programme to be shown [52, 53].

Based on experiences with "The 11", "PEP" (Prevent Injury and Enhance Performance programme) [35, 36] and other exercise-based programmes [15, 31, 32, 34] to prevent football injuries, an advanced version ("FIFA 11+") was developed in 2006 together with the OSTRC and the Santa Monica Orthopaedic and Sports Medicine Research Foundation. "FIFA 11+" is a complete warm-up programme with running exercises at the beginning and end to activate the cardiovascular system and specific preventive exercises focussing on core and leg strength, balance and agility, each of three levels of increasing difficulty to provide variation and progression. It takes about 20 min to be completed and requires a minimum amount of equipment (a set of cones and balls). "FIFA 11+" is time efficient because it replaces the usual warm-up (www.f-marc.com/11plus).

A RCT, conducted by the Oslo Sports Trauma and Research Centre, showed that young female teams performing the "FIFA 11+" at least twice a week (as a standard warm-up before their training) had 37 % fewer training injuries and 29 % fewer match injuries, and severe injuries were reduced by almost 50 % [19]. The compliance with "FIFA 11+" was high in general, and players with a higher compliance had a significantly lower injury risk than others [20]. Recently, a large RCT in male soccer players found significantly lower training and match injuries (−52 % overall) in teams practising "FIFA 11+" as a warm-up routine (yet to be published; Silvers et al. Santa Monica Sports Medicine Foundation, CA, USA) [54].

In another RCT study on Canadian youth female football players, Steffen et al. found that players with higher adherence to "FIFA 11+" showed significant improvements in functional balance and reduced injury risk [55]. Two recent studies in Italian amateur football players showed that the physiological warm-up effects of "FIFA 11+" are similar to or even better than a standard warm-up routine and that it enhances neuromuscular control (core/lower extremity) and knee flexor strength [6, 56]. Other authors have found improvements in static/dynamic balance and thigh muscle strength in male football and futsal players after performing "FIFA 11+" [57–60].

The two nationwide campaigns in Switzerland and New Zealand represent successful examples of injury prevention in amateur football [18, 50]. The success of a prevention programme from a social economic viewpoint was investigated by Gianotti et al. [51] who introduced a pre- and post-implementation cost outcome formulae. The data provided a return on investment for each dollar invested in the programme and cost savings. Since the Soccer Smart Programme (including the "The 11" programme) was introduced in New Zealand in 2004, the Accident Compensation Corporation (ACC) has invested 650,000 NZ dollars into this. Up to June 2011, ACC had saved a total of 5,331,000 NZ dollars, and therefore the return of investment had risen to 8.20 for each invested dollar (personal communication with Dr. S. Gianotti, ACC, New Zealand). These data, together with the published results of the nationwide implementation in Switzerland, reinforce the hypothesis outlined by F-MARC back in 1994: prevention measures or programmes can not only reduce the incidence of football injuries, but have the potential to save billions of dollars in health-related costs worldwide [2] (Fig. 5.2).

5.6 Dissemination/ Implementation of FIFA 11+

For the nationwide campaign in Switzerland, "The 11" was integrated into the coach education of the Swiss Football Association (Schweizerischer Fussballverband (SFV)) using a "teach the teacher" strategy. All instructor coaches of the SFV were educated by sports physical therapists on how to deliver the programme to the coaches participating in licensing or refresher courses. Over a period of 3 years, 5,000 licensed amateur coaches were subsequently instructed on how to perform "The 11" with their teams and received the information material [18]. The same strategy was used in New Zealand, where "The 11" was implemented as part of the "Soccer Smart Programme" [51].

The coach is the key person to promote injury prevention to his/her players. While the coach, especially at a low level, has to consider various aspects in the training (e.g. physical preparation, tactics, fair play, team success), it is important to raise his/her motivation to implement an injury prevention programme with his team.

"FIFA 11+" is best taught to coaches in a course/workshop that includes theoretical background knowledge and practical demonstration of the exercises as recently shown by Steffen et al. [55, 61]. In a cluster randomised trial on different implementation strategies. The authors found that a preseason coach education workshop was more effective in terms of better compliance and decreased injury risk in players than other delivery methods (unsupervised website, additional supervision by a physical therapist) of the programme [3].

In 2009 FIFA began the dissemination of "FIFA 11+" in its 209 Member Associations (MAs). Based on the experience with the nationwide implementation in Switzerland and New Zealand and on the evaluations of other sports injury prevention programme implementations (i.e. rugby) [62, 63], a guideline on how to implement the "FIFA 11+" injury prevention programme at a larger scale in amateur football was developed [3]. The implementation is conducted either in close cooperation with MAs or via FIFA Coaching Instructor courses.

5.7 Challenges I: Injury Prevention to the Pitch

The F-MARC team has gained experience during the years of dissemination of the injury prevention programmes. It has been found that understanding the coach's character and highlighting the importance of the programme to the coach is especially important. By preventing injuries and therefore reducing the number of injured players means that the coach will have more players available for his/her ideal team. Therefore, it is not only information and education about the role of injury prevention which is important but moreover to speak the same language as the coach and to highlight all the advantages of injury prevention. One of keys while conducting a course is "proposing" rather than "imposing" the "FIFA 11+". The dialogue on the pitch with coaches is often more important than the distributed materials, thus allowing for friendly discussion and practical work with the preventive programme. Therefore, the choice of the instructors is crucial, and F-MARC's best experiences have been with sports physiotherapists or athletic trainers who have an active involvement in football, because they already "live and speak the football language". Additionally, the cooperation with famous players and coaches acting as "FIFA 11+" ambassadors (see teaser on https://vimeo.com/45562029 and www.f-marc.com/11plus) has helped significantly in communicating with coaches. "FIFA 11+" has also been presented to the delegates of all MAs at the last two FIFA

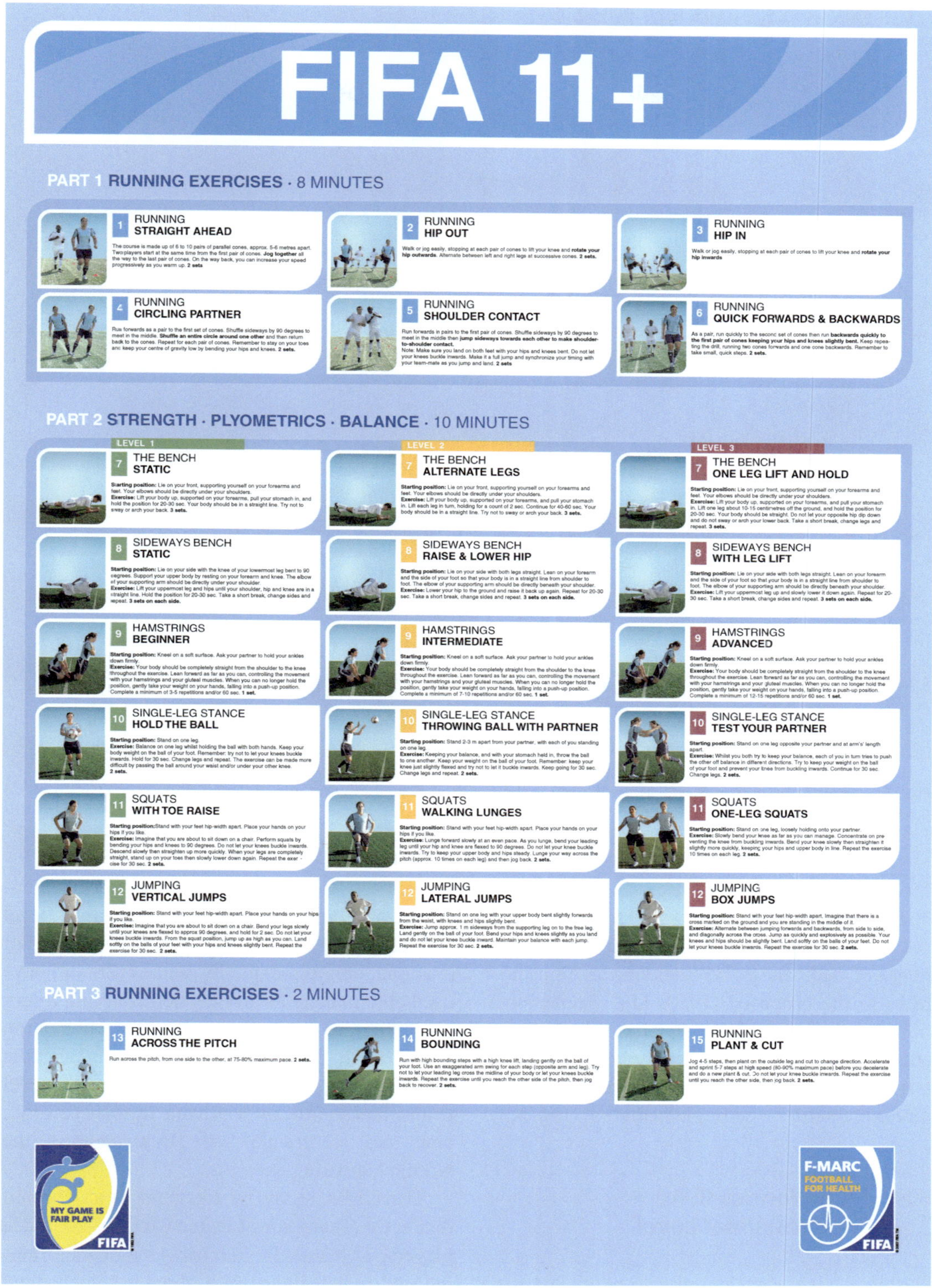

Fig. 5.2 FIFA 11+ warm-up programme to prevent injuries (Courtesy of F-MARC)

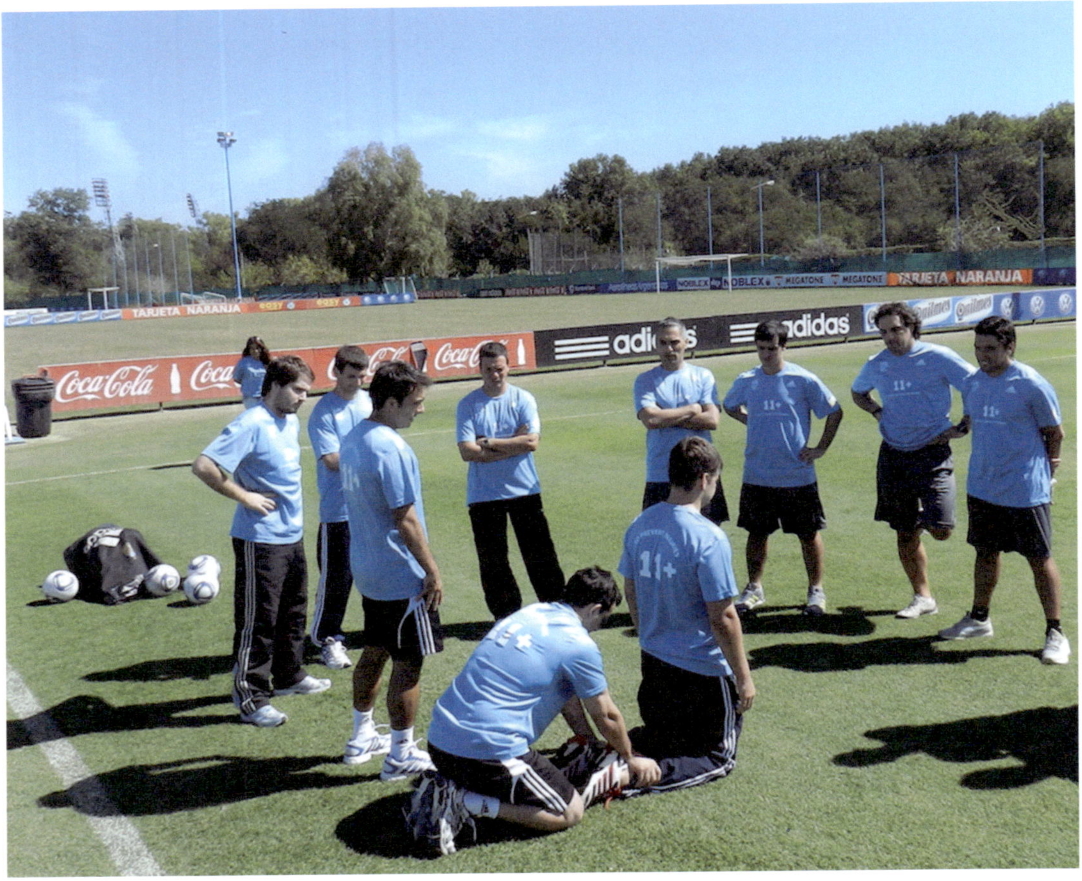

Fig. 5.3 Injury prevention exercises on the pitch: information, education and compliance are the keys (Courtesy of F-MARC)

Medical Conferences (Zürich 2009, Budapest 2012). After initial enthusiasm from the interested MAs, F-MARC has experienced a wide range of dedication and compliance from those MAs to the proposed "FIFA 11+" implementation guidelines. At MA level, it has to be acknowledged that highly motivated people are needed, in order to successfully plan, realise and constantly monitor a nationwide implementation (Fig. 5.3).

5.8 Challenges II: At Professional Level

Despite a significant number of publications on the epidemiology of injuries in professional football, there are very few papers on prevention in professional players [26–30]. Almost all injury prevention studies in football have been conducted in semi-professional (few), lower level (amateur/recreational) and youth football. For example, only three quality studies [26–28] have used elite players to investigate hamstring injury prevention in football. In the best publication [28], Danish professional players, included in the intervention group together with lower level teams, had significant less acute injuries (overall, new and recurrent!) after implementing the Nordic hamstring exercise.

The UEFA study by Ekstrand et al. showed that in the Champions League Clubs (1,743 male players, 27 teams, 10 countries) the overall training and match injury rate remained unchanged over the course of 11 years [64]. Although the injury rate for ligament injury decreased, the rate for muscle and severe injuries remained high or

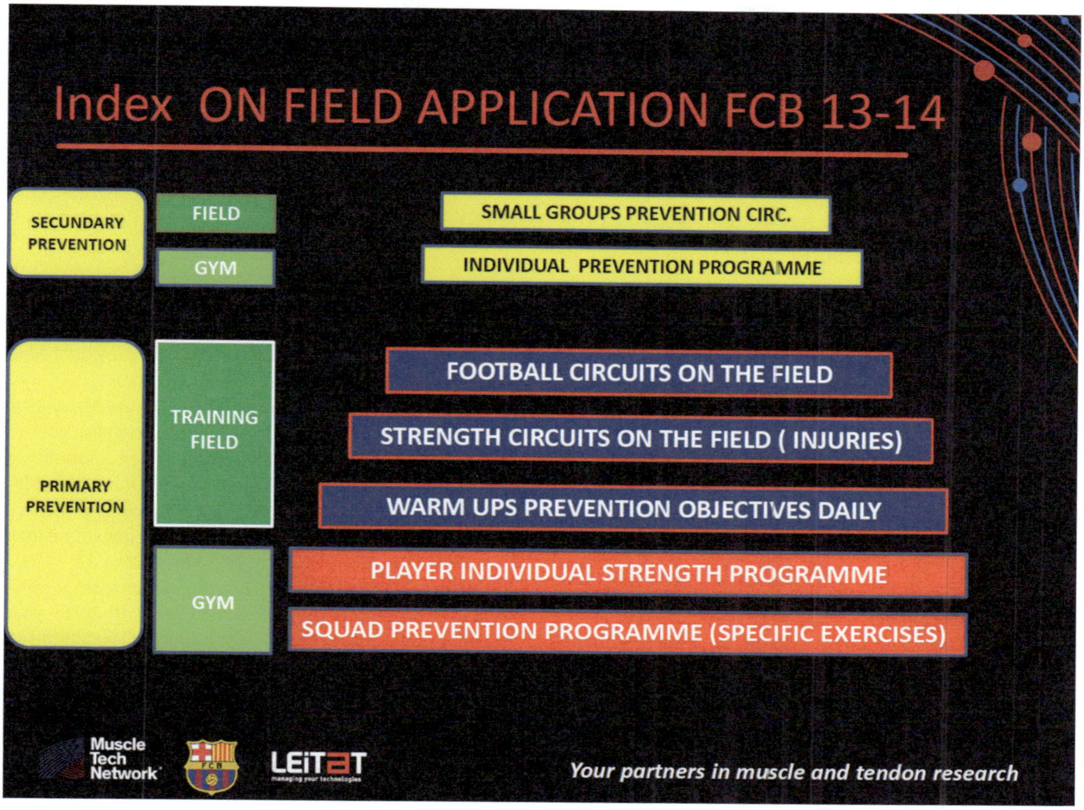

Fig. 5.4 FC Barcelona prevention strategy "on field" 2013–14 (Courtesy of FC Barcelona FIFA medical center of excellence)

even increased, which was found to be associated with the congested calendar of national and international competitions. In another UEFA Champions League injury study, Hägglund et al. found that low injury rates were associated with improved performances at domestic (higher final league ranking) and at European Cups levels (higher UEFA Season Club Coefficient), whereas more injuries had a negative impact on team performance [5]. These figures highlight the importance of optimal medical care and moreover the importance of injury prevention for the players.

Recently McCall et al. conducted a survey ("belief and practice") about preventative strategies for noncontact injuries in 44 professional clubs worldwide (10 countries in 4 continents) and found that mostly physiotherapists were involved in a wide range of injury prevention programmes [65].

The top five exercises used by clubs were (in rank order) eccentric exercises, balance/proprioception, hamstring eccentric, core stability and Nordic hamstring plus gluteus activation. Interestingly these exercises correspond to the components of the FIFA 11+ programme. On a general note, the authors of the survey stated that "additional research is needed to determine the optimal type, timing and prescription of exercises within a multidimensional injury prevention programme for use in the practical setting". Another conclusion from the study was that a club's perceptions and practices are not always evidence based, clearly indicating the gap between the field and the scientific research world [65].

One excellent example on how to integrate injury prevention in the team's training and general planning was provided by FC Barcelona at the ISOKINETIC Football Conference in Milan in 2014. Examples were mandatory pre-activation and adapted warm-ups (based on the contents of FIFA 11+), exercise circuits integrated in the training sessions, supplementary individual sessions (indoor, outdoor) and work in small groups on reinjury prevention (Fig. 5.4).

5.9 Special Group: Referees

An official football match is only possible if the officials are present: the referee and the two assistant referees are responsible for the match control and to ensure that the players follow the laws of the game. Considering the match and training demands and the duration of the career (up to 45 years old), football refereeing entails a certain risk of injury [66]. Research studies have shown that noncontact injuries (with a slight lower incidence than in players) and moreover overuse injuries (with an estimated higher prevalence than in players) are of concern among referees. The most common injuries are hamstring strains, calf strains and ankle sprains, whereas the most frequent locations of musculoskeletal complaints (overuse) are the lower back, hamstring and calf/Achilles tendon [67, 68]. Based on the original FIFA 11+ and on experiences at FIFA tournaments and World Cups, an adapted injury prevention programme was developed and subsequently implemented within the male and female FIFA referee's selections. Since 2014, the "FIFA 11+ REFEREE" is disseminated worldwide through the official FIFA Refereeing courses.

Conclusions

Research has shown that noncontact injuries in football can be prevented by at least one third and up to a half by the means of specific injury prevention programmes, whereas contact injuries can only be prevented by enhanced fair play and stricter refereeing. Although there is still a lack of scientific studies in certain groups (i.e. children, professional players) and in different areas (i.e. influence of the playing surface, role of football shoes), the current evidence clearly supports the implementation of injury prevention programmes at a large scale. Among the 300 million people playing football worldwide, more than 99 % do it at amateur or recreational level, and evidence has shown that less injuries translates into less socio-economic health-related costs. All involved individuals and associations (e.g. federations, clubs, coaches, players, fitness trainers, doctors and physiotherapists) should endorse and promote injury prevention, thus optimising the beneficial health and social effects of football and reducing the economic burden.

References

1. FIFA Big count. http://www.fifa.com/worldfootball/bigcount/2006. Cited 2013 21 Feb 2013
2. Dvorak J (2009) Give Hippocrates a jersey: promoting health through football/sport. Br J Sports Med 43(5):317–322
3. Bizzini M, Junge A, Dvorak J (2013) Implementation of the FIFA 11+ football warm up program: how to approach and convince the football associations to invest in prevention. Br J Sports Med 47(12):803–806
4. Bizzini M, Silvers HJ (2014) Return to competitive football after major knee surgery: more questions than answers? J Sports Sci 32(13):1209–1216
5. Hagglund M et al (2013) Injuries affect team performance negatively in professional football: an 11-year follow-up of the UEFA Champions League injury study. Br J Sports Med 47(12):738–742
6. Bizzini M et al (2013) Physiological and performance responses to the "FIFA 11+" (part 1): is it an appropriate warm-up? J Sports Sci 31(13):1481–1490
7. SUVA Ball sport statistics http://www.suva.ch/startseite-suva/praevention-suva/sichere-freizeit-suva/kampagne-ballsport-fitness-suva/statistik-ballsport-suva.htm
8. van Mechelen W, Hlobil H, Kemper HC (1992) Incidence, severity, aetiology and prevention of sports injuries. A review of concepts. Sports Med 14(2):82–99
9. Sackett D, Strauss S, Richardson W (2000) Evidence-based medicine. How to practice and teach EBM, 2nd edn. Churchill Livingstone, Edinburgh/New York
10. Scherrington C (2012) Integrating evidence into clinical practice to make quality decisions. In: Brukner P et al (ed) Brukner & Khan's clinical sports medicine. McGraw Hill, Sydney, pp 11–13
11. Junge A, Dvorak J (2004) Soccer injuries: a review on incidence and prevention. Sports Med 34(13):929–938
12. Bahr R (2009) No injuries, but plenty of pain? On the methodology for recording overuse symptoms in sports. Br J Sports Med 43(13):966–972
13. Ekstrand J, Gillquist J, Liljedahl SO (1983) Prevention of soccer injuries. Supervision by doctor and physiotherapist. Am J Sports Med 11(3):116–120
14. Junge A et al (2002) Prevention of soccer injuries: a prospective intervention study in youth amateur players. Am J Sports Med 30(5):652–659
15. Heidt RS Jr et al (2000) Avoidance of soccer injuries with preseason conditioning. Am J Sports Med 28(5):659–662
16. Lehnhard R et al (1996) Monitoring injuries in a college soccer team: the effect of strength training. J Strength Cond Res 10:115–119

17. Emery CA, Meeuwisse WH (2010) The effectiveness of a neuromuscular prevention strategy to reduce injuries in youth soccer: a cluster-randomised controlled trial. Br J Sports Med 44(8):555–562
18. Junge A et al (2011) Countrywide campaign to prevent soccer injuries in Swiss amateur players. Am J Sports Med 39(1):57–63
19. Soligard T et al (2008) Comprehensive warm-up programme to prevent injuries in young female footballers: cluster randomised controlled trial. BMJ 337:a2469
20. Soligard T et al (2010) Compliance with a comprehensive warm-up programme to prevent injuries in youth football. Br J Sports Med 44(11):787–793
21. Handoll HH et al (2001) Interventions for preventing ankle ligament injuries. Cochrane Database Syst Rev 3:CD000018
22. Mohammadi F (2007) Comparison of 3 preventive methods to reduce the recurrence of ankle inversion sprains in male soccer players. Am J Sports Med 35(6):922–926
23. Sharpe SR, Knapik J, Jones B (1997) Ankle braces effectively reduce recurrence of ankle sprains in female soccer players. J Athl Train 32(1):21–24
24. Surve I et al (1994) A fivefold reduction in the incidence of recurrent ankle sprains in soccer players using the Sport-Stirrup orthosis. Am J Sports Med 22(5):601–606
25. Tropp H, Askling C, Gillquist J (1985) Prevention of ankle sprains. Am J Sports Med 13(4):259–262
26. Arnason A et al (2008) Prevention of hamstring strains in elite soccer: an intervention study. Scand J Med Sci Sports 18(1):40–48
27. Askling C, Karlsson J, Thorstensson A (2003) Hamstring injury occurrence in elite soccer players after preseason strength training with eccentric overload. Scand J Med Sci Sports 13(4):244–250
28. Petersen J et al (2011) Preventive effect of eccentric training on acute hamstring injuries in men's soccer: a cluster-randomized controlled trial. Am J Sports Med 39(11):2296–2303
29. Croisier JL et al (2008) Strength imbalances and prevention of hamstring injury in professional soccer players: a prospective study. Am J Sports Med 36(8):1469–1475
30. Holmich P et al (2010) Exercise program for prevention of groin pain in football players: a cluster-randomized trial. Scand J Med Sci Sports 20(6):814–821
31. Caraffa A et al (1996) Prevention of anterior cruciate ligament injuries in soccer. A prospective controlled study of proprioceptive training. Knee Surg Sports Traumatol Arthrosc 4(1):19–21
32. Soderman K et al (2000) Balance board training: prevention of traumatic injuries of the lower extremities in female soccer players? A prospective randomized intervention study. Knee Surg Sports Traumatol Arthrosc 8(6):356–363
33. Hewett TE et al (1996) Plyometric training in female athletes. Decreased impact forces and increased hamstring torques. Am J Sports Med 24(6):765–773
34. Hewett TE et al (1999) The effect of neuromuscular training on the incidence of knee injury in female athletes. A prospective study. Am J Sports Med 27(6):699–706
35. Gilchrist J et al (2008) A randomized controlled trial to prevent noncontact anterior cruciate ligament injury in female collegiate soccer players. Am J Sports Med 36(8):1476–1483
36. Mandelbaum BR et al (2005) Effectiveness of a neuromuscular and proprioceptive training program in preventing anterior cruciate ligament injuries in female athletes: 2-year follow-up. Am J Sports Med 33(7):1003–1010
37. Walden M et al (2012) Prevention of acute knee injuries in adolescent female football players: cluster randomised controlled trial. BMJ 344, e3042
38. Kiani A et al (2010) Prevention of soccer-related knee injuries in teenaged girls. Arch Intern Med 170(1): 43–49
39. Hagglund M, Walden M, Ekstrand J (2007) Lower reinjury rate with a coach-controlled rehabilitation program in amateur male soccer: a randomized controlled trial. Am J Sports Med 35(9):1433–1442
40. Fredberg U, Bolvig L, Andersen NT (2008) Prophylactic training in asymptomatic soccer players with ultrasonographic abnormalities in Achilles and patellar tendons: the Danish Super League Study. Am J Sports Med 36(3):451–460
41. Johnson U, Ekengren J, Andersen M (2005) Helping soccer players at risk. J Sport Exerc Psychol 27:32–38
42. Andersen TE et al (2004) Mechanisms of head injuries in elite football. Br J Sports Med 38(6):690–696
43. Arnason A et al (2004) A prospective video-based analysis of injury situations in elite male football: football incident analysis. Am J Sports Med 32(6):1459–1465
44. Fuller CW, Junge A, Dvorak J (2005) A six year prospective study of the incidence and causes of head and neck injuries in international football. Br J Sports Med 39(Suppl 1):i3–i9
45. Fuller CW et al (2004) The influence of tackle parameters on the propensity for injury in international football. Am J Sports Med 32(1 Suppl):43S–53S
46. Tscholl P et al (2007) Causation of injuries in female football players in top-level tournaments. Br J Sports Med 41(Suppl 1):i8–i14
47. Dvorak J et al (2011) Injuries and illnesses of football players during the 2010 FIFA World Cup. Br J Sports Med 45(8):626–630
48. Dvorak J et al (2007) Medical report from the 2006 FIFA World Cup Germany. Br J Sports Med 41(9): 578–581, discussion 581
49. Owoeye OB et al (2014) Efficacy of the FIFA 11+ warm-Up programme in male youth football: a cluster randomised controlled trial. J Sports Sci Med 13(2): 321–328
50. Gianotti S, Hume PA (2007) A cost-outcome approach to pre and post-implementation of national sports injury prevention programmes. J Sci Med Sport 10(6): 436–446
51. Gianotti S, Hume PA, Tunstall H (2010) Efficacy of injury prevention related coach education within netball and soccer. J Sci Med Sport 13(1):32–35

52. Steffen K et al (2008) Preventing injuries in female youth football–a cluster-randomized controlled trial. Scand J Med Sci Sports 18(5):605–614
53. van Beijsterveldt AM et al (2012) Effectiveness of an injury prevention programme for adult male amateur soccer players: a cluster-randomised controlled trial. Br J Sports Med 46(16):1114–1118
54. Silvers H et al The efficacy of the FIFA 11+ program in the collegiate male soccer players (USA) (in press)
55. Steffen K et al (2013) High adherence to a neuromuscular injury prevention programme (FIFA 11+) improves functional balance and reduces injury risk in Canadian youth female football players: a cluster randomised trial. Br J Sports Med 47(12):794–802
56. Impellizzeri FM et al (2013) Physiological and performance responses to the FIFA 11+ (part 2): a randomised controlled trial on the training effects. J Sports Sci 31(13):1491–1502
57. Brito J, Figueiredo P, Fernandes L (2010) Isokinetic strength effects of FIFA's "The 11+" injury prevention training programme. Isokinetics Exerc Sci 18:211–215
58. Daneshjoo A et al (2012) The effects of comprehensive warm-up programs on proprioception, static and dynamic balance on male soccer players. PLoS One 7(12):e51568
59. Daneshjoo A et al (2012) The effects of injury preventive warm-up programs on knee strength ratio in young male professional soccer players. PLoS One 7(12):e50979
60. Reis I et al (2013) Performance enhancement effects of federation internationale de football association's "the 11+" injury prevention training program in youth futsal players. Clin J Sport Med 23(4):318–320
61. Steffen K et al (2013) Evaluation of how different implementation strategies of an injury prevention programme (FIFA 11+) impact team adherence and injury risk in Canadian female youth football players: a cluster-randomised trial. Br J Sports Med 47(8):480–487
62. Chalmers DJ, Simpson JC, Depree R (2004) Tackling Rugby injury: lessons learned from the implementation of a five-year sports injury prevention program. J Sci Med Sport 7(1):74–84
63. Gianotti SM, Quarrie KL, Hume PA (2009) Evaluation of RugbySmart: a rugby union community injury prevention programme. J Sci Med Sport 12(3):371–375
64. Ekstrand J et al (2013) Fewer ligament injuries but no preventive effect on muscle injuries and severe injuries: an 11-year follow-up of the UEFA Champions League injury study. Br J Sports Med 47(12):732–737
65. McCall A et al (2014) Risk factors, testing and preventative strategies for non-contact injuries in professional football: current perceptions and practices of 44 teams from various premier leagues. Br J Sports Med 48(18):1352–1357
66. Weston M et al (2012) Science and medicine applied to soccer refereeing: an update. Sports Med 42(7):615–631
67. Bizzini M et al (2009) Female soccer referees selected for the FIFA Women's World Cup 2007: survey of injuries and musculoskeletal problems. Br J Sports Med 43(12):936–942
68. Bizzini M et al (2009) Injuries and musculoskeletal complaints in referees and assistant referees selected for the 2006 FIFA World Cup: retrospective and prospective survey. Br J Sports Med 43(7):490–497

Preseason Evaluation

6

Fabrizio Tencone

Today the Pre-season Evaluation is one of the topics of greatest interest in sports medicine; one of the primary objectives of the preseason evaluation is to screen for conditions that may predispose a competitive sportspeople to injury or illness. The real objective of the preseason evaluation is to ensure sportspeople that they are medically fit to participate in their sports of choice safely, without harm to themselves or others.

A preseason evaluation is often a mandatory administrative requirement of an athletic association for organized sports participation. There is enormous variation through the world in how these examinations are performed.

For many sportspeople the preseason evaluation serves as an entry point into a healthcare system, especially for adolescent, who may have limited contact with the healthcare system and thus may not have seen physician. Therefore, in many cases, the preseason evaluation allows an opportunity to provide quality and cost-effective healthcare, determine general health, and initiate discussion on health-related topics.

In addition, the preseason evaluation affords the opportunity to screen for conditions that may currently be asymptomatic yet could be potentially life-threatening. Sudden cardiac death, while rare, is known to happen more often in sportspeople compared to those who do not play competitive sports. Developing worldwide uniformity in the approach to a comprehensive preseason evaluation may help define and improve the ability to achieve the goal of identifying these conditions in a typically younger and "healthier" population.

The evaluator should review the sportsperson's medical history in addition to evaluating the present illness or injury. Previous musculoskeletal injuries may not have been adequately rehabilitated, resulting in ongoing weakness, joint laxity, or poor neuromotor control. Identifying such factors enables the evaluator to develop an effective rehabilitation plan for any pre-existing injury.

Concussions can leave the sportsperson with ongoing symptoms, vulnerable to more serious brain injury if continuing to participate in athletics, in particular in contact sports. The evaluator may use this information to determine if the sportsperson is suitable for a certain sports or would benefit from an appropriate protective gear to minimize risk.

Inadequate management of chronic conditions such as asthma can leave a sportsperson with specific impairments that appropriate intervention can target towards improved sports performance. The preseason evaluation can provide a forum for clinicians to advise participants on appropriate sports in which to participate, especially for those sportspeople with disabilities.

F. Tencone
Isokinetic Medical Group Torino,
Via Rosmini 5/A, Torino, 10126, Italy
e-mail: f.tencone@isokinetic.com,
a.giannini@isokinetic.com

P. Volpi (ed.), *Football Traumatology: New Trends*, DOI 10.1007/978-3-319-18245-2_6

There is no literature to support the concept that preseason evaluation predicts who will develop an orthopaedic injury or prevents or reduces the severity of an orthopaedic injury in a sportsperson. However, despite this, there is research regarding individual components that could be included in a preseason evaluation that could guide training in an effort to reduce risk of future injury. For example, in female sportspeople, dynamic knee valgus when landing during a jump was shown to be predictive of anterior cruciate ligament injuries. Thus, early recognition and treatment of factors such as abnormal biomechanics may minimize time lost from training and competition, an important goal of competitive sportsperson.

At higher levels of competition, consider assessing psychological, social, and nutritional factors that may affect performance. Since the list of doping agents change regularly, the assessor should review the sportsperson's medications, if any, to ensure compliance with regulations or to identify a need to request exemption.

The preseason evaluation can serve as vehicle to meet administrative requirements of athletic association or governing body for eligibility to participate in competitive athletics.

In the USA, a preseason evaluation is required in order to participate in organized sports at the high school and collegiate levels. Italy requires compulsory annual medical clearance to compete in organized sports at every competitive level. In addition, there are numerous country-specific legal statutes that govern the rights of sportspeople to participate, as well as the confidentiality of medical records obtained during performance of a Preseason Evaluation.

In the broadest context, all persons who begin a new activity programme should have a preseason evaluation tailored to their age, ability, and anticipated "athletic" endeavour. Ideally, preseason evaluation should take place for competitive sportspeople of all ages, genders, and levels of organized sports competition.

Skills in both musculoskeletal evaluation and cardiac auscultation may require that more than one clinician performs components of the examination. International and professional sportspeople are governed by their athletic organizations as to who is considered qualified to perform a Preseason Evaluation.

Timing of the preseason evaluation ideally should occur in the off-season, at least 2–6 weeks prior to the beginning of the practice season, to allow time for appropriate rehabilitation of injuries or to evaluate and treat medical conditions. The required frequency of the preseason evaluation varies according to the governing bodies of various athletic organizations and the age of the sportsperson.

A thorough medical history is crucial to the preseason evaluation of competitive sportspeople. Various questionnaires have been developed for sportspeople of all ages and levels of competition. The essential components of the history include a thorough system review for acute or chronic medical and orthopaedic conditions. This should include cardiovascular symptoms, pulmonary symptoms, musculoskeletal symptoms, haematological symptoms, allergies, infection/immunology, ear/nose/throat symptoms, dermatological symptoms, genitourinary symptoms, neurological symptoms, endocrine/metabolic symptoms, ophthalmologic symptoms, and dental symptoms. Review the sportsperson's sports participation history, including the use of protective equipment, use of medications and supplements, allergies, and a menstrual history for female sportspeople. Questions regarding immunization status, dietary status, and health-risk behaviours are recommended.

The physical examination component of the preseason evaluation should be performed by skilled clinician (in Italy by physicians specialized in sports medicine) with a particular focus on cardiovascular, neurological, and orthopaedic abnormalities that would identify sportspeople at high risk of injury, disability, or death. Baseline data should also be obtained on blood pressure, weight, height, and organ function in case of injury or illness.

Much interest has been generated in the use of diagnostic testing to assist in screening for cardiovascular conditions that may predispose a sportsperson to sudden cardiac death. Routine diagnostic testing with an ECG/EKG has been performed as a part of the preseason evaluation in Italy for many years and has been found useful in identifying sportspeople with hypertrophic cardiomyopathy in that population. Atherosclerotic coronary disease is the most common form of heart disease in masters athletes, and a routine screening ECG/EKG is recommended for this population as part of their PPE.

Echocardiography and exercise stress testing are not suggested for routine screening; however, these diagnostic tests may be indicated in certain populations such as masters athletes, particularly if they are undertaking sudden vigorous training, and for sportspeople with abnormalities on resting ECG/EKG. It is important to recognize that further testing and referral should be considered for any sportsperson who has a personal or family history of sudden cardiac death or premature coronary disease. Symptoms of syncope, unexplained exertional dyspnea, or chest pain should be thoroughly evaluated as they may be an early sign of one of the genetic cardiovascular diseases. Additional testing should also be undertaken if sportsperson has a heart murmur, hypertension, or abnormalities suggestive of Marfan syndrome or coarctation of the aorta.

In the rare event that findings suggest that participation in sports should be modified or restricted, it is imperative that the sportsperson (and the caregiver if appropriate) be fully informed of findings and associated risks. Some authors suggest that the sportsperson should be involved in the decision-making process wherever possible regarding participation options given the relative risks affecting his or her health or safety; in Italy the medical certification is unquestionable.

Conclusion

Italian sports medical rules can be used as an example to improve preseason evaluation in a well-defined medical evaluation, taking into account both the health of the athletes and the responsibility of the physicians that certify the status of fitness for sports.

Trauma Management in the Field

7

Porcelli Simone, Daniele Casalini,
Alessandro Corsini, Gian Nicola Bisciotti,
and Piero Volpi

7.1 Introduction

Although most sports injuries are relatively minor, life-threatening injuries are unpredictable and can occur during any physical activity and at any level of participation [1]. For this reason prompt care is essential.

In catastrophic injuries time becomes the critical factor, and assistance to the injured athlete must be handled by trained personnel. A mistake in the initial management of injury can prolong the time required for rehabilitation and in rare cases could be fatal. The prime concern of emergency aid is to maintain cardiovascular function and, indirectly, central nervous system function because failure of any of these systems may lead to death [2].

All professionals working in the sports world should be trained and certified in cardiopulmonary resuscitation (CPR), the use of an automatic external defibrillation (AED), and first aid. Besides education and training, preparation should also include maintenance of emergency equipment and supplies, appropriate use of personnel and formation and implementation of an emergency action plan *(EAP),* and continuing education in the area of emergency medicine and planning. A written EAP document defines the standard of care. The absence of an EAP frequently is a basis for claims and lawsuits based on negligence. The EAP should be comprehensive, practical, and flexible enough to adapt to any emergency situation [3].

7.1.1 Emergency Personnel

The first responder in an emergency situation is typically a member of the sports medicine staff, such as a certified athletic trainer. However, the first responder may also be a coach or another member of the staff. Certification in cardiopulmonary resuscitation (CPR), first aid, automated

P. Simone (✉)
Institute of Bioimaging and Molecular Physiology – National Research Council, Segrate (MI), Italy

Medical Staff FC INTERNAZIONALE, Appiano Gentile (CO), Italy
e-mail: simone.porcelli@ibfm.cnr.it; simone.porcelli@inter.it

D. Casalini • A. Corsini • G.N. Bisciotti
Medical Staff FC INTERNAZIONALE, Appiano Gentile (CO), Italy
e-mail: Daniele.casalini@inter.it; bisciotti@libero.it

P. Volpi
Knee Orthopedics and Sport Traumatology Unit, Humanitas Clinical Institute IRCCS, Milan, Italy

Head of Medical Staff FC Internazionale Milan, Milan, Italy
e-mail: piero.volpi@humanitas.it

P. Volpi (ed.), *Football Traumatology: New Trends*, DOI 10.1007/978-3-319-18245-2_7

external defibrillator (AED), prevention of disease transmission, and emergency plan review is required for all athletics personnel associated with practices, competitions, skills instructions, and strength and conditioning [4].

The emergency team may consist of physicians, emergency medical technicians, certified athletic trainers, athletic training student, coaches, managers, and possibly bystanders. Roles of these individuals will vary depending on different factors such as team size, athletic venue, preference of the head athletic trainer, etc.

The four basic roles within the emergency team are:

1. Formation of an emergency team and implementation of specific roles are important.
2. Establish scene safety and immediate care of the athlete: this should be provided by the most qualified individual on the medical team.
3. Activation of emergency medical services: this may be necessary in situations where emergency transportation is not already present at the sporting event.
4. Equipment retrieval: may be done by anyone on the emergency team who is familiar with the types and locations of the specific equipment needed. Coaches may be good choices for this role.

Individuals providing emergency care to the injured athlete must cooperate and act professionally [5]. It is not unusual that rescue team members disagree over exactly how the injured athlete should be handled and transported. To reduce potential conflicts, it is a good idea to establish guidelines and procedures and arrange practice sessions at least once a year [6].

7.1.2 Emergency Communication

Communication is a key to a quick, efficient emergency response. Access to a working telephone line or other devices, either fixed or mobile, should be assured. Cellular or digital phones are recommended. However, a landline should also be available in case cell phone services are not available.

7.1.3 Emergency Equipment

All necessary emergency equipment should be at the site and quickly accessible [7]. Personnel should be familiar with function and operation of each type of emergency equipment. The equipment should be checked on a regular basis to ensure good condition, and equipment use should be rehearsed by all emergency personnel. Creating an equipment inspection logbook is strongly recommended. You should choose a clean, dry, environmentally controlled area, and it should be readily available when emergency situations arise.

This type of equipment could include spine boards and straps, automated external defibrillators (AEDs), AED pads, AED batteries, splinting equipment, bag/valve mask, CPR pocket mask, stretcher, crutches, cervical collar, etc. A bag filled with crushed ice is important to have on hand at all practices and competitions. Ice can be applied to most acute injuries to help reduce swelling and reduce pain. If crushed ice is not available, commercial ice pack can be purchased.

A well-stocked first-aid kit should also be available. First-aid kits need to be inventoried regularly and checked for supplies that have been used and need to be replaced. The first-aid kit should be placed in a location that is readily accessible to the emergency team and not locked in a shed or building.

First-aid kits should include at least the following items:

- Gauze pads
- Assorted bandages
- Protective gloves
- Assorted sizes of Ace bandages (3″, 4″, 6″)
- Roller gauze
- Antibiotic ointment
- Cleaning agent
- Tongue depressors

7.1.3.1 Medical Emergency Transportation

Emphasis is placed on having an ambulance onsite at high-risk sporting events. There should be a designated location with rapid access to the site and cleared route for entering/exiting the venue.

7.2 On-the-Field Injury Assessment

The initial assessment and management of seriously injured patients is a challenging task and requires a rapid and systematic approach. Appropriate medical care cannot be delivered to injured athlete until some systemic assessment has been made. This systematic approach helps to determine the nature of the injury and gives information in the decision-making process. It can be practiced to increase speed and accuracy of the process, but good clinical judgment is also required. It should be remembered that some of the steps may be taken simultaneously even if described in sequence [8].

The aim of good trauma care is to prevent early trauma mortality. Early trauma deaths occur because of failure of oxygenation of vital organs or central nervous system injury or both.

The *primary survey* refers to assessment of potentially life-threatening problems including airway, breathing, circulation, severe bleeding, or shock. Once the condition of the victim is stabilized, the *secondary survey* is used to take a closer look at the injury sustained by the athlete. The secondary survey gathers specific information about the injury from the athlete, systematically assesses vital signs and symptoms, and allows for a more detailed evaluation of the injury. It is done to uncover additional problems in other parts of the body.

The primary survey is usually performed using *DRABC* (danger, response, airway, breathing, circulation – Table 7.1). If emergency treatment is not needed, *TOTAPS* is an effective tool for secondary assessment (Table 7.2). These guidelines do not apply for assessing head injuries, concussion, or suspected spinal injury.

7.2.1 Primary Survey

Life-threatening injuries take precedence over all other injuries sustained by the athletes [9]. The initial assessment consists in:

Forming a General Impression of the Patient

The general impression will help you decide the seriousness of the patient's condition based on his level of distress and mental status.

Assessing the Athlete's Mental Status

Initially this may mean determining if the patient is responsive or unresponsive. The AVPU scale can be useful:

- A – Alert. The alert patient is/will be awake, responsive, oriented, and talking to you.
- V – Verbal. This is a patient who appears to be unresponsive at first, but will respond to a loud verbal stimulus from you – note that the term verbal does not mean that the patient is answering your questions or initiating a conversation. The patient may speak, grunt, groan, or simply look at you.
- P – Painful. If the patient does not respond to verbal stimuli, he or she may respond to painful stimuli such as sternal (breastbone) rub or a gentle pinch to the shoulder.
- U – Unresponsive. If the patient does not respond to either painful or verbal stimuli. The unconscious athlete must always be considered to have life-threatening injury.

Assessing the Athlete's Airway

Is the patient's airway open? If the patient is unresponsive, stabilize the head and neck and use the jaw-thrust maneuver to ensure an open airway. If you do not suspect a spine injury, use the head-tilt/chin-lift maneuver.

Assessing the Athlete's Breathing

Is the patient breathing adequately? With the airway open, place your ear over the patient's nose and mouth and watch for chest movement; note symmetry or lack of symmetry in chest movement. Listen and feel for the presence of exhaled air. Listen to the quality of the breath sounds. Sporadic respirations are called agonal respirations and occur just prior to death.

Assessing the Athlete's Circulation (Pulse and Bleeding)

Does the patient have an adequate pulse? Is there serious bleeding? Did the patient lose a large quantity of blood prior to your arrival?

If the patient is not breathing, check the pulse at the neck (carotid). If the patient is breathing, you can check the carotid or the pulse at the

Table 7.1 DRABC procedure

Danger	Check for *danger*. If someone appears to be unconscious or seriously injured, *first observe the immediate area and check for possible risk* to the injured person, yourself, or anyone else. For example:
Response	Ask the injured person ("the casualty") to respond to you. The *first purpose* of this is to *find out if he or she is conscious*
	To establish if someone is conscious, check if he or she can:
	Speak to you
	Hear your voice
	Move (at all), e.g., open and close his/her eyes
	Respond to being touched
	Caution: Care must be taken if checking for a response to touch. Shaking him/her may cause further injury
Airway	If the athlete does not respond and so appears to be unconscious, check if his or her *airway* is clear, i.e., that his/her throat is not blocked (which could prevent him/her from breathing)
	Blockages in the throat area could be due to:
	Swallowed tongue
	Vomit
	Objects, e.g., mouth guard (if he/she was using one for protection) or false teeth
	Check that the person's head is in a suitable position to allow breathing. It may be sufficient just to tilt the head back gently to clear the person's tongue from his/her airway – but move the casualty as little as possible – just as much as needed to allow breathing while help is on the way
Breathing	Check if the athlete is *breathing*
	If the athlete is breathing it may be appropriate to put her/him into the recovery position while help is on the way. This is not recommended in all cases and especially not if the person has or may have injuries, e.g., broken bones – in which case moving him or her may cause further damage
	If the athlete is *not* breathing even though his/her airway is clear, a trained first aider *might* attempt to "breath for" him/her by blowing air into his/her mouth using a technique called *mouth-to-mouth ventilation* or *mouth-to-mouth resuscitation*
	Caution: The *mouth-to-mouth* technique requires *training*
Circulation	Blood circulation is essential for life. Blood is pumped around the body by the heart. Many first aiders and medical professionals check if blood is circulating around the body by looking for a *pulse*. One good place to check for a pulse is at the carotid artery in the neck
	If the athlete does not have a pulse (i.e., *blood circulation*), first aiders, paramedics, and other qualified personnel may begin *external chest compressions* (which involves applying pressure to the correct part of the chest at appropriate regular intervals)
	Caution: The *external chest compression* technique also benefits from *training* that is included in short courses in first aid, e.g., "First Aid in the Workplace." As for *mouth-to-mouth resuscitation*, people taking part in training courses practice *external chest compressions* on manikins – *not* on real people

wrist (radial). If you document the presence of a carotid pulse but the radial pulse is absent, this may represent a shock situation. A rapid or weak pulse may also represent a shock situation. Assessment of circulation also includes checking skin signs – color, temperature, and moisture. Abnormal findings such as pale cool, moist skin could be indicative of shock.

When CPR is necessary, it must be recorded that coaches, fitness professionals, and even athletic administrators have a "duty to act" given the nature of their job. They are to some extent responsible to the athlete and thus must be willing to provide CPR should it be necessary [14]. It is recommended that first-aid care provider obtains consent from the victim before rendering first aid. In case of unconscious athlete, consent would be implied.

Recognizing Vital Signs Anyone providing emergency care has to be able to evaluate the existing physiological signs and symptoms of injury [10]. Among these vital signs are heart

Table 7.2 Explanation of the TOTAPS injury assessment tool

Keyword	*Action*
Talk	Ask the player what happened Where does it hurt? What kind of pain is it?
Observe	Look at the affected area for redness or swelling Is the injured side different from the other side?
Touch	Touch indicates warmth for inflammation and also assesses pain
Active movement	Ask the injured player to move the injured part without any help
Passive movement	If the player can move the injured part, ask them to try to move it through its full range of motion
Skill test	Did the active and passive movements produce pain? If not, can the player stand and demonstrate some of the skills from the game carefully? If an injury is identified, remove the player from the activity immediately

Table 7.3 Vital signs

Pulse
Descriptors: regular, irregular, strong, or weak
Adult 60–100 beats per minute
Blood pressure
Systolic/diastolic
Adult 90–140 mmHg/60–90 mmHg
Respirations
Descriptors: normal, shallow, labored, noisy, Kussmaul
Adult (normal) 12–20 breaths per minute

rate, breathing rate, blood pressure, temperature, skin color, and pupils of the eye (Table 7.3).

7.2.2 Secondary Survey

If the athlete has no life-threateming injuries, a secondary assessment should be conducted to survey the entire body for injury.

The physical examination of the patient should take no more than two to three minutes and should examine the following parts:

Neck – Examine the patient for point tenderness or deformity of the cervical spine. Any tenderness or deformity should be an indication of a possible spine injury. If the patient's C-spine has not been immobilized immobilize now prior to moving on with the rest of the exam (see below for further details).

Head – Check the scalp for cuts, bruises, swellings, and other signs of injury. Examine the skull for deformities, depressions, and other signs of injury. Inspect the eyelids/eyes for impaled objects or other injury. Determine pupil size, equality, and reactions to light. Look for blood, clear fluids, or bloody fluids in the nose and ears. Examine the mouth for airway obstructions, blood, and any odd odors(11).

Chest – Examine the chest for cuts, bruises, penetrations, and impaled objects. Check for fractures. Note chest movements a look for equal expansion.

Abdomen – Examine the abdomen for cuts bruises, penetrations, and impaled objects. Feel the abdomen for tenderness. Gently press on the abdomen with the palm side of the fingers, noting any areas that are rigid, swollen, or painful. Note if the pain is in one spot or generalized.

Lower Back – Feel for point tenderness, deformity, and other signs of injury. Look for wetness caused by incontinence or bleeding or impaled objects. In male patients check for priapism (persistent erection of the penis). This is an important indication of spinal injury

Lower Extremities – Examine for deformities, swellings, bleedings, discolorations, bone protrusions and obvious fractures. Check for a distal pulse. The most useful is the posterior tibial pulse which is felt behind the medial ankle.

Upper Extremities – Examine for deformities, swellings, bleedings, discolorations, bone protrusions and obvious fractures. Check for the radial pulse (wrist). In children check for capillary refill. Check for motor function and strength.

7.3 Controlling Bleeding

An abnormal external or internal discharge of blood is called a *hemorrhage*. The hemorrhage may be venous, capillary, or arterial and may be external or internal. Venous blood is characteristically dark red with a continuous flow, whereas

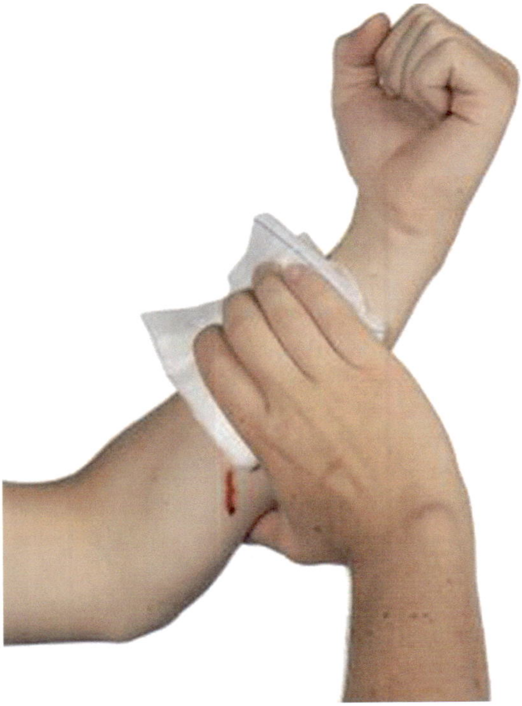

Fig. 7.1 Example of control of external bleeding by use of direct pressure

arterial bleeding flows in spurts and is bright. It is essential to take *universal precautions* to minimize this risk. Disposable non-latex gloves should be used routinely whenever the coach comes in contact with blood or other body fluids.

External Bleeding External bleeding stems from open skin wounds such as abrasions, incisions, lacerations, punctures, or avulsions. The control of external bleeding is most effectively accomplished by use of direct pressure. Elevation and pressure points may also help to control bleeding. *Pressure* applied directly over a wound with the hand over a sterile gauze pad is now recommended as the primary technique for controlling bleeding. The pressure is applied firmly against the resistance of a bone unless there is an underlying fracture (Fig. 7.1). As a gauze pad becomes soaked, additional pads should be placed on top of those already in place to facilitate the clotting process. Pressure may also be applied with a compression bandage holding sterile gauze in place over the wound. *Elevation* could help the reduction of external hemorrhage. Elevating a hemorrhaging part against gravity reduces blood pressure and facilitates venous and lymphatic drainage; consequently, elevating slows bleeding.

When direct pressure combined with elevation fails to slow hemorrhage, the use of pressure points may be the method of choice. The two most commonly used are the brachial artery in the upper limb and the femoral artery in the lower limb. The brachial artery is compressed against the medial aspect of the humerus, and the femoral artery is compressed as it is detected within the femoral triangle.

Internal Hemorrhage Internal hemorrhage is invisible to the eye unless manifested through some body opening and it is very dangerous. When internal hemorrhaging occurs, either subcutaneously, such as in a bruise or contusion, or intramuscularly, in joints, the athlete may be moved without danger. However, the detection of bleeding within a body cavity must be considered as an emergency because it could mean the difference between life and death. Athletes with internal injuries require hospitalization under complete and constant observation by a medical staff to determine the nature and extent of the injuries. All severe hemorrhaging eventually results in shock and should therefore be treated on this premise. The athlete should be kept quiet and body heat should be maintained at a constant and suitable temperature.

7.4 Emergency Splinting

If an athlete appears to have a fracture, an emergency rescue squad should be immediately called and the suspected fracture should be splinted before the athlete is moved [12]. Transporting a person with a fracture without proper immobilization can result in increased tissue damage, hemorrhage, and shock. The application of splints should be a simple process through the use of commercial emergency splints.

The principles of good splinting are [1] to splint from one joint above the fracture to one joint below the fracture and [2] to splint the injury in the position he is found. If at all possible, do not move the athlete until he or she has been splinted.

Evaluation of the injured extremity is usually complicated by protective equipment, such as clothing, padding, or tape, which must be removed to allow complete visualization of the injury. In addition, the athlete will often minimize the injury in an attempt to return to play. It must be considered the mechanism of injury and hazards of the sport to determine the extent of evaluation needed. If there is limb deformity, crepitation, ecchymosis, or swelling, the need for radiographs may be obvious. Other clues include pain with weight bearing, pain with joint manipulation distal and proximal to the injury, pain or abnormal bone motion with applied stress, and bruising distal to the injury site. In addition, any defect in the overlying skin may signal an open fracture, which may require urgent orthopedic referral. The neurologic and vascular status distal to the site of the injury must always be assessed. Assessment of neurologic status should include both motor and sensory components. Motor function is evaluated by observing the range of motion in joints or digits distal to the injury. Sensory examination should include a light touch and two-point discrimination when appropriate. Vascular status of the injured limb is assessed by palpating pulses distal to the injury.

7.4.1 Splinting Principles

Several principles apply in splinting. Splints should be well padded to avoid damage to skin and superficial tissues. This is often accomplished by wrapping elastic bandages around the splint material or by using a soft material such as a cotton prewrap to cover the injured limb.

When possible, the joints above and below the injury should be immobilized with the splint. Elastic bandages are generally used to apply the splint. Care must be taken to avoid applying these dressings too tightly and thus impairing distal perfusion. The treating provider must reassess the neurovascular status after applying the splint and periodically while awaiting definitive care.

Keep in mind that improvisation is often necessary. For example, if no appropriate splinting material is readily available, a lower leg injury can often be protected by "buddy taping" the leg to the uninjured leg. Similarly, an injured finger can be secured to the adjacent finger for temporary protection. Splints can be fashioned from a wide variety of materials, including the athlete's equipment or coach's supplies [13].

An ice bag can be incorporated into the splint by wrapping it in the elastic bandage. Care must be taken to remove the ice periodically to avoid cold injury to soft tissue. In general, the ice should be applied for no more than 10 min at a time. The injured extremity should also be elevated to minimize swelling.

IMPORTANT: On-field reduction should be avoided.

7.4.2 Type of Splinting

The *rapid form vacuum immobilizer* is a new type of splint that is widely used on athletic field (Fig. 7.2). It consists of Styrofoam chips contained inside an airtight cloth sleeve that is pliable. It can be molded to the shape of any joint of angulated fracture using Velcro straps. A handheld pump sticks the air out of the sleeve, giving it a cardboard-like rigidity. An *air splint* is a clear plastic splint that is inflated with air around the affected part. It can be used for extremity splinting, but its use requires some special training. This splint provides support and moderate pressure to the body part. It should not be used if there is risk of alteration of a fracture deformity.

7.4.3 Injury-Specific Splints

The following splints for commonly seen fractures are intended to protect a suspected fracture during transport and while awaiting definitive treatment. They may also be used for short-term immobilization of serious soft tissue injuries before bracing and rehabilitation.

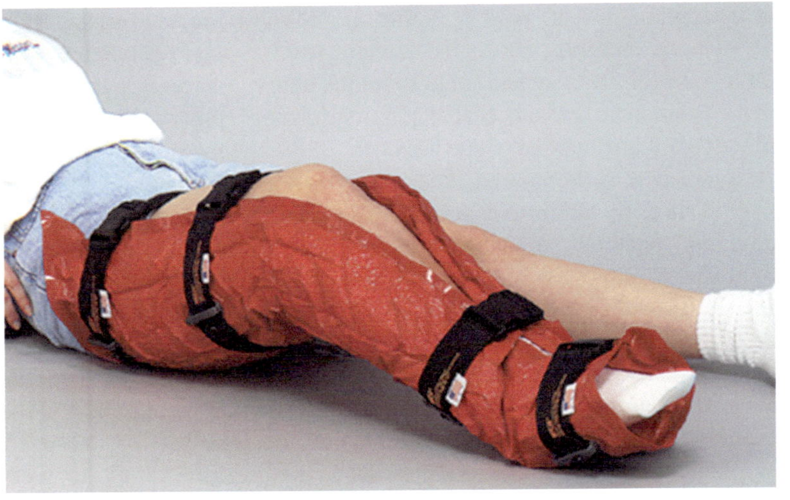

Fig. 7.2 Example of emergency splinting by the rapid form vacuum immobilizer

Femoral Shaft These injuries are rare in team sports but are seen in high-velocity activities such as skiing, cycling, and equestrian sports. Because of the potential for severe vascular injury and the loss of substantial amounts of blood, femoral shaft fractures can represent a true emergency. The first choice is a traction splint, but a long backboard or long rigid splint may also help to stabilize the injury for transport. Athletes who have a suspected femur fracture should be transported as soon as possible for further evaluation and treatment.

Tibial and Fibular Shaft Fractures of the lower leg usually follow a direct blow. Typically these injuries involve ecchymosis, swelling, and tenderness over the fracture site and pain with weight-bearing activities. Suspected lower leg fractures should be immobilized using a plaster, metal, or wire posterior splint or foam leg splint.

Ankle In serious ankle injuries, the mechanism of injury provides substantial clues to the presence and location of a fracture. Inversion (adduction) injuries commonly result in damage to the lateral ligaments, or they can lead to an avulsion fracture of the distal fibula. With eversion (lateral rotation and abduction) injuries, the talus acts as a wedge between the tibia and fibula, resulting in injury to the deltoid ligament, syndesmosis, and, frequently, the proximal fibula (Maisonneuve fracture). The medial malleolus may also be fractured with an eversion injury. The more severe trimalleolar fracture usually occurs with axial loading, as in jumping from a height.

Evaluation of the acutely injured ankle should include palpation of the proximal fibula, particularly with eversion injuries. While debate continues regarding radiographic evaluation of the acutely injured ankle, all but the most mild ankle sprains probably warrant x-rays.

Foot and Toe Fractures of the hindfoot and midfoot include calcaneal, talar, and metatarsal fractures. These injuries are usually splinted using a posterior "L" splint, and the athlete does not bear weight until the evaluation is complete. Nondisplaced fractures of the phalanges can be splinted with "buddy taping" and placing the athlete in a rigid shoe for comfort.

Elbow Fractures of the elbow commonly result from a fall on an outstretched hand with the elbow in extension. These fractures range from the relatively minor radial head fracture to the supracondylar fracture-dislocation, which requires urgent orthopedic referral. In general, suspected fractures of the elbow can be splinted in a posterior elbow splint in 20°–30° of flexion. Alternatively, radial and ulnar straight splints can be applied with elastic bandages. The injured arm is then placed in a sling for comfort until radiographs are obtained.

Forearm and Wrist Shaft fractures of the long bones of the forearm are prone to severe displacement. Thus, all suspected forearm and wrist fractures must be radiographed. The forearm and wrist can be immobilized using a preformed rigid wrist splint or by constructing an ulnar or radial gutter splint from available casting material.

Hand and Finger Metacarpal fractures commonly occur in contact sports. A number of manufactured splints can help immobilize these injuries. Alternatively, an ulnar gutter splint can be constructed using plaster or fiberglass.

Phalangeal fractures occur frequently in ball and contact sports. Care must be taken in the evaluation of these injuries because of the high incidence of associated tendon and ligament injuries. Splinting options for these fractures include preformed plastic orthoses, aluminum and foam moldable splints, and rigid metal immobilizers. Alternatively, the finger can be immobilized by "buddy taping" it to the adjacent finger until the evaluation is complete.

Splinting of the Spine and Pelvis Injuries involving a possible spine or pelvic fracture are best splinted and moved using a spine board (see below, moving and transporting the injured athlete).

7.5 Immediate Treatment Following Acute Musculoskeletal Injury

Musculoskeletal injuries are extremely common in sports. Appropriate first aid must be provided immediately to control hemorrhage and associated swelling. Every initial first-aid effort should be directed toward one primary goal – reducing the amount of swelling resulting from the injury.

If swelling can be controlled initially, the amount of time required for injury rehabilitation will be significantly reduced. Initial management of musculoskeletal injuries should include protection, rest, ice, compression, and elevation (PRICE). It can be used even by someone without first-aid training and should be used immediately when an injury occurs – the earlier, the better – while further medical attention is being sought.

If the athlete experiences too much pain during the process, stop immediately.

The PRICE protocol consists of:

"P" – Protection

Protect the injured person and the area being treated, but also protect yourself. If the injury occurs on the sports field, stop the game.

If the athlete can move, carefully move them to a safer area using a stretcher or a crutch, but if there is any doubt, do not move the injured athlete. If there is a fracture or some joint instability, the injured structure should be immobilized with some type of splint or brace.

"R" – Rest

Rest after any type of injury is an extremely important component of any treatment program. At the time of injury, it immediately begins the healing process. If the injured part is not rested and is subjected to external stresses and strains, the healing process could be delayed.

There are five warning signs of inflammation: pain, redness, tissue hotness, swelling, and loss of function.

Not every injury exhibits all these signs, but if the athlete is in pain, then it is important to stop exercising immediately to avoid further damage. The duration of the resting period necessary to avoid further damage depends on the severity of the injury. Parts of the body that have experienced minor injury should be rested for approximately 48 h to 72 h before the beginning of a rehabilitation program.

"I" – Ice

The initial treatment of acute injuries should use cold. Therefore ice is used for most conditions involving strains, sprains, and contusions.

Ice is the recommended treatment for acute injuries. It is especially helpful to reduce swelling and control pain. Ice is most effective when it is applied early and often for the first 48 h.

Ice should be wrapped in cloth or toweling before being placed onto the skin for an initial period of 5 min; if the skin is red after this time, the ice should be taken off. If the skin is normal color, the ice pack should be placed on the injured area for another 5 or 10 min. Ice should generally not be left on the skin for more than 20 min as this may cause damage to the surface of the skin. A good rule is to repeat the application of cold pack at intervals of 30 min.

Ice pack should be applied to the area for at least 72 h after an acute injury. With many injuries, regular ice treatments may be continued for several weeks. For example, a mild strain will probably require 1–2 days of cold application, whereas a severe knee or ankle sprain may need 3–7 days of intermittent cold.

"C" – Compression

Immediate compression of an acute injury is perhaps more important than ice in controlling swelling and in reducing inflammation. The most significant effect of compression is to reduce internal bleeding in the soft tissue surrounding the injury. Although cold is applied intermittently, the compression wrap should be left in place throughout the day and, if possible, also during the night. This type of compression is *different* from direct pressure applied to control bleeding.

"E" – Elevation

For both upper and lower limb injuries, it is equally important to keep the limb elevated to minimize swelling. Elevation to the level of the heart or above allows for excess fluid to be pumped back into the blood vessel system and will help prevent further swelling from occurring. The greater the degree of elevation, the more effective the reduction in swelling.

7.6 Moving and Transporting the Injured Athlete

Moving, lifting, and transporting the injured athlete must be executed using techniques that prevent further injury. There is no excuse for poor handling of the injured athlete. Planning should take into consideration all the possible transportation methods and the necessary equipment to execute them. Capable and well-trained personnel, spine boards, stretchers, and a rescue vehicle may be needed to transport the injured athlete.

7.6.1 Suspected Spinal Injury

When spinal injuries are suspected, immediately call the emergency and wait until the rescue squad arrives before attempting to move the athlete. The only exception is in cases in which the athlete is not breathing, and logrolling the athlete onto the back is required for CPR.

A suspected spinal injury requires extremely careful handling and is best left to properly trained paramedics or athletic trainers who are more skilled and have the proper equipment for such transport. If such personnel are not available, moving should be done under the express direction of a physician, and a spine board should be used. One danger inherent in moving an athlete with a suspected spinal injury, in particular a cervical injury, is the tendency of the neck and head to turn because of the victim's inability to control his or her movements. Torque so induced creates a possibility of spinal cord or root damage when small fractures are present. The most important principle in transporting an individual on a spine board is to keep the head and neck in alignment with the long axis of the body. In such cases it is best to have one individual whose sole responsibility is to ensure and maintain proper positioning of the head and neck until the head is secured to a spine board (Fig. 7.3).

Placing the Athlete on a Spine Board Once an injury to the neck has been recognized as severe, a physician and rescue squad should be summoned immediately. After the rescue squad has been called, the coach should assume the responsibility for providing primary emergency care that involves maintaining normal breathing, treating for shock, and keeping the athlete quiet and in the position found until medical assistance arrives. Ideally, transportation should not be attempted until the physician has examined the athlete and has given permission to move him or her. Once the rescue squad arrives, they assume responsibility for positioning the athlete on the spine board and carrying the athlete on the spine board to the rescue vehicle. The athlete should be transported while lying on his or her back, with the curve of the neck supported by a rolled-up towel or pad or

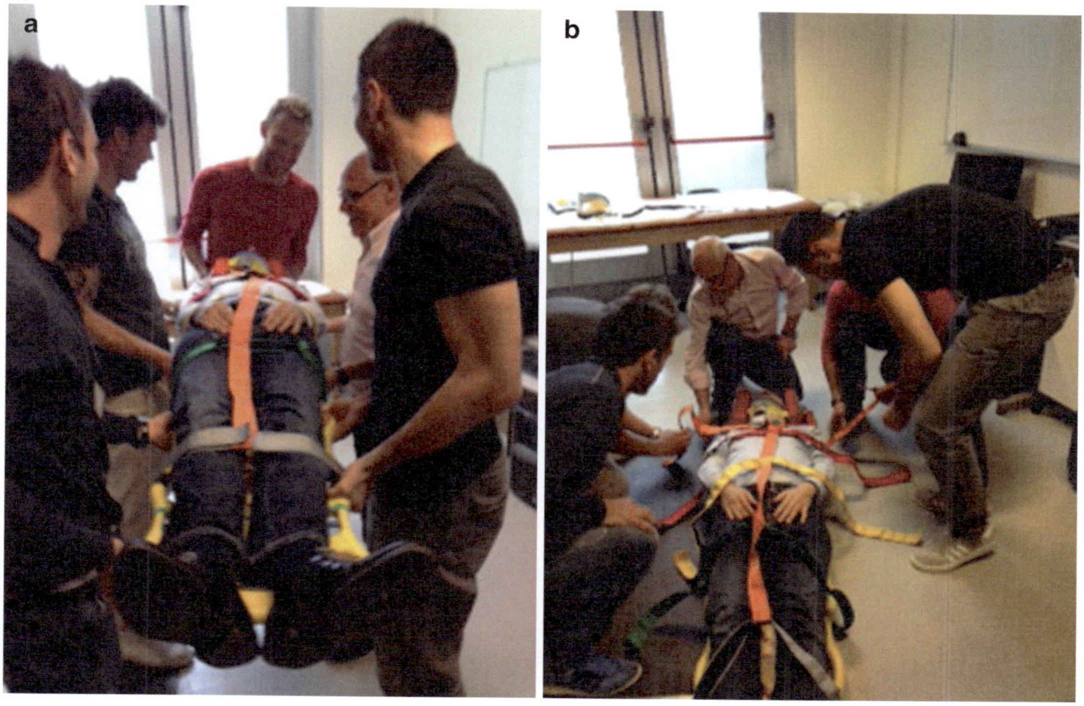

Fig. 7.3 Transportation of an individual on a spine board. These images were taken during a course of primary aid devoted to players of Italian Serie A

encased in a stabilization collar. Neck stabilization must be maintained throughout transportation, first to the emergency vehicle, then to the hospital, and throughout the hospital procedure. If stabilization is not continued, additional spinal cord damage and paralysis may ensue.

7.6.2 Stretcher Carrying

Whenever a serious injury other than a spinal injury is suspected, the best and safest mode of transportation for a short distance is by stretcher; with each segment of the body supported, the athlete is gently lifted and placed on the stretcher and is carried adequately by four assistants, two supporting the ends of the stretcher and two supporting either side (Fig. 7.3). Any person with an injury serious enough to require the use of a stretcher must be carefully examined before being moved. When transporting a person with a limb injury, be certain the injury is splinted properly before transport. Athletes with shoulder injuries are more comfortably moved in a semi-sitting position, unless other injuries preclude such positioning. If injury to the upper extremity is such that flexion of the elbow is not possible, the individual should be transported on a stretcher with the limb properly splinted and carried at the side and with adequate padding placed between the arm and the body.

7.6.3 Ambulatory Aid

Ambulatory aid is support or assistance given to an injured athlete who is able to walk. Before the athlete is allowed to walk, he or she should be carefully scrutinized to make sure that the injuries are minor. Whenever serious injuries are suspected, walking should be prohibited. Complete support should be given on both sides of the athlete by two individuals who are approximately the same height. The athlete's arms are draped over the assistants' shoulders, and their arms encircle his or her back.

7.6.4 Manual Conveyance

Manual conveyance may be used to move a mildly injured individual a greater distance than can be walked with ease. As with the use of ambulatory aid, any decision to carry the athlete must be made only after a complete examination to determine the existence of potentially serious conditions. The most convenient carry is performed by two assistants.

Great care must be taken in moving the seriously injured athlete. The unconscious athlete must be handled as though he or she has a cervical fracture.

7.7 Conclusions: Key Points

The prime concern of emergency aid is to maintain cardiovascular function and, indirectly, central nervous system function. All sports programs should have an emergency action plan that is activated anytime an athlete is seriously injured.

A systematic assessment of the injured athlete should be made to determine appropriate emergency care. A primary survey assesses and deals with life-threatening situations. Once stabilized, the secondary survey makes a more detailed assessment of the injury.

External bleeding can be controlled by direct pressure, applying pressure at pressure points, and by elevation.

Protection, rest, ice, compression, and elevation (PRICE) should be used for the immediate care of a musculoskeletal injury.

Any suspected fracture should be splinted before the athlete is moved.

References

1. American college of sports physicians, sports first injury prevention (2009). Jones and Bartlett, Boston
2. Karren KJ, Limmer D (2007) First aid for colleges and universities. Pearson, Upper Saddle River
3. Leikin JB, Feldman BJ (2000) American medical association handbook of first aid and emergency care. Random House, Philadelphia
4. Magee DJ (2007) Orthopedic physical assessment. W. B. Saunders, Philadelphia
5. Starkey C, Ryan J (2003) Orthopaedic and athletic injuries, evaluation handbook. F.A. Davis, Philadelphia
6. Thygerson A (2004) National safety council: first aid, CPR and AED essentials. Jones and Barlett, Boston
7. Dolan MG (1998) Emergency care: planning for the worst. Athl Ther Today 3(1):12–13
8. Nowlan WP, Davis GA, McDonald B (1996) Preparing for sudden emergencies. Athl Ther Today 1(1):45–47
9. Rubin A (1993) Emergency equipment: what to keep on the sidelines. Phys Sportsmed 21(9):47–54
10. Kleiner DM (1998) Emergency management of athletic trauma: roles and responsibilities. Emerg Med Serv 10:33–36
11. Waeckerle JF (1991) Planning for emergencies. Phys Sportsmed 19(2):35–38
12. American Heart Association (2000) Guidelines 2000 for cardiopulmonary re-suscitation and emergency cardiovascular care: international consensus on science. Curr Emerg Cardiovasc Care 11:3–15
13. Waninger KN (2004) Management of the helmeted athlete with suspected cervical spine injury. Am J Sports Med 32:1331–1350
14. Page RL, Joglar JA, Kowal RC et al (2000) Use of automated external defibrillators. N Engl J Med 343: 1210–1216

Part II

Specific Injuries

Muscle Lesions

8

Ian F.R. Beasley

8.1 Aetiology

Football is a contact, multi-sprint and recovery sport. Muscle injuries are the most common type encountered [1, 2] and can be as a result of contusions, muscle tears, lacerations, ischaemia and drug toxicity. It is imperative that when eliciting a history of this type of injury, one keeps an open mind as to any underlying contribution any of these etiological factors may offer.

Injury risk during match play is approximately seven times that from training [1].

8.1.1 Contusions

These are caused by direct trauma and are part and parcel of contact sport. The contact can cause muscle fibre disruption, leading to bleeding and pain in varying severity. In certain circumstances, an area of bleeding may lead to ectopic calcification (myositis ossificans).

8.1.2 Muscle Tears

According to Ekstrand et al. [1], this is the most common type of injury in football. Indeed, in the review of the UCL injury study [1], 31 % of injuries were due to lower limb muscle injury and caused the biggest injury burden. Injury is caused by overstretching the muscle, and this happens during an eccentric contraction.

The sarcomere is the basic contractile unit of muscle (Fig. 8.1).

I.F.R. Beasley, MBBS, MRCGP, MSc, Dip.Sports Med
Medical Services, The English Football Association,
Wembley Stadium, Harrow HA9 0WS,
United Kingdom
e-mail: Ian.Beasley@thefa.com

P. Volpi (ed.), *Football Traumatology: New Trends*, DOI 10.1007/978-3-319-18245-2_8

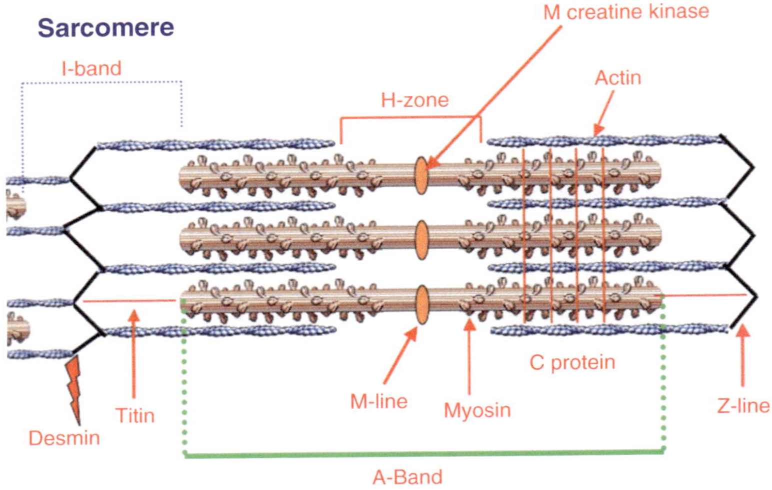

Fig. 8.1 Sarcomere

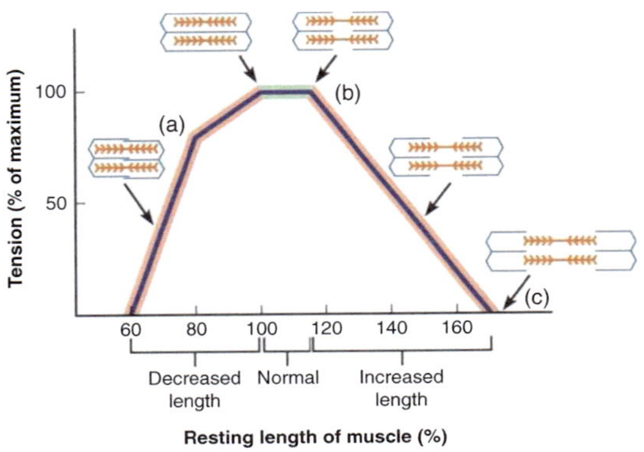

Fig. 8.2 Length-tension curve

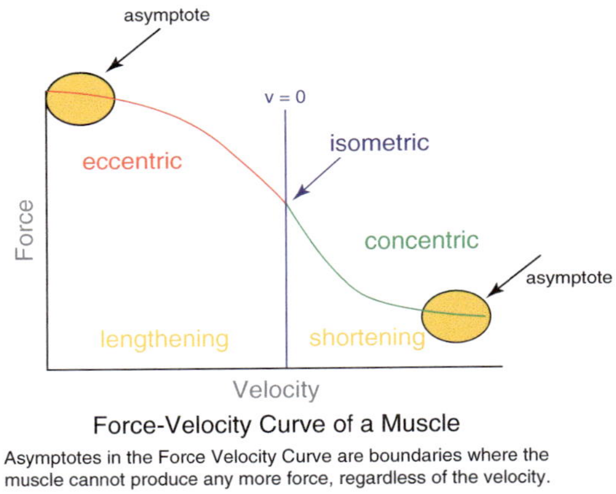

Fig. 8.3 Force – velocity curve of a muscle

The length-tension relationship of a sarcomere determines that there is an optimal length (or tension) that a sarcomere has when it can produce its maximal force (Fig. 8.2).

Once this length is exceeded, the force of contraction falls, and with continued stretch, the sarcomere is unable to engage its actin and myosin to counteract the increasing length. The decline quickens, and the counteractive generative force becomes less (Fig. 8.3).

The sarcomere continues to lengthen, and the fibre eventually becomes disrupted [3, 4]. Damage of the cytoskeletal proteins then occurs as the disruptive force gains momentum. Bleeding and pain ensues, and disruption to the microtubules and sarcoplasmic reticulum causes an increase in local calcium concentration. This and the increased neural signalling that occurs with injury contribute to the local spasm encountered with muscle tears.

8.1.2.1 Lacerations

Muscle lacerations in football are usually associated with contact with footwear. It is mandatory that all players' boots are checked by the referee before they take the field of play. Substitutes are checked on the touchline by the 4th official as they enter the field. In spite of this, lacerations do occur. There has been debate as to whether blades (a type of stud) are responsible for this [5], but no evidence has emerged to confirm this.

8.1.2.2 Ischaemia

Ischaemia usually occurs as a result of pressure build up in a muscle compartment.

Muscles are enclosed in a fascial compartment. As exercise commences, blood flow into the muscle increases; this is a normal physiological response and is enhanced with training. The muscle swells slightly with this engorgement. If the swelling increases to the stage where the fascial casing cannot accommodate, the pressure within the compartment rises. This rise in pressure can be sufficient to inhibit venous drainage, causing pooling of blood in the muscle and a further rise in pressure. Eventually, this process inhibits oxygenation of muscle fibres (by inhibiting arterial flow), causing pain of ischaemia. Ceasing the offending exercise causes a reversal of this process, and the pain subsides. This is compartment syndrome and, in the majority of cases, occurs in the deep posterior compartment of the calf [6].

More seriously, bleeding after a direct blow to a muscle can rapidly increase pressure within a compartment to dangerous levels. Worsening pain that does not settle with inactivity is a feature of this 'acute compartment syndrome' and is an emergency that requires surgical intervention. Failure to do so causes a severe rise in pressure that exceeds local arterial pressure, cuts off any blood supply, and will cause tissue death unless the local pressure is reduced by performing a fasciotomy.

Other causes are constricting dressings/bandages or plaster casts that are applied to injuries. A basic pathological principle of any injury is that it will swell. If, in the acute phase, a dressing or cast is applied to an injury too tightly, this will cause an increase in pressure just as the swelling inevitably occurs. It is imperative that any such dressing or cast be removed if there are any concerns.

8.1.2.3 Drug Toxicity

The treatment of inflammatory illnesses such as bowel disease, asthma and arthropathies can necessitate the use of corticosteroid medication. This type of medication is well known to cause proximal myopathy and has been reported to cause muscle disease in up to 50 % of those on long-term therapy [7].

8.2 Injury Mechanism

Pattern recognition when history taking is an important part of any clinicians' modus operandum. The clinician must have in mind the possibilities that may have resulted in injury, and match these with the findings from the player encounter, and formulate a working diagnosis. This leads to appropriate further investigation and on to treatment planning.

8.2.1 Contusions

The history is usually clear, and a story of a collision or sustaining a kick is almost invariably the case; this may be associated with foul play. The player may need to be substituted when this happens and may not be able to take any further part in the match. There is a tender area around the site of the injury, which may be heralded by skin abrasion if the injury was associated with a kick. Swelling is present. This phenomenon was reported over 100 years ago [8].

8.2.2 Muscle Tears

Following on from the section in *Etiology* above, it is apparent that muscle tears occur when a muscle is stretched beyond the point where the normal resistance to stretch by use of actin and myosin is overcome. With reference to the force-velocity curve (diagram 3), therefore, this occurs during the eccentric (lengthening) phase of muscle contraction.

In order of scale, the four lower limb muscle groups that are reported as injured are hamstrings, groin, quadriceps, and calf [1].

Hamstring muscle injury, being the most common in football [1], has been extensively studied, with the hope that mechanism might lead to a prevention strategy.

Chumanov et al. have examined possible mechanisms of tears of this muscle and have come to the conclusion that it is during the late swing phase of sprinting that this muscle is injured [9–11]. At this time, the hamstring is lengthening. If the muscle contractile tissue cannot resist this, injury occurs.

Groin muscle injuries are common and can be troublesome [12]. In this study, Hölmich et al. found that approximately half of 'groin injuries' were due to muscle injuries, which were more common on the dominant side. Werner et al. [13] found a similar incidence of adductor muscle injury in a study of generic groin injury in professional footballers over seven seasons. Age and previous injury were directly proportional to injury occurrence. The same principle of inability to control overstretching applies to this muscle, with similar muscular and regional anatomical complexities that might expose it to injury.

Quadriceps strain involves the rectus femoris more than the other muscles of this complex [14]. This injury has been reported as being 5 % of the total injury burden (cf 12.8 % for hamstrings, 9.2 % for groin muscle injury), but caused the greatest time absence according to Ekstrand [1].

In a review of injuries to this muscle (Mendiguchia et al. [15]), the mechanism is once more cited as overstretching of the muscle during an eccentric contraction, which is often in the action of kicking a ball. The difference with injuries involving this muscle is that central tendon involvement extends the absence from play [16].

The gastrocnemius is the most commonly injured muscle in the calf, the site of injury being its medial head [17].

Its bi-articular anatomy means that it is more prone to overstretching. Although soleus injury is less common, it often presents with a less dramatic history [17]. Both are more common with age [18].

Due to its position below the knee, the calf is more prone to lacerative injury (from kicks either accidental or deliberate) and is the site for deep posterior compartment syndrome. The mechanism for this particular injury has been explained above.

8.3 Clinical and Diagnostic Examination

Before attempting any examination, a full history should be taken. This will include the injury itself, but also past injury history. Hagglund et al. [19] showed in a study over two seasons in the Swedish professional football league that previous injury is a risk factor that has to be taken into account. The same group [20] confirmed this finding and that older age and kicking leg were also associated with a higher injury rate.

Once a full history has been taken and recorded, the examination can begin. This should take the form of look (inspect), move (active/passive), feel (palpation) and image.

Look for any signs of swelling, bruising or redness that will indicate the site of the injury. Ask the player if the part you think is involved is, in fact, where the pain originates. Players will often have multiple bumps and bruises from matches.

Then start with the 'normal' side!

Ask the player to move the equivalent contralateral, non-injured, part. If they can, then assess the range they can attain, and test the passive range as well. This can then be carried out on the injured side, ensuring that the player is not experiencing pain and spasm that prohibits movement and that there is no possibility of extending any injury that may be present.

Palpation of the injured area can then be carried out. Again, start with the normal side. Heat from inflammation and freezing cold extremities in a possible vascular compromise are important early and easy things to assess. They help the clinician gain the confidence of the player, who may be fearing more pain from heavy handedness, whilst examining an injured, and already painful, area.

Palpation of an injured muscle will demonstrate the site of tenderness and give an idea of where the injury is anatomically. It may be possible to feel a defect, or an area of swelling, giving some indication of severity.

There may be some 'special manoeuvres' that the examiner may want to carry out if it is felt necessary at the time, for instance, straight leg raise or slump testing in a player with hamstring pain. If an exhaustive history and palpation have been carried out, and there is a suspicion that there may be a neural cause rather than a local disruption, straight leg raise or slump test may be carried out with care.

This type of manoeuvre should be carried out with care.

The examination must be done in a calm and stepwise fashion, even in the turmoil of a small post-match dressing room (where the result may not have gone your teams' way!).

If there are any doubts about the findings, ask a member of your multidisciplinary team to re-examine or at least watch whilst you do. Two heads in a difficult situation are often better than one.

If you have a diagnostic ultrasound available, this can be helpful in identifying an inter-/intra-muscular haematoma (Fig. 8.4).

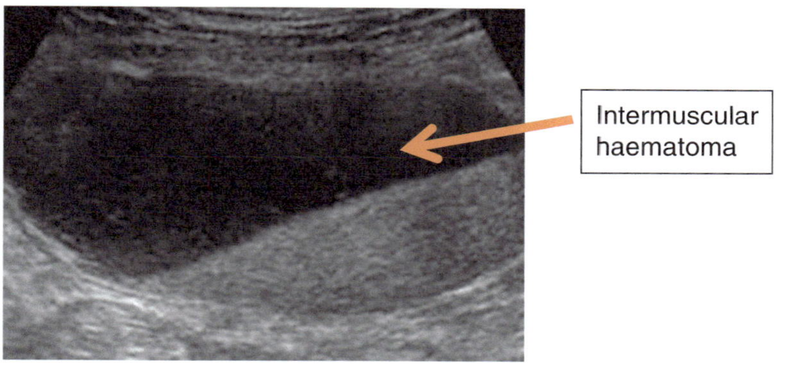

Fig. 8.4 Ultrasound scan image of an intermuscular haematoma

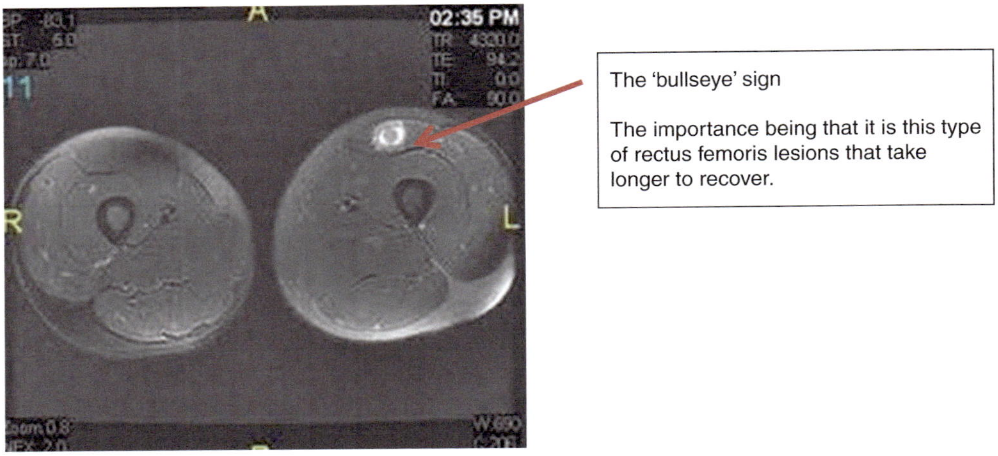

Fig. 8.5 An axial MRI image of a rectus femoris muscle tear

These haematomata may be aspirated under ultrasound guidance. This may not be possible in the acute phase and may be best tackled in the tranquillity of the club medical room.

Diagnostic ultrasound can identify a muscle or tendon rupture, and any acute surgical assessment or intervention can be arranged. It may be possible to identify an interruption in the muscle substance which constitutes a muscle tear. This can be measured and recorded. Muscle tears can be followed with ultrasound, in conjunction with the clinical picture, and consulting the literature on when similar injuries return to play gives the clinician some indication of the timetable involved [1].

Coaching staff must be kept up to date on the state of the evolving injury.

MRI scanning is the gold standard imaging modality for muscle injuries. Many MRI features of muscle injury have aided clinicians in being able to better estimate return to play. The 'bullseye' lesion of the rectus femoris (Fig. 8.5), showing central tendon involvement, was described by Hughes et al. [21].

Orchard [22] makes the point that in the professional arena, it can be difficult to resist an MRI when a player sustains an injury. He cites the study by Moen et al. [23] that the best return to play indicator was how the player felt and the range of straight leg raise, rather than the MRI appearances.

Nonetheless, there have been studies to show that MRI appearances were 'valuable' in prognosticating return to play after lower limb muscle injuries [24].

It is to be expected that clinicians will try to use all possible imaging modalities as well as clinical abilities to assess and grade injuries with a view to accurate prognostication, thereby enabling an accurate return to play prediction. In professional football, this can save a club millions of pounds/euros in transfer fees and wages if there is more certainty regarding player availability.

In this vein, many classification and/or grading systems have emerged [25–27].

Of course, originally, and going as far back as the ***1960s***, these were based on clinical findings only [28], and Hamilton [29] asserts 'categorical scales for grading muscle injuries are pragmatic and popular with clinicians and patients'. Hence the number of such systems that have been devised and proposed.

The aim is to reach a conclusion on the magnitude of injury and prognosis that is reproducible; it follows that this lends itself to a more accurate idea of return to play.

8.4 Treatment Strategy

After a careful and full history has been taken, examination and investigations have been carried out and a diagnosis has been reached, a treatment strategy should be formulated.

All members of the multidisciplinary team should be involved in this. The strategy should include timescales that are realistic. Team management should be kept up to date as the plan is formulated and as the player recovers. Reference to the literature on the type of injury incurred is an integral part of this process.

This type of approach enables audit of the treatment and rehabilitation process. Comparison with 'norms' and player to player variations can be made and examined with a view to streamlining the process.

Treatment should be split into three main areas:

Acute
1st 48 h
Ongoing

Acute

The protection, rest, ice, compression, elevation (PRICE) protocol is standard, but often impossible to follow. If a player sustains a lower limb muscle injury and has to travel home, the rest part of this acronym is difficult to apply. A slightly different approach has been proposed by Bleakley et al. [30]. POLICE substitutes 'R' for 'OL' and indicates optimum loading as the more pragmatic, and realistic, tactic.

This approach allows that all that could be done is done. Although insidious extension of an injury can occur, preventing this completely may be impossible.

Standard therapy is to apply ice and compression to the area [31].

This can be carried out using compression bandages or using a proprietary product that supplies pressure and cryotherapy concurrently. Decreasing the temperature of a cellular system means it will require less oxygen, and in an injured state, where oxygenation of tissues is less than optimum, this affords some protection to (further) hypoxic damage and cell death. It is important to continue this treatment whilst travelling from a playing venue.

Although cryotherapy is a part of the standard treatment in muscle injuries, Bleakley et al. [32] and Bizzini [33] point out that there is a dearth of scientific evidence supporting its use. Animal studies have shown reduction in tissue temperature after injury with ice application, but similar evidence is lacking in humans; the point is made that reductions in tissue temperature may be less in humans given the deeper siting of some muscle injuries.

Compression of the area should be applied [34]. After a working diagnosis has been made, and ice has been applied, the player will need to shower and dress. Minimising oedema and bleeding at this time is an important part of the 'protection', as the injured muscle, almost always dependant (w.r.t. gravity) during this period, will be at risk of excessive swelling. Compression will decrease the local tissue pressure, by decreasing oedema and lymphatic and capillary 'leak' – a normal feature of inflammation. This will limit disruption to the normal vascular physiology, which optimises oxygenation to tissues

In a similar way, elevation of the injured part will decrease cellular pressure, by helping any fluid of oedema to drain proximally rather than pool around the injured part.

All these strategies aim to minimise further damage and pain for the player: the gain may be small, but may mean a return to play 1 or 2 days earlier.

This treatment should continue for 24 h, with icing for 10 min per 30 for the first 12 h. 10 min per hour is reasonable after this.

In the acute phase, and if available, ultrasound examination may be able to give an early idea of the extent of the injury.

During this phase of treatment, any further investigations should be planned and performed. With all investigations, and a summary of the clinical findings as the injury has evolved, it is now possible to formulate a treatment and rehabilitation protocol. As mentioned above, this should involve the medical, sports science and strength and conditioning of staff working with the team. Milestones can be estimated. Devising a strategy for treatment in this way ensures that all staff, including coaching staff, will have an idea of when a return to play might be possible.

After the first 48 h of treatment, a graduated exercise programme should begin.

At all times, it is imperative that staff keep an open mind on how a player is progressing against the milestones laid out in the treatment strategy. Any doubts should herald a reassessment of the original diagnosis, investigations and whether the strategy was unrealistic.

Audit of the process and outcomes, with feedback, is essential.

Trying to modify the physiological response to injury, in an effort to promote healing and effect an early return to play, is a natural urge for all concerned in player care. To this end, a number of treatments have been proposed. Traumeel and Actovegin use in the acute phase of injury have been employed for many years, and Lee et al. [35] describe a pilot study where 4 players in a treatment group with grade 1 (hamstring) injuries returned to play 8 days sooner (Actovegin only) than controls. Another group [36] suggest that Traumeel and Actovegin use should be the preserve of those experienced in its use. Reurink et al. [37] conclude that there is limited evidence to support its use and suggest that further research should be undertaken in their use.

PRP has gained a lot of attention. The fact that it is autologous and has some logic attached to its use has meant that its use in injury management has mushroomed. The IOC [38] published a consensus on its use and concluded that there is a lack of evidence to support its use, but made a final recommendation that more research should be carried out on the basic science leading to its therapeutic use. Reurink et al. [39] conducted a clinical trial of 80 athletes with hamstring tears and found no difference in resuming sport between the treatment with PRP and non-PRP groups.

Nonsteroidal anti-inflammatories are commonly used in football, and Tscoll et al. have identified their excessive use [40]. However, there have been many studies that have shown that early use of these drugs can lessen the strength of muscle fibres once healing has taken place [41], and their use in the first 48 h of a muscle being injured should be avoided.

Muscle contusions should follow the same early treatment regimen. To avoid heterotopic calcification excessive movement and massage to the injured area should be avoided. If calcification does occur, Indomethacin is effective in restricting its genesis.

Compartment syndrome can be troublesome, although uncommon in footballers. Surgery to decompress the offending compartment may be necessary if symptoms persist, and the diagnosis is confirmed. Acute compartment syndrome requires urgent surgical intervention (see above).

8.4.1 Rehabilitation and Return to Play

There is an overlap between treatment and rehabilitation that starts as soon as the treatment/recovery strategy has been decided upon.

Treatment time will decrease as the injury recovers and return to play looms. Rehabilitation in all its forms will become more and more prominent. With progression, reinjury prevention must be addressed. At the beginning of the process, all those involved in the care of the player are aware of this, but spend a small amount of time addressing this particular aspect. As time moves on, it becomes more and more important.

De Vos [42] states how important it is for the team physician to accelerate recovery and get athletes playing again as quickly as possible.

There are some basic physiological principles that one should consider, beginning with how a muscle injury heals. Muscle tissue contains satellite cells, without which it cannot regenerate. These are basically muscle stem cells [43].

It is also reported that eccentric exercise encourages satellite cells to multiply [44, 45] and affect muscle regeneration in the face of damage caused by injury.

The use of this pathophysiological process is important in the rehabilitation and return to play pathway. In other words, the route to recovery from muscle injury is via exercise. The Dreyer and Parise studies, mentioned above, used aerobic exercise and eccentric contractions to examine satellite cell proliferation and find it present in they types of exercise.

In the therapeutic phase of a muscle injury and assuming the whole process is on track, range of motion of the injured part should reattain its pre-injury state (it is therefore important that this is understood, by having screened/profiled players before the season starts and at midseason). Central (core) stability is an integral part of this process [37].

It must be remembered that the muscle is just a part of the player and that a holistic approach should be taken when rehabilitating a player to a position where they are available for selection again.

Cardiovascular fitness is important to maintain and may require rehabilitation involving water immersion/swimming. Other parts of the musculoskeletal system can become deconditioned, and this should be kept in mind; the player should be given programmes to offset this possibility. It is well known that players may have emotional difficulties, especially with longer-term injuries. POMS (**P**rofile **O**f **M**ood **S**tates) questionnaires are a useful tool to follow mood during the rehabilitation period. Spending time at a club training ground, *not* training with your teammates, and doing extra sessions when only staff are present can be demotivating for the player and interfere with physical progress.

8.4.2 Return to Play

The question that the team physician and everyone else in the multidisciplinary team is asked on a daily basis, by the club manager and coach, or by a fan in the street! This is why the 'business end' of injury management is studied so avidly and is of high pressure.

There is no doubt that investigations are useful [29, 46].

Correlation of MRI findings with return to play via accurate diagnosis and knowledge of MRI features that may denote a more, or less, problematic injury can only be helpful.

Together with the various classification systems [25–27], there are now more tools to aid accurate diagnosis and prognosis than there has ever been. As in the rest of medicine, SEM suffers that no system is perfect, and this is demonstrated by the study carried out by Moen et al. [23]. Taking a thorough history, with reference to the known predisposing factors (see above), and performing an adequate examination will augment the newer tools that we have to diagnose the grade of a muscle injury more accurately and offer a prognosis that is credible. Setting out time frames and milestones is helpful, but is a guide rather than 'the law'. Auditing this process will enable the multidisciplinary team to reflect (it must be done in an open meeting) on the outcomes and improve on the process for the inevitable 'next time'. Delvaux et al. [47] outline the parameters used in France and Belgium for return to play following a hamstring injury. There, a seven-part assessment is made (complete pain relief, normalised muscle strength assessment, subjective feeling reported by the player, normalised flexibility and achievement of a specific soccer test).

Tol et al. [48] report that two thirds of clinically recovered hamstring injuries in football players showed 'at least one isokinetic hamstring deficit of more than 10 %'. This apparent lack of full recovery is backed up by the findings of Reurink et al. [49], whose group demonstrated that almost 9 out of ten clinically recovered hamstrings showed increased fluid signal intensity on MRI.

De Vos et al. [50] report some clinical features that have some predictive value of re-injury.

Despite all this returning to play is always a risk; football is an unpredictable game. The risk can be stratified by using information from the literature, knowledge of the original injury (including all examinations and investigations), and the status of the player with respect to their rehabilitation. There will be occasions when the team manager/coach may wish to select a player who may not be optimally rehabilitated. The team physician must make the manager/coach aware of the players' status to encourage a safe return to play.

References

1. Ekstrand J et al (2013) Fewer ligament injuries but no preventive effect on muscle injuries and severe injuries: an 11-year follow-up of the UEFA Champions League injury study. Br J Sports Med 47:732–737
2. Drawer S et al (2002) Evaluating the level of injury in English professional football using a risk based assessment process. Br J Sports Med 36:446–451
3. Morgan DL, Allen DG (1999) Early events in stretch-induced muscle damage. J Appl Physiol. 87: 2007–2015

4. Proske U, Morgan DL (2001) Muscle damage from eccentric exercise: mechanism, mechanical signs, adaptation and clinical applications. J Physiol 537(Pt 2):333–345
5. Blades of gory: the story of 'lethal' hybrid boots that caused injury to Wayne Rooney. The independent, 27.09.13
6. Micheli LJ (ed) Encyclopaedia of sports medicine, pp 476–477. ISBN 978.1-4129-6115-8
7. Valiyil R, Christopher-Stine L (2010) Drug-related myopathies of which the clinician should be aware. Curr Rheumatol Rep 12(3):213–220
8. Makins GH (1911) Traumatic Myositis Ossificans. Proc R Soc Med 4(Surg Sect):133–142
9. Chumanov ES et al (2011) Hamstring musculotendon dynamics during stance and swing phases of high-speed running. Med Sci Sports Exerc 43:525–532
10. Chumanov ES et al (2007) The effect of speed and influence of individual muscles on hamstring mechanics during the swing phase of sprinting. J Biomech 40:3555–3556
11. Chumanov E et al (2012) Hamstrings are most susceptible to injury during the late swing phase of sprinting. Br J Sports Med 46:90
12. Hölmich P et al (2014) Incidence and clinical presentation of groin Injuries in sub-elite male soccer. Br J Sports Med 48:1245–1250
13. Werner J et al (2009) UEFA injury study: a prospective study of hip and groin injuries in professional football over seven consecutive seasons. Br J Sports Med 43:1036–1040
14. Garrett WE (1996) Muscle strain injuries. Am J Sports Med 24:S2–S8
15. Mendiguchia J (2013) Rectus femoris muscle injuries in football: a clinically relevant review of mechanisms of injury, risk factors and preventive strategies. Br J Sports Med 47(6):359–366
16. Balius R et al (2009) Central aponeurosis tears of the rectus femoris practical sonographic prognosis. Br J Sports Med 43:818–824
17. Dixon JB (2009) Gastrocnemius vs. soleus strain: how to differentiate and deal with calf muscle injuries. Curr Rev Musculoskelet Med 2(2):74–77
18. Ekstrand J et al (2011) Epidemiology of muscle injuries in professional football. Am J Sports Med 39(6):1226–1232
19. Hagglund M et al (2006) Previous injury as a risk factor for injury in elite football: a prospective study over two consecutive seasons. Br J Sports Med 40: 767–772
20. Hagglund M et al (2013) Risk factors for lower extremity muscle injury in professional soccer:the UEFA injury study. Am J Sports Med 41(2):327–335
21. Hughes C, Hasselman CT, Best TM et al (1995) Incomplete, intrasubstance strain injuries of the rectus femoris muscle. Am J Sports Med 23:500–506
22. Orchard J (2014) What role for MRI in hamstring strains? An argument for a difference between recreational and professional athletes. Br J Sports Med 48(18):1337–1338
23. Moen MH et al (2014) Predicting return to play after hamstring injuries. Br J Sports Med 48:1358–1363
24. Hallen A, Ekstrand J (2014) Return to play following muscle injuries in professional footballers. J Sports Sci 32:1229–1236
25. Pollock N et al (2014) British athletics muscle injury classification: a new grading system. Br J Sports Med 48:1347–1351
26. Mueller-Wohlfahrt H-W, Haensel L, Mithoefer K et al (2013) Terminology and classification of muscle injuries in sport: the Munich consensus statement. Br J Sports Med 47:342–350
27. Chan O, Del Buono A, Best TM et al (2012) Acute muscle strain injuries: a proposed new classification system. Knee Surg Sports Traumatol Arthrosc 20: 2356–2362
28. Verrall G (2013) Aspetar sports. Med J 47:342–350
29. Hamilton B et al (2014) Excellent reliability for MRI grading and prognostic parameters in acute hamstring injuries. Br J Sports Med 48:1385–1387
30. Bleakly CM et al (2012) PRICE needs updating, should we call the POLICE? Br J Sports Med 46: 220–221
31. Meeusen R, Lievens P (1986) The use of cryotherapy in sports injuries. Sports Med 3(6):398–414, Springer
32. Bleakley CM et al (2012) Cooling an acute muscle injury: can basic scientific theory translate into the clinical setting? Br J Sports Med 46:296–298
33. Bizzini M (2012) Ice and modern sports physiotherapy: still cool? Br J Sports Med 46:219
34. Kraemer WJ (2004) Compression in the treatment of acute muscle injuries in sport. Int Sport Med J 5(3): 200–208
35. Lee P et al (2011) Our experience on Actovegin, is it cutting edge? Int J Sports Med 32(4):237–241. doi:10.1055/s-0030-1269862, Epub 2011 Jan 26
36. Hamilton B, Robinson M (2013) Aspetar sports. Med J 462–266
37. Reurink G et al (2012) Therapeutic interventions for acute hamstring injuries: a systematic review. Br J Sports Med 46:103–109
38. Lars E, Kathrin S, Joseph A, Eduardo A et al (2010) IOC consensus paper on the use of platelet-rich plasma in sports medicine. Br J Sports Med 44:1072–1081
39. Reurink G (2014) Platelet-rich plasma injections in acute muscle injury. N Engl J Med 370(26): 2546–2547
40. Tscholl P (2008) The use of medication and nutritional supplements during FIFA World Cups 2002 and 2006. Br J Sports Med 42:725–730
41. Mackey A et al (2012) Rehabilitation of muscle after injury – the role of anti-inflammatory drugs. Scand J Med Sci Sports 22(4):e8–e14
42. de Vos R-J (2014) Knowledge is only rumour, until it is in the muscle. Br J Sports Med 48(18):1335
43. Relaix F, Zammit PS (2012) Satellite cells are essential for skeletal muscle regeneration: the cell on the edge returns centre stage. Development 139(16): 2845–2856

44. Dreyer HC et al (2006) Satellite cell numbers in young and older men 24 hours after eccentric exercise. Muscle Nerve 33(2):242–253
45. Parise G et al (2008) Muscle satellite cell and atypical myogenic progenitor response following exercise. Muscle Nerve 37(5):611–619
46. Ekstrand J et al (2012) Hamstring muscle injuries in professional football. Br J Sports Med 46:112–117
47. Delvaux F et al (2013) Return to play criteria after hamstring injury: actual medical practice in professional soccer teams. Br J Sports Med 47:e3
48. Tol JL et al (2014) At return to play following hamstring injury the majority of professional football players have residual isokinetic deficits. Br J Sports Med 48:1364–1369
49. Reurink G et al (2014) MRI observations at return to play of clinically recovered hamstring injuries. Br J Sports Med 48:1370–1376
50. De Vos R-J et al (2014) Clinical findings just after return to play predict hamstring re-injury, but baseline MRI findings do not. Br J Sports Med 48: 1377–1384

Hamstring Injuries

9

Gianluca Melegati and Davide Tornese

9.1 Hamstring Strain Injuries

Muscle injuries are common in football and soccer [1–4]. A recent epidemiological study of injuries in professional football (soccer) reported that muscle injuries account for over 30 % of all injuries and are the cause of injury-related absence in about one-fourth of cases [5]. Muscle injuries pose numerous challenges for the team sports physician. The team medical staff is under considerable pressure, particularly in elite football clubs, to release players to return to play before biological healing is complete. Furthermore, players may often remain absent from training and matches for extended periods, incurring economic losses for their clubs [6].

Over 90 % of muscle strains in soccer involve four major muscle groups: the hamstrings, adductors, quadriceps, and gastrocnemius. Volpi et al. [7] conducted a 5-year survey of the incidence and site of muscle strains in an Italian major league team between 1995 and 2000 (five sports seasons) and found that the muscle group most frequently injured was the quadriceps (33 %), followed by the hamstrings (29 %), the adductors (19.4 %), and the sural triceps (13 %). In their epidemiological study of professional soccer players, Ekstrand et al. [5] reported muscle injury rates by site: hamstrings (37 %), adductors (23 %), quadriceps (19 %), and gastrocnemius (13 %). Very recently, Melegati et al. [8] reported on muscle injuries and reinjuries in an Italian professional male soccer team (Series A Italian championships) during the 2010–2011 sports season. The total hours of exposure were 8,041, of which 7,165 (89 %) hours were spent in training and 876 (11 %) hours in matches, with a training-match ratio of 3.8 for that season. A total of 64 injuries occurred, 36 (56 %) of which during training and 28 (44 %) during matches. Muscle strains accounted for 31.3 % (n=20) of all injuries, 14 (70 %) of which occurred during training and 6 (30 %) during matches. The muscle groups most often involved were the hamstrings (femoral biceps and semimembranosus; 55 %), adductors (long and short adductors; 15 %), quadriceps (rectus femoris; 10 %), and gastrocnemius (10 %).

Since the publication of Volpi et al.'s survey in 2004, more recent studies have revealed a shift in the distribution of leg muscle injuries. Our study published in 2014 found that hamstring strains were the most common muscle injuries, followed by injury to the quadriceps, adductors, and sural triceps. The high number of quadriceps injuries Volpi et al. reported may have been due to the

G. Melegati (✉)
Rehabilitation Unit,
IRCCS Galeazzi Orthopaedic Institute,
Via Riccardo Galeazzi 4, Milan, MI 20161, Italy
e-mail: gianluca@melegati.it

D. Tornese
Center for Sports Rehabilitation,
IRCCS Galeazzi Orthopaedic Institute,
Via Riccardo Galeazzi 4, Milan, MI 20161, Italy
e-mail: davidzai@tin.it

P. Volpi (ed.), *Football Traumatology: New Trends*, DOI 10.1007/978-3-319-18245-2_9

training program the team followed, a regimen that favors aggressive quadriceps strength training using isotonic and isokinetic exercises, possibly leading to overloading of the anterior thigh muscles.

In their 5-year epidemiological survey (2003–2007), the Barcelona FC medical staff [9] found that hamstring injuries were the most prevalent type of muscle strains: 396 hamstring pulls (14 %) occurred far more often than injury to the adductors (260; 9 %), quadriceps (160; 6 %), or sural triceps (124; 4 %). Of note, however, is that adductor muscle strains again ranked second in prevalence, which may be related to the training program the team followed.

Currently, the hamstrings are the muscle group most often injured in soccer. In professional soccer, hamstring strain injuries account for 12 % of all injuries. The factors contributing to injury include player age, climate, prevention program, match schedule, muscle fatigue, and type of playing field turf among many others [5, 10]. In addition, reinjury rates are high [11, 12]. Hägglund et al. [13], reporting the results of the UEFA Injury Study, found that 30 % of hamstring injuries will recur, creating frustration for the injured player and the team medical staff and increasing treatment costs and days absent from training and matches. Therefore, a better understanding of hamstring injury prevention and treatment strategies is needed.

Among the muscles of the posterior compartment of the thigh (hamstring), the femoral biceps is most often susceptible to injury [8]. In their study involving professional football players, Ekstrand et al. [14] reported that of the 180 hamstring injuries diagnosed by magnetic resonance imaging (MRI), 84 % involved the femoral biceps, 11 % the semimembranosus, and 5 % the semitendinosus. These observations are consistent with findings by Koulouris et al. [15] who assessed the risk of recurrent hamstring injuries: Of 31 hamstring injuries, 84 % involved the femoral biceps, 10 % the semimembranosus, and 6 % the semitendinosus. The biarticular structure of the femoral biceps and other muscles of the posterior compartment of the thigh is thought to be a common factor potentially predisposing to injury in these muscles. This notion is corroborated by the observation that other muscles crossing two joints, i.e., gastrocnemius, adductors, and rectus femoris, are often injured during sports [16].

The mean time absent, as classified by hamstring injury grade in professional soccer players, is estimated to be 17 ± 10 days for grade I injuries, 22 ± 11 days for grade II injuries, and 73 ± 60 days for grade III injuries [14]. The overwhelming majority (97 %) of hamstring strains in soccer are classified as grade I and grade II injuries [7, 17]. Complete muscle rupture is rare, accounting for about 1 % of all hamstring injuries. Grade III hamstring injuries involve the muscle belly or, more often, the proximal myotendinous junction and can result in an avulsion fracture of the ischial tuberosity or rupture of the conjoined tendon off its ischial tuberosity bony origin. When this occurs, the injury is complete and is sometimes misdiagnosed as a simple hamstring pull and treated inadequately, leading to the risk of chronic pain and potentially severe functional impairment [18].

Hamstring strains are common in sports requiring high-speed running and multidirectional acceleration, with alternating rhythm of movement and frequent changes in direction [19–22]. Ekstrand et al. [5] found that hamstring strains most often occur during fast running or sprinting. Woods et al. [23] reported that over 60 % of hamstring strains in professional English football occurred during running. Similarly, Brooks et al. [24] found that 68 % of hamstring strains in professional rugby union in the UK occurred during running.

9.2 Mechanisms of Causes of Injury

The hamstring muscles extend the hip and flex the knee. In terms of muscle strength, speed, and power, the biomechanical requirements for walking and jogging are far less demanding than for sprinting [25]. Experimental musculoskeletal models have shown that peak hamstring torque and tension occur during the late swing phase in running and that the torque increases with faster running speed [26]. It has also been shown that eccentric hamstring activation increases markedly during running or kicking. Eccentric overloading during the late swing phase is thought to be a possible cause of mechanism of injury [27, 28] since the hamstrings generate maximum tension as they lengthen to decelerate knee extension. Wood [29] reported electromyographic data on peak torque, power, and activation and hamstring length during sprinting. The data show that eccentric contraction occurs during both the late swing phase, before initial contact with the ball (foot strike), and the late stance phase before the foot is raised and the beginning of takeoff, thus confirming that hamstring strain can occur before both foot strike and takeoff. However, hamstring strains are more likely to occur during the late swing than during the late stance phase because during the late swing phase the hamstrings are lengthened and, consequently, under tension near at the limit of their mechanical resistance [30]. In brief, the hamstrings act eccentrically to slow knee extension during deceleration in running. Furthermore, deceleration during high-speed running is often accompanied by leaning the trunk forward, which places additional eccentric overload on the hamstrings and increases the risk of hamstring strain. The trunk is typically inclined forward during dribbling or handling the ball in tight spaces, two situations which require rapid multidirectional changes in movement, quick turns, and leaning the trunk forward to maintain control of balance.

Hamstring strains can also be caused by kicking. Brooks [24] reported that about 10 % of hamstring muscle injuries in professional rugby union occur during kicking and that such injuries were associated with longer injury-related absence. However, because rugby differs from soccer and the mechanisms of cause of injury differ from one sport to another, knowledge about mechanisms of injury cannot be translated indiscriminately. Muscle activation in kicking is described by the "soccer paradox": the extensor muscles are activated during flexion and the flexor muscles during extension. DeProft et al. reported that activation of the quadriceps and hamstring muscles is greatest when they oppose limb movement: the quadriceps during the loading phase and the hamstring muscles during the forward swing phase [31]. Further confirmation of this observation comes from a study by Robertson and Mosher [32] who found no knee extensor activity immediately before ball contact. During this phase, eccentric hamstring activity predominates, thus reducing the angular velocity of the knee and preventing hyperextension. Electromyographic studies [33, 34] have shown that the eccentric peak torque of the hamstring muscles occurs just before the foot kicks the ball, which protects against knee hyperextension but places enormous stress on the hamstrings [35].

9.3 Diagnosis

The diagnosis of hamstring strains is based on clinical signs and symptoms, as well as knowledge of the mechanisms of the causes of injury. Imaging studies with MRI and ultrasonography are essential for confirming the clinical diagnosis. Two types of acute hamstring strain are distinguished: the one typically occurs during sprinting, while the other results from movements that overstretch the hamstrings, as occur during simultaneous hip flexion and knee extension, for example, during kicking. Woods et al. [23], in their audit of injuries in professional football and analysis of hamstring injuries, reported that stretch injuries accounted for 17 % of all injuries, whereas injuries that occurred during high-speed running accounted for 57 % of all hamstring strains.

Sprinting injuries typically occur at the myotendinous junction proximal to the long head of the femoral biceps, whereas stretch injuries occur near the proximal origin near the ischial tuberosity and often involve the semimembranosus tendon. Though sprinting injuries may more severely limit joint function, they normally heal faster than stretch injuries. The site can usually be located by the worst pain elicited on palpation and from MRI findings obtained within the first 2 weeks following injury. In their study on the assessment of acute hamstring strain by MRI and clinical examination in sprinters, Askling et al.

[36] found that the closer the hamstring strain is to the ischial tuberosity, the longer the rehabilitation time. The study also showed that thorough clinical examination performed during the first 3 weeks following injury can provide useful information for the prognosis of hamstring strain injuries.

Clinical examination will include evaluation of muscle strength and pain elicited during active muscle contraction, first with isometric then concentric movement with the patient in the prone position, to determine the range of motion. Also useful is to evaluate muscle contraction with the knee flexed at 90°, with intrarotation and extrarotation of the tibia to determine whether the medial or lateral hamstring muscle is involved. Other tests (active knee extension test, straight leg raise) are performed to evaluate hamstring muscle flexibility and maximum length. Such tests do not always yield reliable information in cases of acute injury, however. Palpation discloses important clues about the injury site and so may give an initial rough estimate of recovery time. Palpation should be carried out proximal to distal along the medial and lateral muscle belly, starting from the ischial tuberosity, while measuring the distance from the tuberosity to the site of maximum pain on palpation. During the clinical exam, differential diagnosis is key to identifying the various different hamstring structures that may be the site of posterior pain. Thorough biomechanical evaluation of the lumbopelvic core will disclose whether the pain is caused by damage to a nerve root or disc or is correlated with a degenerative condition or lumbar instability, all situations commonly encountered in soccer players.

While radiography is important for revealing bone avulsion of the ischial tuberosity in young players, sonography and MRI are appropriate for visualizing the area of the injury, which is characterized by edema and sometimes blood accumulation, both of which can be readily revealed by ultrasound and high-intensity signal MRI (T2-weighted images). MRI is preferable for evaluating deep injuries and to identify residual scar tissue from a previous injury, a clinical picture often misdiagnosed as an acute injury on sonography. Studies [37, 38] have reported that MRI is essential for accurately defining the length and area of injury, two elements directly correlated with the time required for recovery but not useful for identifying players at risk for potential reinjury.

9.4 Prognosis

Hamstring strain injury site and severity, based on clinical and MRI examinations, are useful criteria for determining the duration of rehabilitation and estimating return to play. The injuries requiring long recovery times include injury of the free proximal tendon and injuries near the ischial tuberosity. A direct correlation has been shown between lesion length and duration of recovery [39]. Although injuries involving the myotendinous junction and the muscle fibers adjacent to it are clinically more severe because of greater pain elicited on palpation and less flexibility, they tend to heal faster than injuries involving only the proximal tendon.

9.5 Risk Factors

Recent clinical studies [5, 40] involving professional soccer players have reported several factors that can predispose players to hamstring strains, including previous muscle injuries, diminished flexibility, diminished concentric and eccentric strength, imbalanced strength between agonists and antagonists, muscle fatigue, inadequate rehabilitation, player age, and ethnic origin. One of the most widely recognized risk factors is a history of an identical previous hamstring strain. Hägglund et al. [13] reported that the risk of recurrent injury was three times higher in players who had sustained a similar injury during the previous playing season than players who had not. Engebretsen et al. [40], in a prospective cohort study involving 508 players from 31 amateur clubs during the 2004 playing season, evaluated the potential risk factors by means of a questionnaire survey investigating the history of previous injuries, clinical examination of hamstring strains, and functional tests. They found that previous injury was the risk factor that contributed most to recurrence of hamstring injury.

A previous history of injury involving other muscle groups can raise the risk of recurrent injury of the quadriceps and gastrocnemius in professional football players, but no published studies have reported that this may also be so in hamstring injuries. Orchard [41] reported that in Australian football players, hamstring strains are associated with a previous gastrocnemius injury. Verrall et al. [42] found that a clinical history of previous knee injuries or groin pain raised the risk of hamstring injury. They identified an alteration in the biomechanics of the lower limbs as the probable cause for the increased incidence of hamstring strains. Following an initial problem involving the joint, the muscle, or the tendon insertion point, the athlete may not be able to recover normal biomechanical balance even after an adequate rehabilitation program. Although such has not been described in football, it may hold true for soccer since soccer and Australian football involve similar game situations characterized by sprinting, changes in direction, and acceleration, all of which can lead to hamstring muscle strains.

In their study using animal models, Nikolaou et al. [43] suggested that the fibrous scar tissue within the muscle seen on histological evaluation at 7 days after initial injury might explain the elevated risk of reinjury. Other studies have reported that previous muscle strain injury can set the stage for biomechanical imbalance between the lumbopelvic girdle and the lower limbs. Brockett et al. [44] found that previous injury can lead to hamstring shortening, resulting in higher risk of recurrent injury. Diminished agility and ability to stabilize the trunk, as well as sacroiliac joint dysfunction have also been suggested as factors contributing to hamstring injury [45, 46].

Another factor predisposing players to muscle injury, and hamstring strain in particular, is age [1, 42, 47]. Older players appear, in fact, to be at greater risk of muscle injuries, as demonstrated in samples of semiprofessional and amateur soccer players but, interestingly, not in elite professional players. Hägglund et al. [13], in their survey of Champions League teams, found a twofold higher incidence of gastrocnemius injuries in older players but no association between older age and the occurrence of injury to the adductors, quadriceps, or hamstrings.

Hamstring strain may be correlated with lower back problems. Mooney et al. [48] found increased electrical activity and diminished hamstring flexibility in patients with lower back pain. This means that lower back pain can trigger a perturbation in the hamstring muscles which manifests as increased muscle tension and may be associated with injury. In their retrospective study, Hennessey et al. [49] reported a marked prevalence of lumbar lordosis among athletes with hamstring strain, indicating a possible association between muscle strain and lumbar posture. In a recent clinical study involving athletes with and without hamstring strain, Emami et al. [50] described activity patterns of the lumbopelvic muscles and found that altered core biomechanics can lead to the recurrence of hamstring injury.

In clinical practice, lower back pain often manifests with an increase in pain in the posterior compartment of the thigh, though this does not necessarily indicate muscle injury. The reason is that the hamstrings act as target organs and that their state of tension is modulated by the motor component of the corresponding spinal nerve. Spinal nerve irritation due to discal problems, joint instability, or degeneration can irritate the muscle and thus increase muscle tone. Lower back pain is common in sports in general and in soccer in particular. It typically results from nerve root compression at the last two intervertebral discs and manifests with pain in the hamstrings, gastrocnemius, or peroneal muscles, restricting flexibility and potentially mimicking muscle injury [51]. However, there is no anatomic damage of the muscle fibers in this clinical situation. Recent clinical classifications of muscle injuries in sports, such as those devised by Mueller-Wohlfahrt et al. [52] and the Italian Society of Muscles, Ligaments, and Tendons (ISMu.LT) [53] identify this clinical presentation as a "functional dysfunction" or "nonstructural injury."

The importance of diminished flexibility as a cause of hamstring strain is controversial. Orchard et al. [54] found no correlation between a deficit in hamstring flexibility and the risk of injury, whereas Witvrouw et al. [55], in their prospective study involving professional Belgian soccer players over one competitive season, found that as compared with uninjured players, the players that had sustained a hamstring or quadriceps injury early in the season showed significantly lower flexibility in these muscle group. Since previous muscle injury is a recognized intrinsic risk factor, players that had sustained muscle injury during the previous two seasons were excluded from the study. Specific tests were applied to evaluate the flexibility of the quadriceps, hamstring, adductor, and gastrocnemius muscles. Quadriceps flexibility was measured by means of goniometry with the subject lying prone on the examination table, the contralateral leg resting on the floor, and the maximum passive knee flexion measured with the hip flexed at 90°. The hamstring test was performed with the subject supine, with passive hip flexion, and with extension of the knee to the point at which it indicated the limit of hamstring flexibility. As defined by the study protocol, flexibility less than 90° was significantly correlated with a risk of injury. Adductor flexibility was measured by means of goniometry, with the subject supine, passive hip abduction with the knee extended to the point where femoral rotation indicated the limit of adductor flexibility. Gastrocnemius flexibility was evaluated with the subject standing and the limb to be assessed positioned behind the contralateral limb and the sole of the foot resting on the floor in the sagittal axis; dorsal tibiotarsal flexion was performed and the maximum angle measured. Owing to the small number of adductor and gastrocnemius injuries, no conclusions could be drawn as to the role of diminished flexibility in these muscles and risk of injury, leaving the debate open on whether a correlation exists [56] or not [57].

Ekstrand et al. [58] reported that, in addition to diminished muscle flexibility, another factor predisposing to muscle injury is inadequate warm-up. Hamstring strains are known to occur more often when stretching exercise programs are not correctly followed; quadriceps strains in particular occur when players practice goal shots before a warm-up session. Gabbe et al. [59] noted that diminished quadriceps flexibility can contribute to hamstring strain.

Since muscle injuries often occur during eccentric muscle activation, it is thought that microscopic damage from eccentric exercises can sometimes produce macroscopic damage. The extent of microscopic damage depends on the optimum muscle length for the development of active tension, i.e., the joint angle at which peak torque is produced. Brockett et al. [44] reported that peak torque values could be recorded in previously injured hamstrings that were significantly shorter than the uninjured hamstrings in the contralateral limb and in the group of athletes without hamstring injury. In the healthy athletes, the optimal work angle was 16–34° in knee flexion. Taking an angle of about 20° as a typical value of healthy hamstrings, subjects with a greater angle will be at a higher risk of injury. The small sample size did not allow for considering this as a predictor of injury.

As mentioned above, the hamstrings dissipate kinetic energy through eccentric activation during the forward swing in kicking. Since eccentric contraction can produce microscopic muscle damage, repeated stress can weaken anatomic structures and trigger greater damage [60]. Nonuniform sarcomere lengthening is the putative pathogenic mechanism which occurs above the optimum length on the length-tension curve [61]. Because hamstring muscles adapt to eccentric exercise by changing optimum length, it is believed that there exists a phase of instability of sarcomere length [33]. Beyond this optimum length, the sarcomere units differ in length and the longer sarcomere units adapt more rapidly to lengthening by eccentric contraction. A muscle with a suboptimum length for developing tension is at greater risk of injury because it has a wider work angle in the area where microscopic damage occurs. It has been hypothesized that muscles adapt to microscopic damage from eccentric exercise by increasing the number of sarcomeres in series in the muscle fibers. This adaptation relies on increasing the optimum length to higher values, thus reducing the risk of injury [62]. In contrast, concentric exercise tends to reduce the number of sarcomeres in the muscle fibers, with a subsequent shift to a shorter length at which peak torque is produced [62].

Eccentric hamstring training is justified by the fact that eccentric activation is an integral part of this muscle group's functional repertoire [63, 64]. Because hamstring strains often occur during the eccentric phase, this is just one among other important aspects to consider when designing a rehabilitation program. Equally important are angular velocity and joint angle. Angular velocity of the knee during sprinting may reach 600–700°/s or more. We have mentioned above that the pathogenetic mechanism of hamstring strain has been identified during maximum eccentric activation for decelerating forward swing during the late swing phase so that leg excursion does not exceed knee flexion of about 30°.

Muscle weakness and imbalance between agonist and antagonist muscle strength are factors predisposing to hamstring strain. One of the most widely used methods to measure hamstring strength is by eccentric and concentric isokinetic dynamometry to determine the difference in peak torque between the right and left limbs and the hamstring-quadriceps ratio in the same limb. An imbalance in strength as obtained from these two measures is considered a risk factor for hamstring strain. Opinions diverge on this issue, however. Orchard et al. [41] reported that hamstring strain was significantly associated with a decrease in peak torque in Australian football players and with an altered flexor-extensor ratio on isokinetic dynamometry. Benelli et al. [65], in contrast, found that isokinetic strength testing does not predict hamstring injury in Australian Rule footballers. This observation is shared by Grace et al. [66] who found no correlation between isokinetic dynamometry test results before the beginning of the competition season and the risk of hamstring injury during the following months in American footballers.

Muscle strengthening has been suggested as a preventive measure to reduce hamstring strain [67]. This suggestion derives from animal models in which it was shown that a stronger muscle has a higher rupture load than a weaker muscle [21]. Askling et al. [12] found that a program of eccentric hamstring strengthening during preseason preparation reduces the incidence of hamstring strain during the following competition season in 30 professional Swedish soccer players. This observation is shared by Petersen et al. [68] in their study on the preventive effect of eccentric training on acute hamstring injuries. In their prospective study involving 100 professional soccer players, Fousekis et al. [69] reported that asymmetrical eccentric hamstring strength is the most reliable predicator of hamstring strain. Croisier et al. [70], in their prospective study involving professional Brazilian, Belgian, and French soccer players, reported a correlation between strength imbalances in quadriceps and flexors, as measured by isokinetic dynamometry, and the risk of hamstring strain. Recovery of normal strength values, as expressed by a normal concentric and eccentric function ratio between quadriceps and flexors, led to a reduction in the incidence of hamstring strains. Schache et al. [71] reported a 10 % deficit in isometric hamstring strength of the right leg as compared to the left leg 5 days before a hamstring strain in the right leg occurred. They suggested that a simple maximal isometric strength test could indicate a predisposition to hamstring strain.

Although there is no universal agreement on a correlation between strength deficit and hamstring strain, Nordic hamstring exercises for eccentric hamstring strengthening have been scientifically demonstrated as the best type of exercise for preventing hamstring injury as it has been proven highly effective in increasing eccentric hamstring strength [11]. It is precisely the efficacy of this type of exercise in preventing hamstring strain that allows us to correlate, at least theoretically, eccentric strength deficit and hamstring injury. Nordic hamstring exercises require no special equipment; can be reasonably offered to all soccer players, whatever their level, but especially to those with a history of hamstring strain; and can be included in exercise routines during training [12].

The tendency of muscle injury to recur warrants greater attention to the management of players with previous muscle strain. The main goal of rehabilitation is, therefore, not to hasten recovery but to prevent injury recurrence. Also to be kept in mind is that, unlike spontaneous tissue healing, a previous or residual biomechanical function deficit will resolve only with adequate rehabilitation therapy.

Muscle fatigue can play a determinant role in hamstring strain. The peak torque of eccentric hamstring strength diminishes progressively during physical activity and particularly at the end of the match half-times and return to play after the half-time interval [72]. Hamstring flexibility decreases, reducing the angle of hip flexion and knee extension during the late swing phase, thus increasing the risk of injury. In addition, fatigue can alter the normal neuromuscular activity of the hamstring muscles, predisposing them not only to muscle injury but also to joint injury. The slower sprinting speed some studies have reported for players at the beginning of the second match time, immediately after the half-time interval, has been imputed to a decrease in core body temperature, with a reduction in flexibility, flexion angles, and hip and knee extension [73, 74]. It is therefore recommended that players maintain their body temperature during the half-time interval by performing warm-up exercises to prevent against muscle strain. Finally, a nonmodifiable factor contributing to the risk of hamstring injury is ethnic origin. Woods [23] found a higher incidence of hamstring strain in black or Caribbean soccer players.

9.6 Prevention

An ample literature documents that maximum hamstring strength and tension develop during eccentric braking to slow the rate of movement during the late swing phase in running. The eccentric action increases as the running speed increases [26]. Because the risk of hamstring strain increases during this phase of running, theoretically, the best way to prevent hamstring strain is to increase eccentric hamstring strength through exercises that lengthen the hamstring muscles while they are activated and contracted. Brockett et al. [44] described a simple exercise method for eccentric hamstring lengthening called Nordic hamstring exercise. It was subsequently developed by Mjølsnes et al. [75] who conducted a 10-week randomized trial comparing eccentric versus concentric hamstring strength training in soccer players. The results showed that Nordic hamstring exercise is effective in increasing eccentric hamstring strength. In their randomized controlled trial (RCT), Petersen et al. [68] demonstrated that a 10-week program combining Nordic hamstring exercise and conventional training in professional and amateur soccer players can significantly reduce the incidence of first-time and recurrent hamstring injury, as compared with a control group of soccer players who had not participated in a Nordic hamstring strengthening program. Askling et al. [12] conducted a study involving 30 professional soccer players divided into two groups: one group trained twice a week for 10 weeks with a yo-yo device designed to increase eccentric and concentric hamstring strength; the other group received conventional training. Both groups underwent isokinetic dynamometry to evaluate eccentric hamstring strength and maximum velocity testing. The results showed a significantly lower incidence of hamstring strain (3/15) in the group that received yo-yo training and a marked increased in eccentric strength and velocity in the treatment group. Overall, the results show the usefulness of eccentric hamstring strengthening in soccer players.

Melegati et al. [8] conducted a study investigating the effectiveness of a prevention program during one competition season (2010–2011) in an elite Italian soccer team. The program included two types of prevention intervention: collective and individual. Collective intervention was composed of core stability exercises the entire team performed before each training session. Individual intervention consisted of personalized interventions based on the results of clinical, kinesiologic, and isokinetic evaluation at the beginning of the season and the player's history of acute or overload injuries recorded on clinical history taking. The program was carried out, either with the assistance of a physiotherapist when needed or self-managed, two to three times a week usually before the daily technical-athletic collective training session. The goals were individualized for each player. The team medical staff diagnosed all injuries that occurred during the study period. Diagnosis was based on clinical examination and imaging with a 1.5 tesla MRI system. An injury was defined as an event that occurred during training or competition and excluded the player from the next training session or match [76]. Adherence to the prevention program was good overall and was supported by strict principles of muscle strain treatment and application of rigorous criteria for return to play. The results showed that the program was highly effective in reducing the number of muscle injuries (−26 %) and the injury recurrence rate (from 18.5 % to 0 %) as compared with the previous season. No recurrent injuries were recorded, whereas three recurrent injuries occurred in players who had sustained an injury during the previous season. Muscle injuries accounted for 31 % of all injuries, as compared with 59 % of all injuries recorded during the previous season. The number of injuries per 1,000 h of exposure was cut in half (from 5.6 to 2.5) and the number of days absent per 1,000 h of exposure was reduced from 106 to 37.

9.7 Basic Principles of Treatment

Mild hamstring muscle strains are repaired by mononuclear satellite cells that differentiate into myoblasts. In more severe injuries, the formation of scar repair tissue predominates, and the progression of functional recovery is essential for guiding the repair of the newly forming tissue. Chronologically, three repair phases are distinguished: acute, remodeling, and functional recovery [77, 78].

Repair phases of a grade 2 hamstring strain

Acute phase	Time since injury
Stage I. Injury	0–6 h
Stage 2. Inflammatory reaction	6–24 h
Stage 3. Phagocytosis	24–48 h
Tissue remodeling	
Stage 4. Initial repair	3–6 days
Stage 5. Advanced repair	7–14 days
Functional recovery	
Stage 6. Functional recovery	15–60 days

9.8 Acute Phase

Immediately following injury, an elastic compression bandage and local cryotherapy (20 min every hour) should be applied. This phase is characterized by local bleeding, myofibril retraction, and edema due to increased capillary permeability. The objective is to limit local tissue damage as much as possible. Opinions diverge on the real utility of applying compressive bandages. A prospective study by Thorsson et al. [79] involving 19 subjects who received external compression within 5 min after thigh and calf muscle injury showed that immediate compression therapy was not effective in reducing muscle hematoma or hastening recovery, as compared with 20 subjects who received only cryotherapy and raising the injured leg or, in some cases, in combination with compression bandage applied 10–30 min after the injury event.

We do not normally administer nonsteroidal anti-inflammatory drugs (NSAIDs), muscle relaxants, or other medications since the pain is generally not so severe as to require analgesics. Controversy surrounds the use of NSAIDs to reduce inflammation in pain fatigue and muscle pulls [80]. Although biochemical and histochemical studies [81] have shown that indomethacin can reduce local muscle damage, Reynolds et al. [82] reported that NSAIDs fail to enhance healing of acute hamstring injuries. The use of corticosteroids has been found to impede healing of such injuries [80]. Furthermore, analgesics can mask important pain symptoms during the healing phase, leading to more aggressive treatment than is necessary or appropriate at this critical stage of healing.

Around 24–48 h postinjury, edema becomes more pronounced, with mechanical weakening of muscles due to massive macrophage migration to the injury site. Adequate management at this point is essential since aggressive treatment can cause further tissue damage, prolong the inflammatory phase, and delay tissue repair. Transcutaneous electrical nerve stimulation, because of the beneficial neuroreflexive response it elicits, can be safely and effectively applied to counteract pain symptoms [83]. Ambulation with weight bearing and two Canadian crutches is allowed as tolerated based on pain. Important during this phase is to protect the injured muscle as it heals.

Walking with the assistance of one Canadian crutch is permitted starting from day 3. The compression bandage is removed for ultrasound or MRI examination. Walking without aids can be started as soon as the gait pattern has normalized and no localized pain is present. Hydrotherapy in decreasing pool depths can facilitate a more normal walking pattern. The benefits with hydrotherapy derive from its hydrostatic, hydrodynamic, proprioceptive [84], and thermal effects and allow early active mobilization, with all the advantages this has for the next phase of recovering joint function.

9.9 Remodeling Phase

During the initial remodeling phase (3–6 days postinjury), fibroblastic activity is characterized by the deposition of collagen. Healing is promoted by capillary neovascularization which provides centripetal supply of oxygen and nutrients required for regenerative tissue metabolism [85]. Tissue repair can be enhanced with the use of physical therapies, including neodymium-doped yttrium aluminum garnet (Nd-YAG) laser or transfer energetic capacitive and resistive (TECAR) therapy [86] according to specific protocols depending on sonographic findings. Importantly, however, physical therapies lack adequate evidenced-based support. When gait pattern has normalized and pain is absent, cautious use of passive stretching can be initiated to relax the muscle fibers in the perilesional zone. No massaging is done at this time. Appropriate exercises for recovering lumbopelvic neuromuscular control and exercises to improve one-leg standing balance are started. Neuromuscular control of the pelvic region is believed necessary for optimal hamstring function during sports.

Sherry and Best [45] reported a significant reduction in injury recurrence in subjects with hamstring strain who underwent a core stability exercise program, as compared with those who received conventional rehabilitation with concentric strengthening and stretching. Isometric contraction of the injured muscle involves submaximal exercising below the pain threshold. During the advanced repair phase (7–14 days postinjury), concomitant with muscle fiber regeneration, muscle weakness is about 50 % that prior to injury. This deficit is thought to be due more to the inflammatory phase of the healing process, accompanied by edema and pain, rather than a real decrease in muscle contractility. The risk of reinjury during this phase is high because pain is diminished and function has improved, though the site of injury remains structurally vulnerable. When hamstring elasticity has improved, concentric isotonic exercises are started, followed by submaximal eccentric exercises, both of which are performed with manual resistance. Tissue elasticity is maintained and/or regained with passive stretching exercises. As regards the timing of static stretching, Bandy et al. [87–89] reported that daily passive stretching sessions for 30 s provide optimal results and that longer sessions of up to 60 s do not produce a greater increase in flexibility. At this point, aerobic exercise on a cycle ergometer or step machine is introduced, delaying running to the next phase of functional recovery. Proprioceptive rehabilitation is then gradually introduced in three progressive stages: joint positioning/repositioning (cortical), one- and two-leg balance training with eyes open and eyes closed (subcortical), and dynamic reflexive stabilization exercises and sport-specific activities (spinal) [90].

9.10 Functional Recovery Phase

During the functional recovery phase (15–60 days postinjury), following collagen maturation and complete recovery of voluntary muscle control, the rehabilitation goal is to regain complete recovery of muscle strength and function. Generally, normal gait and muscle elasticity have been attained by the third or fourth week, and prolonged maximal isometric contraction does not elicit pain. At this stage, sonography is obtained to determine the progression of fiber remodeling in the muscle scar tissue.

Heiser et al. [91] recommend initiating running when the peak torque at an angular velocity of 60°/s is at least 70 % that of the contralateral limb. This presumes that maximal isokinetic testing has been performed, which, however, carries the risk of reinjury during the procedure. Importantly, isokinetic dynamometry is useful for evaluating muscle strength expressed during open kinetic chain exercise without loading. Therefore, it is impossible to reproduce joint kinematics in a closed kinetic chain system with loading. This means that the test is inappropriate for evaluating the role the muscles play in dynamic joint stabilization. Aagaard et al. [92] suggested interpolating the peak eccentric hamstring torque value from the peak concentric hamstring torque value (eccentric Ham/concentric Quad), thus defining the result as the "functional ratio of the knee extensors." In this case, the peak hamstring torque is directly proportional to the angular velocity of the exercise and is inversely proportional to the degree of knee flexion. In their study involving professional soccer players, Dauty et al. [93] reported that an eccentric Ham/concentric Quad ratio less than 0.6 will identify players who, though returned to play, had experienced a previous hamstring strain. However, the ratio was not a predictive indicator for future injuries.

Hamstring strain typically occurs during the eccentric phase of muscle contraction; therefore, rehabilitation with eccentric strengthening exercise is warranted. Eccentric contraction can stimulate intense protein synthesis in the myotendinous junction, promoting myofibrillogenesis with remodeling of the myotendinous junction. The intensity of eccentric contraction should be gradually increased to reach maximum exercise intensity by the fourth or fifth session. The angular velocity of exercise should also be progressively increased since elevated angular velocity increases muscle tension.

The high risk of recurrent hamstring strain can be attributed to alterations in the length-tension ratio in the injured muscle: because muscle tension is greater in shorter muscles, they are at higher risk of injury due to the limited reserves available. This biomechanical alteration can result from predominantly concentric exercises during this rehabilitation phase or due to the presence of residual scar tissue in the myotendinous junction [44, 94]. In healthy subjects, eccentric exercise has been shown to facilitate the recovery of a normal muscle length-tension ratio [60]. It may be speculated that eccentric strengthening in the rehabilitation of hamstring strain can restore an optimal muscle length-tension ratio and thus reduce the risk of injury recurrence.

Eccentric isokinetic exercise at increasing speeds (starting at 60°/s), beginning at submaximal intensity, should not be performed more than three times a week in order to avoid overloading which could cause muscle fatigue. The success of rehabilitation hinges on exercise performed at high angular velocity. Jonhagen et al. [22] reported that recurrent hamstring strain in athletes engaging in sports characterized by high angular speeds, as seen in sprinters, is often attributable to a strength deficit in the eccentric phase. The most important aspect of eccentric strengthening is to have a proper lengthening position during exercising that can help to restore eccentric strength at the normal limits of muscle lengthening. Eccentric hamstring training for hamstring stretching is begun with the use of resilience bands or pulleys during isokinetic dynamometry, with the patient's hips flexed. The exercise is then carried out on the isokinetic dynamometer, making sure that hip is kept flexed [95].

Athletes can be returned to unrestricted training when muscle strength is at least 80 % that of the contralateral limb and when muscle fatigue is absent after prolonged running. Athletes who have sustained a hamstring strain should continue with eccentric exercising for the remainder of their professional career. The common tendency of muscle injuries, and hamstring strains in particular, to recur poses additional challenges for the team physician to find the right balance between preventing injury recurrence and ensuring rapid recovery. Return to play will depend on adequate recovery of muscle strength, resistance, and flexibility, as well as neuromuscular control [2]. The site and extent of muscle damage, the athlete's motivation and general psychophysical condition, appropriate rehabilitation techniques, and seamless coordination of the entire medical staff are the requisites for providing complete functional recovery. Recurrence of injury within 2 months after return to play is a clear sign of inadequacies in the rehabilitation program.

One approach to acute muscle injuries that has garnered interest from the international sports medicine community stems from work by Mueller-Wohlfahrt and colleagues [52], which is now widely recognized as a seminal approach to muscle injuries in sports. Although injection therapy, as long practiced by Mueller-Wohlfahrt, lacks the evidenced-based support of RCTs, it has become the mainstay of treatment in Germany where an increasing number of elite soccer players and other athletes have undergone therapy. The therapy protocol calls for the injection of a local anesthetic, followed by the administration of Actovegin [96, 97], a deproteinized hemoderivative of calf blood, which appears to markedly accelerate myofibril synthesis in the injured muscle and diminish muscle tone, in combination with Traumeel S, a homeopathic product that modulates inflammatory response and the release of anti-inflammatory cytokines. The drugs are injected at the site of the injury, along the involved muscle and in the lumbar region (epidural and paravertebral). The first injection is given the day of the injury and then at 2 and 4 days postinjury.

As mentioned, scientific evidence demonstrating the efficacy of this treatment is patchy. Lee et al. [96] reported a significant reduction in recovery time in athletes with acute hamstring strain treated with Actovegin, as compared with subjects who had received conventional physiotherapy. According to a systematic review of the literature [98], the study has a high risk of bias owing to flawed methodology: no randomization, no blinded control, and allocation of patients who refused therapy to the control group. There exists, however, a certain analogy between Mueller-Wohlfahrt's theories about how injured muscles heal and studies from basic science that found that aggressive control of the inflammatory process can reduce tissue damage and enhance functional recovery [99]. Beyond the question whether the therapy can be considered best practice in the treatment of elite and amateur athletes, the use of injectable Traumeel and Actovegin is not approved in many countries.

References

1. Arnason A, Sigurdsson SB, Gudmundsson A, Holme I, Engebretsen L, Bahr R (2004) Risk factors for injuries in football. Am J Sports Med 32(suppl 1):S5–S16
2. Ekstrand J, Hagglund M, Walden M (2011) Injury incidence and injury pattern in professional football—the UEFA injury study. Br J Sports Med 45(7):553–558
3. Ekstrand J, Gillquist J (1983) Soccer injuries and their mechanisms: a prospective study. Med Sci Sports Exerc 15:267–270
4. Inklaar H (1994) Soccer injuries, I: incidence and severity. Sports Med 18:55–73
5. Ekstrand J, Hägglund M, Waldén M (2011) Epidemiology of muscle injuries in professional football (soccer). Am J Sports Med 39(6):1226–1232
6. Woods C, Hawkins R, Hulse M, Hodson A (2002) The football association medical research programme: an audit of injuries in professional football-analysis of preseason injuries. Br J Sports Med 36:436–441
7. Volpi P, Melegati G, Tornese D, Bandi M (2004) Muscle strains in soccer: a five-year survey of an Italian major league team. Knee Surg Sports Traumatol Arthrosc 12:482–485
8. Melegati G, Tornese D, Gevi M, Trabattoni A, Pozzi G, Schonhuber H, Volpi P (2014) Reducing muscle injuries and reinjuries in one italian professional male soccer team. Muscles Ligaments Tendons J 3(4): 324–330, eCollection 2013
9. Rodas G, Pruna R, Til L, Martín C (2009) Clinical practice guide for muscular injuries. Epidemiology, diagnosis, treatment and prevention. Apunts Med Esport 164:179–203
10. Ekstrand J, Timpka T, Hagglund M (2006) Risk of injury in elite football played on artificial turf versus natural grass: a prospective two -cohort study. Br J Sports Med 40:975–980
11. Arnason A, Andersen TE, Holme I, Engebretsen L, Bahr R (2008) Prevention of hamstring strains in elite soccer: an intervention study. Scand J Med Sci Sports 18:40–48
12. Askling C, Karlsson J, Thorstensson A (2003) Hamstring injury occurrence in elite soccer players after preseason strength training with eccentric overload. Scand J Med Sci Sports 13:244–250
13. Hagglund M, Waldèn M, Ekstrand J (2013) Risk factors for lower extremity muscle injury in professional soccer. The UEFA injury study. Am J Sports Med 41:327–335, AJSM PreView
14. Ekstrand J, Healy JC, Waldén M et al (2012) Hamstring muscle injuries in professional football: the correlation of MRI findings with return to play. Br J Sports Med 46(2):112–117

15. Koulouris G, Connell DA, Brukner P et al (2007) Magnetic resonance imaging parameters for assessing risk of recurrent hamstring injuries in elite athletes. Am J Sports Med 35:1500–1506
16. Orchard J, Best TM, Verrall GM (2005) Return to play following muscle strains. Clin J Sport Med 15(6):436–441
17. Schneider-Kolsky ME, Hoving JL, Warren P, Connell DA (2006) A comparison between clinical assessment and magnetic resonance imaging of acute hamstring injuries. Am J Sports Med 34(6):1008–1015, Epub 2006 Feb 13
18. Gidwani S, Bircher MD (2007) Avulsion injuries of the hamstring origin – a series of 12 patients and management algorithm. Ann R Coll Surg Engl 89: 394–399
19. Askling CM, Tengvar M, Saartok T et al (2007) Acute first-time hamstring strains during high-speed running: a longitudinal study including clinical and magnetic resonance imaging findings. Am J Sports Med 35:197–206
20. Elliott MC, Zarins B, Powell JW et al (2011) Hamstring muscle strains in professionalfootball players: a 10-year review. Am J Sports Med 39:843–850
21. Garrett WE Jr (1990) Muscle strain injuries: clinical and basic aspects. Med Sci Sports Exerc 22: 436–443, 34
22. Jönhagen S, Németh G, Eriksson E (1994) Hamstring injuries in sprinters. The role of concentric and eccentric hamstring muscle strength and flexibility. Am J Sports Med 22:262–266
23. Woods C, Hawkins RD, Maltby S, Hulse M, Thomas A, Hodson A (2004) The football association medical research programme: an audit of injuries in professional football e analysis of hamstring injuries. Br J Sports Med 38:36e41
24. Brooks JH, Fuller CW, Kemp SP, Reddin DB (2006) Incidence, risk, and prevention of hamstring muscle injuries in professional rugby union. Am J Sports Med 34:1297e306
25. Schache AG, Wigley TV, Baker R, Pandy MG (2009) Biomechanical response to hamstring muscle strain injury. Gait Posture 29:332–338
26. Chumanov ES, Heiderschelt BC, Thelen DG (2007) The effect of speed and influence of individual muscles on hamstring mechanics during the swing phase of sprinting. J Biomech 40:3555–3562
27. Mann R, Sprague P (1980) A kinetic analysis of the ground leg during sprint running. Res Q Exerc Sport 51:334e48
28. Mann RV (1981) A kinetic analysis of sprinting. Med Sci Sports Exerc 13:325e8
29. Wood GA (1987) Biomechanical limitations to sprint running. Med Sport Sci 25:58e71
30. Yu B, Queen RM, Abbey AN, Liu Y, Moorman CT, Garrett WE (2008) Hamstring muscle kinematics and activation during overground sprinting. J Biomech 41:3121e6
31. DeProft E, Clarys JP, Bollens E et al (1988) Muscle activity in the soccer kick. In: Reilly T, Lees A, Davids K et al (eds) Science and football. E & FN Spon, New York, pp 434–440
32. Robertson DGE, Mosher RE (1985) Work and power of the leg muscle in soccer kicking. In: Biomechanics. Human Kinetics Publishers, Champaign
33. Asami T, Nolte V (1983) Analysis of powerful ball kicking. In: Matsui H, Kobayashi K (eds) Biomechanics VIII-B. Human Kinetics Publishers, Champaign, pp 695–700
34. Lindbeck L (1983) Impulse and moment of impulse in the leg joints by impact from kicking. J Biomech Eng 105:108–111
35. Roberts EM, Metcalfe A (1968) Mechanical analysis of kicking. In: Wartenweiler J, Jokl E, Hebbelinck M (eds) Biomechanics I. University Park Press, Baltimore, pp 315–319
36. Askling C, Saartok T, Thorstensson A (2006) Type of acute hamstring strain affects flexibility, strength, and time to return to pre-injury level. Br J Sports Med 40:40–44
37. Connell DA, Schneider-Kolsky ME, Hoving JL et al (2004) Longitudinal study comparing sonographic and MRI assessments of acute and healing hamstring injuries. AJR Am J Roentgenol 183:975–984
38. Slavotinek JP, Verrall GM, Fon GT (2002) Hamstring injury in athletes: using MR imaging measurements to compare extent of muscle injury with amount of time lost from competition. AJR Am J Roentgenol 179:1621–1628
39. Gibbs NJ, Cross TM, Cameron M, Houang MT (2004) The accuracy of MRI in predicting recovery and recurrence of acute grade one hamstring muscle strains within the same season in Australian rules football players. J Sci Med Sport 7(2):248–258
40. Engebretsen AH, Myklebust G, Holme I, Engebretsen L, Bahr R (2010) Intrinsic risk factors for hamstring injuries among male soccer players: a prospective cohort study. Am J Sports Med 38(6):1147–1153
41. Orchard JW (2001) Intrinsic and extrinsic risk factors for muscle strains in Australian football. Am J Sports Med 29(3):300–303
42. Verrall GM, Slavotinek JP, Barnes PG, Fon GT, Spriggins AJ (2001) Clinical risk factors for hamstring muscle strain injury: a prospective study with correlation of injury by magnetic resonance imaging. Br J Sports Med 35(6):435–439
43. Nikolaou PK, Macdonald BL, Glisson RR, Seaber AV, Garrett WE (1987) Biomechanical and histological evaluation of muscle after controlled strain injury. Am J Sports Med 15:9e14
44. Brockett CL, Morgan DL, Proske U (2004) Predicting hamstring strain injury in elite athletes. Med Sci Sports Exerc 36:379e87
45. Sherry MA, Best TM (2004) A comparison of 2 rehabilitation programs in the treatment of acute hamstring strains. J Orthop Sports Phys Ther 34: 116–125, 91
46. Cibulka MT, Rose SJ, Delitto A, Sinacore DR (1986) Hamstring muscle strain treated by mobilizing the sacroiliac joint. Phys Ther 66:1220e3

47. Henderson G, Barnes CA, Portas MD (2010) Factors associated with increased propensity for hamstring injury in english premier league soccer players. J Sci Med Sport 13(4):397–402
48. Mooney V, Robertson J (1976) The facet syndrome. Clin Orthop Relat Res 115:149–156
49. Hennessey L, Watson AW (1993) Flexibility and posture assessment in relation to hamstring injury. Br J Sports Med 27:243–246
50. Emami M, Massoud Arab A, Ghamkhar L (2014) The activity pattern of the lumbopelvic muscles during prone hip extension in athletes with and without hamstring strains injury. IJSPT 9(3):312–319
51. Orchard JW, Farhart P, Leopold C (2004) Lumbar spine region pathology and hamstring and calf injuries in athletic: is there a connection? Br J Sports Med 38:502–504
52. Mueller-Wohlfahrt HW et al (2012) Terminology and classification of muscle injuries in sport: the Munich consensus statement. Br J Sports Med 0:1–9
53. Maffulli N, Oliva F, Frizziero A, Nanni G, Barazzuol M, Giai Via A, Ramponi C, Brancaccio P, Lisitano G, Rizzo D, Freschi M, Galletti S, Melegati G, Pasta G, Testa V, Valent A, Del Buono A (2013) ISMuLT guidelines for muscle injuries muscles. Ligaments Tendons J 3(4):241–249
54. Orchard J, Marsden J, Lord S et al (1997) Preseason hamstring weakness associated with hamstring muscle injury in Australian footballers. Am J Sports Med 25:81–85
55. Witvrouw E, Danneels L, Asselman P, D'Have T, Cambier D (2003) Muscle flexibility as a risk factor for developing muscle injuries in male professional soccer players. A prospective study. Am J Sports Med 31(1):41–46
56. Ekstrand J, Gillquist J (1983) The avoidability of soccer injuries. Int J Sports Med 4:124–128
57. Tyler TF, Nicholas SJ, Campbell RJ et al (2001) The association of hip strength and flexibility with the incidence of adductor muscle strains in professional ice hockey players. Am J Sports Med 29:124–128
58. Ekstrand J, Gillquist J, Moller M et al (1983) Incidence of soccer injuries and their relation to training and team success. Am J Sports Med 11:63–67
59. Gabbe BJ, Bennell KL, Finch CF, Wajswelner H, Orchard JW (2006) Predictors of hamstring injury at the elite level of Australian football. Scand J Med Sci Sports 16:7–13, PubMed: 16430675
60. Brockett CL, Morgan DL, Proske U (2001) Human hamstring muscles adapt to eccentric exercise by changing optimum length. Med Sci Sports Exerc 33:783–790
61. Morgan DL (1990) New insights into the behavior of muscle during active lengthening. Biophys J 57: 209–221
62. Gordon AM, Huxley AF, Julian FJ (1966) The variation in isometric tension with sarcomere length in vertebrate muscle fibres. J Physiol 184:170–192
63. Nilsson J, Thorstensson A, Halbertsma J (1985) Changes in leg movements and muscle activity with speed of locomotion and mode of progression in humans. Acta Physiol Scand 123:457–475
64. Mann RA, Morgan GT, Dougherty SE (1986) Comparative electromyography of the lower extremity in jogging, running and sprinting. Am J Sports Med 14:501–510
65. Bennell K et al (1998) Isokinetic strenght testing does not predict hamstring injury in Australian rules footballers. Br J Sports Med 32:309–314
66. Grace TG et al (1984) Isokinetic muscle imbalance and knee-joint injuries. A prospective blind study. J Bone Joint Surg Am 66:734–740
67. Stanton P, Purdam C (1989) Hamstring injuries in sprinting. The role of eccentric exercise. J Orthop Sports Phys Ther 10:343–349
68. Petersen J, Thorborg K, Nielsen MB, Budtz-Jørgensen E, Hölmich P (2011) Preventive effect of eccentric training on acute hamstring injuries in men's soccer: a cluster-randomized controlled trial. Am J Sports Med 39:2296–2303
69. Fousekis K, Tsepis E, Poulmedis P, Athanasopoulos S, Vagenas G (2011) Intrinsic risk factors of non-contact quadriceps and hamstring strains in soccer: a prospective study of 100 professional players. Br J Sports Med 45:709e14
70. Croisier JL, Ganteaume S, Binet J, Genty M, Ferret JM (2008) Strength imbalances and prevention of hamstring injury in professional soccer players: a prospective study. Am J Sports Med 36(8):1469–1475
71. Schache AG, Crossley KM, Macindoe IG, Fahrner BB, Pandy MG (2011) Can a clinical test of hamstring strength identify football players at risk of hamstring strain? Knee Surg Sports Traumatol Arthrosc 19:38e41
72. Greig M, Siegler JC (2009) Soccer-specific fatigue and eccentric hamstrings muscle strength. J Athl Train 44(2):180–184
73. Mohr M, Krustrup P, Nybo L, Nielsen JJ, Bangsbo J (2004) Muscle temperature and sprint performance during soccer matches–beneficial effect of re-warm-up at half-time. Scand J Med Sci Sports 14(3): 156–162
74. Small K, McNaughton LR, Greig M, Lohkamp M, Lovell R (2009) Soccer fatigue, sprinting and hamstring injury risk. Int J Sports Med 30(8):573–578
75. Mjølsnes R, Arnason A, Østhagen T, Raastad T, Bahr R (2004) A 10-week randomized trial comparing eccentric vs. concentric hamstring strength training in well-trained soccer players. Scand J Med Sci Sports 14(5):311–317
76. Ekstrand J (1982) Soccer injuries and their prevention. Thesis, Linköping University, Linköping
77. Reid DC (1992) Muscle injury: classification and healing. In: Sport injury. Assessment and rehabilitation. Churchill Livingstone, New York, pp 85–101
78. Fisher BD et al (1990) Ultrastructural events following acute muscle trauma. Med Sci Sports Exerc 22:185–193
79. Thorsson O et al (1997) Immediate external compression in the management of an acute muscle injury. Scand J Med Sci Sports 7:182–190

80. Almekinders LC (1999) Anti-inflammatory treatment of muscular injuries in sport. Sports Med 28:383–388
81. Salimen A, Kihlstrom M (1987) Protective effects of indomethacin against exercise induced effects of injury in mouse skeletal muscle fibers. Int J Sports Med 8:46
82. Reynolds JF et al (1995) Non-steroidal anti-inflammatory drugs fail to enhance healing of acute hamstring injuries treated with physiotherapy. S Afr Med J 85:517–522
83. Wolf SL (1978) Perspectives on central nervous system responsiveness to transcutaneous electrical nerve stimulation. Phys Ther 58:1443–1449
84. Speer KP et al (1993) A role for hydrotherapy in shoulder rehabilitation. Am J Sports Med 21:850–853
85. Benazzo F et al (1989) Attuali orientamenti nella patogenesi, evoluzione e trattamento degli ematomi muscolari negli atleti Italian. J Sports Traumatol 4:273
86. Mondardini P et al (1999) Nuove metodologie nel trattamento della patologia traumatica dell'atleta: la T.E.C.A.R. terapia. Med Sport 52:201–213
87. Bandy WD, Irion JM (1994) The effect of time on static stretch on the flexibility of the hamstring muscle. Phys Ther 74:845–850
88. Bandy WD, Irion JM, Briggler M (1997) The effect of time and frequency of static stretching on flexibility of the hamstring muscles. Phys Ther 77: 1090–1096
89. Bandy WD, Irion JM, Briggler M (1998) The efect of static stretch and dynamic range of motion training on the flexibility of the hamstring muscles. J Orthop Sports Phys Ther 27:295–300
90. Lephart SM, Pinciviero DM et al (1997) The role of proprioception in the management and rehabilitation of athletic injuries. Am J Sports Med 25(1):130–137
91. Heiser TM et al (1984) Prophylaxis and management of hamstring muscle injuries in intercollegiate football players. Am J Sports Med 12:368–370
92. Aagaard P et al (1998) A new concept for isokinetic hamstring: quadriceps muscle strength ratio. Am J Sports Med 26:231–237
93. Dauty M, Potiron-Josse M, Rochcongar P (2003) Consequences et prediction des lesions musculaires des ischiojambiers a partir des parametres isocinetiques concentriques et excentriques du joueur de football professionel. Ann Readapt Med Phys 46:601–606
94. Proske U, Morgan DL, Brockett CL, Percival P (2004) Identifying athletes at risk of hamstring strains and how to protect them. Clin Exp Pharmacol Physiol 31:546–550, PubMed: 15298549
95. Schmitt B, Tyler T, McHugh M (2012) Hamstring injury rehabilitation and prevention of reinjury using lenghtened state eccentric training: a new concept. Int J Sports Phys Ther 7(3):333–341
96. Lee P, Rattenberry A, Connelly S, Nokes L (2011) Our experience on Actovegin, is it cutting edge? Int J Sports Med 32(4):237–241
97. Wright-Carpenter T, Klein P, Schäferhoff P, Appell HJ, Mir LM, Wehling P (2004) Treatment of muscle injuries by local administration of autologous conditioned serum: a pilot study on sportsmen with muscle strains. Int J Sports Med 25(8):588–593
98. Reurink G, Goudswaard GJ, Tol GL, Verhaar JAN, Weir A, Moen MH (2012) Therapeutic interventions for acute hamstring injuries: a systematic review. Br J Sports Med 46:103–109. doi:10.1136/bjsports-2011-090447
99. Brickson S, Ji LL, Schell K, Olabisi R, St Pierre Schneider B, Best TM (2003) M1/70 attenuates blood-borne neutrophil oxidants, activation, and myofiber damage following stretch injury. J Appl Physiol (1985) 95(3):969–976. Epub 2 May 2003

Patellar and Quadriceps Tendinopathy

10

Andrea Ferretti

10.1 Introduction

Quadriceps and patellar tendinopathies are known as "jumper's knee," similarly following a tradition of reference to the etiology of a pathology, such as "tennis elbow" or "thrower's shoulder."

Even though patellar tendinopathy had already been described in Italy [1], the term "jumper's knee" was due to a study published in 1973 by Blazina [2], one of the coworkers of the famous sports physician Frank Jobe, Chief of the Sports Medicine Center in Inglewood (California, USA), located near the sports center where the prestigious Los Angeles Lakers team now plays. It was certainly to the basketball players that Blazina was referring when he wisely described the painful syndrome "jumper's knee."

Successively, many other studies have focused on this so far unclear pathology which deserves to be known by sports physicians who, considering the frequency of this pathology in some types of players, will have to face this pathology during their career.

A. Ferretti
Faculty of Medicine,
Orthopaedic and Traumatology Department,
"Kirk Kilgour" Sports Traumatology Center,
University "La Sapienza" S. Andrea Hospital,
00189 Rome, Grottarossa St. 1037, Italy
e-mail: aferretti51@tiscali.it

In this chapter, we will discuss the different aspects of patellar and quadriceps pathologies according to the most recent experiences and the newest types of treatments.

10.2 Epidemiology and Predisposing Factors

As cited above, patellar and quadriceps tendinopathies are very common among athletes involved in jumping activities or whose activity is based on the use of the lower limb's extensor apparatus (such as weight lifters). It has been estimated that up to 40 % of volleyball players suffer or have suffered from this pathology during their career [3].

In the sport of soccer, jumper's knee syndrome was unknown until the eighties, when coaches started putting more attention on basic training with weight-lifting exercises, jumping (plyometric), eccentric strengthening, and so forth. Therefore, with this particular attention given to quadriceps muscle strengthening came consequent repercussions or stress on the patellar tendon. Nowadays, patellar tendinopathy affects about 2.5 % of soccer athletes, data which is still lower compared to athletes of other sports who comprise the highest percentage of incidence (volleyball, basketball) [4, 5].

Predisposing factors to the onset of such a pathology are classified as "intrinsic" and "extrinsic;" intrinsic factors are those related to the

P. Volpi (ed.), *Football Traumatology: New Trends*, DOI 10.1007/978-3-319-18245-2_10

athlete, and extrinsic are those due to environmental stresses.

Besides sex incidence, which is higher in male patients, many epidemiologic studies have shown no correlation between morphologic characteristics of patients and jumper's knee syndrome. In particular, it has never been shown that varus or valgus malalignment of the knee, a malalignment of the extensor apparatus, a patellar hypermobility, or a high or low patella syndrome might be predisposing factors and, aside from the knee area, nor are valgus hindfoot deformity, pronated foot valgus, cavus foot, or even others. Researchers' interest therefore focused more on peculiar characteristics of the patellar tendon tissue and on its collagen composition.

However, the results about extrinsic factors were different. The first data, which is also the most obvious, concerns the correlation between the number of training sessions and matches per week and the incidence of jumper's knee syndrome. This strict positive correlation clearly confirms the importance of overuse in the onset of such a type of tendinopathy. Conversely less significant was the type of training (if carried out with weights, therabands, or jumps) [6].

Training fields have been widely studied with the result that the harder the field the higher the incidence. Regarding soccer games, however, there do not seem to be significant differences between players who usually train on natural fields and those who train on artificial fields [7].

Other factors predisposing patellar tendinopathy, which might be considered both intrinsic and extrinsic, regard jumping capability with a higher incidence among athletes with higher explosive strength [8].

10.3 Symptomatology and Classification

The main symptom of jumper's knee is pain, with varying intensity, but always localized in one of the typical places which represent the fulcrum of the extensor apparatus. The most frequent localization is the origin of the patellar tendon at the lower site of the patella (70 % of the cases), followed by the insertion of the quadriceps tendon at the superior site of the patella (20 %) and by the insertion of the patellar tendon on the anterior tibial tuberosity (10 %). The most recent classifications are based on the intensity of the pain with jumper's knee which, compared to the first classification proposed by Blazina, focus more attention on evaluating the effect of the pain on sports performance.

Jumper's Knee Classification According to Symptoms (Ferretti and Coworkers [9]**)**

STADIUM 0 - No pain
STADIUM I - Rare pain with no sports restriction
STADIUM II - Moderate pain during sports activity with no restriction on sports performance (normal performance)
STADIUM III - Pain with slight qualitative and quantitative restriction on performance (reduced number of training sessions or minor intensity)
STADIUM IV - Pain with severe restriction of sports performance
STADIUM V - Pain during daily activity; sports activity impossible

As we can see, the classification above described does not take into account rupture of the patellar tendon (catastrophic jumper's knee) [10] which cannot be considered the evolution of the insertional patellar tendinopathy but an acute event as a consequence of a chronic tendinous degeneration, which is totally different from an anatomo-pathology point of view. Indeed the discrepancy between pain (severe) and tendinous damage (moderate) seen in jumper's knee forces the athlete to suspend the activity much earlier before the pathology lead to rupture; the exact opposite happens with tendinosis degeneration where the tendinous damage is severe and progressive with a painful symptomatology usually moderate or even absent. By an objective point of view, local digital pain represents the only important factor. Locally, in some cases, we can observe a mild swelling of the soft tissue but never an articular effusion. Knee articular semeiotic, as well as the one concerning the extensor apparatus, is negative.

10.4 Radiological Findings

Radiological evaluation consists of X-rays, ultrasound evaluations, and magnetic resonance imaging. Standard X-rays might show insertional calcifications (spurs) which show the exact localization of the pathology. Ultrasound may show a thickening of the patellar tendon close to the insertion and even a loss of the normal fibrillar pattern. Recently ultrasound has also been used to study patellar tendon vascularization (ecocolordoppler): This methodology might show cases with hypervascularization as well as cases of normal or reduced vascularization, even though these patterns are not adequately understood [11]. Magnetic resonance allows better definition of the tendon morphology which often shows a tendon modification at the insertional site. However, MRI rarely ever changes therapeutic protocol.

10.5 Anatomo-pathology

With regard to anatomo-pathologic classification of overuse tendinopathy as proposed by Perugia et al. [12], jumper's knee might be included in the insertional tendinopathies.

On the other hand, an anatomo-pathologic pattern of subcutaneous ruptures usually represents the consequence of a chronic degenerative process (tendinosis) which is often totally asymptomatic and which usually occurs, abruptly, with an acute rupture. In these cases, tendinous tissue shows wide areas of degeneration with lack of the normal fibrillar pattern and an important reduction in the cellular component.

With regard to jumper's knee, peculiar data which surgeons detected in the seventies was the discrepancy between painful symptomatology, which was often very restricting in daily activities, and the lack of tendinous damage. Research of the "nidus" of tendon degeneration, as proposed by Basset, was often useless in a surgical approach, with the consequence that many surgical procedures were performed with the aim of treating different pathologies (menisci, patellar chondral damages). In a previous histological study, we showed the presence of microscopic insertional alteration consisting of a disruption of the *blue line* along with a microcystic area full of granulation tissue, suggesting microinsertional detachments with an attempt of reparation, which nowadays represents one of the most plausible pathogenetic hypothesis of this pathology [13]. Obviously, spots of degenerative tendinous tissue can come together even though their role in the painful symptomatology is not yet clear.

10.6 Treatment

Patellar tendinopathy treatment is basically conservative and consists of medical and physical therapy.

Medical therapy is based on the use of NSAIDs. Their use is not justified though since at the level of the tendinous degeneration a phlogistic process has never been shown. For this reason, the success of such a type of therapy, widespread even though there is a lack of scientific studies supporting their use, is perhaps dependent more on their analgesic effect than their anti-phlogistic effect.

What is certainly efficient is the use of local infiltration of corticosteroids, even though there is a big debate about their use. While it was once considered the gold standard, it was progressively abandoned and afterward criminalized because of its potential effect on the tendinous tissue leading to rupture [14]. Actually in specific and well-selected cases and especially during some period of the athletic season and of the career of an athlete, corticosteroid infiltration may be a valid therapeutic option for the sports physician, in particular in those cases in which radiological exams do not show a significant degenerative process. Beneficial effects of corticosteroid injections are usually immediate even though temporary; this pain-free period should be used in adjunct to other physical therapies for better long-time follow-up results. Recently corticosteroid injections have been duplicated in more diluted preparations with satisfactory preliminary results even with restrictions similar to the traditional steroidal infiltration [15].

Other infiltrative drugs have recently been proposed but major literature about them is still missing [16].

A promising but not yet adequately understood type of treatment for tendinopathies is represented by the infiltration of autologous PRP. It consists of the use of growth factors present within platelets, potentially able to facilitate the cellular differentiation toward a fibroblastic line with the aim of promoting tissue healing [17]. The methodology for using PRP was introduced about 10 years ago, and it reached a high popularity after its use on professional athletes with very satisfactory results documented in scientific studies; this apparent success has created a big economic interest around its use with sometimes criticizable implications. However, it is a matter of fact that its use has a solid biological base, it seems without related risks, and, even without picturing this type of treatment as a miraculous option, it may be a valid alternative for sports physicians. In our experience, the use of PRP for patellar tendinopathy consisting of three injections, one each week, provided better medium- and long-term results compared to the use of ESWT [18]. Besides radial and focalized ESWT [19], many other types of conservative treatments (ultrasound, laser, TENS, magnetotherapy, TECAR) have been used for the treatment of patellar tendinopathy, but always with uncertain and sometimes unsatisfactory results.

Kinesitherapy, whose main aim would consist of improving the mechanical properties of the tendon through selective training, nowadays represents the gold standard in the treatment of jumper's knee. It is based on the practice of different types of muscular exercises, isotonic, isometric, isokinetic, and eccentric; in particular eccentric exercises are recommended in any phase of the pathology, both alone and with all other types of exercises [20]. The knowledge of kinesitherapy as a valid option for the cure and prevention of jumper's knee is so widespread among athletes, volleyball players in particular, that they usually practice it themselves as soon as they feel the onset of the symptomatology.

The use of elastic bandages or braces at the level of the patellar tendon has been practiced by many athletes with the aim of reducing painful symptomatology during sports practice. Despite the fact that their use has been documented to reduce insertional stresses, their real efficacy has never been totally demonstrated [21].

Surgical treatment is indicated in a very small number of cases (less than 10 %) [22], usually in the advanced phases of the pathology, when all other conservative options have failed, and at the end of the agonistic season. Surgery has the aim of promoting a valid healing at the level of tendon insertion and consists of different steps: deepest tendon fiber disinsertion, removal of the damaged tissue (*Basset's nidus*) when present, plastic of the lowest part of the patella or apicoectomy, patella drilling, or tendinous scarifications [9].

Postoperative protocol consists of a short period of immobilization (2–4 weeks) followed by a progressive recovery of range of motion and then of muscular trophism and usually requires about 4–6 months before the return to specific training and professional matches. Results of surgical procedures, even though usually satisfactory, are not always brilliant, especially in athletes involved in high-performance jumps with percentages of total lack of pain not higher than 65 % and with a little higher percentage in those athletes affected by quadriceps rather than patellar insertional pathology. The abovementioned surgical steps may also be carried out arthroscopically but with more difficulties, a longer learning curve, and most of all, with no advantage in terms of final results and recovery time [23, 24].

10.7 Patellar Tendon Rupture

Patellar tendon rupture will be presented here in a different chart because it is usually a consequence of a different tendinous pathology which involves the middle part of the tendon and not the insertional end. Patellar tendon rupture, which usually occurs abruptly, involves a dramatic clinical feeling of a tear in the anterior part of the knee, immediate fall, and complete lack of capability of weight-bearing, walking, or actively extending the knee followed by severe swelling, hemarthrosis, and wide ecchymosis; it is hardly ever preceded by the typical jumper's knee symptoms. It is commonly the final event of a progressive degenerative process involving the tendon itself which leads to a progressive weakening of the tendon until the final rupture, similarly to what happens with the Achilles tendon. The pattern of severe tendinous damage detected in the surgery room is significantly different than the one observed in cases of insertional tendinopathy where the tendon itself looks macroscopically normal, despite an intense clinical symptomatology with severe restrictions. Diagnosis of patellar tendon rupture is easy and is based on the anamnesis and the evidence of a gap below the apex of the patella which also appears higher than the contralateral knee. Quadriceps tendon rupture has a similar clinical onset even though the gap in these cases is localized above the patella. X-ray exam shows a high patella (or low in cases of quadriceps rupture), while ultrasound and MRI exams may give some more details in regard to the tendinous pathology even though they do not change the type of therapy needed which is surgery. Surgical procedure consists of suturing the tendon and in some cases reinforcement with transosseous sutures. As is well known, since tendon biology is prosperous and has a high capability of healing, it is hardly ever necessary to use autologous, homologous, or synthetic tissue reinforcement; on the contrary, we recommend to only and always use reabsorbable suture. Postoperative follow-up consists of knee immobilization in full extension for 5 weeks, with the first two with no weight-bearing, followed by a physical rehabilitation aimed at recovering range of motion first and strengthening the quadriceps muscle later. Return to sports is not allowed before 6 months. Postoperative rehabilitation is usually easier and faster in quadriceps suture. Not common but even more dramatic are the cases of bilateral simultaneous rupture of the tendons, the so-called catastrophic jumper's knee, which obviously requires the same type of surgical treatment but with a less favorable prognosis in regard to return to sports activity.

References

1. Maurizio E (1963) la tendinite rotulea nei giocatori di pallavolo. Arch Soc Tosco Umbra Chir 24:443–452
2. Blazina ME, Kerlan RK, Jobe FW, Carter VS, Carlson GJ (1973) Jumper's knee. Orthop Clin North Am 4(3):665–678
3. Ferretti A (1986) Epidemiology of jumper's knee. Sports Med 3(4):289–295
4. Zwerver J, Bredeweg SW, van den Akker-Scheek I (2011) Prevalence of Jumper's knee among nonelite athletes from different sports: a cross-sectional survey. Am J Sports Med 39(9):1984–1988. doi:10.1177/0363546511413370, Epub 2011 Jul 7
5. Lian OB, Engebretsen L, Bahr R (2005) Prevalence of jumper's knee among elite athletes from different sports: a cross-sectional study. Am J Sports Med 33(4):561–567, Epub 2005 Feb 8
6. Ferretti A et al (1984) Jumper's Knee: an epidemiological study in volleyball players. Phys Sportsmed 12:97–103
7. Hägglund M, Zwerver J, Ekstrand J (2011) Epidemiology of patellar tendinopathy in elite male soccer players. Am J Sports Med 39(9):1906–1911
8. Visnes H, Aandahl H, Bahr R (2013) Jumping ability and change of jumping ability as risk factors for developing jumper's knee. Br J Sports Med 47(9):e2. doi:10.1136/bjsports-2013-092459.22
9. Ferretti A, Conteduca F, Camerucci E, Morelli F (2002) Patellar tendinosis: a follow-up study of surgical treatment. J Bone Joint Surg Am 84-A(12):2179–2185
10. Tarsney FF (1981) Catastrophic jumper's knee. A case report. Am J Sports Med 9(1):60–61
11. Hoksrud A, Ohberg L, Alfredson H, Bahr R (2008) Color Doppler ultrasound findings in patellar tendinopathy (jumper's knee). Am J Sports Med 36(9): 1813–1820
12. Perugia L, Ippolito E, Postacchini F I tendini. In: Masson (ed)
13. Ferretti A, Ippolito E, Mariani P, Puddu G (1983) Jumper's knee. Am J Sports Med 11(2):58–62
14. Meissner A, Tiedtke R (1985) Tendon rupture of the extensor muscles of the knee. Aktuelle Traumatol 15(4):170–174
15. Crisp T, Khan F, Padhiar N, Morrissey D, King J, Jalan R, Maffulli N (2008) Frcr OC High volume ultrasound guided injections at the interface between the patellar tendon and Hoffa's body are effective in chronic patellar tendinopathy: a pilot study. Disabil Rehabil 30(20–22):1625–1634
16. van Ark M, Zwerver J, van den Akker-Scheek I (2011) Injection treatments for patellar tendinopathy. Br J Sports Med 45(13):1068–1076
17. Ferretti A (2011) PRP treatment in football players. UEFA Direct 107(4):8–13
18. Vetrano M, Castorina A, Vulpiani MC, Baldini R, Pavan A, Ferretti A (2013) Platelet-rich plasma versus focused shock waves in the treatment of jumper's knee in athletes. Am J Sports Med 41(4):795–803. doi:10.1177/0363546513475345, Epub 2013 Feb 13
19. Furia JP, Rompe JD, Cacchio A, Del Buono A, Maffulli N (2013) A single application of low-energy radial extracorporeal shock wave therapy is effective for the management of chronic patellar tendinopathy. Knee Surg Sports Traumatol Arthrosc 21(2):346–350. doi:10.1007/s00167-012-2057-8
20. Visnes H, Bahr R (2007) The evolution of eccentric training as treatment for patellar

tendinopathy (jumper's knee): a critical review of exercise programmes. Br J Sports Med 41(4): 217–223
21. Lavagnino M, Arnoczky SP, Dodds J, Elvin N (2011) Infrapatellar straps decrease patellar tendon strain at the site of the Jumper's Knee Lesion: a computational analysis based on radiographic measurements. Sports Health 3(3):296–302
22. Ferretti A, Puddu G, Mariani PP, Neri M (1985) The natural history of jumper's knee. Patellar or quadriceps tendonitis. Int Orthop 8(4):239–242
23. Pascarella A, Alam M, Pascarella F, Latte C, Di Salvatore MG, Maffulli N (2011) Arthroscopic management of chronic patellar tendinopathy. Am J Sports Med 39(9):1975–1983
24. Marcheggiani Muccioli GM, Zaffagnini S, Tsapralis K, Alessandrini E, Bonanzinga T, Grassi A, Bragonzoni L, Della Villa S, Marcacci M (2013) Open versus arthroscopic surgical treatment of chronic proximal patellar tendinopathy. A systematic review. Knee Surg Sports Traumatol Arthrosc 21(2):351–357. doi:10.1007/s00167-012-2100-9, Epub 2012 Jun 20

11 Return to Play After a Muscle Lesion

Gian Nicola Bisciotti

11.1 Introduction

The return of an athlete to sporting activity after a muscular lesion is a critical moment in the overall rehabilitation program. The medical staff has the responsibility of evaluating whether an effective rehabilitation process has been carried out, although there may be little objective data available to aid such a decision. The objective of sports medicine is for the athlete to recuperate, in the minimum time possible, while minimizing the risk of recurrence. This often means having to balance the needs of the sporting activity and the necessity to carry out a therapeutic course that guarantees anatomical healing and optimal function.

The concepts of anatomical healing and functional healing warrant further discussion. In a sedentary person or a person with reduced functional requirements, the end of the rehabilitative process after a muscular lesion may coincide with anatomical healing of the injured site. For an athlete, this may not be the case. Athletes, especially professional athletes, have extremely high functional requirements, and the rehabilitative process may not be considered concluded until there is optimal recovery of muscular function. Therefore, in the athlete, *restituito ad integrum* after muscular lesion must necessarily incorporate both anatomical healing and functional healing.

The true skill of the medical staff is the contextual minimization of recovery time and of recurrence risks. This difficult job is further complicated by the fact that the risk factors for recurrence are not clear, even if they may be traced to the same intrinsic and extrinsic factors responsible for the original trauma. In addition to the original risk factors, after the first muscular lesion, others will be added: an increase in muscle rigidity, a decrease in the muscles' levels of force, formation of fibroses, alteration of the muscles' biomechanic function, or a possible state of muscular inhibition. In addition, there may be consequences linked to an accelerated or aggressive rehabilitation program or even an incorrect one. For these reasons, the decision to reintegrate a professional athlete after a muscular lesion should be based on, to the extent possible, objective data that assist and reassure the medical staff making this difficult decision.

In our rehabilitative experience, we have developed a protocol of guidelines to provide objective data to help in the decision to return

G.N. Bisciotti, MSc, PhD
FIFA Center of Excellence, Qatar Orthopaedic and Sports Medicine Hospital, Doha, Qatar

Kinemove Rehabilitation Centers, Via Veterani dello Sport no 1, Parma, La Spezia (I), Pontremoli 54027, Italy
e-mail: bisciotti@libero.it, giannicola.bisciotti@aspetar.com

P. Volpi (ed.), *Football Traumatology: New Trends*, DOI 10.1007/978-3-319-18245-2_11

an athlete to agonistic activity. This chapter presents these guidelines and provides the scientific rationale for their use. Obviously, such guidelines differ depending on the function of the muscle group under consideration. Specific examples are presented describing the return to sporting activity after a muscular lesion. These show the points of "fundamental objectivity" that allow us to minimize the risks of recurrence and returning the athlete to an agonistic context while trying to respect the goal previously mentioned: minimizing both recuperation time and risk.

11.2 Indirect Lesion of the Hamstring

The biceps femoris (BF) is a flexor of the knee and an extensor of the hip, and, like all the other flexors of the leg, prevents, if the leg is extended, the force of elevation of the inferior limb or flexing forward of the upper body. Indeed, the flexor muscles may not be lengthened further than a certain point, which represents their limit of extension. The BF is one of the most insulted muscles in sport. In Australian football, for example, damage to the BF represents 13 % of all traumas and causes a loss of work equal to 16 % of the total training time [1]. Sprinters may also experience recurring damage to the BF [2]. A study by Askling et al. [3] demonstrated that, in football (also known as soccer), 47 % of indirect muscular traumas suffered during competition or training involve the flexor muscles of the thigh (biceps femoris, semitendinosus, and semimembranosus, which are collectively called, in English language literature, the hamstring). Other studies of football have found that injuries of the hamstring account for 12–15 % of injuries and an average of six accidents per professional club during a season [4–6]. Injuries to the hamstring are particularly recurrent in sporting activities that require sprinting, acceleration, deceleration, rapid changes of direction, and jumping [2, 7].

11.3 Hamstring Lesion and Risk of Recurrence

The hamstring, in addition to being the most insulted muscle in sports, also is subject to a high incidence of injury recurrence; in professional football, for example, the recurrence rate is about 12 % [6, 8]. In other sports, such as professional Australian football,[1] the recurrence rate may reach 30 % [8–10]. One-third of these recurrences occurs during the first two weeks after the return to sporting activity [11]. This suggests that a rehabilitation program may have been inadequate or that an athlete returned too early to full sporting activity; it is also possible that these both the case [11]. However, it is possible that this high rate of recurrence can be traced to intrinsic factors, such as a low ratio of tissue healing, which is typical of the hamstring, or an original factor risk [12, 13].

It should be noted that lesions of the BF present a worse prognosis with respect to lesions of the semimembranosus, semitendinosus, or both [14]. It is furthermore interesting to underline the fact that if the entity of the lesion presents a strong link with recovery time [14–16], otherwise may not be said regarding the risk of recurrence [17].

The literature reports that a shortfall in strength is an important parameter in the risk of

[1] Australian football: Australian football (Australian rules, aussie rules, footy) is the national Australian sport and the most practiced and followed athletic activity in Australia. It is played between two teams of 18 players (with four reserves with flying substitutions) on cricket fields or other fields of an oval form. These fields vary in dimension; they may be as long as 185 m, and as wide as 155 m. They thus represent the largest game fields used in the different forms of football and almost four times larger than a football pitch. The players may pass the ball in two ways: with a kick or a handball pass. A kick is the propulsion of the ball with any part of the leg below the knee; a handball pass is done by holding the ball in one hand and hitting it with the other, closed in a fist. Any other way of passing the ball is forbidden, unless it is constricted by the game situation (e.g., acquiring a stray ball from other players). Game out does not exist; thus, the passes may occur in any direction, just as the players may position themselves on the field wherever they like.

injury recurrence in the hamstring [2, 18–23]. To minimize the risk of recurrence in our daily practice, we focus on a protocol of return to the field that is based on a series of variations that provide interpretable signs, with positive signs representing a "green light" regarding return to the field and negative signs representing a "red light" with respect to a resumption of sporting activity. Every type of injury, whether to a muscle or tendon, presents parameters of evaluation regarding the return to extremely specific functionality. Many, if not all, of the parameters we use in the functional evaluation of the hamstring represent points of specific evaluation regarding the injury to this exclusive functional district. It must be stressed that, in the exhaustive post-injury rehabilitation plan of an athlete, healing of the anatomical damage represents only one stage, which is necessary to allow full recuperation of the functionality of the injured muscular district in general and specific terms. Only at this point may a rehabilitation plan be considered concluded.

The points on which we base our judgment regarding an athlete's return to the field after an injury of the hamstring are represented by four steps that may be described as follows.

11.4 Clinical Examination

During the clinical examination, the athlete is tested with

i. Maximal isometric contractions carried out from different articular angles (generally three: 180, 90, and 45° and in function of the anatomical location of the lesion);
ii. Maximal concentric contractions by complete range of motion (ROM);
iii. Maximal eccentric contractions by complete ROM; and
iv. Eccentric-flash contractions of maximal intensity by reduced ROM.

During each test, subjective pain symptoms on the part of the athlete, referred to on a VAS scale, must be equal to zero. The presence of residual pain symptoms in one of the tests above imposes a delay in the return to the field.

Passive and active lengthening tests are also carried out on the damaged flexor muscle, which should show the same elongating capacity as the contralateral muscle [19]. A diagram of the clinical exams is presented in Table 11.1.

11.5 Imaging Examination

In our rehabilitative experience, return of the athlete to the field is conditional on a first-level (echography) or second-level (magnetic resonance imaging) imaging examination that shows that the lesion is completely repaired and stabilized from an anatomical point of view. A dynamic scan is particularly useful in discovering shortfalls of the sliding myofascial or areas of altered functional shortfalls. To this end, we have elaborated and adopted a specific table (Table 11.2) that allows us to classify the functional behavior of the examined muscular sector in dynamic scans. Levels 1 and 2 in this table allow a return to sport whereas levels 3 and 4 preclude it. Elastography has allowed us to carry out quality evaluations of healing muscle tissue [24], however, this method is still in the development phase. Table 11.3 presents the red and green lights that are relative to imaging exams.

11.6 Dynamometric Evaluation

The dynamometric evaluation we have adopted is based on different types of tests of function in different types of injury, carried out in both concentric and eccentric ways (through both isokinetic and isoinertial tests). We have found that one dynamometric test alone will not exhaustively account for the functional behavior of a muscular group such as the hamstring. Different tests, each one providing detailed and specific information on the dynamic behavior of the muscle, must be interpreted as a part of the whole

Table 11.1 The clinical exam is composed of four strength tests and two lengthening tests, which have either red or green lights

Clinical examination	Red light	Green light	Notes
Maximum isometric contractions performed at different joint angles	Pain symptoms ≥1 on VAS scale	Absence of pain symptoms	Parameter used to access to the dynamometry tests
Maximum concentric contractions performed at full ROM	Pain symptoms ≥1 on VAS scale	Absence of pain symptoms	Parameter used to access to the dynamometry tests
Maximum eccentric contractions performed at full ROM	Pain symptoms ≥1 on VAS scale	Absence of pain symptoms	Parameter used to access to the dynamometry tests
Maximum flash-eccentric contraction performed at reduced ROM	Pain symptoms ≥1 on VAS scale	Absence of pain symptoms	Parameter used to access to the dynamometry tests
Passive stretch test	Difference in ability to stretch in comparison to the contralateral limb with or without associated pain symptoms	Same ability to stretch in comparison to the contralateral limb and absence of pain	Parameter used to access to the dynamometry tests
Active stretch test	Difference in ability to stretch in comparison to the contralateral limb with or without associated pain symptoms	Same ability to stretch in comparison to the contralateral limb and absence of pain	Parameter used to access to the dynamometry tests

Table 11.2 A dynamic scan allows evaluation of the sliding of muscular fibers, which is classified into four levels of reference. Levels 1 and 2 allow return to the field, levels 3 and 4 impose a delay in return to the field

Level	Definition
1	Normal sliding
2	Light slight deficit
3	Slight deficit
4	Very important slight deficit

[25]. In addition to this fundamental concept, the parameters to which we refer during the interpretation of the various torque tests are as follows:

i. No return to running activity until the strength of the flexors has reached a value of at least 70 % of the baseline, or a value of flexor/extensor ratio equal to at least 0.55 [19].
ii. No return to specific sporting activity before the value of strength of the injured flexors (both in eccentric and concentric ways) has returned to 90–95 % of the value of the flexors of the contralateral limb [2, 23].

Table 11.3 Summarizing diagram of the imaging examination and the relative red and green lights

Imaging examination	Red light	Green light	Notes
US	Not complete anatomic repair / injury not yet stabilized	Complete anatomic repair / stabilized injury	Parameter used to access to the dynamometry tests
MRI	Not complete anatomic repair / injury not yet stabilized	Complete anatomic repair / stabilized injury	Parameter used to access to the dynamometry tests
Dynamics US	Sliding level 3 and 4	Sliding level 1 and 2	Parameter used to access to the dynamometry tests

iii. The peak of measured strength, both in concentric and eccentric ways, should be produced, in the injured limb, to the same articular angle in which the contralateral is registered [26, 27].

Furthermore, the protocol of the isokinetic test that we have adopted is

i. Concentric modality 60 and 300°/s
ii. Eccentric modality 60°/s

The data is normalized in relation to the body weight of the subject. This protocol conforms to the protocol used by the QFA (Qatar Football Association) in the FIFA Center of Excellence of Doha (Qatar). The reference data, regarding football, is inferred from a database exclusively populated by data from professional footballers.

Specifically, the "reference data" we use are

Relationship hamstring in eccentric modality/ Quadriceps in concentric modality – 60°/s (dominant limb[2]) : 0.84 ± 0.19 N.m^{-1}.kg^{-1}.
Relationship hamstring in eccentric modality/ Quadriceps in concentric modality – 60°/s (nondominant limb) : 0.78 ± 0.14 N.m^{-1}.kg^{-1}.
Hamstring concentric peak torque/kg – 60°/s (dominant limb) : 1.78 ± 0.14 N.m^{-1}.kg^{-1}.
Hamstring concentric peak torque/kg – 60°/s (nondominant limb) : 1.66 ± 0.3 N.m^{-1}.kg^{-1}.
Difference %: 5.12 ± 0.25 %
Hamstring concentric peak torque/kg – 300°/s (dominant limb) : 1.32 ± 0.26 N.m^{-1}.kg^{-1}.
Hamstring concentric peak torque/kg – 300°/s (nondominant limb) : 1.29 ± 0.24 N.m^{-1}.kg^{-1}.
Difference %: 2.27 ± 0.25 %
Hamstring eccentric peak torque/kg – 60°/s (dominant limb) 2.59 ± 0.45 N.m^{-1}.kg^{-1}.
Hamstring eccentric peak torque/kg – 60°/s (nondominant limb) 2.52 ± 0.40 N.m^{-1}.kg^{-1}.
Difference %: 2.70 ± 0.55 %

The data reference relative to the set of isokinetic tests are summarized in Table 11.4.

11.7 Field Tests

Tests on the field are carried out only after the first three evaluation steps (i.e., the clinical evaluation, imaging, and the torque evaluation) have registered all results in the "green light" area. The field tests represent a "programmed risk" in the rehabilitation program. The execution of a sprinting braking test or an Illinois test, carried out in an all-out manner, represents a degree of risk greater than that of a maximal isokinetic test. For this reason, we begin the administration of field tests assured by maximum positivity of registered results during the previous tests.

[2] In football, by dominant limb we mean the limb usually used by the athlete to kick (QFA National Test Protocol).

Table 11.4 Summarizing diagram of the reference data concerning the isokinetic testing protocol and consequent red and green lights

Test	Red light	Green light	Notes
Concentric isokinetic test	Value < 70% of the base line or <70% of the contralateral	Value ≥ 70% of the base line or ≥ 70% del contralateral	Parameter used only for the resumption of run
Concentric isokinetic test	Value < 90% of the contralateral hamstring value	Value ≥ 90% of the contralateral hamstring value	Parameter used to access to the field tests
Eccentric isokinetic test	Vallue < 90% of the contralateral hamstring value	Value ≥ 90% of the contralateral hamstring value	Parameter used to access to the field tests
Concentric force peak	Produced at a joint angle ≠ in comparison to the contralateral limb	Produced at a joint angle = in comparison to the contralateral limb	Parameter used to access to the field tests
Eccentric force peak	Produced at a joint angle ≠ in comparison to the contralateral limb	Produced at a joint angle = in comparison to the contralateral limb	Parameter used to access to the field tests
Hamstring concentric peak torque/kg - 60°/sec	Difference ≥ 15% in comparison to the contralateral limb	Difference < 15% in comparison to the contralateral limb	Parameter used to access to the field tests
Hamstring concentric peak torque/kg - 300°/sec	Difference ≥ 15% in comparison to the contralateral limb	Difference < 15% in comparison to the contralateral limb	Parameter used to access to the field tests
Hamstring eccentric peak torque/kg - 60°/sec	Difference ≥ 15% in comparison to the contralateral limb	Difference < 15% in comparison to the contralateral limb	Parameter used to access to the field tests

The tests carried out on the field in our protocol are

i. Sprinting braking test [28], the minimal reference value of which regarding the power expressed by the muscles of the inferior limbs is 12 W. kg $^{-1}$;
ii. Illinois agility test (Fig. 11.1), the reference values of which are indicated in Table 11.5.

The data reference relative to the set of field tests are summarized in Table 11.6.

11.8 General Parameters

In evaluating whether an athlete (specifically a football player) is able to return to the field, we also take into account a series of general parameters, summarized as follows.

i. Experimental evidence exists that shows core stability, in the area of injuries to the flexors, significantly reduces the risk of recurrence [29].

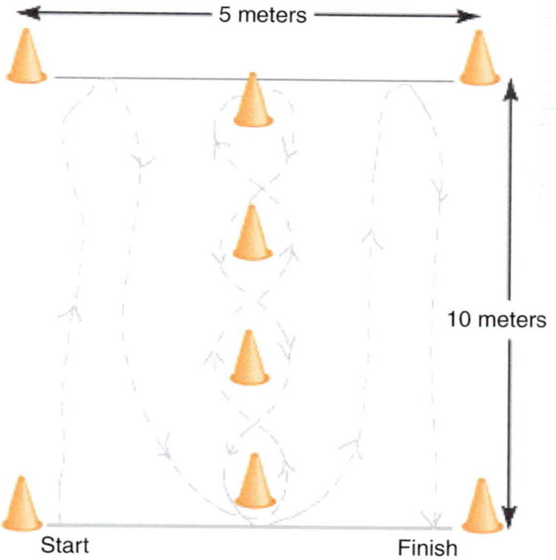

Fig. 11.1 Illinois Agility Test. The length of the test – or the distance between the start point and the stop point – is 10 m. The athlete must follow the entire distance at maximum speed according to the indicated diagram. The start is freely decided by the athlete. The stopwatch results represent the final result of the test

Table 11.5 Reference values concerning the Illinois Agility Test

Rating	Lap result (sec)
Excellent	< 15.2
Good	16.1-15.2
Medium	18.1-16.2
Insufficient	18.3-18.2
Very insufficient	> 18.3

Table 11.6 Note (*): in the case of a value equal to the "medium" recorded during the Illinois testing, the latter must be accompanied (to represent a "green light") by a value ≥15 $W.kg^{-1}$ recorded during the sprinting braking test; otherwise, a value of "medium" represents a "red light"

Test	Red light	Green light	Notes
Sprinting braking test	Value < 12 $W.kg^{-1}$	Value ≥ 12 $W.kg^{-1}$	Parameter used to return to sports (reintegration with the team)
Illinois agility test	Recorded value : very insufficient or insufficient	Recorded value: excellent, good or medium*	Parameter used to return to sports (reintegration with the team)

Table 11.7 Different factors that may suggest either a conservative program or a swift return to sporting activity (Modified from Orchard et al. [31])

Factors which indicate a following of conservative treatment	Factors which give evidence of a rapid return to sporting activity
Persistent shortfall of strength	The expression of strength is equal to that of the contralateral limb
Persistent shortfall of flexibility	The flexibility is superimposable to that of the contralateral limb
Impossibility to totally finish a training session without pain symptoms or limping	Being able to totally finish a traing session
Extended area of abnormality in imaging	Negative imaging (USorRM)
Practising of one of the disciplines particularly at risk below: -Speed discipline in the area of athletics - Football -Australian football - Rugby	Playing a low risk sport of muscular lesion
Advanced chronological age	Player with young chronological age but already in possession of sufficient experience to be able to play also in non optimal conditions
Getting an injury at the beginning of the sporting season	Having to play a decisive match at the end of the season (for example play off or play out) without having the possibility of a valid substitute
Anatomical dislocation of the lesion in a high risk area (biceps femoris, rectus femoris medial calf, adductor longus, adductor magnus)	Anatomical dislocation of the injury in a low risk area (semimembranosus, vastus medialis, lateral calf , gluteus muscles)

ii. A correct preventive strategy may drastically lower the risk of recurrences of hamstring injuries. An eloquent demonstration of this is given by the Australian Football League, which, through its specific prevention program, reduced the percentage of hamstring injury recurrence from 37 % to 22 % in the period between 1997 and 2004 [10].

iii. Some authors [30] have suggested a causal association between the recurrence of injuries of the hamstrings and the twin muscles and anatomical damage on the level of L5/S1 that causes a trapping of the relative nerve root.

Table 11.7 [31] presents the different factors that may suggest either the adoption of a conservative rehabilitation program or a swift return to sporting activity.

11.9 Aerobic Aspects

Recurrences may happen even when the athlete seems to have perfectly satisfied all the various steps in the evaluation process. It is difficult, given the multifactorial etiology of muscles injuries and, consequently, of the recurrences, to precisely identify the factor responsible for an unsuccessful rehabilitation. However, it is often the case that, in such situations, the athlete's general physical conditions, especially aerobic, may be the main cause of the recurring event.

It is reasonable to hypothesize that an insufficient level of aerobic conditioning may represent a risk factor regarding indirect muscle lesions [32] or recurring lesions. For this reason, the athlete should start agonistic activity after having reached levels of maximal aerobic velocity (VAM) close to the values registered in the pre-lesion period. The value of VAM represents the speed, expressed in km/h, at which the maximal consumption of oxygen is reached (VO_2 max) and is the best indicator of aerobic fitness. A program specifically addressed to the *restituito ad integrum* of a muscular lesion should include a specific plan for the recuperation of aerobic fitness to minimize the risk of recurrence related to a possible shortfall in this important aspect of athletic performance.

Conclusions

The return of an athlete to the field represents the final and, probably, most delicate stage of the rehabilitation process. For this reason, precise and trustworthy criteria are needed for reference in making the decision to allow the return to sporting activity and to minimize the risk of injury recurrence.

It is objectively impossible to achieve "zero risk" of muscle injury recurrence, even with a conservative treatment program and the adoption of prevention strategies. From the author's experience in the sport of football, the economics are also of fundamental importance, and the reader is invited to reflect on the following statement by Orchard [31]: "It is preferable to have a medium return time to the field of three weeks with a percentage of success of 90 % rather than eight weeks with a percentage of success equal to 100 %."

References

1. Sewar H, Orchard J, Hazard H, Collinson D (1993) Football injuries in Australia at the elite level. M J Aust 159(5):298–301
2. Drezner J (2003) Practical management of hamstring injuries. Clin J Sport Med 13:48–52
3. Askling C, Karlsson J, Thorstensson A (2003) Hamstring injury occurrence in elite soccer players after preseason strength training with eccentric overload. Scand J Med Sci Sports 13:244–250
4. Dvorak J, Junge A, Chomiak J, Graf-Baumann T, Peterson L, Rösch D, Hodgson R (2000) Risk factor analysis for injuries in football players. Possibilities for a prevention program. Am Ortho Soc Sports Med 28(5):69–74
5. Hawkins RD, Hulse MA, Wilkinson C, Hodson A, Gibson M (2001) The association football medical research programme. An audit of injuries in professional football. British J Sport Med 35:43–47
6. Woods C, Hawkins RD, Maltby S, Hulse M, Thomas A, Hodson A (2004) The football association medical research programme: an audit on injuries in professional football analysis of hamstring injuries. British J Sport Med 38:36–41
7. Devlin L (2000) Recurrent posterior thigh symptoms detrimental to performance in rugby union. Predisposing factor. Sport Med 29(4):273–287
8. Orchard J, Best T (2002) The management of muscle strain injuries: an early return versus the risk of recurrence. Clin J Sport Med 12:3–5
9. Orchard J, Seward H (2000) Epidemiology of injuries in the Australian Football League, seasons 1997–2000. Br J Sports Med 36:39–45
10. Orchard J, Seward H (2004) AFL injury report 2003. J Sci Med Sport 7:264–265
11. Heiderscheit BC, Sherry MA, Silder A, Chumanov ES, Thelen DG (2010) Hamstring strain injuries: recommendations for diagnosis, rehabilitation, and injury prevention. J Orthop Sports Phys Ther 40(2):67–81
12. Upton PA, Noakes TD, Jurits JM (1996) Thermal pants may reduce the risk of recurrent hamstring injuries in rugby players. British J Sport Med 30:57–60
13. Arnason A, Sigurdsson SB, Gudmundsson A, Holme I, Engebretsen L, Bahr R (2004) Risk factors for injuries in football. Am J Sports Med 32:5S–16S
14. Connell D, Schneider-Kolsky M, Hoving J (2004) Longitudinal study comparing sonographic and MRI assessments of acute and healing hamstring injuries. AJR Am J Roentgenol 183:975–984
15. Pomeranz SJ, Heidt RS Jr (1993) MR imaging in the prognostication of hamstring injury: work in progress. Radiology 189:897–900
16. Slavotinek J, Verrall G, Fon G (2002) Hamstring injury in athletes: using MR imaging measurements to compare extent of muscle injury with amount of time lost from competition. AJR Am J Roentgenol 179:1621–1628
17. Gibbs N, Cross T, Cameron M (2004) The accuracy of MRI in predicting recovery and recurrence of acute grade one hamstring muscle strains within the same season in Australian Rules football players. J Sci Med Sport 7:248–258
18. Burkett LN (1970) Causative factors in hamstring strains. Med Sci Sports Exerc 2:39–42

19. Heiser TM, Weber J, Sullivan G et al (1984) Prophylaxis and management of hamstring muscle injuries in intercollegiate football players. Am J Sports Med 12:368–370
20. Yamamoto T (1993) Relationship between hamstring strains and leg muscle strength: a follow-up study of collegiate track and field athletes. J Sports Med Phys Fitness 33:194–199
21. Jonhagen S, Nemeth G, Eriksson E (1994) Hamstring injuries in sprinters: the role of concentric and eccentric hamstring muscle strength and flexibility. Am J Sports Med 22:262–266
22. Orchard J, Marsden J, Lord S (1997) Preseason hamstring muscle weakness associated with hamstring muscle injury in Australian footballers. Am J Sports Med 25:81–85
23. Croisier J, Forthomme B, Namurois M (2002) Hamstring muscle strain recurrence and strength performance disorders. Am J Sports Med 30:199–203
24. Lv F, Tang J, Luo Y, Ban Y, Wu R, Tian J, Yu T, Xie X, Li T (2012) Muscle crush injury of extremity: quantitative elastography with supersonic shear imaging. Ultrasound Med Biol 38(5):795–802
25. Bisciotti GN (2000) Per ritrovare la funzionalità. Sport e medicina 6:43–47
26. Brockett C, Morgan D, Proske U (2001) Human hamstrings adapt to eccentric exercise by changing optimum length. Med Sci Sports Exerc 33:783–790
27. Brockett C, Morgan D, Proske U (2004) Predicting hamstring strain injury in elite athletes. Med Sci Sports Exerc 36:379–387
28. Bisciotti GN. (2003). A avaliação funcional dos atletas. Faculty of Sport Sciences and Physical Therapy, University Estacio de Sa de Puerto Alegre (BR). October 15th 2003. Lecture notes, Estacio de Sa (Ed). Vol 3, p 35
29. Sherry M, Best T (2004) A comparison of 2 rehabilitation programs in the treatment of acute hamstring strains. J Orthop Sports Phys Ther 34:116–125
30. Orchard J, Farhart P, Leopold C (2004) Lumbar spine region pathology and hamstring and calf injuries in athletes: is there a connection? Br J Sports Med 38:502–504
31. Orchard J, Best TM, Verral GM (2005) Return to play following muscle strain. Clin J Sport Med 15:436–441
32. Chomiak J, Junge A, Peterson L, Dvorak J (2000) Severe injuries in football players. Influencing factors. Am J Sports Med 28(5 Suppl):S58–S68

Shoulder Injuries in Goalkeepers 12

Raffaele Garofalo, Piero Volpi, Giacomo Delle Rose, Dario Pitino, and Alessandro Castagna

12.1 Aetiology

Soccer is the world's game, played by more than 120 million people around the world. Soccer is a contact sport characterised by short and quick movements such as sprinting, sudden acceleration or deceleration, cutting, pivoting, shooting and kicking. Tackling and collision are also common [1]. Shoulder injuries in soccer are not nearly as common as lower limb injuries such as the hip, knee or ankle. The incidence in the reported literature is approximately in a percentage between 2 % and 13 % of all football injuries [11, 17]. However, shoulder injuries are generally more serious than many of the other more common injuries sustained and result in a longer off-play time than other joint injuries.

R. Garofalo
Shoulder Service, Miulli Hospital,
Acquaviva delle Fonti, Bari, Italy

P. Volpi
Knee Orthopedics and Sport Traumatology Unit,
Humanitas Clinical Institute IRCCS,
Milan, Italy

Head of Medical Staff FC Internazionale Milan,
Milan, Italy

G.D. Rose • D. Pitino
A. Castagna, M.D. (✉)
Shoulder and Elbow Unit,
IRCCS Humanitas Institute,
Rozzano, Milano, Italy
e-mail: alex.castagna@tin.it

In the last years, shoulder injuries have represented an increasing health problem in football players. The modern soccer has been characterised by high-speed game, "aggressive" tactical solutions such as pressing and marking, and increased number of legal and illegal physical contacts. FIFA injury reports show the high incidence of contact injuries compared with non-contact injuries (World Cup 2002 [11] and World Cup 2006 [6], 73 % vs. 27 %).

The percentage of shoulder injuries (injuries per year/total shoulder injuries) increased from 35 % in the 2006–2007 season to 89 % in the 2009–2010 season [15].

In literature, mostly the shoulder injuries are reported associated to contact during matches. Chomiak et al. [5] in their series reported six shoulder injuries including three separations of the acromioclavicular joint (grade I or II), one fracture and one refracture of the clavicle and one dislocation of the glenohumeral joint. The majority of the injuries were caused by foul play, and two were non-contact injuries. Very interesting to note is that in that series, no goalkeepers suffered a severe injury of the shoulder girdle.

Differently from the previous study, research from Norway found that 36 % of goalkeeper injuries are to the upper extremity. This is in stark contrast to outfield positions where most injuries are to the lower extremity. In practice, goalkeepers are more likely to be injured during goalkeeper-specific training versus standard soccer training. The Norwegian study revealed that

P. Volpi (ed.), *Football Traumatology: New Trends*, DOI 10.1007/978-3-319-18245-2_12

23.6 injuries occur per 1,000 h of goalkeeper-specific training versus 9.1 injuries per 1,000 h of standard soccer training. 27.9 injuries occur per 1,000 h of goalkeeping during matches, making matches the most likely time for an injury [16].

In an unpublished data, one of the authors (Volpi P.) observed during his activity as team doctor of a major league team that training for professional goalkeepers will end up to 200 dives per week.

Because of this paucity of literature, Hart and Funk [8] undertook a study to analyse the incidence and treatment of shoulder injuries in professional soccer. Data was provided over a 3-year period from January 2007 to January 2010. There were 35,000 claimed injuries in this period, of which 3.3 % was shoulder injuries. This is a total of 1,155 shoulder injuries or 385 serious shoulder injuries per year, which represent a significant number of injuries. In this paper, authors reported that the majority of serious shoulder injuries in soccer players occur at a positional extreme of external rotation and abduction in high-energy situations, while a significant number occur in low-energy situations away from this position. Most serious shoulder injuries in professional soccer are dislocations. Ekstrand et al. [7] in a recent epidemiologic study focused on upper extremity injuries in male elite football players, noted that upper extremity injuries are uncommon among male elite football players. Goalkeepers, however, are prone to upper extremity injury, with a five times higher incidence compared to outfield players.

12.2 Injury Mechanism

Goalkeepers are more likely to be injured at shoulder joint because of goalkeeper-specific gestures and trauma. Statistically, goalkeepers are most likely to be injured during aerial duels defending crosses. The risk of injury appears to be increasing as the modern game is evolving. Teams are requiring more and more from their goalkeepers. These players are expected to clear balls swinging into the box, intercept long through balls outside the box and receive back passes. This aggressive play was not seen in decades past. Goalkeepers are exposed to frequent overhead use of both arms and repetitive lateral falls over the lateral aspect of the shoulder. On the other hand, they also can suffer a traumatic event on the shoulder during a contact with another player.

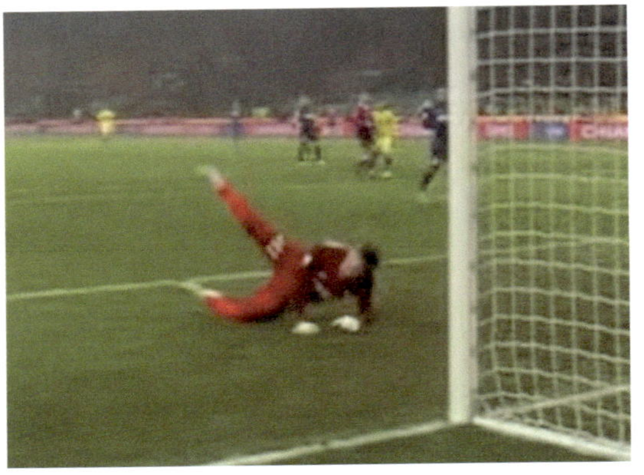

Fig. 12.1 A traumatic injury on the left shoulder in a professional goalkeeper falling on the ground with the arm in abduction and slight forward flexion. In this case, this athlete sustained a traumatic anterior subluxation associated with massive cuff tear (supra and infraspinatus)

As mentioned before, goalkeepers suffer on average 200 shoulder ground contacts per week, which are generally kept under control without damage.

Nevertheless, the same observer (Volpi P.) reported that exercising a sliding fall instead of direct impact is protecting the joint by distributing the trauma to many different parts of the shoulder. In consequence, it is very important for the goalkeeper to improve training skills about how to fall, technical gesture and external rotator strengthening. A fully trained goalkeeper in fact does not land directly on the shoulder but curves it to spread the impact over a round surface. When in some exceptional circumstances this protection is not possible or the impact on the ground is abnormal or more violent with an associated posterior impact on the ground, joint dislocation can occur (Fig. 12.1). With a fall directly on the shoulder with the arm adducted, an acromion-clavicular dislocation can occur.

Another shoulder injury that can occur specifically in goalkeeper is the rotator cuff tear. The severity of injury can widely vary. Many injuries could be classified as minor impingement, where injury and irritation cause pain in the shoulder during certain movements like overhead motions or reaching behind the back. If untreated, shoulder impingement associated to rotator cuff insufficiency can lead to inflammation, and the painful shoulder long-standing irritation and inflammation can result in a tear of the rotator cuff. However, tears can also result from the trauma of landing on outstretched arms or on the shoulder.

When landing on the arm, the humerus typically can subluxate anteriorly (upper arm bone misaligns towards the front of the shoulder). The rotator cuff muscles attach to the humerus, so abnormal position of the arm, in the shoulder socket, can result in added stress to the muscles and other tissues. For that reason, adjustment of the shoulder is critical to prevent injury.

Goalkeepers use their rotator cuff muscles for throwing, catching, deflecting balls and often landing on the arms and shoulders which results in injury to the muscles, tendons and ligaments of the shoulder. However, a significant trauma is not the only way the rotator cuff is damaged. The nature of goalkeeping is repetitive. Keepers dive and land on the arms and shoulders. They jump in the air and come down on their arms and shoulders. During these repetitive gestures, the rotator cuff could be overstressed and then result in an injury. Another but very rare shoulder girdle injury in a goalkeeper is the pectoralis major tear. This injury could be related to training, just because soccer require more and more physical performance, and goalkeeper makes some weightlifting particularly bench pressing during training [14]. This activity could be responsible to predispose to muscle/tendon injury. Another mechanism of injury is a direct blow such as during a football tackle or during a contact with another player with the arm in abduction and external rotation [12].

According to literature, taken into account all the soccer players, labral injuries represented the most common injury type affecting 21 (84 %) subjects, two rotator cuffs (8 %) and two combined labral/rotator cuffs (8 %) [8]. However, goalkeeper suffered more rotator cuff injury than field players, whether field player had more Bankart lesion [8]. Often, rotator cuff and labral tear are associated.

Pectoralis major tear could be another shoulder injury in goalkeeper as we observed in our experience too.

12.3 Clinical and Diagnostic Examination

The clinical examination in an athlete with an acute or chronic sports-related shoulder injury is used to confirm or strengthen the suspected diagnosis. In consequence, shoulder clinical signs depend from type of injury and lesions occurred. In case of an acute glenohumeral dislocation, the athlete will complain of absolute loss of shoulder function, and normally the injured arm is supported by contralateral arm in a position of slight abduction and internal rotation. The elbow is flexed and the forearm lifted against the trunk. The neck is inclined towards the side of the injury to give an analgesic effect. A compliant at the level of acromion-clavicular joint associated with tenderness and loss of function can be related to a trauma on the AC joint. Usually patients with this injury showed the arm with the elbow extended along the trunk. In case of acute injury of the pectoralis major tendon, athlete will complain of intense pain in the anterior aspect of the shoulder associated with swelling and early appearance of ecchymosis over the axilla and/or down the arm. About rotator cuff tear, it could be very rare to have a real traumatic tear. Normally an acute or chronic tear can occur following a trauma. In this case, the athlete could complain a loss of function with an inability to actively lift the arm associated with a very important pain.

The next step in the physical examination of the shoulder is testing the active and passive range of motion present in the joint.

In case of acute trauma, of course, as mentioned, any active or passive shoulder movement could be very painful. In case of acute shoulder dislocation, clinician will enable to move the arm and shoulder of the athlete. In case of AC joint trauma, a certain grade of passive movement is always possible, and very important is possible to obtain a passive external rotation of the arm with the elbow at the side. This clinical sign is very important to exclude an anterior and overall posterior shoulder dislocation. In case of AC trauma, tenderness on the top of AC joint is found, and passive movements with the arm across the chest position are impossible to realise.

A different clinical scenario could be observed in case of chronic shoulder injury. In this case, of course, clinical findings will be related to the type of lesion.

An athlete with shoulder instability can show a limited active motion because of apprehensive/protective attitude. In other cases, the motion could be normal and patient can show a positivity of the apprehension tests. Also in case of a rotator cuff injury, the athlete will show a limited active motion because of muscle weakness. The clinician should always assess the strength of the shoulder joint and should seek to isolate individual muscle whenever possible. Subacromial impingement test (Neer, Hawkins) should be also evaluated, taking care that particularly in young athlete patients, these signs could be positive also in case of subtle shoulder instability and could be confounding [13]. These athletes present a complex clinical scenario because they do not have any history of shoulder dislocation or subluxation, but they refer just a painful shoulder. During clinical examination, classic apprehension tests are negative, and the only clinical sign could be a pain reproduced with the arm in an anterior apprehension position and relieved by a relocation test. These athletes very often are hyper lax, and during clinical examination, impingement sign could be also positive [3].

About pectoralis major injury, clinical scenario in acute cases has been already described. When the athlete is observed once, the ecchymosis and swelling subsides; a loss of the anterior axillary fold and normal pectoralis contour could be observed (Fig. 12.2). Palpation of the anterior axillary wall will reveal decreased thickness compared with the contralateral side. As the patient forcefully presses the hands against one another in front of the chest "prayer position", asymmetry of the chest wall can be seen. Often a distinct deformity or hollow exists where the pectoralis muscle will move medially. Loss of strength is particularly notable to internal rotation of the arm when tested at neutral.

Initial workup of the shoulder injuries should include plain radiographs to exclude bony abnormality. These imaging could be enough in case of acute AC or glenohumeral dislocation. X-rays are also important to exclude fracture associated with dislocation. MRI investigation is indicated for all the shoulder injuries in which there is a suspect of shoulder instability, rotator cuff tear or pectoralis major rupture. The use of direct or indirect gadolinium enhancement may facilitate the assessment of labral and capsular injury pattern as well as capsular volume. A Bankart lesion is present in most part of case of traumatic shoulder instability. This pathology is best observed on axial and coronal views. Of course, also ALPSA lesion or Perthes lesion could be observed with MRI. Most surgeons recommend the use of CT scan in case of recurrent instability or in case with acute traumatic dislocation to exclude any glenoid bone defect or associated fracture.

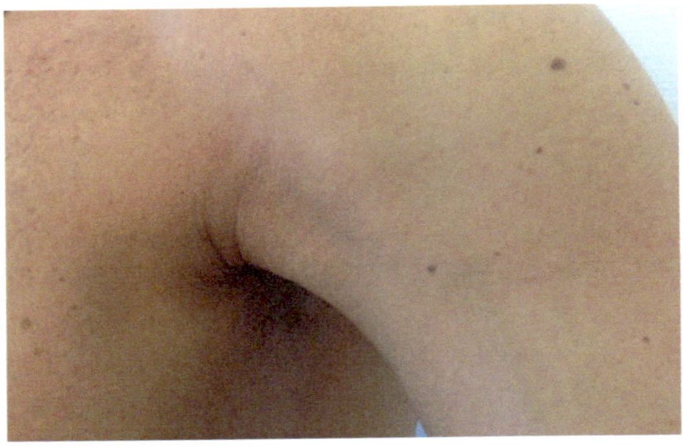

Fig. 12.2 Clinical examination of a complete acute left pectoralis major muscle rupture. Note the deformity and loss of contour of the anterior left chest wall and axilla

MRI is useful to also evaluate rotator cuff tear. In case of partial articular rotator cuff tear, an arthro-MRI is the gold standard.

12.4 Treatment Strategy

Treatment will depend from the type of injury. In this section, we will focus on treatment of the more common shoulder injuries found in goalkeeper.

Most athletes with a labral injury and associated pathologies require surgical repair. Some may be able to cope through the season and can be repaired at the end of the season or they can be treated conservatively. These are usually the less significant injuries with lesser pathology on MRI

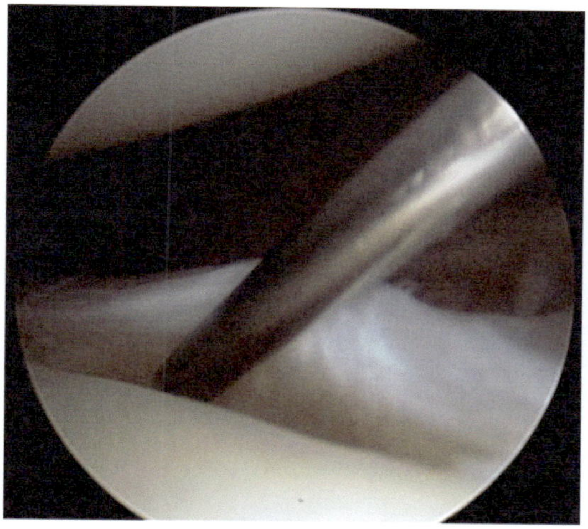

Fig. 12.3 Left shoulder as viewed from a classic posterior portal. The probe shows the anterior Bankart lesion

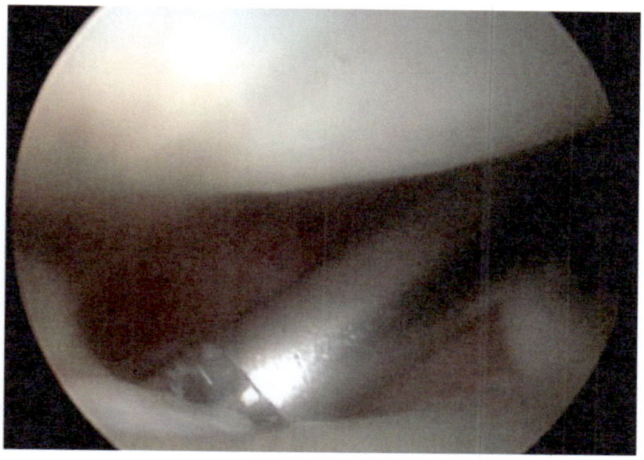

Fig. 12.4 Once the lesion is identified, a shaver is used to abrade the glenoid neck and also the capsulolabral tissue avoiding to use suction

(like subtle instabilities). Large structural lesions such as bony Bankart injuries, rotator cuff tears and large Hill-Sachs lesion or pectoralis major tear generally require early surgical repair. Treatment of rotator cuff pathologies depend on the severity of the pathology as well as the significance of the symptoms of the athlete. Mild impingement symptoms with bursitis are treated with rehabilitation and subacromial steroid injection if required. If the athlete fails 3 months of physical therapy course, an indication to surgery is done.

In case of arthroscopic surgery, we prefer a lateral decubitus position with the right arm placed in a foam sleeve traction system. Four kilogrammes of balanced suspension are used with the arm in 70° of abduction and 20° of forward flexion. The scope is introduced through a standard posterior portal for diagnostic arthroscopy. A classic anterosuperior portal just anterior to the long head of the biceps tendon is made. Normally we used only two portals to perform labral repair. Most of the procedure is carried out with the scope in posterior portal, although we switch at the beginning portals to perform a diagnostic procedure of the posterior part of shoulder looking with the scope through the anterior-superior portal.

Once the labral lesion is identified, we start the glenoid labral preparation (Fig. 12.3). With an elevator, the labrum is freed from the glenoid neck until the fibres of subscapularis muscle can be observed under the labrum. Sometimes it could be difficult to understand when the labrum is sufficiently mobilised. A useful test is to insert the shaver into the joint, open the window and turn the section on. If the labrum floats up to anatomic position, mobilisation is complete. A further step is using the shaver to abrade a little bit the surface of the glenoid neck near the articular surface (Fig. 12.4). The tear configuration is evaluated, and the plan for suture anchor placement is established. Normally we suggest to use at least two double-loaded suture anchors to repair an anterior instability [2].

We place at the beginning the most inferior anchor. The anchor should be placed at average 45° angle to the glenoid face and just up on the glenoid face (Fig. 12.5). The position of insertion is related to the tear so to realise a south to north and east to west capsulolabral shift.

The spectrum (Conmed Linvatec, LARGO FL) suture hook is used to pass the suture through the tissue. A PDS (polydioxanone) No. 0 is used as a shuttle relay. The soft tissue penetrates capsulolabral tissue 5–10 mm inferior and lateral to the labral edge so to realise the above-mentioned shift (Fig. 12.6).

After the first anchor insertion and inferior capsulolabral repair, sequential anchor is placed in identical fashion. The capsulolabral tissue should be continually advanced superiorly for retention of the capsulolabral complex.

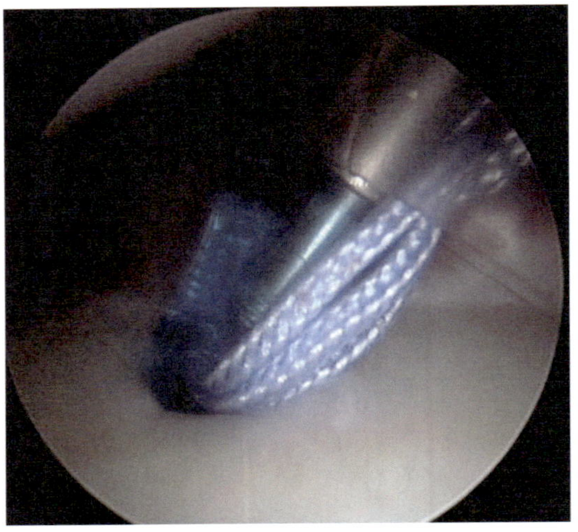

Fig. 12.5 A bio-absorbable suture anchor is inserted on the glenoid face, 5 mm from the glenoid edge and average 10 mm superior from the most inferior part of the capsulolabral detachment

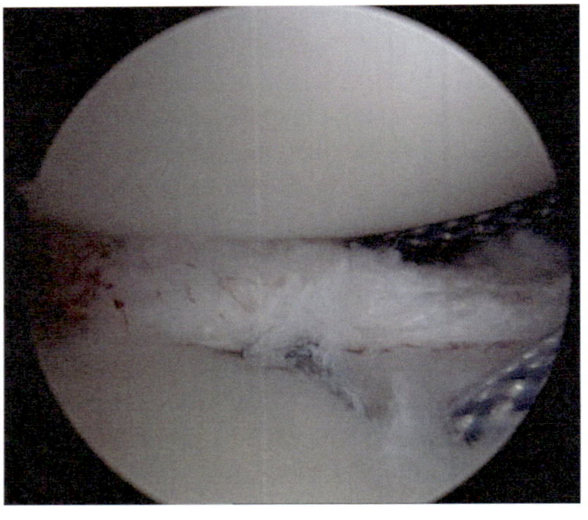

Fig. 12.6 We can observe as the capsulolabral tissue is grasped most inferiorly in respect to the point where the anchor was inserted. This realise a south-north capsulolabral shift

In case of a rotator cuff tear, surgical technique depends from the type of tear (partial or full thickness tear).

In case of partial articular tear, we prefer to use a transtendon technique using suture anchors [4]. The anchor is placed percutaneously through the remaining tendon into the bone of the decorticated rotator cuff footprint. A spinal

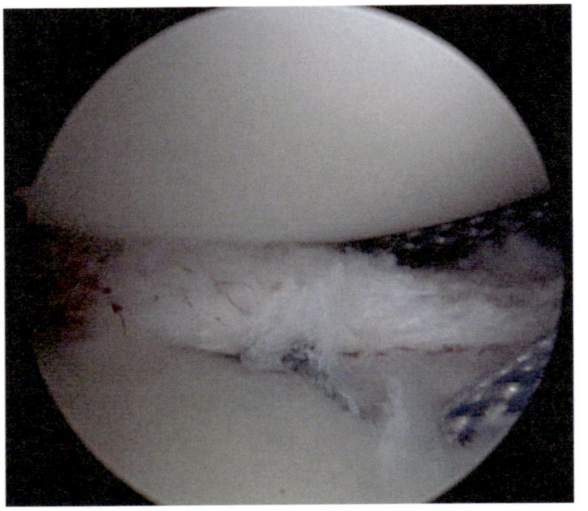

Fig. 12.7 A left shoulder observed intra-articularly from a posterior portal. All the three sutures coming from the anchor have been passed through the articular part of the supraspinatus tendon using a spinal needle and monofilament suture as shuttle. This goalkeeper had also an antero-superior labral tear that was fixed with a suture anchor technique

needle loaded with a No. 1 monofilament absorbable suture (PDS; Ethicon, Norwood, Massachusetts) is introduced percutaneously lateral to the edge of the acromion. It is passed through the bursal side of the remaining cuff and through a healthy portion of the articular portion of tendon. The suture is used to "shuttle" the two or three anchored sutures through the edge of the partial cuff tear (Fig. 12.7). The sutures are retrieved and tied in the subacromial space.

In case of full thickness RCT, normally we use a standard posterior portal, a lateral portal and an anterior-superior portal. We prefer a single row technique using triple-loaded suture anchors so to maximise the strength of repair (PW [10]). The tendon edges are debrided with a shaver, the bony bed of the repair is prepared with a burr, and the cuff is mobilised. Anchors are inserted at 45° angle (dead men angle) and between cartilage edges of humeral head in the foot print of the cuff tendon avoiding overtensioning of the tendon. In athletes, we prefer to use nonmetallic anchor (Fig. 12.8). Suture is passed through the tendons using different tools and different configurations according to surgeon's preference but taking care

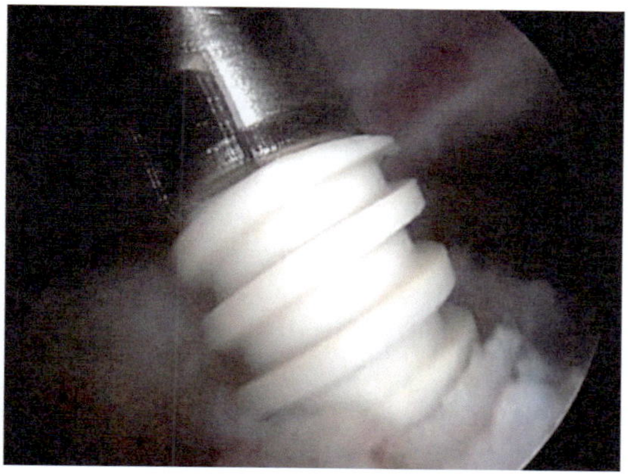

Fig. 12.8 A left shoulder observed in the subacromial space from a classic posterior portal. A nonmetallic anchor is inserted with an average 45° angle on the footprint area of the superior cuff

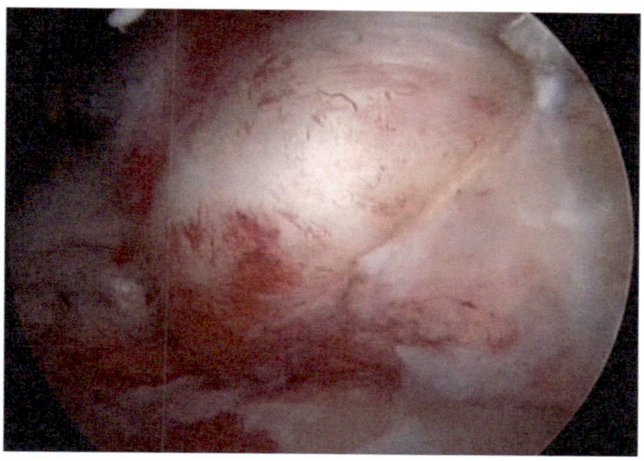

Fig. 12.9 Final view of a left shoulder observed in the subacromial space from lateral portal. A repaired rotator cuff with a single row technique is shown

to keep all the delaminated part of the tendon. At the end of repair, the sutures are tied from the lateral portal (Fig. 12.9).

12.4.1 Tricks and Tips

In case of associated lesions (labral and RCT), we suggest the following steps.

In case of labral tear associated with partial RCT, we prepare the labral lesion, then we move to the cuff; we put the anchor and then we pass the sutures through the tendon (transtendon repair); we do not tie the knot. We move back to labral tear, we repair the labral lesion, and then we move in the subacromial space to tie the knots of the previously passed suture through the tendon.

In case of labral tear associated with full thickness RCT, we suggest to repair the labral tear first and then move in the subacromial space to repair the cuff tendon.

12.4.2 Pectoralis Major Tear

In case of pectoralis major tear, primary repair should be done within 3 weeks from the tear. Patients are in beach chair position, and distal part of deltopectoral approach is made. A careful dissection is carried out until the torn end of the tendon is identified and retrieved. The pectoralis major has a long narrow footprint requiring a broad repair site. The tendon is secured with two or three nonabsorbable sutures and then is attached to the humerus adjacent to the lateral side of the intertubercular groove. A variety of techniques have been described. We use two triple-loaded titanium anchors and the sutures are passed with a Mason-Allen configuration.

12.5 Rehabilitation and Return to Play

The rehabilitation will depend on different factors, particularly by type of pathologies and procedure performed. As rule, in the immediate postoperative period, the emphasis is on protecting the healing tissue, controlling pain and inflammation and minimising the negative effects of immobilisation. We allow according to the type of repair a safe passive motion of the operated shoulder in the first week after surgery.

12.5.1 Rotator Cuff Repair

In case of rotator cuff repair, a supine exercise in passive forward flexion until 90° and external rotation until 60° is allowed. Primary importance after the rotator cuff repair surgery is avoiding the development of shoulder stiffness through initiation of early shoulder mobility without possibly compromising the repair. Time of sling depends by the size of repaired lesion and normally is variable between 28 and 35 days. In the subacute or intermediate phase, the exercise emphasis is on improving strength and neuromuscular control of the scapulothoracic muscle. The purpose of the movements in this phase is to improve continuously the passive ROM and start to correct problems such as muscle imbalances or specifically weak points. The progression is to active-assisted ROM exercise once adequate tissue healing occurs and for us not before than 8 weeks after surgery. At 3 months, we start dynamic strengthening phase; the objective of the exercise protocol is to improve strength, power and muscular endurance. These parameters need to be reestablished in parallel with the functional activities to which the athlete will return. Therapeutic exercises are provided to further enhance and integrate targeted rotator cuff, deltoid and scapular muscles. At 4 months, the clinician can advance the exercises to include more functional sport-specific ranges. At this point, the objective of the therapeutic exercise is to progressively implement functional demands on the shoulder complex and help the athlete return to full participation in sport activities.

12.5.2 Anterior Capsulolabral Procedure

In case of surgery for anterior instability, passive motion in forward flexion until 90° and external rotation until 30° is started after 2 weeks from surgery. External rotation is held less than 30° until 3 weeks and then progressed to 45° by the sixth postoperative week [9]. About forward flexion, this is limited to 90° until 3 weeks and then is gradually increased to 135° through postoperative week 6. Time of sling is 35 days.

After 6 weeks, we start to improve the passive ROM and start to correct problems such as muscle imbalances or specifically weak points. The goal is to achieve full ROM in all planes at 3 months after surgery. Scapular isolation exercises with arms below shoulder level in pain-free and safe ranges are prescribed. Even though the rotator cuff does not require specific protection after arthroscopic stabilisation procedures, shoulder active ROM and rotator cuff strengthening are purposefully delayed because of the potentially detrimental effect to the healing tissues. The strengthening programme should integrate the appropriate ROM progression. At 3 months, we start dynamic strengthening phase. At 4 months, we advance the sport-specific exercises to include more functional sport-specific ranges.

In case of combined injuries (anterior instability and cuff), we favour the protocol for instability.

About the time to come back to full sports activities, we suggest a time around 5 months. However, some published series reported a return to full sport activities after surgery for the goalkeepers after a mean time of 11.1 weeks after surgery also in case of combined injuries [8].

12.5.3 Pectoralis Major Repair

In case of pectoralis major repair, the athlete will wear the sling for 5 weeks. After 1 week, he is allowed to start passive forward flexion up to 130° on supine position with the arm adducted. For the first 5 weeks, any active abduction, forward elevation and external rotation are to be avoided.

After 6 weeks, the sling should be discontinued, and a programme of a passive range of motion can begin in all the plane of shoulder motion according to the pain. No active internal rotation is allowed until 8 weeks. Scapular isolation exercises with arms below shoulder level in pain-free are started at this time. At 3 months, a progressive programme of strengthening is started. At 6 months, the athlete can start slowly to perform lightweight with high-repetition bench press and push-up. We assume the resumption of sport at a mean time of 9 months after surgery.

References

1. Amason A, Gudmundson A, Dahl HA et al (1996) Soccer injuries in Iceland. Scand J Med Sci Sports 6(1):40–45
2. Boileau P, Villalba M, Hèry JY et al (2006) Risk for recurrence of shoulder instability after arthroscopic Bankart repair. J Bone Joint Surg Am 88(8): 1755–1763

3. Boileau P, Zumstein M, Balg F, Penington S, Biknell RT (2011) The unstable painful shoulder (UPS) as a cause of pain from unrecognised anteroinferior instability in the young athlete. J Shoulder Elbow Surg 20(1):98–106
4. Castagna A, Delle Rose G, Conti M et al (2009) Predictive factors of subtle residual shoulder symptoms after transtendinous arthroscopic cuff repair: a clinical study. Am J Sports Med 37(1): 103–108
5. Chomiak J, Junge A, Peterson L, Dvorak J (2000) Severe injuries in football players influencing factors. Am J Sports Med 28(5):S58–S68
6. Dvorak J, Junge A, Grimm K et al (2007) Medical report from the 2006 FIFA world cup Germany. Br J Sports Med 41(9):578–581, discussion 81
7. Ekstrand J, Hagglund M, Tornqvist H et al (2013) Upper extremity injuries in male elite football players. Knee Surg Sport Traum Arthrosc 21(7): 1626–1632
8. Hart D, Funk L (2013) Serious shoulder injuries in professional soccer; return to participation after surgery. Knee Surg Sports Traum Arthrosc. Br J Sports Med 2011;45:A15. doi:10.1136/bjsports-2011-090606.48
9. Itoi E, Hatakeyama Y, Urayama M et al (1999) Position of immobilization after dislocation of the shoulder. A cadaveric study. J Bone Joint Surg Am 81:385–390
10. Jost PW, Khair M, Chen DX et al (2012) Suture number determines strength of rotator cuff repair. J Bone Joint Surg 94(14):e100
11. Junge A, Dvorak J, Graf-Baumann T (2004) Football injuries during the world cup 2002. Am J Sports Med 32(1 Suppl):23S–27S
12. Manske RC, Prohaska D (2007) Pectoralis major tendon repair post surgical rehabilitation. N Am J Sports Phys Ther 2(1):22–33
13. Nordenson U, Garofalo R, Conti M et al (2011) Minor or occult shoulder instability: an intra-articular pathology presenting with extra-articular subacromial impingement symptoms. Knee Surg Sports Traumatol Arthrosc 19(9):1570–1575
14. Petilon J, Carr DR, Sekiya JK et al (2005) Pectoralis major muscle injuries: evaluation and management. J Am Acad Orthop Surg 13:59–68
15. Pritchard C, Mills S, Funk L, Batty P (2011) Incidence and management of shoulder injuries in premier league professional football players. Br J Sports Med 45:A15. doi:10.1136/bjsports-2011-090606.48
16. Strand E, Krosshaug T, Andersen TE (2011) Injury risk for goalkeepers in norwegian male professional football. Br J Sports Med 45:331. doi:10.1136/bjsm.2011.084038.59
17. Tegnander A, Olsen OE, Moholdt TT et al (2008) Injuries in Norwegian female elite soccer: a prospective one-season cohort study. Knee Surg Sports Traumatol Arthrosc 1682:194–198

13 Acromioclavicular Dislocation

Gianezio Paribelli, Stefano Boschi,
Alfonso Massimiliano Cassarino, and F. Leonardi

Abbreviations

AC Acromioclavicular
AP Anteroposterior
CC Coracoclavicular
SC Sternoclavicular

13.1 Epidemiology and Incidence

Acromioclavicular (AC) joint dislocations account for 3–10 % of all shoulder injuries [1, 2] and 40 % of sports-related shoulder injuries [2] and are more likely to affect young males owing to their greater involvement in sporting activities. The sports most at risk are those with a high risk of falls such as cycling and contact sports such as basketball, rugby, and, obviously, football (or soccer). A nation's tendency to practice one sport rather than another also explains the geographical differences in the incidence of this injury.

G. Paribelli (✉) • A.M. Cassarino • F. Leonardi
Struttura accreditata S.S.N. Maria Cecilia Hospital,
Via Corriera, 1, Cotignola (RA) 48010, Italy
e-mail: geparibelli@libero.it; cassarinomass@tiscali.it

S. Boschi
Ospedale Privato Accreditato Prof. Fogliani Modena,
Via Lana, 1, Modena, 41124, Italy
e-mail: s.boschi@iol.it

13.2 Etiopathogenesis

AC joint dislocations more commonly result from a direct trauma [3], even though indirect traumas are also possible [4].

Direct Trauma Frequent injuries include a fall onto the top of the shoulder with arm adducted, as occurs in falls from a bicycle or in *football*, especially in *outfield playing positions*, or a blow to the upper surface of the acromion with respect to the clavicle, as occurs in contact sports such as, again, *outfield playing positions in football*.

Direct traumas involve the development of a vertical force on the upper surface of the acromion with respect to the clavicle: as the upper extremity and scapula are displaced inferiorly, the clavicle cannot follow because it is obstructed by the first rib, which acts as a pivot. Moreover, because the AC joint is characterized by poor soft tissue coverage, it has limited ability to absorb shock forces. If the force is not absorbed by the upper limb, it is transmitted to the clavicle and then to the sternoclavicular (SC) joint. Owing to the significant stability of the SC joint, the energy of the impact is entirely re-transferred to the AC joint. The severity of the lesion and effect on affected structures depends on the direction and intensity of the forces [5, 6]. The force is initially transferred to the AC ligaments and capsule, then to the coracoclavicular (CC) ligaments, and finally to the deltotrapezial fascia.

P. Volpi (ed.), *Football Traumatology: New Trends*, DOI 10.1007/978-3-319-18245-2_13

Indirect Trauma This is typically described as a force impacting an outstretched adducted arm or an adducted elbow and directed superiorly such that the humerus is pushed upwards against the acromion, as occurs during a fall. In this situation, the force impacts above all the AC joint, as the CC distance is decreased with the coracoid and clavicle coming closer together, and their respective ligaments are released.

Rockwood's type VI dislocations are another matter. Here, there is a force acting on the distal end of the clavicle with the arm adducted and the clavicle retracted.

This etiological differentiation also applies to football players, although the goalkeeper's position requires special attention. In addition to the risk of falls and direct injury common to all players, goalkeepers perform voluntary dives with arm at maximum adduction and elevation, which makes them similar to overhead athletes, with important implications in terms of pathoanatomy, diagnostics, treatment, and rehabilitation.

13.3 Pathoanatomical Classification

The severity of the dislocation is clearly related to the energy of the impact: this can lead to a spectrum of injuries that range from a simple sprain to tearing of the affected structures. Although several classifications exist, the most commonly used is the Rockwood classification, which distinguishes among six classes of injury, based on the extent and direction of clavicular displacement:

- Type I: low energy, simple sprain of the AC ligaments, intact CC ligaments, no displacement
- Type II: greater energy, rupture of AC ligaments and capsule, intact CC ligaments, horizontal instability, up to 50 % vertical displacement of the clavicle with <20 % increase in CC distance
- Type III: high energy, rupture of AC ligaments and capsule, rupture of CC ligaments, intact deltotrapezial fascia, up to 100 % vertical displacement of clavicle with 20–100 % increase in CC distance
- Type IV: rupture of AC ligaments and capsule, rupture of CC ligaments, disinsertion of deltotrapezial fascia, posteriorly displaced clavicle in or through the trapezius muscle. Necessary to assess SC for possible alterations
- Type V: rupture of the AC ligaments and capsule, rupture of the CC ligaments, complete detachment of the deltotrapezial fascia from the distal end of clavicle, >300% clavicular displacement, 100–300 % increase in CC distance compared to normal
- Type VI: rupture of AC ligaments and capsule, rupture of CC ligaments, clavicle displaced inferiorly to the acromion or coracoid

The literature reports one case of acromion displaced inferiorly to the clavicle, suggesting an inferomedially directed force being applied to the upper surface of the acromion; this led the authors to propose the addition of a type VII injury to the Rockwood classification [7].

13.4 Clinical Examination

History Obtaining a thorough history with details of the symptoms and causative event is mandatory: involvement of the AC joint should be suspected in any *football player* with shoulder trauma and a history of the typical mechanism of injury.

Inspection This will reveal swelling or prominence of the distal clavicle. It is important to assess the patient while he is sitting or standing, as this will allow the weight of the limb to exaggerate the deformity. The relative position of the clavicle with respect to the acromion can provide an indication as to the direction of the trauma. Although we believe clavicular elevation to be inevitable given the bone's mobility, we are convinced that the prominence is mostly the result of downward sagging of the shoulder and arm due to gravity. Often, in the acute phase, the patient will present supporting his shoulder with the contralateral hand: this, combined with the swelling, can in part mask the prominence. As the initial swelling subsides, the finding will become more appreciable.

Palpation Palpation exacerbates pain as does active and passive motion and allows testing of joint stability.

- Pain. The nature of the pain may be variable, given that the AC joint is supplied by the lateral supraclavicular, lateral pectoral, axillary, and suprascapular nerves [8]. In the case of type I dislocations, the pain will be the only symptom: a local infiltration of lidocaine can help to establish the diagnosis [8].
- Stability. In higher-grade dislocations, once the swelling and pain have subsided, joint stability can be tested, and the direction of possible instability, anteroposterior or superoinferior, can be established.
- Tests. Depending on lesion severity, the movement that most exacerbates pain is abduction or cross arm adduction: in less severe forms, the same movements should be tested against resistance. To this end, the cross arm test (with arm adducted and flexed to 90°, and elbow flexed to 90°, an additional adduction force is applied) and the Paxinos test (double pressure, thumb on acromion posteriorly, and index finger on clavicle anteriorly) are particularly useful [8]. The O'Brien active compression test is done with the operator standing behind the patient, who may be standing or sitting. The patient is instructed to forward flex his arm to 90°, with elbow completely extended and internally rotated with thumb pointing downwards: he is then invited to adduct the arm 10–15° and hold that position against resistance. He is then asked to repeat the maneuver in external rotation, that is, with the thumb pointing upwards: reduction or disappearance of the pain indicates a positive test. The test has 41 % sensitivity and 94 % specificity [8]. The presence of pain inside the shoulder during the test is indicative of labrum disorders rather than AC dysfunction [8]. A useful test for assessing the integrity of the deltotrapezial fascia in suspected higher-grade dislocations is the shoulder shrug: reduction of the dislocation indicates fascial integrity and permits differentiation between a grade III and grade V dislocation [8].

More in detail:

Grade I: pain and swelling are mild and often the athlete does not interrupt activity. Pain is exacerbated only by palpation and flexion and adduction.

Grade II: pain and swelling are moderate to intense. If the patient is examined before the swelling arises or after has subsided, running of a finger along the clavicle as far as the joint will reveal a step deformity. In addition, anteroposterior instability can be tested by grasping the clavicle itself and moving it anteriorly and posteriorly. There may also be moderate pain at the CC space.

Grade III: moderate to intense pain in both the AC and CC space and swelling. Visible clavicular displacement, which can be reduced with arm elevation, performed by the patient to relieve tension and thus pain or by the examiner. Pain is exacerbated by active and passive mobility and by the tests. By grasping the distal end of the clavicle, both horizontal and vertical stability can be assessed.

Grade IV: more intense pain in both the AC and CC space and greater swelling compared to grade III. When the swelling subsides, posterior displacement through the trapezoid muscle becomes evident. As in grade III, there is no horizontal fluctuation.

Grade V: intense pain and displacement, greater than in the previous grades. Tear of the deltotrapezial fascia accounts for the vertical fluctuation of the clavicle, the so-called "piano key" sign, which is much more evident than in the previous grades.

Grade VI: because of the inferior displacement of the clavicle, the shoulder has a flattened profile (the acromion forms a step and there is a depression at the clavicle). Given the inferior displacement and the violence of the trauma, assessment of possible associated nervous or thoracic lesions is necessary.

13.5 Diagnosis

Imaging investigations are required not only to confirm the diagnosis but also to plan the treatment.

13.5.1 Radiography

Recommended views for assessment of the AC joint are the anteroposterior (AP) and axillary (or axial) views (Figs. 13.1 and 13.2).

AP View This is fundamental for assessing superior dislocation. The extent of dislocation can be quantified by (a) measuring the percentage of displacement of the clavicle with respect to the acromion, (b) using the distal edge of the clavicle as a reference, and (c) measuring the CC distance. The difference in the position of the structures should not exceed 4 mm [9]: the normal distance between the acromial and clavicular joint surfaces ranges from 1 to 3 mm and may decrease with age. The CC distance is assessed in terms of percentage compared to the contralateral side. A Zanca view, i.e., an AP view with a 15° cephalic tilt, may be indicated to avoid superimposition of the joint with the spine of the scapula.

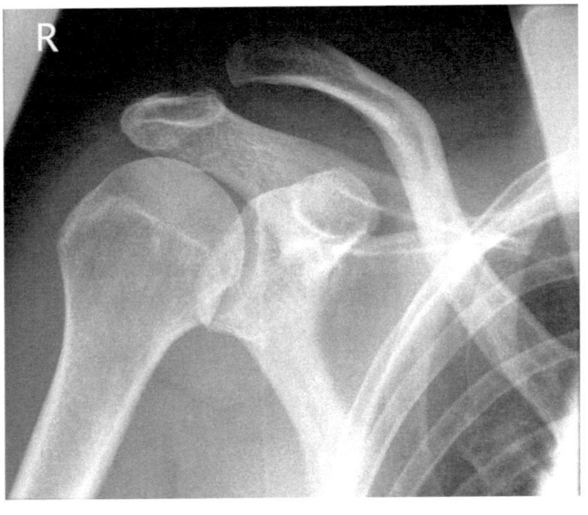

Fig. 13.1 Grade III acromioclavicular dislocation

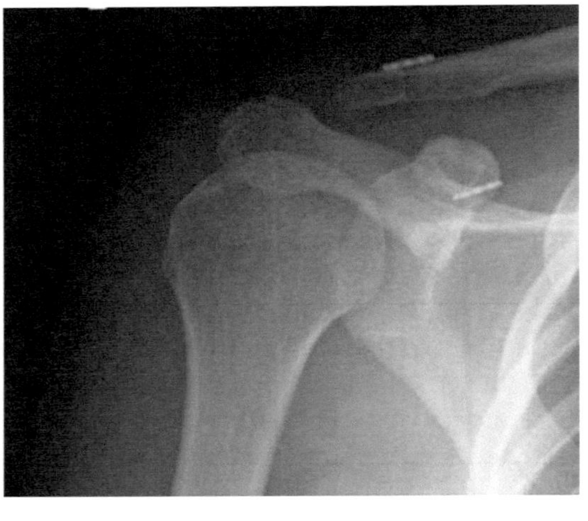

Fig. 13.2 Reduction using a suspension system and biological boost

Axillary View This is required for evaluating any dislocations in the AP direction (type IV). This view provides better depiction of the joint which appears quadrilateral in shape.

Radiographically, the AC joint is considered to be stable if it shows no dislocation compared to the contralateral joint, subluxated if the dislocation is ≤50 % of the contralateral joint, or dislocated if there is complete dislocation accounting for ≥100 % of the AC joint surface.

Other aspects that may be assessed, in the various views, are ossification of the CC space (complete or incomplete), arthritis (attested by osteophytes, sclerosis, or space narrowing), and osteolysis of the distal portion of the clavicle (if there are signs of bone demineralization).

In some cases, despite the suspected injury, CC distances on the two sides may appear identical: in order to rule out a fracture, a Stryker notch view can be used, in which the patient lies supine on the table, with arm elevated parallel to the body axis, palm behind the neck, and beam oriented 10° cranially [1]; alternatively, the previously described Zanca view can be used.

Stress radiograms, useful for differentiating grade II from grade III dislocations, are less commonly used than in the past owing to the tendency not to treat grade III and because of their poor clinical yield and the discomfort felt by the patient.

13.5.2 Computed Tomography (CT)

Although not a first-line examination, CT can be useful in the event of hidden fractures or multiple traumas.

13.5.3 Magnetic Resonance (MR) Imaging and MR Arthrography

These can be important for the detection of capsular-ligamentous abnormalities, possible distal clavicle edema, or concomitant lesions to nearby structures. Although MR imaging is not routinely recommended, it should be borne in mind that certain specific situations will warrant its use.

As previously stated, goalkeepers, for example, should be considered overhead athletes in view of their most frequent athletic movements; for this reason, in addition to the traumas described so far, they are also prone to tendon and glenoid labrum traumas, which require imaging investigations capable of revealing soft tissue injuries.

In detail:

Grade I: AP and axillary views, normal radiographic findings compared to contralateral joint.

Grade II: AP view, slight widening of AC joint space compared to the contralateral joint and preservation of CC space, even on stress radiography; axillary view, normal radiographic findings.

Grade III: AP view, evident disruption of the AC and CC joint; axillary view, no posterior displacement of the clavicle.

Grade IV: AP view, evident AC and CC disruption; axillary view, posterior displacement of the clavicle. When a good axillary view cannot be obtained, as in cases of polytrauma, a CT examination is recommended.

Grade V: AP and axillary view, major disruption of the AC and CC joints.

Grade VI. AP view, evident inferior displacement of clavicle. Owing to the violence of the trauma, attention should be given to possible associated lesions.

13.6 Treatment

Treatment decisions are driven by the Rockwood classification, which recommends surgery for high-grade dislocations.

Grade I–II (conservative treatment): Cryotherapy, pain relief, and immobilization with an ultrasling brace. Early mobilization is advised to promote return to play, but only after the pain has subsided. Return to play is usually possible after 7–14 days, provided anatomy and range of motion are normal. Players of contact sports and therefore also *football players are advised to use a padded splint for a few days after resuming athletic activity*. Complications of conservative treatment are residual instability, arthritic degeneration, distal clavicular osteolysis and pain [1], arthritis, and ossification of the CC ligaments [10].

Grade III: The most appropriate treatment is widely debated in the literature, as there is no clear evidence of the superiority of one over the others [4, 11]. Almost 90 % of patients treated either conservatively or surgically achieve satisfactory results, even though surgery is associated with a greater risk of complications such as repeat surgery, infections, and deformity, but also a faster return to play [4, 11, 12]. The advantages of surgical treatment appear to be greater strength, less residual pain, or deformity [13]. Conservative treatment could have a negative impact on scapular biomechanics: less-than-perfect reduction of the dislocation, by negatively influencing scapulohumeral biomechanics, is often associated with effects on the cervical spine, probably as a result of secondary hyperlordosis or postural changes or because of the increased tension of the upper trapezius produced by the changed insertion on the AC [12]. Surgery based on biomechanical reasons alone is not recommended, since anatomical reduction by itself is not considered sufficient to provide optimal results [14]. The current tendency is to opt for surgery only in the event of failed conservative treatment or in athletes with high-level functional demands. The persistence of pain 3 months after the end of conservative treatment is generally regarded as a failure. Waiting, however, could prove to be a risk. Subjects who underwent surgery within 3 weeks of the trauma had better results [15, 16], but not all authors have come to the same conclusion [17]:

In football players, grade III dislocations require different approaches depending on whether the player is a goalkeeper or an outfield player.

AC dislocation in a goalkeeper requires immediate surgical treatment and interruption of athletic activity for at least 3 months, if during the season.

AC dislocation in an outfield player allows for a wider choice of management strategies:

(a) *Conservative treatment and interruption of athletic activity for at least 40 days.*
(b) *Surgical treatment and 40–60 days' interruption. This may clearly be done in the immediate post-trauma period, but if in season, it may also be postponed to after the end of the season. The player will nonetheless require a resting period of 40–60 days.*

We tend to support immediate surgical treatment which allows us to exploit the biological repair response. Should we decide, in agreement with the athlete, to put off surgery until after the end of the season, we prefer to associate CC ligament reconstruction with tissue-bank tendons so as to boost the biological repair processes, as will be described below.

The modalities for functional recovery are the same, although we prefer to delay return to play by one month compared to the normal postoperative period for this type of procedure.

Grades IV, V, and VI, and grade III with failed conservative treatment or patients with high-level functional demands: surgical treatment.

Many different, open or closed, surgical procedures have been described, and despite the wide range of surgical techniques, it is difficult to achieve excellent results. The intrinsic mobility of the clavicle, scapula, and AC joint is a contraindication for rigid stabilization systems. The ideal system preserves the joint biomechanics and tries to reproduce the normal anatomy of the damaged ligaments, in terms of stiffness and resistance, while paying attention to the distribution of tensions, so as to avoid complications such as cutting of the suture materials over the bony structures.

The literature does not help to choose the most effective technique as comparative studies are few and most authors simply report the results of a single treatment.

Below we describe the most widespread approaches:

Dynamic Muscle Transfer This involves transferring the tip of the coracoid process, with the conjoint tendon attached, to the undersurface of the clavicle, thereby creating a dynamic depressor and a vertical stabilization force. Often the stabilization obtained is inadequate, and the lack of stability leads to failure to repair the lesion. In addition, patients often complain of continued articular pain [18].

Primary Stabilization of the AC Joint This can be performed with stiff devices such as Kirschner wires, Steinmann pins or screws, bioabsorbable materials, or plates. However, in view of some undoubted disadvantages, these treatments are not recommended in athletes.

CC Stabilization This is achieved by securing the clavicle to the coracoid process. Several techniques have been described including the Bosworth screw and cerclage wires.

- The tightrope is a nonrigid stabilization technique which, through a minimally invasive procedure, aims at stabilizing the joint until healing of the CC ligament. The most obvious advantages are no need for re-intervention and limited tissue damage. At 12 months, 40 % of patients complained of discomfort due to the knot on the upper clavicular surface and returned to play after 4 months on average. Complications are infrequent and include erosion of the synthetic material and bony resorption [13] and, in subjects with hyperlaxity, residual horizontal instability [19]. Biomechanical studies have shown the tightrope to have the same resistance as homologue implants (semitendinosus), but with the advantage of being less rigid, a feature that could promote normal scapula biomechanics. Furthermore, compared to other stabilization systems, the tightrope provides better distribution of forces thanks to the presence of buttons. Another, non-negligible, aspect is the economic advantage compared to other stabilization systems demonstrated by some studies [13].

Ligament Reconstruction With or Without Clavicle Excision Recreating a vertical constraint between the undersurface of the clavicle and the coracoid process is the primary goal of ligament reconstruction. To this end, several techniques and materials have been described. The techniques can broadly be subdivided into:

- Transfer of the CC ligament with or without augmentation (not anatomical). These are usually associated with greater anterior translation of the clavicle compared to normal anatomy [20].
- Reconstruction of the CC ligament (anatomical).
- Combination of the above [8].

The typical nonanatomical reconstruction is the Weaver-Dunn technique, first described in 1972. This has major contraindications in athletes, including detachment of the coracoacromial ligament from the acromion, resection of the lateral end of the clavicle, and a biomechanically demonstrated stabilization strength equal to 25 % of the original, all reasons why we do not use this approach in our practice.

Reconstruction of the CC Ligament This is done with a technique similar to the Weaver-Dunn method and involves autograft or allograft CC reconstruction though two tunnels drilled into the clavicle. In this context, biomechanical studies focusing on the position of the ligaments on the clavicle are particularly interesting; these found fixed relationships between the length of the clavicle and the distance of the insertions on the articular lateral margin (30 % of clavicle length for the conoid and 17 % for the trapezoid) [8, 21]. In addition, the biomechanical superiority of anatomical reconstructions compared to other techniques has also been demonstrated [22]. The most commonly used grafts are the doubled semitendinosus (autograft) and the anterior tibialis (allograft).

Arthroscopic Repair Firstly, this should be referred to as endoscopy/arthroscopy given that the treatment is performed inside the extra-articular cavity. This technique was first reported in 2001, when the authors described placing, via a guidewire, of a suture thread through the clavicle and coracoid to stabilize the reduction and reproduce the CC ligaments [23]. The mechanism of injury underlying AC dislocations can also cause injuries to the rotator cuff, especially in the over 40s, as well as to other structures, as in goalkeepers, which is why we believe arthroscopic repair to be necessary. According to some authors, rotator cuff injuries are associated in 20 % of cases: for this reason, they recommend an arthroscopic phase to obtain a complete assessment [24].

In football players, we recommend the immediate use of a "suspension" or "pulley" system, with or without biological support. In our opinion, this technique ensures major primary stability and does not require reoperation for the removal of the fixation device. We believe the pulley system to be sufficient when used in the acute stage, as we consider football players to have a satisfactory spontaneous biological healing stimulus related to the temporal closeness of the trauma. In patients with chronic dislocations who, for athletic needs, wish to postpone the procedure to after the end of the season, we advise the addition of biological support. This is because the capability for spontaneous repair in these patients may be exhausted or inadequate. The most frequently used grafts are semitendinosus and gracilis allografts (Fig. 13.2).

Timing of Treatment Another difficult problem is the choice of the best timing for surgery in the athlete. Despite many studies demonstrating that the best clinical results are achieved when surgery is carried out in the acute stage, it may sometimes be preferable, or necessary for the athlete's career, to postpone surgery to the off-season period. In this case, one needs to carefully evaluate the biological repair capability of ligaments and the possible use of grafts able to provide a stimulus to the repair process itself.

Postoperative Care Although protocols vary depending on the surgical technique used, they all involve one night's hospitalization, early passive mobilization and pendulum movement 7–10 days postoperatively, and sling immobilization for 3–8 weeks, depending on the authors. We recommend the use of an ultrasling brace for 4 weeks with removal after radiographic assessment; progressive restoration of first passive and then active mobility, even by means of exercise in water as soon as this is possible; and return to play after 3 months for outfield players.

We adopt a more cautious strategy in goalkeepers and recommend return to play 3 months after surgery provided that no associated lesions are present: otherwise, return to play is delayed to 6 months after surgery. Active movements are started when the sling is removed and a good biological repair is assumed and after total passive range of movement is restored. Return to play is expected after 6–8 months.

References

1. Wei HF, Chen YF, Zeng BF, Zhang CQ, Chai YM, Wang HM, Lu Y (2011) Triple endobutton technique for the treatment of acute complete acromioclavicular joint dislocations: preliminary results. Int Orthop 35(4):555–559
2. Tavakoli Darestani R, Ghaffari A, Hosseinpour M (2013) Acromioclavicular joint fixation using an acroplate combined with a coracoclavicular screw. Arch Trauma Res 2(1):36–39. Published online 1 June 2013
3. Lee KW, Debski RE, Chen CH, Woo SL, Fu FH (1997) Functional evaluation of the ligaments at the acromioclavicular joint during anteroposterior and superoinferior translation. Am J Sports Med 25(6):858–862
4. Chillemi C, Franceschini V, Dei Giudici L, Alibardi A, Salate Santone F, Ramos Alday L, Osimani M (2013) Epidemiology of isolated acromioclavicular joint dislocation. Emerg Med Int 2013:171609
5. Bearn JM, Hughston JC, Whatley GS (1973) Acromioclavicular dislocation: method of treatment. Am J Sports Med 1:5–17
6. Nuber GW, Bowen MK (1997) Acromioclavicular joint injuries and distal clavicle fractures. J Am Acad Orthtop Surg 5:11–18
7. Elamin SE, Sinha A, Webb M (2013) Locked superior dislocation of the acromioclavicular joint. Case Rep Orthop 2013:508219
8. Epstein D, Day M, Rokito A (2012) Current concepts in the surgical management of acromioclavicular joint injuries. Bull NYU Hosp Jt Dis 70(1):11–24
9. Chen W, Zhagn Q, Su YL, Zhang ZK, Hou ZY, Pan JS, Zhang XL, Zhang YZ (2012) Axial and tangential views of the acromioclavicular joint: the introduction of new projections. Chin Med J (Engl) 125(14):2493–2498
10. Cox JS (1981) The fate of the acromioclavicular joint in athletic injuries. Am J Sports Med 9(1):50–53
11. Smith T, Chester R, Pearse EO, Hing CB (2011) Operative versus non-operative management following Rockwood grade III acromioclavicular separation: a meta-analysis of the current evidence base. J Orthop Traumatol 12(1):19–27
12. Gumina S, Carbone S, Arceri V, Rita A, Vestri AR, Postacchini F (2009) The relationship between chronic type III acromioclavicular joint dislocation and cervical spine pain. BMC Musculoskelet Disord 10:157
13. Horst K, Dienstknecht T, Andruszkow H, Gradl G, Kobbe P, Pape HC (2013) Radiographic changes in the operative treatment of acute acromioclavicular joint dislocation – tight rope technique vs. K-wire fixation. Pol J Radiol 78(4):15–20. doi:10.12659/PJR.889615. Epub 19 Nov 2013
14. Calvo E, López-Franco M, Arribas IM (2006) Clinical and radiologic outcomes of surgical and conservative treatment of type III acromioclavicular joint injury. J Shoulder Elbow Surg 15(3):300–305
15. Weinstein DM, McCann PD, McIlveen SJ, Flatow EL, Bigliani LU (1995) Surgical treatment of complete acromioclavicular dislocations. Am J Sports Med 23:324–331
16. Li H, Wang C, Wang J, Wu K, Hang D (2013) Restoration of horizontal stability in complete acromioclavicular joint separations: surgical technique and preliminary results. Eur J Med Res 18(1):42. doi:10.1186/2047-783X-18-42. Published online 13 Nov 2013
17. Dumontier C, Sautet A, Man M, Apoil A (1995) Acromioclavicular dislocations: treatment by coracoclavicular ligamentoplasty. J Shoulder Elbow Surg 4:130–134
18. Ferris BD, Bhamra M, Paton DF (1989) Coracoid process transfer for acromioclavicular dislocations. A report of 20 cases. Clin Orthop Relat Res 242:184–187
19. Motta P, Maderni A, Bruno L, Mariotti U (2011) Suture rupture in acromioclavicular joint dislocations treated with flip buttons. Arthroscopy 27(2):294–298
20. Rolf O, von Weyhern AH, Ewers A, Boehm TD, Gohlke F (2008) Acromioclavicular dislocation Rockwood III–V: results of early versus delayed surgical treatment. Arch Orthop Trauma Surg 128(10):1153–1157
21. Rios CG, Arciero RA, Mazzocca AD (2007) Anatomy of the clavicle and coracoid process for reconstruction of the coracoclavicular ligaments. Am J Sports Med 35(5):811–817
22. Ad M, Arciero RA, Bicos J (2007) Evaluation and treatment of acromioclavicular joint injuries. Am J Sports Med 35(2):316–329
23. Wolf EM, Pennington WT (2001) Arthroscopic reconstruction for acromio-clavicular joint dislocation. Arthroscopy 17:558–563
24. Takase K, Yamamoto K, Imakiire A (2004) Therapeutic results of acromioclavicular joint dislocation complicated by rotator cuff tear. J Orthop Surg (Hong Kong) 12(1):96–101

Knee Medial Collateral Ligament Injuries

14

Luis Pedro Duarte Silva, C. Desai, N. Loureiro, H. Pereira, and J. Espregueira-Mendes

14.1 Etiology/Epidemiology/Anatomy and Biomechanics

The medial collateral ligament (MCL) is a common site of injury in sports and so it is very important to have great knowledge of all the parts involved for prevention, treatment, and rehabilitation. MCL injury is more common in sports that require contact and male athletes are at greater risk [1, 2].

In a paper that studied the epidemiology of knee injuries, which included 17,397 patients with 19,530 sports injuries over a 10-year period, MCL lesion corresponded to 7.9 % and soccer was the main activity leading to this injury [3].

MCL injuries sometimes are associated to other lesions such as meniscal tear and anterior or posterior cruciate ligaments tears [4].

The MCL (Fig. 14.1*) is considered a static stabilizer of the knee and is a strong ligament that is attached to the medial meniscus and capsule. It is divided into two portions, superficial MCL and deep MCL. The posterior oblique ligament (POL) is also a structure that is often neglected but has an important role in static knee stabilization, and since its anatomy and functions are correlated with the MCL, it also has to be mentioned. The anatomy of the medial side of the knee is classically described in three layers, with the superficial MCL and posterior oblique ligament (POL) being in the second layer and the deep MCL in the third, and this division was described in a dissection study of 154 knees* [5].

The superficial MCL has an average width of 1.5 cm and length of 11 cm, it originates in the medial femoral epicondyle and inserts distal to the joint line on the medial aspect of the proximal tibia with two different attachments, the first 1 cm

L.P.D. Silva (✉)
Dragon Clinic, Espregueira-Mendes Sports Centre – FIFA Medical Centre of Excellence – FIFA Medical Centre of Excellence – Dom Henrique Research Center, Via Futebol Club do Porto Estadio Entrada nascente –Piso 3, Porto 4350-415, Portugal

Local Health Unit Guarda, Guarda, Portugal
e-mail: luisduartesilva1985@gmail.com

C. Desai • N. Loureiro
Dragon Clinic, Espregueira-Mendes Sports Centre – FIFA Medical Centre of Excellence – FIFA Medical Centre of Excellence – Dom Henrique Research Center, Via Futebol Club do Porto Estadio Entrada nascente –Piso 3, Porto 4350-415, Portugal

H. Pereira
Dragon Clinic, Espregueira-Mendes Sports Centre – FIFA Medical Centre of Excellence – Dom Henrique Research Center, Via Futebol Club do Porto Estadio Entrada nascente –Piso 3, Porto 4350-415, Portugal

Hospital Póvoa de Varzim, Braga, Portugal

3 B's Research Group Minho University, ICVS/ 3B's associated Laboratory Minho University, Braga, Portugal

J. Espregueira-Mendes
Dragon Clinic, Espregueira-Mendes Sports Centre – FIFA Medical Centre of Excellence – Dom Henrique Research Center, Via Futebol Club do Porto Estadio Entrada nascente –Piso 3, Porto 4350-415, Portugal

Minho University, School of Health sciences 3 B's/ ICVS, Braga, Portugal

P. Volpi (ed.), *Football Traumatology: New Trends*, DOI 10.1007/978-3-319-18245-2_14

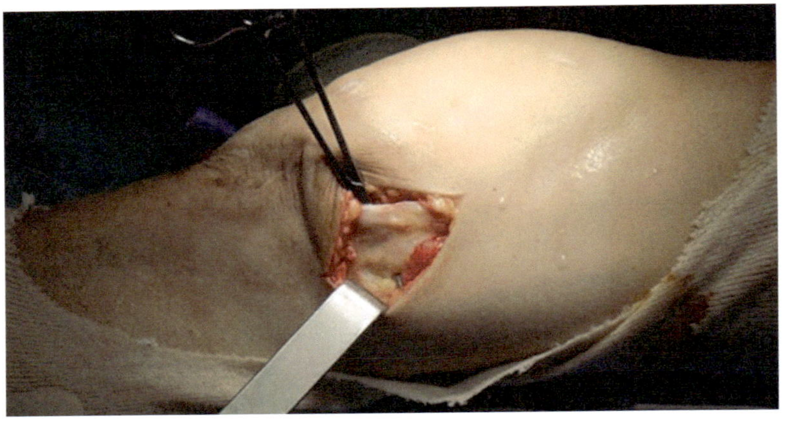

Fig. 14.1 MCL

distal to the joint line and the other approximately 6 cm (this attachment is the strongest) [2, 6, 7].

The deep MCL also called "middle capsular ligament" since it isn't a distinct structure; classically it is divided in two portions: meniscofemoral and meniscotibial. It extends from the femur (1 cm distal to the origin of the superficial MCL) then courses distally to attach the medial meniscus and finally inserting in the tibia 3–4 mm distal to the joint line [2, 7].

The posterior oblique ligament is a structure often misunderstood and neglected. Its origin arises from the adductor tubercle and has three distal attachments: (1) posterior tibia, (2) posterior capsule, and (3) sheath of the semimembranosus tendon [2, 7].

In terms of biomechanics, the MCL and related structures are mainly referred in the literature has valgus restraining structures, but recent studies have reported that the superficial MCL is also implicated in rotational stability [8]. *A study tested the maximum load supported by these structures, and the results were 534 N for the superficial MCL, 194 N for the deep MCL, and 425 N to the posterior oblique ligament. In the same study, the momentum of failure was also analyzed for the three structures; the results were 10,2 mm to the superficial MCL, 7.1 mm for the deep MCL, and 12 mm to the posterior oblique ligament* [9].

14.2 Injury Mechanism

The injury mechanism is typically one of the two mechanisms: direct valgus blow to the lateral side of the knee (typically this mechanism causes more severe lesions) and a noncontact rotational injury. Noncontact rotational injury can be a valgus force (most common); despite this commonly used reference in the literature, the normal mechanism generally includes a combination of movement: flexion/valgus/external rotation (Fig. 14.2) [10–13]. This can occur when a player tries to change direction quickly or when the shoe stays stuck to the ground. In a cadaver study, femoral attachment was the most common location of failure for the superficial MCL, but interstitial failure was more common in the posterior oblique ligament and deep MCL [9].

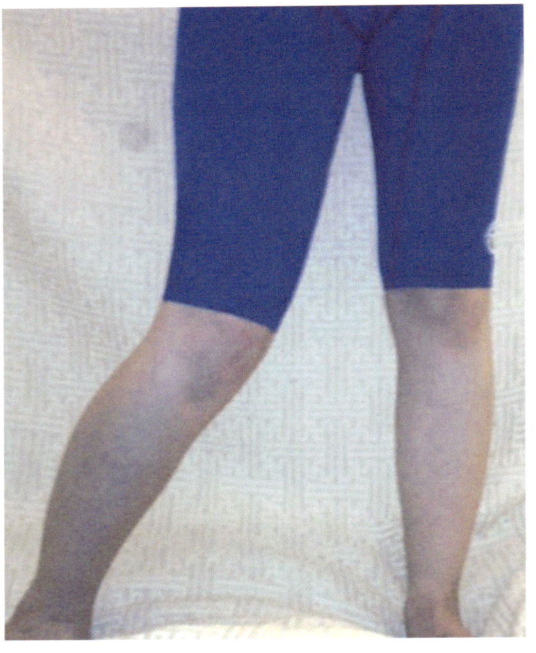

Fig. 14.2 Flexion/valgus/external rotation of the knee

Table 14.1 MCL injury classification, based on: [14]

Severity/grade 1	Involves a few fibers; tenderness; no instability		
Severity/grade 2	Disruption of more fibers; broad tenderness; no instability		
Severity/grade 3	Complete disruption of the ligament; *with* instability	Laxity/grade 1+	3–5 mm of absolute medial separation
		Laxity/grade 2+	*6–10 mm* of absolute medial separation
		Laxity/grade 3+	*>10 mm* of absolute medial separation

14.3 Clinical and Diagnostic Examination

The classification of MCL injuries could cause confusion, but since Hughston in 1994 optimizes the classification in terms of severity and laxity, it became more obvious [2, 14] (the laxity grading is inserted on grade 3 of severity) (Table 14.1).

A full knee examination should be performed to rule out associated injuries. In this chapter, the main aspects related to MCL injury will be referred. In the acute injury, the ideal timing to the physical examination is immediately after the injury so that the pain, swelling, and muscular spasm don't make the assessment less reliable and difficult [2]. Some important information regarding the injury are ability to walk immediately after the event, sensation of pop or tear, and time and onset of swelling [15].

The physical exam should start with inspection, including stance and gait. Swelling, deformity, and ecchymosis can be present. Since more severe injuries can also involve the anterior cruciate ligament, meniscus, or the posterior cruciate ligament, joint effusion can occur [2]. Comparing the range of motion of the two knees is important because a wide variation among individual exists. If the patient has a limited active knee (flexion/extension), passive motion should be tried to exclude a block.

Palpation should be performed since it can help identify other pathologies; bony and soft tissue landmarks should be inspected; a 78 % of accuracy in detecting MCL injury when tenderness is present at the joint line in the place of the MCL has been reported [15].

Valgus stress tests should be performed in 0° and 30° of flexion and compared to the other knee. Any laxity at 0° of flexion should lead to suspect injury to other structures such as the posterior cruciate ligament [16, 17]. Isolated laxity at 30° suggests injury of the superficial portion of the MCL.

The use of Porto Knee Testing Device (PKTD®) in MRI is useful to evaluate and measure the rotation instability (especially if associated with ACL injury) inside MRI [18].

In chronic MCL injuries, the patient often complains of medial knee pain and instability [12, 19] that can be confirmed by physical exam.

For a complete assessment of MCL injuries, imaging studies are often necessary such as radiographs, magnetic resonance imaging (MRI), and ultrasound. The plain x-rays should only be obtain if the requirements on the Ottawa knee rules are fulfilled, exceptions are to stress x-rays in the individuals with immature skeleton [20, 21]. Ultrasound can be a useful tool in evaluating isolated medial collateral ligament injuries and also predicting the outcome on the basis of the location of the injury [22], but more studies are needed to confirm these allegations. MRI is rarely necessary to evaluate low-grade MCL injuries, but it can have an important role in the exclusion of other associated injury and to a preoperative planning [2].

14.4 Treatment Strategy

Injuries categorized as grade 1, 2, or 3 (without associated injuries) are treated nonoperatively and will be discussed at the end of the chapter. Changes have been made during the last decades in the approach for isolated grade 3 injuries. When comparing isolated grade 3 injuries treated nonoperatively versus surgically, some reports present better results in subjective scores and earlier return to play in the cases where conservative treatment was applied [12]. Due to better results with the conservative treatment of isolated grade 3 MCL injury, this is now the standard approach. The use of a brace with protection of the valgus stress is a good option.

Surgical options are indicated in acute grade 3 injuries with multiligament injuries or other situations such as presence of intra-articular ligamentous entrapment, large bony avulsion, or an acute complete tear of the tibial insertion [7, 19, 23, 24]. In grade III, MCL lesions associated with ACL injury in football players, we perform more and more MCL repairs.

There are many different surgical techniques described in the literature, and some include the use of allografts or autografts with good results [25, 26].

14.4.1 Acute Injury Grade 3 MCL Injury

14.4.1.1 Technique

Clinical grade of the injury can be more accurately determined under anesthesia. A diagnostic arthroscopy is mandatory to diagnose associated meniscus and cartilage injuries. This also helps to determine the site of deep MCL injury, which may be above or below the meniscus. Care is necessary to preserve the infrapatellar branch of the saphenous nerve which lies 5 ± 1 cm from the adductor tubercle [27]. The sartorial fascia is identified. A longitudinal incision is taken on the fascia. The superficial MCL can be identified beneath the gracilis and semitendinosus tendons. The deep MCL is examined. Any tear in the deep MCL must be identified and the medial meniscus should be examined simultaneously for injuries. Repair the deeper structures first. The meniscofemoral ligament repair can be done using sutures or suture anchors. However, the meniscotibial part should be addressed using suture anchors preferably. The posterior oblique ligament repair can be done by direct suture to the femur. The knee is positioned in varus and extension to finish the repair. The superficial MCL end should be repaired when avulsed. Interrupted absorbable sutures are used to repair the semimembranosus portion of the posterior oblique ligament. After repairing the MCL, the anterior border of the torn posterior oblique ligament can be sutured to its posterior border [2].

Augmentation procedures have been studied to repair the superficial medial collateral ligament with similar results to anatomic reconstruction [28], and according to some authors, if the superficial MCL is extensively injured, they can be performed [29].

14.4.2 Surgical Treatment Chronic Injury

Those patients who remain with chronic knee pain and instability with isolate grade 3 injury can be candidates for surgery [19].

Some precautions have to be taken in these patients, and a careful radiological study is indicated so that patients with valgus alignment can be identified and if necessary submitted to a corrective osteotomy (that can in fact reduce the functional limitations but is a bad option for football players and that can also reduce the stress in a soft tissue graft if it is necessary to apply it). The patients that don't improve and have a genu varum or neutral alignment can be indicated for surgery. According to LaPrade, a technique that can be used for acute and chronic severe medial knee injuries is composed of two independent grafts in four tunnels. The superficial MCL reconstruction graft is inserted distally 6 cm to the tibial joint line after being fixed on the femur (at the anatomic attachment site); this graft is tightened at 20° of knee flexion and in neutral rotation. To replicate the proximal tibial attachment site, a suture anchor is used in the native location. The graft that is used for the reconstruction of the POL is also inserted in the tunnels (femoral and tibial) that are placed in the original anatomical locations of the POL; this graft is then tightened with the knee extended and in neutral rotation [7].

14.4.2.1 Complications

Some complications that are described in the literature are infection, arthrofibrosis, saphenous nerve lesion, and recurrent valgus laxity [12].

14.5 Rehabilitation and Return to Play

Since the majority of MCL injuries are managed conservatively, this topic will focus more on this subject.

The type of rehabilitation treatment indicated for a medial collateral ligament (MCL) injury depends on the severity of the injury. Platelet-rich plasma (PRP) can be used with ongoing promising results as it has been referred in the literature [30, 31]. Recommendations for treatment that are followed in our group include the following:

14.5.1 Mild MCL Injury

In this case usually, there may be mild tenderness on the inside of the knee over the ligament and usually no swelling. The rehabilitation guidelines can be split into four phases:

Phase 1 (0–1 Week)

Aims: patient education, reduce swelling if there is any, allow +15° extension and +100° flexion, and begin pain-free strengthening exercises.

Physiotherapy treatment: cold therapy and a compression support to limit any swelling, electrotherapy, and manual therapy.

Exercise program: gentle range of motion (ROM) (flexion mainly), static strengthening exercises can begin as soon as pain is tolerable, isometric quadriceps exercises, calf raises with both legs, and resistance band exercises for the hamstrings, hip abductors, and hip extension but not for adduction as this will stress the medial ligament.

Activity: rest from activities that cause pain. If pain is tolerable, progress to full weight bearing and normal gait pattern [32–39].

Phase 2 (1–2 Weeks)

Aims: eliminate any swelling completely, full flexion ROM, allow +10° extension, continue strengthening exercises, and return to slow jogging.

Physiotherapy treatment: cold therapy and a compression support to limit any swelling, electrotherapy, manual therapy, exercise modification, and supervision.

Exercise program: introduce dynamic strengthening exercises (knee flexion, half squats, step-ups, single leg calf raise, bridging, and leg press are suitable exercises if is pain bearable) and balance and proprioceptive drills (single leg).

Activity: with hinged knee brace, rest from painful activities; however, the athlete may be able to do straight line jogging (slowly as long as it is not painful), swimming (light kick), and road bike [32–39].

Phase 3 (2–4 Weeks)

Aims: full ROM, equal strength of both legs, full squat, dynamic proprioceptive training, and return to running and some sports-specific training.

Physiotherapy treatment: cold therapy after training sessions and manual therapy.

Exercise program: Build on dynamic strengthening exercises such as leg extension and leg curls exercises as well as squats to horizontal and lunges. Increase the intensity, weight lifted, and number of repetitions until the strength is equal in both legs.

Activity: in addition to straight running, start to include sideway and backward running, swimming, agility drills, and plyometric exercises. Increase speed to sprinting and changing direction drills [32–39].

Phase 4 (3–6 Weeks)

Aims: return to full sports-specific training and competition.

Physiotherapy treatment: cold therapy after training sessions and manual therapy.

Exercise program: high-level sports-specific strengthening as required.

Activity: with hinged knee brace, return to sports-specific drills, restricted training, and match play [32–39].

14.5.2 Moderate-to-Severe MCL Injury

For this kind of injury, it is important that the ends of the ligament are protected and left to heal without continually being disrupted. The rehabilitation guidelines can be split also into four phases:

Phase 1 (0–4 Weeks)

Aims: patient education, control swelling, allow +30°extension and +90° flexion, and begin pain-free strengthening exercises.

Physiotherapy treatment: cold therapy and a compression support to limit swelling, electrotherapy, manual therapy, and limited motion knee brace.

Exercise program: exercises done in brace; gentle flexion ROM, extension ROM to 30° only; if pain is tolerable, static quads and hamstring exercises, double leg calf raises, and hip abduction and extension; and maintain aerobic fitness on stationary cycle as soon as pain is bearable.

Activity: rest from all painful activities, wear a hinged or stabilized knee brace to protect the medial ligament, use crutches initially, non-weight bearing to start with, and then partial weight bearing from week 2 and by end of week 4 aim to be walking normally [32–39].

Phase 2 (4–6 Weeks)

Aims: eliminate swelling, full weight bearing on the injured knee, full ROM, injured leg almost as strong as the good one.

Physiotherapy treatment: remove the knee brace at this stage, but it is important to use a simple stabilized knee support at this stage to apply compression to the knee, cold therapy, electrotherapy, manual therapy, exercise modification, and supervision.

Exercise program: range of motion exercises should continue along with isometric quadriceps exercises. Mini squats, lunges, double leg press, hamstring curls, step-ups, bridges, hip abduction, hip extension, and single leg calf raises can begin or be continued.

Activity: swimming (light kick), road bike, and walking [32–39].

Phase 3 (6–10 Weeks)

Aims: aims to regain full ROM, strength and endurance of affected limb, return to sports-specific drills, and restricted training, and match play.

Physiotherapy treatment: cold therapy after training sessions, manual therapy.

Exercise program: strengthening exercises as above increasing intensity and moving double leg exercises to single jump and land drills.

Activity: straight line jogging with hinged knee brace (no earlier than 6 weeks); after week 8, begin to run sideways and backwards, so by week 10, the athlete is able to begin to change direction at speed. For footballers, kicking may now be possible. When confident enough, plyometric drills, hopping, box jumps, and agility drills can begin [32–39].

Phase 4 (8–10/12 Weeks)

Aims: return to full sports-specific training and competition.

Physiotherapy treatment: cold therapy after training sessions, manual therapy.

Exercise program: high-level sports-specific strengthening as required.

Activity: with hinged knee brace for the first 2–4 weeks, return to sports-specific drills, restricted training, and match play [32–39].

14.6 Complications of Nonoperative Treatment

The two main complications are medial knee pain and residual valgus laxity [12].

14.6.1 Postoperative Care

There are many rehabilitation techniques related to this subject, and they depend on the surgical procedure that is performed and that is also true for the knee brace.

The main goals are a pain-free range of motion to obtain an increase in muscular strength along with a correct proprioceptive training, culminating in a gradual return to play.

References

1. Roach CJ et al (2014) The epidemiology of medial collateral ligament sprains in young athletes. Am J Sports Med 42(5):1103–1109
2. Phisitkul P et al (2006) MCL injuries of the knee: current concepts review. Iowa Orthop J 26:77–90

3. Majewski M, Susanne H, Klaus S (2006) Epidemiology of athletic knee injuries: a 10-year study. Knee 13(3):184–188
4. Azar FM (2006) Evaluation and treatment of chronic medial collateral ligament injuries of the knee. Sports Med Arthrosc 14(2):84–90
5. Warren LF, Marshall JL (1979) The supporting structures and layers on the medial side of the knee: an anatomical analysis. J Bone Joint Surg Am 61(1):56–62
6. LaPrade RF et al (2007) The anatomy of the medial part of the knee. J Bone Joint Surg Am 89(9):2000–2010
7. Laprade RF, Wijdicks CA (2012) The management of injuries to the medial side of the knee. J Orthop Sports Phys Ther 42(3):221–233
8. Wijdicks CA et al (2009) Medial knee injury: part 2, load sharing between the posterior oblique ligament and superficial medial collateral ligament. Am J Sports Med 37(9):1771–1776
9. Robinson JR, Bull AM, Amis AA (2005) Structural properties of the medial collateral ligament complex of the human knee. J Biomech 38(5):1067–1074
10. Hayes CW et al (2000) Mechanism-based pattern approach to classification of complex injuries of the knee depicted at MR imaging. Radiographics 20 Spec No: S121–S134
11. Perryman JR, Hershman EB (2002) The acute management of soft tissue injuries of the knee. Orthop Clin North Am 33(3):575–585
12. Macmahon P (2007) Current diagnosis & treatment in sports medicine, in Lange medical book. Lange Medical Books/McGraw Hill Medical Pub, New York, pp 73–77
13. Jesse C, DeLee DD, Miller MD (2003) DeLee & Drez's orthopaedic sports medicine: principles and practice. Saunders, Philadelphia
14. Hughston JC (1994) The importance of the posterior oblique ligament in repairs of acute tears of the medial ligaments in knees with and without an associated rupture of the anterior cruciate ligament. Results of long-term follow-up. J Bone Joint Surg Am 76(9):1328–1344
15. Indelicato PLR (2003) DeLee & Drez's orthopaedic sports medicine. Saunders, Philadelphia
16. Fetto JF, Marshall JL (1978) Medial collateral ligament injuries of the knee: a rationale for treatment. Clin Orthop Relat Res 132:206–218
17. Grood ES et al (1981) Ligamentous and capsular restraints preventing straight medial and lateral laxity in intact human cadaver knees. J Bone Joint Surg Am 63(8):1257–1269
18. Espregueira-Mendes J, Pereira H, Sevivas N, Passos C, Vasconcelos JC, Monteiro A, Oliveira JM, Reis RL (2012) Assessment of rotatory laxity in anterior cruciate ligament-deficient knees using magnetic resonance imaging with Porto-knee testing device. Knee Surg Sports Traumatol Arthrosc 20(4):671–678. doi:10.1007/s00167-012-1914-9
19. Marchant MH Jr et al (2011) Management of medial-sided knee injuries, part 1: medial collateral ligament. Am J Sports Med 39(5):1102–1113
20. Stiell IG et al (1995) Use of radiography in acute knee injuries: need for clinical decision rules. Acad Emerg Med 2(11):966–973
21. Zionts LE (2002) Fractures around the knee in children. J Am Acad Orthop Surg 10(5):345–355
22. Lee JI et al (1996) Medial collateral ligament injuries of the knee: ultrasonographic findings. J Ultrasound Med 15(9):621–625
23. Lobenhoffer, P., [Complex instability of the anterior knee]. Orthopade, 2002. 31(8): p. 770–7
24. Lind M et al (2009) Anatomical reconstruction of the medial collateral ligament and posteromedial corner of the knee in patients with chronic medial collateral ligament instability. Am J Sports Med 37(6):1116–1122
25. Liu X et al (2013) Surgical treatment of subacute and chronic valgus instability in multiligament-injured knees with superficial medial collateral ligament reconstruction using Achilles allografts: a quantitative analysis with a minimum 2-year follow-up. Am J Sports Med 41(5):1044–1050
26. Wijdicks CA et al (2010) Sartorial branch of the saphenous nerve in relation to a medial knee ligament repair or reconstruction. Knee Surg Sports Traumatol Arthrosc 18(8):1105–1109
27. Noyes FR, Barber-Westin SD (1995) The treatment of acute combined ruptures of the anterior cruciate and medial ligaments of the knee. Am J Sports Med 23(4): 380–389
28. Wijdicks CA et al (2013) Superficial medial collateral ligament anatomic augmented repair versus anatomic reconstruction: an in vitro biomechanical analysis. Am J Sports Med 41(12):2858–2866
29. Bosworth DM (1952) Transplantation of the semitendinosus for repair of laceration of medial collateral ligament of the knee. J Bone Joint Surg Am 34-A(1):196–202
30. Eirale C, Mauri E, Hamilton B (2013) Use of platelet rich plasma in an isolated complete medial collateral ligament lesion in a professional football (soccer) player: a case report. Asian J Sports Med 4(2):158–162
31. Yoshioka T et al (2013) The effects of plasma rich in growth factors (PRGF-Endoret) on healing of medial collateral ligament of the knee. Knee Surg Sports Traumatol Arthrosc 21(8):1763–1769
32. Quarles JD, Hosey RG (2004) Medial and lateral collateral injuries: prognosis and treatment. Prim Care 31(4):957–975, ix
33. Hastings DE (1980) The non-operative management of collateral ligament injuries of the knee joint. Clin Orthop Relat Res 147:22–28
34. Indelicato PA (1995) Isolated medial collateral ligament injuries in the knee. J Am Acad Orthop Surg 3(1):9–14
35. Lundberg M, Messner K (1996) Long-term prognosis of isolated partial medial collateral ligament ruptures. A ten-year clinical and radiographic evaluation of a prospectively observed group of patients. Am J Sports Med 24(2):160–163
36. Lundberg M, Messner K (1997) Ten-year prognosis of isolated and combined medial collateral ligament ruptures. A matched comparison in 40 patients using clinical and radiographic evaluations. Am J Sports Med 25(1):2–6
37. Reider B (1996) Medial collateral ligament injuries in athletes. Sports Med 21(2):147–156

38. Reider B et al (1994) Treatment of isolated medial collateral ligament injuries in athletes with early functional rehabilitation. A five-year follow-up study. Am J Sports Med 22(4):470–477
39. Lundblad M et al (2013) The UEFA injury study: 11-year data concerning 346 MCL injuries and time to return to play. Br J Sports Med 47(12): 759–762

Injuries of the Lateral Collateral Ligament and Posterolateral Corner of the Knee

15

Andrea Campi and Stefano Campi

15.1 Introduction

The lateral collateral ligament (LCL) is a crucial part of the posterolateral corner. Therefore, it can be treated exclusively in the context of the musculoligamentous complex to which it belongs.

The posterolateral corner (PLC) consists of various structures. Even if the PLC is not well defined in the literature, most of the authors include in its description the lateral collateral ligament, the popliteal tendon (PT), the popliteofibular ligament (PFL) and the posterolateral capsule that is reinforced by the arcuate ligament (AL) and the fabellofibular ligament (FFL).

The PLC is responsible for the posterolateral stabilization of the knee, resisting to varus angulation, posterior translation and external rotation forces [1].

Injuries to the LCL and PLC are uncommon, representing less than 2 % of all acute knee ligamentous injuries, while the incidence in association with other ligamentous injuries, such as the anterior cruciate ligament (ACL) and/or the posterior cruciate ligament (PCL), is much higher (43–40 %) [2, 3]. Isolated lesions of the LCL are even more rare.

The most common mechanism of injury of the PLC is a combined, high-energy hyperextension and varus force [4].

Interest in PLC injuries is recently increasing, since several studies have highlighted its importance in knee stability. As a consequence, together with improvements in diagnostic imaging, the recognition of these injuries is rising. Several studies have demonstrated superior results with immediate surgical intervention [3–6], whereas untreated or improperly treated PLC injuries are recognized as a cause of morbidity. Furthermore, unidentified lesions can negatively affect the outcome of other surgeries as ACL and PCL reconstruction [7, 8].

15.2 Anatomy

The anatomy of the posterolateral corner is intricate and complex. Most authors describe the lateral collateral ligament, the popliteus tendon and the popliteofibular ligament as the most important static stabilizers of the posterolateral side of the knee (Fig. 15.1).

The lateral collateral ligament attaches proximally on the femur in a small depression about

A previous version of this chapter included an incorrect affiliation for Andrea Campi and Stefano Campi. For this reason an erratum has been published, correcting the mistake in the previous version and showing the correct affiliation (see DOI:10.1007/978-3-319-18245-2_15).

Andrea Campi (✉)
Department of Orthopaedic Surgery
Azienda Ospedaliera San Giovanni - Addolorata
Rome, Italy
e-mail: and.campi@gmail.com

Stefano Campi
Università Campus Bio-Medico, Rome, Italy
e-mail: stefano.campi@gmail.com

P. Volpi (ed.), *Football Traumatology: New Trends*, DOI 10.1007/978-3-319-18245-2_15

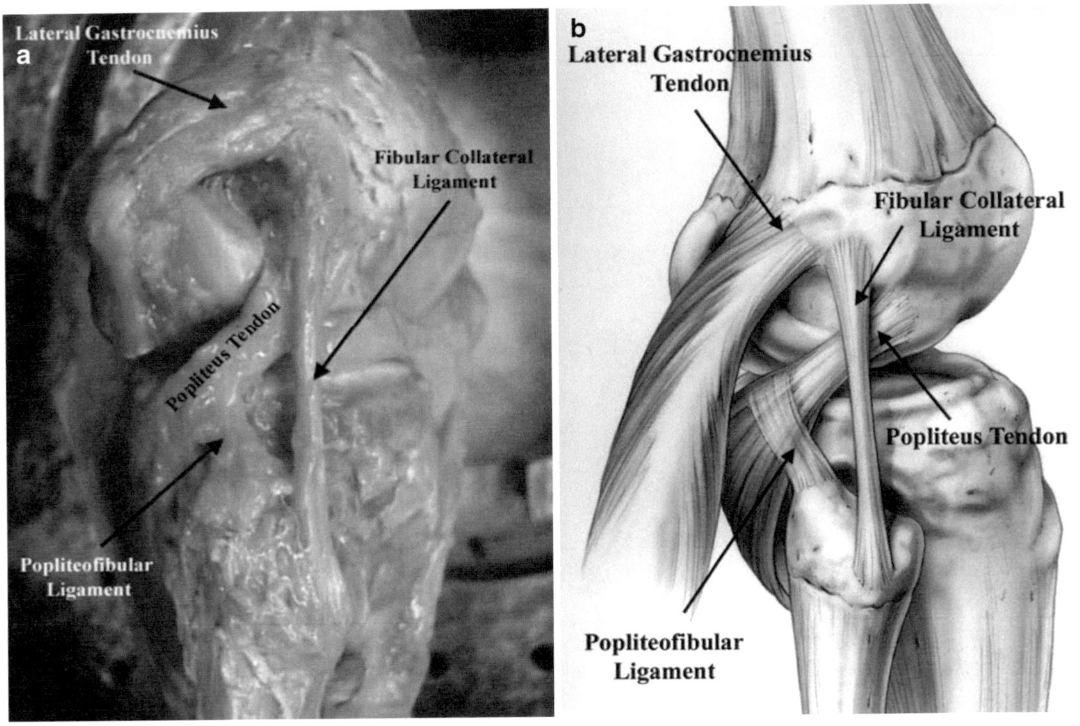

Fig. 15.1 Photograph (**a**) and illustration (**b**) showing the anatomy of the posterolateral corner. (Reprinted from LaPrade et al. [13] with permission of SAGE Publications)

1.4 mm proximal and 3.1 mm posterior to the lateral epicondyle and distally on the fibular head 8 mm posterior to the anterior cortex and 28 mm distal to the tip of the fibular styloid process [9, 10]. The lateral collateral ligament is mainly responsible for the stabilization to varus opening of the knee, especially during the first 30° of knee flexion [11].

The popliteus muscle originates on the posteromedial portion of the proximal tibia. Its tendon curses in a proximolateral direction becoming intra-articular, passes deep to the LCL and popliteofibular ligament and reaches the lateral femoral condyle, where it attaches in the sulcus popliteus. This is on average 18.5 mm away from the LCL attachment.

Three popliteomeniscal fascicles (anteroinferior, posterosuperior and posteroinferior) connect the popliteal tendon to the lateral meniscus [9].

The popliteofibular ligament originates at the musculotendinous junction of the popliteus muscle and courses laterally and distally, where it forms an anterior and a posterior portion that insert on the anteromedial and posteromedial aspect of the proximal fibula, respectively. Expansions also attach to the lateral tibia and the proximal tibiofibular joint capsule. The popliteofibular ligament acts as a stabilizer of external rotation of the knee [12].

A thickening of the lateral capsule forms the mid-third lateral capsular ligament, composed by a meniscofemoral and a meniscotibial portion. The mid-third lateral capsular ligament is thought to be an important stabilizer to varus forces. The meniscotibial component is more frequently injured with a bony avulsion (Segond fracture) [11].

Further structures provide static and dynamic stability to the posterolateral corner. Among these, the iliotibial band, the biceps tendon, the lateral gastrocnemius tendon and the lateral meniscus are the most relevant.

The iliotibial band is a lateral thickening of the fascia lata in the thigh. It inserts distally on the Gerdy's tubercle on the anterolateral face of the proximal tibia and conflates with an expansion of the biceps tendon forming an anterolateral sling about the knee. During knee extension, the iliotibial band is tightened and anterior to the flexion axis of the knee, acting against varus opening of the knee. This function vanishes as the knee is flexed and the iliotibial band moves posteriorly.

The biceps tendon inserts distally on the styloid process of the fibula, embracing the lateral collateral ligament, and acts as a dynamic stabilizer of the knee.

The lateral gastrocnemius tendon inserts into the posterior aspect of the lateral femoral condyle and merges to the posterolateral joint capsule [13].

Finally, the lateral meniscus acts as a stabilizer increasing the conformity of the convex surfaces of the lateral compartment of the knee.

15.3 Biomechanics

The structures of the posterolateral corner primarily work as a static restraint to varus opening, external rotation and posterior tibial translation [14].

Previous biomechanical studies have underlined the role of each component of the PLC by selective sectioning of the structures. Specifically, the isolated sectioning of the PLC produces an increased varus laxity and tibial external rotation. At 90° of knee flexion, this external rotation is partially reduced if the posterior cruciate ligament is intact. Conversely, isolated sectioning of the PCL has no effect on external tibial rotation, suggesting its role as a secondary constraint.

These biomechanical findings justify the rationale for performing the dial test at 30° and 90° of flexion to discern an isolated PLC or combined PLC/PCL injury [15].

Section of the LCL leads to an increase of varus opening up to 5 mm at 15° of flexion. Further sectioning of the popliteus tendon and the popliteofibular ligament implies an additional varus opening that is limited in full extension by the cruciate ligaments [16].

In knee full extension, the LCL reaches its maximal tension, and between 5° and 25° of flexion, it acts as the main restraint to varus opening of the knee. Beyond 30°, the LCL becomes progressively loose, and the surrounding structures relieve its role of varus stabilizer. However, the LCL still contributes to external rotatory stability of the tibia in knee flexion [17].

The stability against external rotation of the tibia is also provided by the popliteus muscle, that generates an internal rotational force on the tibia, and by the popliteofibular ligament, that is the primary restraint to tibial external rotation at all flexion angles, remaining isometric throughout the whole range of motion of the knee.

Therefore, the LCL and the popliteus complex have complementary functions as stabilizers to external rotation, with a primary role of the lateral collateral ligament at lower knee flexion angles and a primary role of the popliteus complex at higher knee flexion degrees [3, 18].

Finally, the lateral structures offer resistance to posterior translation of the tibia in knee extension. During progressive knee flexion, the posterior cruciate ligament progressively undertakes this function [17, 19].

15.4 Clinical Diagnosis

A thorough knee examination is essential for a correct diagnosis of posterolateral instability, as well as a precise history and the mechanism of injury evaluation.

The most common mechanisms of injury include combined external rotation and hyperextension, direct trauma on the anteromedial aspect of the proximal tibia resulting in hyperextension, direct trauma on flexed knee or high-energy trauma [15, 20].

Associated ligamentous tears, such as the posterior cruciate ligament, may sometimes hide posterolateral corner injuries. Therefore, during knee examination, it is paramount to suspect and investigate the presence of these lesions, especially in case of a suggestive mechanism of injury.

In high-energy traumas and complex injuries, the possibility of a knee dislocation that spontaneously reduced before examination should be considered. Thus, it is important to assess the neurovascular status, focusing on the peroneal nerve and popliteal vessels integrity [3].

Limb alignment and gait should be assessed first. In chronic setting the evaluation of gait and alignment could reveal an asymmetric standing varus alignment and a varus or hyperextension-varus thrust under bearing. In the acute setting, limping and antalgic gait are usually prevalent.

In the acute traumas, swelling and/or ecchymosis about the posterolateral aspect of the knee may be revealed, as well as tenderness to palpation that can be better assessed in a figure-of-four position.

The evaluation of range of motion may reveal an asymmetric hyperextension in the affected knee.

Specific examination should be performed on both knees and comprises the varus stress test, the dial test, the external rotation recurvatum, the reverse pivot-shift and the posterolateral drawer test.

Varus stress testing must be performed at 0° and 30° of knee flexion. Generally, an evident varus opening with the knee in full extension is highly suggestive of a severe posterolateral corner injury with an associated lesion of cruciate ligaments injury, since they act as secondary varus stabilizers in full extension. In presence of isolated posterolateral injuries, the higher varus opening is at 30° of flexion. However, in some PLC injury patterns such as PFL or popliteus lesions, the varus deformity can be minimal with a predominant rotational instability [3, 20]. On the other hand, isolated lesion of the lateral collateral ligament may result in a positive varus stress with no posterolateral rotation instability. In the latter setting, the LCL could not be found on palpation in figure-of-four position [21].

The dial test is performed with the patient in supine or prone position. The examiner places one hand behind the proximal tibia to keep it in a reduced position and with the other hand holds and externally rotates the patient's foot, both at 30° and 90° of knee flexion.

A minimum difference of 10° in external rotation at 30° of knee flexion suggests a significant PLC injury. A decrease of the external rotation at 90° of knee flexion (compared with 30° of flexion) indicates an isolated lesion of the PLC, while an increase of external rotation implies a combined PLC/PCL injury [3, 22].

The external rotation recurvatum test is performed with the patient in supine position. The examiner lifts the patient's heels off the table at the same time holding his great toes. The hyperextension of the affected leg, often associated with external rotation into relative varus of the tibia, is suggestive of a significant posterolateral corner injury. Alternatively, the examiner can perform the test by holding the heel of the patient with one hand and placing the other hand behind proximal tibia to keep the knee at 30° of flexion. The test is positive when progressive extension of the knee reveals a relative hyperextension and external rotation of the tibia [23].

The posterolateral drawer test is performed with the knee at 90° of flexion and the foot externally rotated by 15°. As a posterior load is applied to the proximal tibia, a significant increase in posterior translation and external rotation suggests a deficient PLC. A positive test frequently indicates a popliteal tendon or popliteofibular ligament injury [23, 24].

The reverse pivot-shift test starts with the knee at 90° of flexion and the foot externally rotated. The knee is then progressively taken into extension under a valgus force. When the test is positive, at the starting point the lateral tibia plateau is posteriorly subluxated and quickly reduces at about 20° of flexion as the iliotibial band force vector changes from a flexor to an extensor of the knee. Occasionally the test may be positive in normal knees; therefore, a comparison to the contralateral knee is always needed [24, 25].

15.5 Imaging

X-rays are usually negative in patients with posterolateral corner lesions, but they can occasionally reveal abnormal findings including the arcuate sign or fibular styloid fracture, the widening of the lateral joint space, the Segond fracture, the medial Segond fracture or the Gerdy's tubercle avulsion [6].

Stress radiography can be useful both in acute and chronic setting to confirm the clinical suspect of a posterolateral corner injury. The widening of the lateral compartment can be revealed by the application of a slight varus stress to the knee. In a cadaveric biomechanical study, LaPrade et al. [26] have demonstrated that an increased opening of approximately 2.7 mm on clinician-applied varus stress radiographs suggests an isolated lateral collateral ligament injury, whereas an increase by approximately 4.0 mm indicates a grade III posterolateral corner injury.

The Segond fracture is an avulsion of the lateral capsule attachment from the lateral tibial plateau, and it can be found in isolated posterolateral corner injuries or in association with cruciate ligament tears. Occasionally, a medial or "reverse" Segond fracture may be associated to isolated posterolateral corner, combined PLC/PCL injuries and meniscal tears. This small anteromedial tibial plateau fracture has been hypothesized as the result of a valgus and external rotation force on the flexed knee or from impingement of the anterior femoral condyle on the anteromedial tibial plateau in hyperextension and varus stress [27–30].

The "arcuate sign" is a radiographic finding representing an avulsion of the "arcuate complex" insertion on the fibular styloid from the proximal head of fibula. The arcuate complex is composed by the popliteofibular, fabellofibular and arcuate ligaments and inserts on the fibular styloid of the fibular head. Therefore, the arcuate sign is pathognomonic for posterolateral corner injuries. The detached fragment is usually small (1–8 mm) and displaced medially and superiorly. Larger fragments (15–25 mm) are generally the result of a conjoined tendon avulsion. The conjoined tendon (composed by the LCL and biceps femoris tendon) inserts anteriorly and inferiorly to the styloid process, on the lateral aspect of the fibular head [24, 30–33].

Magnetic resonance imaging (MRI) is the gold standard for diagnosis of the multiligamentous injuries of the knee. The imaging of the structures of the posterolateral corner, like arcuate ligament, fabellofibular ligament and popliteofibular ligament, is difficult, and many authors recommend the use of high strength magnets (1.5 T or higher) and the addition of coronal oblique series [34, 35]. The advent of 3-Tesla, high-definition MRI significantly improved the visualization of the ACL, PCL, LCL, biceps femoris, iliotibial band, posterolateral capsule, popliteofibular ligament and the popliteus tendon. Moreover, MRI can reveal associated condition like chondral damage and meniscal tears [21].

15.6 Treatment Strategy

15.6.1 Nonoperative Treatment

Partial injuries (grades I and II) of posterolateral corner can be usually addressed with conservative treatment. The nonoperative treatment consists in knee immobilization in full extension for 3–4 weeks, followed by tolerance weight-bearing and progressive exercises for range of motion recovery. After 6–8 weeks from injury, closed chain exercises can be performed, avoiding hamstring exercises until at least 10 weeks. After progressive strengthening, return to full activity is usually allowed 12–14 weeks after injury [11, 35].

15.6.2 Operative Treatment

Grade III injuries often require surgical treatment, since conservative measures generally lead to poor outcome. The operative treatment of posterolateral corner injuries is strictly related to the timing and to the presence of associated lesion. According to these parameters, it is possible to identify four categories: isolated acute posterolateral injuries, combined acute posterolateral injuries, isolated chronic posterolateral injuries and combined chronic posterolateral injuries [11].

The aim of this chapter is to treat isolated injuries of lateral collateral ligament and posterolateral corner, both in acute and chronic settings.

According to numerous studies, anatomic repair of the acute posterolateral corner injuries produces superior outcome when compared to reconstruction of chronic lesions [5, 11].

Primary repairs should be performed within 3 weeks of injury, as the scar tissue makes it difficult to identify anatomic structures and confuses the planes of the posterolateral aspect of the knee. Within the first days after injury, the musculotendinous structures tend to proximal retraction and may preclude an anatomic repair. The fibrous tissue can conceal the peroneal nerve, with higher risks of iatrogenic lesions. Furthermore, in the early period, tissue quality is usually superior and more suitable to be sutured [2].

For all the above reasons, many authors recommend to perform anatomic repair of the posterolateral structures within 1–2 weeks after injury [11, 35]. On the other hand, early surgery on a severely injured knee is associated with higher risk of arthrofibrosis, especially in patients with large effusion and limited preoperative range of motion. Therefore, some authors recommend full motion recovery with controlled ROM exercises before surgery to avoid severe postoperative stiffness [2].

15.6.2.1 Surgical Approach

Anatomic landmark include the Gerdy's tubercle, the lateral joint line and the fibular head. Skin incision extends about 10 cm proximal and 5 cm distal to the joint line. Proximally, it is performed along the posterior margin of the iliotibial band and then curves and extends distally between the fibular head and the Gerdy's tubercle.

The internervous plane lies between the iliotibial band and the biceps femoris. In alternative, dissection can be performed sectioning central portion of the iliotibial band, parallel to the fibres. The common peroneal nerve must be identified along the posterior aspect of the biceps femoris and the fibular head and gently retracted.

By mobilization of the iliotibial band, popliteofibular ligament, popliteus tendon and muscle, biceps femoris and lateral collateral ligament can be identified [36, 37].

15.6.2.2 Primary Repair

When torn tissues are sufficient, each component of the posterolateral corner should be anatomically repaired. The repair should be performed at 60°–70° of knee flexion in neutral or slight internal rotation [38].

The popliteus tendon is the first structure to be assessed. The popliteus tendon is frequently torn at the myotendinous junction rather than being avulsed from the femur. In this case, the tendon is generally sutured or fixed by cancellous screws to the posterolateral aspect of the tibia, converting the tendon into a static stabilizer of the knee and imitating the popliteofibular ligament function.

In case of avulsion from the femur, the popliteus tendon can be fixed at his proximal insertion site by drilling parallel transosseous tunnels through the femoral condyles from lateral to medial. The tendon is then sutured and the sutures passed through the drill holes and fastened over a button.

Many authors have underlined the important role of the popliteofibular ligament as stabilizer in external rotation and posterior translation of tibia. In case of a popliteofibular ligament tear, the tenodesis of the popliteus tendon (if intact) to the posterior aspect of the fibula can replace its function [5, 36].

The LCL is generally avulsed at the femoral insertion. In this case it can be sutured and reinserted using transosseous drill holes through the femoral condyles. The avulsion from fibular head can be repaired either by transosseous drill holes or screw fixation [38].

Midsubstance tears of PCL components are more difficult to repair than avulsion or proximal and distal lesions. When tissue is sufficient, they can be treated by end-to-end suture with the knee positioned in 60°–70° of flexion.

In presence of capsular tears or redundancy, repair or imbrication should be executed [36].

15.6.2.3 Augmentation

Whether the tissues are not suitable for primary repair or this is considered not adequate, it is possible to consider an augmentation with autogenous or allogeneic tissue grafts.

The popliteus tendon can be augmented using the central portion of the iliotibial band by harvesting a longitudinal strip about 2 cm wide without detaching the insertion on the Gerdy's tubercle. A tunnel is then drilled in the tibia inferiorly to the iliotibial band insertion and directed towards the posterolateral portion of the tibia. The graft is then passed through the tunnel and sutured to the popliteus tendon remnant. Part of the biceps tendon can be used to augment or reconstitute the popliteofibular ligament and the popliteus tendon. The central portion of the tendon is harvested leaving the distal insertion attached. The graft is then passed beneath the remaining portion of the biceps tendon and inserted on the lateral aspect of femoral condyle [5, 36].

The biceps tendon can be either used to replace an insufficient LCL by performing a tenodesis on the lateral femoral condyle. Moreover, the biceps tendon tenodesis eliminates the external rotation and flexion force exercised by the biceps. Integrity of the posterolateral capsule is required for a successful tenodesis. The augmentation of LCL can also be performed using free hamstring grafts [36, 39].

The fibular-based figure-of-eight reconstruction is the most widespread non-anatomic technique for posterolateral corner reconstruction. The reconstruction can be performed with several graft including hamstrings, tibialis anterior and tibialis posterior, either autograft or allograft. A tunnel is drilled in the middle of the fibular head from anterior to posterior, protecting the common peroneal nerve. The LCL and popliteus tendon insertions on the lateral femoral epicondyle are then identified, and a K wire is positioned in the isometric point. The graft is then passed through the tunnel on the fibular head and fixed on the isometric point on the femur with an interference screw, with the anterior band passing beneath the iliotibial band and the posterior band beneath the biceps tendon and the iliotibial band. The anterior band of the graft reproduces the LCL, while the posterior band reconstructs the popliteofibular ligament. The graft should be fixed with the knee at 30° of flexion in slight valgus and internal rotation [5, 40].

Several authors have modified this technique to better reproduce the posterolateral corner anatomy. Arciero proposed a modified technique adjusting the positions of the graft on the femur and the fibular head to match the anatomic insertions of LCL and PFL. The fibular tunnel is directed slantwise from the anterolateral to the posteromedial aspect of fibular head, and two tunnels placed on the anatomical footprints of LCL and PFL substitute the isometric femoral tunnel. The technique also implies the insertion of an additional interference screw in the fibular tunnel to improve the stability of the construct [40, 41]. Several authors have described other construct configurations based on similar principles, with variable clinical outcomes (Fig. 15.2) [2, 42–44].

In 1985 Hughston et al. proposed an operative approach that consisted in the advancement of the posterolateral corner structures insertion on the femur. The popliteus, the LCL, the arcuate ligament, the lateral gastrocnemius tendon and the capsule are advanced proximally and fixed to the lateral femoral condyle to increase posterolateral stability. This technique is helpful when the tissues are not suitable for primary repair, even though it involves a substantial modification of the normal anatomy of the posterolateral corner. The authors reported high percentage of satisfactory results with a follow-up of 2–13 years. Alternatively, the isolated advancement of the popliteus tendon can be performed if the tendon is strained but not torn. This technique respects more the anatomy, but implies a higher risk of failure [36, 45].

15.6.2.4 Proximal Tibial Osteotomy

The mechanical alignment is a central contributor to knee stability, and the effects of varus or valgus malalignment become even more evident in presence of ligamentous injuries. The evaluation and treatment of limb malalignment are therefore crucial in PLC deficient knees, especially in case of prior failed reconstructions. Many authors have reported that failure to correct varus alignment can frequently result in failure of the posterolateral knee repair or reconstruction.

In presence of a varus malalignment, a proximal tibial medial opening wedge osteotomy should be performed before ligament repair or reconstruction [2, 46, 47]. After realignment, the eventual joint laxity can be treated successfully with secondary ligamentous reconstruction [2, 46, 48], even though in selected cases tibial osteotomy can result as a definitive treatment.

In a biomechanical study on cadaveric knees, LaPrade concluded that a proximal tibial medial opening wedge osteotomy reduced varus and external rotation laxity in posterolateral corner deficient knees. However, the authors observed

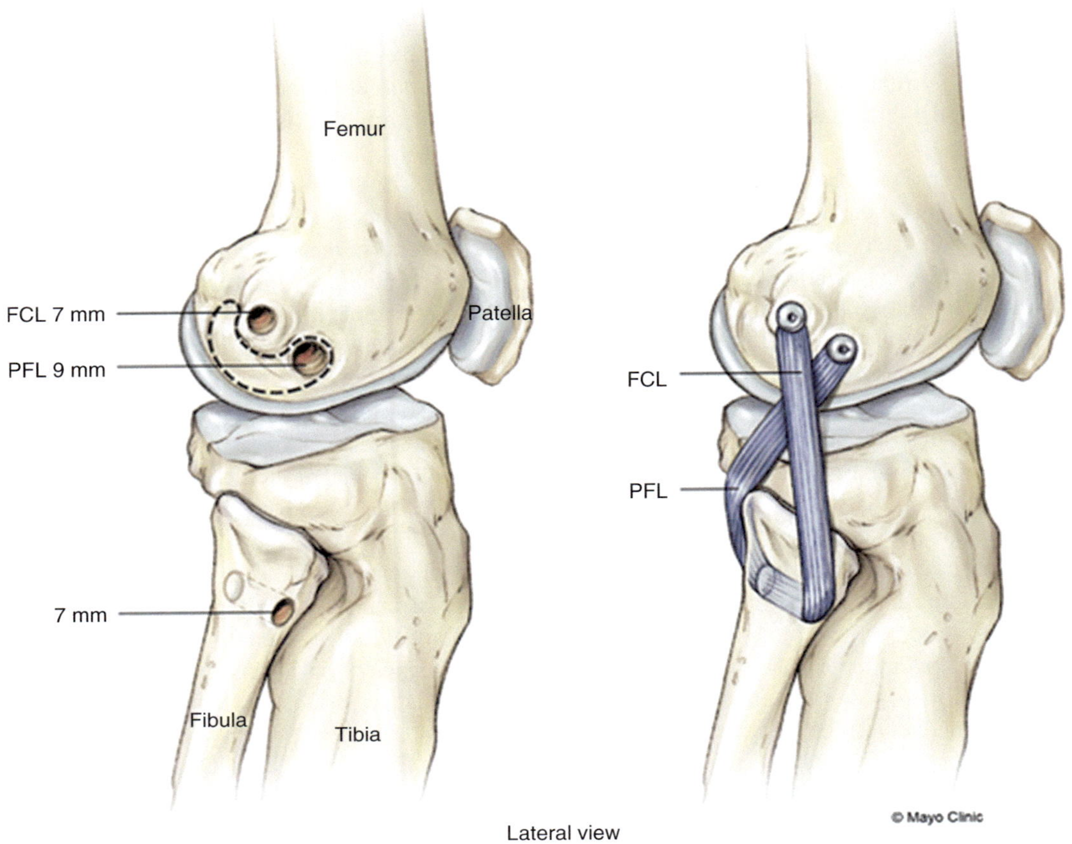

Fig. 15.2 Modified figure-of-eight reconstruction of the posterolateral corner (Reprinted from Schechinger et al. [44] with permission from Elsevier)

an increased stress on the superficial medial collateral ligament, with uncertain long-term consequences [49].

15.6.3 Postoperative Rehabilitation

The postoperative rehabilitation of PLC injuries is controversial. A brace immobilization in full extension is generally indicated for about 6 weeks. Indications for weight-bearing are variable. Most authors suggest non-weight-bearing for at least 6 weeks, even though some surgeons allow early partial weight-bearing. Quadriceps exercises are usually considered the cornerstone of rehabilitation, including quadriceps sets, mini squats and straight leg raises. Some authors suggest immediate initiation of ROM, while others suggest delaying up to 3–4 weeks postoperatively. Active hamstring exercises should not be performed during the first 4 months. Open-chain hamstring-strengthening exercises are generally delayed for 4–6 months. Return to sport and/or work activities is generally allowed around 9–12 months after surgery [2, 3, 50].

References

1. Bolog N, Hodler J (2007) MR imaging of the posterolateral corner of the knee. Skeletal Radiol 36: 715–728
2. Levy BA, Stuart MJ, Whelan DB (2010) Posterolateral instability of the knee: evaluation, treatment, results. Sports Med Arthrosc 18:254–262

3. Ranawat A, Baker CL, Henry S, Harner CD (2008) Posterolateral corner injury of the knee: evaluation and management. J Am Acad Orthop Surg 16:506–518
4. Baker CL, Norwood LA, Hughston JC (1983) Acute posterolateral rotatory instability of the knee. J Bone Joint Surg Am 65:614–618
5. Veltri DM, Warren RF (1994) Operative treatment of posterolateral instability of the knee. Clin Sports Med 13:615–627
6. Covey DC (2001) Injuries of the posterolateral corner of the knee. J Bone Joint Surg Am 83-A:106–118
7. Harner CD, Vogrin TM, Höher J et al (2000) Biomechanical analysis of a posterior cruciate ligament reconstruction. Deficiency of the posterolateral structures as a cause of graft failure. Am J Sports Med 28:32–39
8. LaPrade RF, Resig S, Wentorf F, Lewis JL (1999) The effects of grade III posterolateral knee complex injuries on anterior cruciate ligament graft force. A biomechanical analysis. Am J Sports Med 27:469–475
9. Terry GC, LaPrade RF (1996) The posterolateral aspect of the knee. Anatomy and surgical approach. Am J Sports Med 24:732–739
10. Laprade RF, Griffith CJ, Coobs BR et al (2014) Improving outcomes for posterolateral knee injuries. J Orthop Res 32:485–491
11. Cooper JM, McAndrews PT, LaPrade RF (2006) Posterolateral corner injuries of the knee: anatomy, diagnosis, and treatment. Sports Med Arthrosc 14:213–220
12. Maynard MJ, Deng X, Wickiewicz TL, Warren RF (1996) The popliteofibular ligament. Rediscovery of a key element in posterolateral stability. Am J Sports Med 24:311–316
13. LaPrade RF, Ly TV, Wentorf FA, Engebretsen L (2003) The posterolateral attachments of the knee: a qualitative and quantitative morphologic analysis of the fibular collateral ligament, popliteus tendon, popliteofibular ligament, and lateral gastrocnemius tendon. Am J Sports Med 31:854–860
14. Gollehon DL, Torzilli PA, Warren RF (1987) The role of the posterolateral and cruciate ligaments in the stability of the human knee. A biomechanical study. J Bone Joint Surg Am 69:233–242
15. Veltri DM, Warren RF (1994) Anatomy, biomechanics, and physical findings in posterolateral knee instability. Clin Sports Med 13:599–614
16. Grood ES, Stowers SF, Noyes FR (1988) Limits of movement in the human knee. Effect of sectioning the posterior cruciate ligament and posterolateral structures. J Bone Joint Surg Am 70:88–97
17. Sugita T, Amis AA (2001) Anatomic and biomechanical study of the lateral collateral and popliteofibular ligaments. Am J Sports Med 29:466–472
18. LaPrade RF, Tso A, Wentorf FA (2004) Force measurements on the fibular collateral ligament, popliteofibular ligament, and popliteus tendon to applied loads. Am J Sports Med 32:1695–1701
19. Bowman KF, Sekiya JK (2010) Anatomy and biomechanics of the posterior cruciate ligament, medial and lateral sides of the knee. Sports Med Arthrosc 18: 222–229
20. Hughston JC, Andrews JR, Cross MJ, Moschi A (1976) Classification of knee ligament instabilities. Part II. The lateral compartment. J Bone Joint Surg Am 58:173–179
21. Levy BA, Boyd JL, Stuart MJ (2011) Surgical treatment of acute and chronic anterior and posterior cruciate ligament and lateral side injuries of the knee. Sports Med Arthrosc 19:110–119
22. Veltri DM, Deng XH, Torzilli PA et al (1995) The role of the cruciate and posterolateral ligaments in stability of the knee. A biomechanical study. Am J Sports Med 23:436–443
23. Hughston JC, Norwood LA (1980) The posterolateral drawer test and external rotational recurvatum test for posterolateral rotatory instability of the knee. Clin Orthop Relat Res 147:82–87
24. Bahk MS, Cosgarea AJ (2006) Physical examination and imaging of the lateral collateral ligament and posterolateral corner of the knee. Sports Med Arthrosc 14:12–19
25. Cooper DE (1991) Tests for posterolateral instability of the knee in normal subjects. Results of examination under anesthesia. J Bone Joint Surg Am 73:30–36
26. LaPrade RF, Heikes C, Bakker AJ, Jakobsen RB (2008) The reproducibility and repeatability of varus stress radiographs in the assessment of isolated fibular collateral ligament and grade-III posterolateral knee injuries. An in vitro biomechanical study. J Bone Joint Surg Am 90:2069–2076
27. Hall FM, Hochman MG (1997) Medial Segond-type fracture: cortical avulsion off the medial tibial plateau associated with tears of the posterior cruciate ligament and medial meniscus. Skeletal Radiol 26: 553–555
28. Bennett DL, George MJ, El-Khoury GY et al (2003) Anterior rim tibial plateau fractures and posterolateral corner knee injury. Emerg Radiol 10:76–83
29. Cohen AP, King D, Gibbon AJ (2001) Impingement fracture of the anteromedial tibial margin: a radiographic sign of combined posterolateral complex and posterior cruciate ligament disruption. Skeletal Radiol 30:114–116
30. Gottsegen CJ, Eyer BA, White EA et al (2008) Avulsion fractures of the knee: imaging findings and clinical significance. Radiographics 28:1755–1770
31. Shindell R, Walsh WM, Connolly JF (1984) Avulsion fracture of the fibula: the "arcuate sign" of posterolateral knee instability. Nebr Med J 69:369–371
32. Lee J, Papakonstantinou O, Brookenthal KR et al (2003) Arcuate sign of posterolateral knee injuries: anatomic, radiographic, and MR imaging data related to patterns of injury. Skeletal Radiol 32:619–627
33. Huang G-S, Yu JS, Munshi M et al (2003) Avulsion fracture of the head of the fibula (the "arcuate" sign): MR imaging findings predictive of injuries to the posterolateral ligaments and posterior cruciate ligament. AJR Am J Roentgenol 180:381–387
34. Yu JS, Salonen DC, Hodler J et al (1996) Posterolateral aspect of the knee: improved MR imaging with a coronal oblique technique. Radiology 198:199–204

35. LaPrade RF, Wentorf F (2002) Diagnosis and treatment of posterolateral knee injuries. Clin Orthop Relat Res 402:110–121
36. Murphy KP, Helgeson MD, Lehman RA (2006) Surgical treatment of acute lateral collateral ligament and posterolateral corner injuries. Sports Med Arthrosc 14:23–27
37. Hoppenfeld S, deBoer P, Buckley R (2012) Surgical exposures in orthopaedics: the anatomic approach. Wolters Kluwer Health, Philadelphia
38. Chen FS, Rokito AS, Pitman MI (2000) Acute and chronic posterolateral rotatory instability of the knee. J Am Acad Orthop Surg 8:97–110
39. Jackson D (2008) Reconstructive knee surgery. Wolters Kluwer Health/Lippincott Williams & Wilkins, Philadelphia
40. Dickens C (2011) The posterolateral corner: surgical approach and technique overview. Knee Surg 24(3): 151–158
41. Arciero RA (2005) Anatomic posterolateral corner knee reconstruction. Arthroscopy 21:1147
42. Fanelli GC, Edson CJ (2004) Combined posterior cruciate ligament-posterolateral reconstructions with Achilles tendon allograft and biceps femoris tendon tenodesis: 2- to 10-year follow-up. Arthroscopy 20: 339–345
43. Strobel MJ, Schulz MS, Petersen WJ, Eichhorn HJ (2006) Combined anterior cruciate ligament, posterior cruciate ligament, and posterolateral corner reconstruction with autogenous hamstring grafts in chronic instabilities. Arthroscopy 22:182–192
44. Schechinger SJ, Levy BA, Dajani KA et al (2009) Achilles tendon allograft reconstruction of the fibular collateral ligament and posterolateral corner. Arthroscopy 25:232–242
45. Hughston JC, Jacobson KE (1985) Chronic posterolateral rotatory instability of the knee. J Bone Joint Surg Am 67:351–359
46. Arthur A, LaPrade RF, Agel J (2007) Proximal tibial opening wedge osteotomy as the initial treatment for chronic posterolateral corner deficiency in the varus knee: a prospective clinical study. Am J Sports Med 35:1844–1850
47. Badhe NP, Forster IW (2002) High tibial osteotomy in knee instability: the rationale of treatment and early results. Knee Surg Sports Traumatol Arthrosc 10: 38–43
48. Phisitkul P, Wolf BR, Amendola A (2006) Role of high tibial and distal femoral osteotomies in the treatment of lateral-posterolateral and medial instabilities of the knee. Sports Med Arthrosc 14:96–104
49. Laprade RF, Engebretsen L, Johansen S et al (2008) The effect of a proximal tibial medial opening wedge osteotomy on posterolateral knee instability: a biomechanical study. Am J Sports Med 36:956–960
50. Stannard JP, Brown SL, Robinson JT et al (2005) Reconstruction of the posterolateral corner of the knee. Arthroscopy 21:1051–1059

Anterior Cruciate Ligament (ACL) Lesions

16

Pier Paolo Mariani, Guglielmo Cerullo, Germano Iannella, and Marco Giacobbe

16.1 Epidemiology

Soccer is currently the most popular sports with over 240 million participants worldwide, and unfortunately, soccer-related knee injuries are very common. The anterior cruciate ligament (ACL) is the most common ligament knee injury during soccer activity and usually causes long layoff from soccer [1]. The annual prevalence of ACL injury is reported to be between 0.5 % and 6.0 % of all female players and between 0.6 % and 8.5 % of all male players, respectively [2]. The frequency of ACL ruptures, whether expressed as an incidence or as an absolute value, is probably higher because the gathering of data on a large number of athletes with different age, gender, or level is actually impossible. Moreover, many other extrinsic factors such as differences of training, climate zones, exposure time to match play, and team level may reduce the statistical power of epidemiological analyses. Despite our little knowledge regarding incidence of ACL injury, soccer has a high rate of injury especially when compared to other types of sports. The etiology of ACL injuries includes a variety of intrinsic and extrinsic factors. The intrinsic factors, race and gender specific, are not modifiable and include hormonal issues, lower limb alignment, intercondylar notch size, ACL size, and joint laxity. In addition to these, there exist a variety of extrinsic factors such as environmental conditions, equipment, and athlete strength and conditioning.

16.1.1 Age

Injuries in young male soccer player are a major problem, and previous studies have observed that the injury rate is higher when compared to other team sports. There is a low frequency of ACL ruptures in elite young soccer players due to contact mechanism probably because the younger players develop less force during game situations. In nonelite young player, there is higher incidence of noncontact injuries. Low age at injury seems to be a special concern among female players, and the risk seems to be highest during the late pubertal or first postpubertal years [3].

16.1.2 Match Play

In soccer, match play is associated with a considerably higher ACL injury risk than training (10–27 times higher) [2]. The contact injury is the main mechanism of injury, and this occurs

P.P. Mariani (✉)
Università degli Studi di Roma "Foro Italico", Piazza L. De Bosis 15, 00194 Rome, Italy
e-mail: ppmariani@virgilio.it, ppmariani@uniroma4.it

G. Cerullo • G. Iannella • M. Giacobbe
Villa Stuart Sport Clinic, FIFA Medical Center, Rome, Italy

P. Volpi (ed.), *Football Traumatology: New Trends*, DOI 10.1007/978-3-319-18245-2_16

significantly more in matches than in training sessions. It has been supposed that congested periods of match play increases injury risk, but no association is observed between the time delay separating games and injury rate. Carling et al. [4] have shown that injury rate and layoff time in consecutive games separated by a short interval (≤3 days) are comparable to those after a longer interval (≥4 days). Interestingly, the injury rates and patterns varied substantially over the course of the playing season with overall injury incidence peaking in March that is the month with a busy match schedule. In addition, fatigue and lack of concentration may play a role. Match injuries resultant from player-to-player contact occurred significantly more in the second than in the first half. Playing position seems to be not a discriminatory factor influencing the risk of sustaining a rupture of the ACL [5, 6] even if Roos et al. [7] reported a greater risk of injury in forwards compared to midfielders and defenders.

16.1.3 Gender

Female football players have been shown to be more susceptible to an ACL injury in several cohort studies with an increased average risk among females of between two and eight times. Interestingly, this difference becomes significant only after the pubertal age. Several factors justify this increased rate of ACL injury: differences of dynamic knee stability, muscular strength, and an increased anteroposterior translation across the menstrual cycle. Moreover, gender difference in muscle activation patterns is present during running, jumping, landing, and cutting. Possible reasons for this significant incidence include extrinsic factors, such as muscle strength and hormonal differences, and intrinsic factors, such as joint laxity. Joint laxity is a heritable trait; increased magnitudes of anterior knee laxity, genu recurvatum, and general joint laxity have been consistently associated with a greater risk of ACL injury. Bell et al. [8], in a study on 50 males and 74 females, reported a relationship between presence of several collagen gene variants and anterior cruciate ligament injury, but the mechanism of these relationship is still unclear. Joint laxity may constitute an important intermediate phenotype for the genetic association with ACL injury that can be measured clinically. Other biomechanical studies suggest that the valgus knee is a factor of injury risk due to the torque applied to the knee joint. Kobayashi et al. [9] analyzed the data of more than 1,700 athletes (838 males and 880 females) with an ACL injury in order to confirm the relationship between the ACL injury occurrence and the dynamic alignment of the lower extremity. The number of the subjects with the alignment of "knee-in and toe-out" was the largest (793/1,603), followed by "unclear" and "knee-out and toe-in" and "hyperextension" in this order.

16.1.4 Level

In some studies, ACL injury risk has been reported to be higher at the elite level of play compared to lower levels [10–13]: a men's team at the highest playing level can expect around 0.4 ACL injuries per season.

16.1.5 Ground

In recent years, the number of soccer field with artificial turf has increased dramatically. Currently, there are over 256 million soccer players of both genders worldwide [14]. This increase is mainly due to that more fields are available throughout the year independent of the weather conditions. Beyond the seasonal advantages, there are financial benefits, such as reduced maintenance costs and the development of mixed-use sports facilities in which different events (training or competition, young or senior, male or female) can take place. However, soccer players frequently voice their criticisms toward artificial turf for difficulty with ball control and perceive higher physical effort when playing on artificial turf compared to natural grass [15]. Additionally, there is a general perception that the risk of injury is higher on artificial turf than on natural grass, a feeling that has not been fully confirmed in epidemiological investigations [16,17]. From the literature, the injuries in the lower extremity, resultant from both body contact and noncontact situations, affected mostly the dominant compared to the non-dominant side. When playing on artificial turf, fewer sliding tackles are expected [18], but the dominant lower limb is still at increased risk of injury, mainly because it is preferentially used for kicking, pushing off, jumping, and landing. Nonetheless, the proportion of traumatic and overuse injuries observed on artificial turf is similar to the values reported on natural grass [16, 19].

16.2 Injury Mechanism

Several studies have attempted to identify factors predisposing to ACL injury, and the mechanism of injury during competition is the subject of intense and ongoing researches. There are two different injury mechanisms: contact and noncontact. The first mechanism is mainly the result of a direct blow applied to the proximal tibia with anteroposterior direction. Typical examples of this mechanism are front or side tackles in soccer. Most soccer-related ACL injuries seem to result from a noncontact injury mechanism with reported frequencies up to 84 %. In noncontact mechanism, the two most commonly described injury situations in soccer are turning of the trunk with the foot fixed to the ground (pivoting) or landing awkwardly from a jump [20]. In earlier studies, the frequency of contact injuries in male soccer players was shown to be similar to that of injuries without contact between players [10,21]. It is difficult to suggest reasons for this decrease over recent years in the rate of contact injuries leading to an ACL rupture. Modifications in the rules of the game concerning serious foul play may have led to an increased level of protection and therefore to a reduced risk of injury. The risk of sustaining an ACL injury during other locomotor activities such as acceleration/cutting movements was common in groups at lower standards of play such as in under 15, veteran, and leisure-time players. This finding suggests that players with lesser physical and/or technical ability are more susceptible to ACL injury in certain match situations.

In a review of literature from 1950 through 2007, Griffin et al. [22] demonstrated noncontact ACL injuries are likely to happen during deceleration and acceleration motions with excessive quadriceps contraction and reduced hamstrings cocontraction at or near full knee extension. The ACL loading is higher when a valgus load is combined with internal rotation as compared with external rotation. However, because the combination of knee valgus and external rotation motions may lead to ACL impingement, these combined motions cannot be excluded from the noncontact ACL injury mechanisms. Further, decelerating activities increase ACL loading for excessive valgus knee loads applied during weight-bearing. Anterior cruciate ligament injuries often happen when an individual attempts to decelerate the body from a jump or forward running while the knee is in a shallow flexion angle. The ACL has been widely known to be loaded with anterior tibial shear forces [23–25]. Unopposed quadriceps muscle forces produce anterior shear forces, possibly damaging the ACL, especially near full extension [26, 27]. On the other hand, hamstrings cocontraction forces are protective to the ACL, increasing knee stability while the quadriceps are contracting. An ACL injury often occurs when the body is positioned with the weight back on the heel, which may increase the quadriceps contraction force and reduce the efficacy of the hamstrings [27]. Because a combination of knee external rotation and valgus motions may impinge the ACL against the femoral intercondylar notch and because these motions have been often observed during noncontact ACL injury, knee external rotation remains an important consideration for ACL injury [28]. At this point, it is not possible to definitively conclude which motions are more problematic for ACL injuries. Yet the results of studies to date demonstrate the importance of focusing not only on the combination of knee valgus and external rotation motion but also on knee internal rotation motion during dynamic motion [29–31].

16.3 Clinical and Diagnostic Examination

Evaluation of the patient starts with the history. An acute ACL tear history is very familiar to the knee surgeon and usually the athlete refers of a "pop" or "crack" with pain in a pivoting movement, often in noncontact type, while playing the sports and also describes the knee as "coming apart." Mild or marked effusion occurs within 6–12 h after trauma. However, some ACL tears happen with minor trauma, no internal sensation, and no or minimal effusion and mild pain. An athlete with a chronic ACL history often refers of pain from a meniscal tear or cartilage damage, with minimal instability in pivoting activities and mild effusion after training or competition. However, a top-level athlete refers very unusual a history of chronic instability as in case of ACL injury he is promptly treated with surgical reconstruction. Chronic instability can occur more often after ACL if not a good stability was achieved with surgical operation.

16.3.1 Lachman Test

Lachman test is considered the most reliable and reproducible method of investigation to confirm an ACL tear, as it has in acute a sensitivity of 78–99 % [32]. In acute injuries of top-level athletes, with large muscular thigh or hamstrings spasm, the Lachman test is not simple to perform and often is unpredictable unless a firm end-point is felt to exclude an ACL tear. We prefer to perform also the prone Lachman test [33] in which gravity assists the forward movement of the tibia, hip extension stabilizes the femur, and relaxation is enhanced by the contact of quadriceps with the table. The patient is prone, the knee is held 20° or 30° flexed and the examiner's hands grasp the tibia, and the fingers are positioned in the joint line. Anteroposterior tibiofemoral movement is attempted; its interpretation and the quality of end-point are no different from that when the patient is supine.

16.3.2 Pivot Shift

Pivot shift is a specific but very insensitive test for acute ACL injury in the non-anesthetized patient [34, 35] and also subject to interobserver error, and we use it in operating room under anesthesia to evaluate rotatory instability. In soccer player, we perform an additional anterolateral plasty in case of marked positivity. Valgus, varus, and posterior laxity are also examined in the routine manner.

For instrumental evaluation of anteroposterior translation, we routinely use an **arthrometer**. In the past, we have used for many years the KT-1000 or KT-2000 (MED Metric Corp, San Diego, Ca, USA) arthrometer, but we are now using GNRB (GeNouRob, Laval, France) that some studies have demonstrated to have a superior intra- and interexaminer reproducibility over the KT-1000 and examiner independency [36]. With this later arthrometer, it is possible to differentiate also a partial tear of ACL [37].

16.3.3 Magnetic Resonance Imaging (MRI)

Magnetic resonance imaging (MRI) is an invaluable test to the diagnosis of an ACL injury as it has a specificity of 95 % and a sensibility of 86 % with normal coronal, axial, and sagittal views [38]. We are routinely using the oblique coronal and oblique sagittal images for their improved accuracy [39] in the evaluation of the ACL. Normal ACL is distinctly seen while when acutely injured appears as indistinct and/or lax structure. MRI is also useful in ruling out other internal derangements detect [40]. Segond's fracture, visible also in anteroposterior X-ray, reveals avulsion of the anterolateral ligament [41, 42] that in some case needs to be refixed or reconstructed.

16.4 Treatment Strategy

16.4.1 Indications

In soccer activity that requires cutting, jumping, and pivoting stress, it is mandatory to carry out the reconstruction after an ACL tear. It is well documented in literature that early ligament reconstruction reduces the risk of subsequent meniscal injury, especially in athletic population. Sports activity predisposes early damage of all static structures. Therefore, in ACL tear, surgical treatment is our indication for all athletes who want to continue playing soccer. Despite the natural history of partial ACL tears is quite good over the medium term in the patients that limit their sports activities, functional instability seems to progress with time, especially in athletic population [43]. Therefore, also in case of ACL partial tear, our indication is an ACL reconstruction.

16.4.2 Timing

In the past, initial concern existed over early reconstruction of ACL injury because of the increased risk for arthrofibrosis, and the surgery was delayed until minimal swelling, good leg control, and full range of motion were achieved. Top-level athletes request early surgery in order to reduce the time of layoff from their activity. Moreover, in presence of associated injuries such as meniscal or collateral ligaments tears, immediate suture repair gives better results than delayed repair. For these reasons, we prefer a surgical reconstruction in all athletes, and we pay careful attention to postoperative pain control and to a more aggressive rehabilitative protocol with early continuous passive motion and active muscles exercises [44].

16.4.3 Graft

The central third of patella tendon (bone-patellar tendon-bone) is our first autograft choice in top-level athletes both in male and female. The main reason of this choice is the achievement of biological fixation, bone to bone, that allows an accelerated protocol of rehabilitation when a prompt return to sports is required. In soccer players who are frequently subjected to hamstring lesions, concerns have been raised that harvesting the semitendinosus (ST) tendon may result in an increased risk for subsequent muscular injuries. For this reason, this graft is harvested only in the revisional surgery. We don't use allografts in our primary ACL reconstruction for concern regarding time of return to play. Moreover, recently on the basis of their large retrospective cohort, Krych et al. [45] recommend the use of autogenous grafts in active patients because the proportion of subjects able to return to their preinjury activity levels is higher among autografts compared with allografts.

16.4.4 Surgical Procedure

Surgical treatment of ACL tears has evolved over the past century. Several techniques and methods of fixation have been described, and a detailed description of all procedures is impossible. Our preferred method of ACL reconstruction is a single-bundle arthroscopic transtibial technique. Following an initial arthroscopic examination that confirms ACL rupture, the meniscal lesions are searched and treated. When possible, a meniscal suture is always carried out. A vertical central skin incision is made from the center of the patella to the tibial tubercle. The deep fascia is incised and divided to expose the patella tendon that is harvested 10 mm in width with patellar (20 mm in length) and tibial (30 mm in length) bone plugs. During the harvesting, the knee is held in flexion so that the tendon fibers are straight due to tension. An oscillating saw is used to make the bone cuts, and in the professional athletes, we perform an oblique cut in order to avoid abnormal stress and the potential risk of patellar fracture (Fig. 16.1). The tibial tunnel is drilled with the knee in full extension using a Howell tibial guide (Arthrotek Inc., Warsaw, IN, USA). An impingement rod is used to avoid the femoral roof to impinge on the graft and notchplasty performed, if necessary, with an abrader. The femoral tunnel is drilled through the tibial tunnel with the knee flexed at 90° on a pin guide located in the center of the anatomical ACL insertion (at 10 o'clock for right knee and 2 o'clock for left knee, 7 mm anterior to the

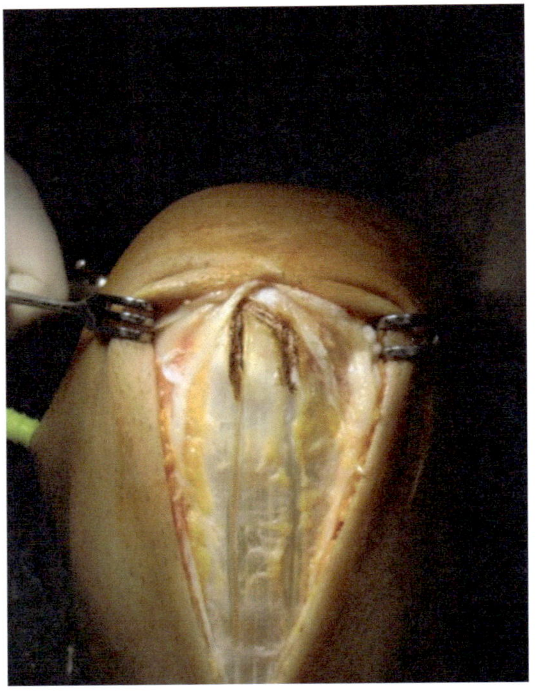

Fig. 16.1 Oblique cut of patellar bone block in order to reduce risk of patellar fracture after ACL reconstruction

posterior margin of the lateral femoral condyle) [46]. Sometime it is difficult to reach the anatomical point with the femoral transtibial guide. In this case, after the first pin was positioned with the guide, the second pin is positioned lower, in the right place, with the aid of a cannulated transtibial corrector. Another possibility is to drill the femoral tunnel through the anteromedial portal. The graft, armed at the patellar plug with X-endobutton (Smith & Nephew) and at the tibial plug with two sutures, is passed through the tunnels and the button flipped over the lateral femoral cortex. The knee is repeatedly extended and flexed to allow stress relaxation of the graft. With the knee flexed at 20°, the graft is tensioned at 80 N and fixed with an absorbable interference screw in the tibial tunnel. In case of gross anterolateral rotatory instability (jerk test +++), we are currently using a lateral additional procedure to improve knee stability. Our preferred techniques are the ITB extra-articular tenodesis described by Noyes [47] or by Christel and Djian [48].

16.4.5 Rehabilitation After ACL Reconstruction

The importance of a rehabilitation program cannot be underestimated, and although there is no one rehabilitation program proven to be superior to others, the speed and safety with which an athlete returns to play are more dependent upon the rehabilitation program than whether the patient had arthroscopically assisted or two-incision technique or what type of graft or fixation was used. Rehabilitation has undergone a relatively rapid and global evolution over the past years. Traditionally, rehabilitation is divided into three distinct phases based on experimental study performed by Amiel et al. [49] on biological process of graft implanted into a joint, process called *ligamentization*. For this reason, after surgery many rehabilitative protocols have relied on protection of the reconstructed ligament by limiting knee extension, weight-bearing, and the return to strenuous activities. On contrary, some amounts of strain and force applied to the ACL are necessary to enhance the process of graft maturation. Question regarding the ideal amount of load that could be necessary is still without answer. Moreover, only few studies on the ligamentization process of the grafts have been conducted in humans, and this prevents to draw conclusions on when the process ends in the human. Current rehabilitative programs following ACL reconstruction are now more aggressive than those utilized in the 1980s. Presently, in soccer players we employ an accelerated protocol that can be administrated only if the athlete may follow the protocol under the supervision of an expert therapist. The progression through the various phases of rehabilitation and the period of time necessary prior to running and sports is based more on achievement of specific and tailored drills than on a time frame.

Our current program emphasizes full passive knee extension, immediate motion, immediate full weight-bearing, and functional exercises mainly during the first postoperative period. As demonstrated by Zech et al. [50], it is during the first postoperative month that voluntary activation and quadriceps weakness show significant deficit. For this reason, we believe that an aggressive rehabilitation is important mainly during the 1st month.

16.4.5.1 Active and Passive Motion

After the surgery, the athlete starts to perform passive and active knee extension exercises. Immediate motion decreases pain and postoperative joint effusions, aids in the prevention of adhesions, and decreases muscle disuse effects.

16.4.5.2 Full Weight Bearing

It is permitted without crutches. If no other procedures have been performed, the weight-bearing is permitted and facilitates quicker return of quadriceps function and subsequent decrease in anterior knee pain and without deleterious effect on knee stability [51].

16.4.5.3 Brace

Despite conflicts in the literature, we recommend to discharge as soon as possible the use of postoperative brace in full extension. Immobilization has deleterious effects on muscle and synthesis of new collagen, and for this reason, the brace is allowed while ambulating and sleeping only during the first 2 weeks after surgery, and the athlete is encouraged to discharge the brace as soon as possible.

16.4.5.4 Functional Exercises

Strengthening is performed during this phase using both *closed-chain exercises (CKC)* and selective use of *open-chain exercises (OKC)*. It is generally thought that the biomechanical environment of the healing graft can be optimized by prescribing CKC exercises and avoiding OKC exercises because in cadaveric studies isolated quadriceps exercises produce harmful forces on healing ACL graft [52, 53] and that the range of 0° to 30° should be avoided during the rehabilitation. CKC exercises have been justified because they: (1) increase tibiofemoral compressive forces, (2) increase cocontraction of the hamstrings, (3) mimic functional activities more closely than OKC exercises, and (4) reduce the incidence of patellofemoral complications [54]. On contrary, clinical evidence have shown that the addition of OKC quadriceps training after ACL reconstruction results in a significantly better improvement in quadriceps torque without reducing knee joint stability at 6 months and also leads to a significantly higher number of athletes returning to their previous activity earlier and at the same level as before injury [55]. In our protocol, we prescribe OKC and CKC exercises in the early phase of rehabilitation, and athletes are encouraged to progress by increasing resistance or duration as soon as they are able to perform exercises without demonstrating an extension lag or discomfort. Neuromuscular training, including proprioceptive and balance training, is added and progressed as tolerated. Once strength and neuromuscular control have been demonstrated, neuromuscular control drills are gradually advanced to include dynamic stabilization and controlled perturbation training. Functional activities such as running and cutting may begin 4–6 weeks after surgery. On the 2nd or the 3rd month after surgery, the last phase of ACL rehabilitation that involves the restoration of function through sports-specific training is allowed. Some sports-specific running and agility drills include side shuffling, cariocas, sudden starts and stops, zigzags, 45° cutting, and 90° cutting.

In order to ensure a safe progression, we carry out tests throughout all rehabilitative course in order to provide objective criteria for advancement from one phase to the following. Testing procedures also follow a progression, which begins with basic measures after the 1st month and progresses to functional tests of increasing difficulty that include sports-specific testing before returning to field play. Table 16.1 summarizes the progression of evaluations performed throughout all different phases.

16.4.6 Return to Play

We do not release players until muscle and functional objective measurements have been achieved regardless of the amount of time that

Table 16.1 Progression of evaluations performed during the different phases of postoperative rehabilitation

	15 days	30 days	45 days	60 days	90 days	6 m.
ROM	+	+				
Single limb squat	+	+	+			
Sit-to-stand test	+	+	+			
Vertical jump			+	+	+	+
MVIC		+	+	+	+	+
Squat jump			+	+	+	+
Y balance			+	+	+	+
Riva test			+	+	+	+
GeNouRob					+	+
Single-leg hop					+	+
Triple hop					+	+
Isokinetic					+	+
Pro-shuttle test					+	+
MAT					+	+

has passed since surgery. Standardized criteria for return to play after ACL injury are still missing, and no one single outcome criterion has been correlated with successful return to sports. Most clinicians use a combination of criteria, namely, functional, clinical, and subjective testing. In our practice, we use two different criteria: first is general criteria such as achievement of full range of motion, negative pivot-shift test, absence of swelling or pain, and stability as measured by an arthrometer. A 3 mm, side-to-side difference is associated with an unstable knee. Arthrometric results do not necessarily correlate with subjective or objective outcome criteria. However, increased knee laxity is a cause for concern, because it is associated with altered contact loading of the articular surfaces and possible inferior structural properties of the graft. Decisions regarding return to play should not be made solely on arthrometric data. We routinely recommend an MRI evaluation of the graft at 3 months postoperatively. The specific functional criteria include three different types of evaluations: muscular, neuromuscular, and athletic. The tests for the muscular strength include the MVIC (maximal voluntary isometric contraction) test that we consider satisfactory if it is 80 % or more of that of the contralateral side and the isokinetic evaluation. The general rule is that in an athlete's hamstrings, mean LSI (limb symmetry index) values for isokinetic knee flexion should be in the range of 80–90 % at 6 months and near normal values at 1 year. For isokinetic knee extension, the values should be in the 75 % range at 6 month, but they remain below 90 % at or after 1 year [56]. The most common functional tests are the one-leg single hop for distance, the one-leg triple hop for distance, the one-leg timed hop, and the one-leg cross-over hop for distance. The one-leg single hop is an indicator of power, whereas the other three tests indicate both power and endurance. The results are compared with the uninjured leg. The results of hoping tests are an objective measurement of knee function, but have not correlation with RTP [57]. Review of the literature supports that a measurement of 80–85 % of the uninjured leg is advisable before returning to sports. Objective assessment of static and dynamic balance may be performed using computerized instrumentation on the Biodex Balance System that provides a high degree of statistical validity and reliability in determining postural sway differences between limbs. Star excursion balance test (SEBT) has been shown to be reliable and valid in determining postural deficits and is used to evaluate dynamic balance (Fig. 16.2) [58, 59]. For the functional on-field tests, we prescribe the MAT (modified agility test) that may accurately identify the differences between the involved and not involved limb. The player should attain a 10 % of symmetry in the time taken to complete the test.

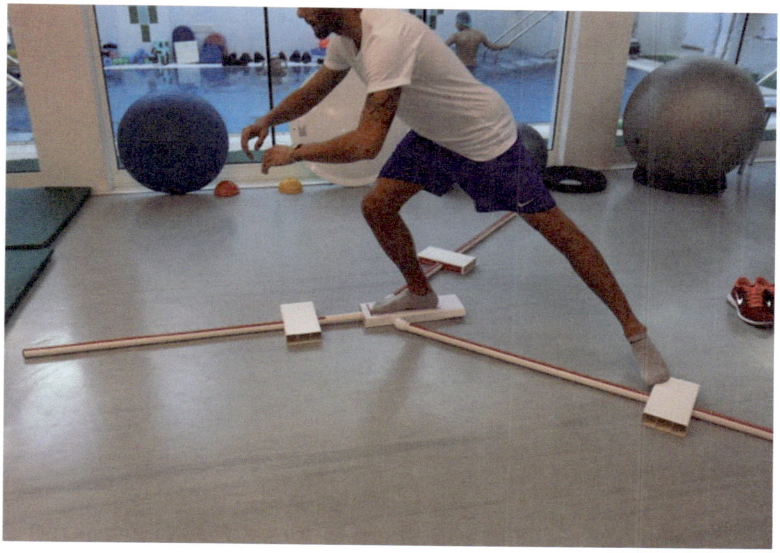

Fig. 16.2 Star excursion balance test form to assess dynamic postural control

References

1. Linko E, Harilainen A, Malmivaara A et al (2005) Surgical versus conservative interventions for anterior cruciate ligament ruptures in adults. Cochrane Database Syst Rev 18(2):CD001356
2. Waldèn M, Hagglund M, Werner J et al (2011) The epidemiology of anterior cruciate ligament injury in football (soccer): a review of the literature from a gender-related perspective. Knee Surg Sports Traumatol Arthrosc 19:3–10
3. Shea KG, Pfeiffer R, Wang JH et al (2004) Anterior cruciate ligament injury in pediatric and adolescent soccer players: an analysis of insurance data. J Pediatr Orthop 24:623–628
4. Carling C, Orhant E, Le Gall F (2010) Match injuries in professional soccer: inter-seasonal variation and effects of competition type, match congestion and positional role. Int J Sports Med 31:271–276
5. Ekstrand J, Gillquist J, Moller M (1983) Incidence of soccer injuries and their relation to training and team success. Am J Sports Med 11:63–67
6. Faude O, Junge A, Kindermann W et al (2006) Risk factors for injuries in elite female soccer players. Br J Sports Med 40:785–790
7. Roos H, Ornell M, Gardsell P et al (1995) Soccer after anterior cruciate ligament injury: an incompatible combination? Acta Orthop Scand 66:107–112
8. Bell RD, Shultz SJ, Wideman L et al (2012) Collagen gene variants previously associated with anterior cruciate ligament injury risk are also associated with joint laxity. Sports Health 4:312–318
9. Kobayashi H, Kanamura T, Koshida S et al (2010) Mechanisms of the anterior cruciate ligament injury in sports activities: a twenty-year clinical research of 1,700 athletes. J Sports Sci Med 9:669–675
10. Bjordal JM, Arnöy F, Hannestad B et al (1997) Epidemiology of anterior cruciate ligament injuries in soccer. Am J Sports Med 25:341–345
11. Azubuike SO, Okcjie OH (2009) An epidemiological study of football (soccer) injuries in Benin City, Nigeria. Br J Sports Med 43(5):382–386
12. Rochcongar P, Laboute E, Carling C (2009) Ruptures of the anterior cruciate ligament in soccer. Int J Sports Med 30:372–378
13. Hagglund M, Walden M, Ekstrand J (2009) UEFA injury study-an injury audit of European Championships 2006 to 2008. Br J Sports Med 43(7):483–489
14. FIFA (2011) Fédération internationale de football association e quality concept for football turf. consult. 10 Jun 2011. disponível em. http://www.fifa.com
15. Andersson H, Ekblom B, Krustrup P (2008) Elite football on artificial turf versus natural grass: movement patterns, technical standards, and player impressions. J Sports Sci 26(2):113–122
16. Aoki H, Kohno T, Fujiya H et al (2010) Incidence of injury among adolescent soccer players: a comparative study of artificial and natural grass turfs. Clin J Sport Med 20(1):1–7
17. Bjorneboe J, Bahr R, Andersen T (2010) Risk of injury on third-generation artificial turf in Norwegian professional football. Br J Sports Med 44(11):794–798
18. Ekstrand J, Hagglund M, Fuller C (2011) Comparison of injuries sustained on artificial turf and grass by male and female elite football players. Scand J Med Sci Sports 21(6):824–832
19. Arnason A, Tenga A, Engebretsen L et al (2004) A prospective video-based analysis of injury situations in elite male football: football incident analysis. Am J Sports Med 32(6):1459–1465
20. Faunø P, Wulff Jakobsen B (2006) Mechanism of anterior cruciate ligament injuries in soccer. Int J Sports Med 27:75–79

21. Arendt E, Dick R (1995) Knee injury patterns among men and women in collegiate basketball and soccer. Am J Sports Med 23:694–701
22. Griffin LY, Agel J, Albohm MJ et al (2000) Noncontact anterior cruciate ligament injuries: risk factors and prevention strategies. J Am Acad Orthop Surg 8(3): 141–150
23. McNair PJ, Marshall RN, Matheson JA (1990) Important features associated with acute anterior cruciate ligament injury. N Z Med J 103(901):537–539
24. Livesay GA, Rudy TW, Woo SL et al (1997) Evaluation of the effect of joint constraints on the in situ force distribution in the anterior cruciate ligament. J Orthop Res 15(2):278–284
25. Sakane M, Livesay GA, Fox RJ et al (1999) Relative contribution of the ACL, MCL, and bony contact to the anterior stability of the knee. Knee Surg Sports Traumatol Arthrosc 7(2):93–97
26. Draganich LF, Vahey JW (1990) An in vitro study of anterior cruciate ligament strain induced by quadriceps and hamstring forces. J Orthop Res 8(1):57–63
27. Markolf KL, O'Neill G, Jackson SR et al (2004) Effects of applied quadriceps and hamstrings muscle loads on forces in the anterior and posterior cruciate ligaments. Am J Sports Med 32(5):1144–1149
28. Fung DT, Zhang LQ (2003) Modeling of ACL impingement against the intercondylar notch. Clin Biomech (Bristol, Avon) 18(10):933–941
29. Shimokochi Y, Shultz SJ (2008) Mechanisms of noncontact anterior cruciate ligament injury. J Athl Train 43(4):396–408
30. Burkhart B, Ford KR, Myer GD et al (2008) Anterior cruciate ligament tear in an athlete: does increased heel loading contribute to ACL rupture? J Sports Phys Ther 3(3):141–144
31. Boden BP, Griffin LY, Garrett WE (2000) Etiology and prevention of noncontact ACL injury. Phys Sportsmed 28:53–60
32. Torg JS, Conrad W, Kalen V (1976) Clinical diagnosis of anterior cruciate ligament instability in the athlete. Am J Sports Med 4(2):84–93
33. Feagin JA, Cooke TD (1989) Prone examination for anterior cruciate ligament insufficiency. J Bone Joint Surg Br 71(5):863
34. Benjaminse A, Gokeler A, van der Schans CP (2006) Clinical diagnosis of an anterior cruciate ligament rupture: a meta-analysis. J Orthop Sports Phys Ther 36(5):267–288
35. van Eck CF, van den Bekerom MP, Fu FH et al (2013) Methods to diagnose acute anterior cruciate ligament rupture: a meta-analysis of physical examinations with and without anaesthesia. Knee Surg Sports Traumatol Arthrosc 21(8):1895–1903
36. Robert H, Nouveau S, Gageot S et al (2009) A new knee arthrometer, the GNRB: experience in ACL complete and partial tears. Orthop Traumatol Surg Res 95(3):171–176
37. Collette M, Courville J, Forton M et al (2012) Objective evaluation of anterior knee laxity; comparison of the KT-1000 and GNRB arthrometers. Knee Surg Sports Traumatol Arthrosc 20(11):2233–2238
38. Spindler KP, Wright RW (2008) Clinical practice. Anterior cruciate ligament tear. N Engl J Med 359(20):2135–2142
39. Kosaka M, Nakase J, Toratani T et al (2014) Oblique coronal and oblique sagittal MRI for diagnosis of anterior cruciate ligament tears and evaluation of anterior cruciate ligament remnant tissue. Knee 21(1):54–57
40. Dimond PM, Fadale PD, Hulstyn MJ et al (1998) A comparison of MRI findings in patients with acute and chronic ACL tears. Am J Knee Surg 11(3): 153–159
41. Irvine GB, Dias JJ, Finlay DB (1987) Segond fractures of the lateral tibial condyle: brief report. J Bone Joint Surg Br 69(4):613–614
42. Vincent JP, Magnussen RA, Gezmez F et al (2012) The anterolateral ligament of the human knee: an anatomic and histologic study. Knee Surg Sports Traumatol Arthrosc 20(1):147–152
43. Pujol N, Colombet P, Cucurulo T et al (2012) Natural history of partial anterior cruciate ligament tears: a systematic literature review. Orthop Traumatol Surg Res 98(Suppl8):S160–S164
44. Andernord D, Karlsson J, Musahl V et al (2013) Timing of surgery of the anterior cruciate ligament. Arthroscopy 29(11):1863–1871
45. Krych AJ, Jackson JD, Hoskin TL et al (2008) A meta-analysis of patellar tendon autograft versus patellar tendon allograft in anterior cruciate ligament reconstruction. Arthroscopy 24(3):292–298
46. Cain EL Jr, Clancy WG Jr (2002) Anatomic endoscopic anterior cruciate ligament reconstruction with patella tendon autograft. Orthop Clin North Am 33(4):717–725
47. Noyes FR (2010) ITB extra-articular tenodesis. In: Noyes FR (ed) Noyes' knee disorders: surgery, rehabilitation, clinical outcomes. Saunders/Elsevier, Philadelphia, pp 170–172
48. Christel P, Djian P (2002) Plastie extra articulaire antero latérale du genou utilisant une ténodèse courte au fascia-lata. Rev Chir Orthop Rep Appar Mot 88: 508–513
49. Amiel D, Kleiner JB, Roux RD, Harwood FL et al (1986) The phenomenon of "ligamentization": anterior cruciate ligament reconstruction with autogenous patellar tendon. J Orthop Res 4:162–172
50. Zech A, Awiswu F, Pfeifer K (2009) Longitudinal changes of neuromuscular quadriceps function after reconstruction of the anterior cruciate ligament. Curr Orthop Pract 20(3):276–280
51. Tyler TF, McHugh MP, Gleim GW et al (1998) The effect of immediate weightbearing after anterior cruciate ligament reconstruction. Clin Orthop Relat Res 357:141–148
52. Grood ES, Suntay WJ, Noyes FR et al (1984) Biomechanics of the knee-extension exercise. Effect of cutting the anterior cruciate ligament. J Bone Joint Surg Am 66(5):725–734
53. Mikkelsen C, Werner S, Eriksson E (2000) Closed kinetic chain alone compared to combined open and closed kinetic chain exercises for quadriceps

strengthening after anterior cruciate ligament reconstruction with respect to return to sports: a prospective matched follow-up study. Knee Surg Sports Traumatol Arthrosc 8(6):337–342

54. Perry MC, Morrissey MC, King JB et al (2005) Effects of closed versus open kinetic chain knee extensor resistance training on knee laxity and leg function in patients during the 8- to 14-week post-operative period after anterior cruciate ligament reconstruction. Knee Surg Sports Traumatol Arthrosc 13(5):357–369
55. Seto JL, Orofino AS, Morrissey MC et al (1988) Assessment of quadriceps/hamstring strength, knee ligament stability, functional and sports activity levels five years after anterior cruciate ligament reconstruction. Am J Sports Med 16:170–180
56. Thomeé R, Kaplan Y, Kvist J et al (2011) Muscle strength and hop performance criteria prior to return to sports after ACL reconstruction. Knee Surg Sports Traumatol Arthrosc 19(11):1798–1805
57. Schmitt LC, Paterno MV, Hewett TE (2012) The impact of quadriceps femoris strength asymmetry on functional performance at return to sport following anterior cruciate ligament reconstruction. J Orthop Sports Phys Ther 42(9):750–759
58. Kinzey SJ, Armstrong CW (1998) The reliability of the star-excursion test in assessing dynamic balance. J Orthop Sports Phys Ther 27(5):356–360
59. Plisky PJ, Rauh MJ, Kaminski TW et al (2006) Star excursion balance test as a predictor of lower extremity injury in high school basketball players. J Orthop Sports Phys Ther 36(12):911–919

17 Anterior Cruciate Ligament Lesions in Adolescent

Corrado Bait, Matteo Denti, A. Orgiani, G. Carimati, and Piero Volpi

17.1 Introduction

Football is acknowledged as the most popular sport worldwide with more than 270 million active players, of whom 10 % are females (data report from *The Big Count* survey, 2006 http://www.fifa.com). Anterior cruciate ligament (ACL) injury is a rather unusual football injury rarely constituting more than 5 % of all time loss injuries regardless of the playing level [1].

But in the last two decades, the increased involvement of children and adolescents beginning at an early age to play an organized sport raises concern regarding risk and severity of sport injury, mostly ligament injuries.

C. Bait (✉) • M. Denti, MD • A. Orgiani
G. Carimati
Knee Surgery and Sport Traumatology,
Humanitas Research - IRCCS,
Milan, Italy
e-mail: corrado.bait@humanitas.it;
matteo@denti.ch.it

P. Volpi
Knee Orthopedics and Sport Traumatology Unit,
Humanitas Clinical Institute IRCCS,
Milan, Italy

Head of Medical Staff FC Internazionale Milan,
Milan, Italy
e-mail: piero.volpi@humanitas.it

In the child-adolescent age group, an intrinsic risk factor for this type of pathology is the increased capsular ligament laxity that is constitutional in children. In addition, the physical stress associated with frequent and intense training as well as participation in contact sports (soccer, basketball, rugby) or other high-risk sports (alpine-ski, volleyball) is an extrinsic risk factor for ACL injuries.

17.2 Risk Factors

ACL injury risk in young athletes is probably multifactorial. Injury data from many fields demonstrate that numerous physical and psychological parameters affect ACL injury rates. Although ACL injury rates increase with age in both genders, girls have higher rates immediately after their growth spurt. It is likely that increases in body weight, height, and bone length during pubertal development underlie the mechanism of increased risk of ACL injury with increasing age. During puberty, the tibia and femur grow at a rapid rate. This growth of the two longest levers in the human body translates into greater torques on the knee. In pubertal boys, testosterone mediates significant increases in muscular power, strength, and coordination, which affords them with greater neuromuscular control of these larger body dimensions. Pubertal girls do not experience this same growth spurt in muscular power, strength, and coordination, which might

P. Volpi (ed.), *Football Traumatology: New Trends*, DOI 10.1007/978-3-319-18245-2_17

explain their higher rates of ACL injuries compared with pubertal boys. Hormonal factors are also likely to play a role; however, results from studies investigating hormonal factors are both equivocal and controversial. Although the female knee appears to get slightly more lax, on the order of 0.5 mm, at midmenstrual cycle, injuries tend to cluster near the start of menses at the polar opposite time in the cycle [2]. Activation of the quadriceps before the hamstrings, a pattern more frequently seen in female individuals, increases the anterior shear force that directly loads the ACL and also could be related to increased dynamic valgus alignment at initial contact during cutting and landing maneuvers. Although fatigue is often cited as a potential risk factor for ACL injury, there are relatively few published studies to support or refute this [3, 4], certainly a greater weight and BMI have been associated with increased risk of ACL injury. A narrow intercondylar notch, where the ACL is housed, is proposed to increase ACL injury risk, because a narrow notch tends to be associated with a smaller, weaker ACL and also could cause increased elongation of the ACL under high tension. Some studies have shown that a narrow notch increases risk of ACL injury. However, others have shown no association between notch width and ACL injury [5, 6]. Subtalar joint overpronation,*flat foot,* has been associated with noncontact ACL injuries, probably because overpronation increases anterior translation of the tibia with respect to the femur, thereby increasing the strain on the ACL [7]. Generalized joint laxity and knee hyperextension were found to significantly increase the risk for ACL injury in female soccer players. Patients with ACL injury have significantly more knee recurvatum at 10° and 90° of hip flexion and an increased ability to touch palms to floor. Athletes with generalized joint laxity had a 2.7 times greater risk of ACL injury than did those without generalized laxity, and those with increased anterior-posterior laxity of the knee, as measured by a knee arthrometer, had an approximately three times greater risk of ACL injury than those without such laxity. Joint laxity affects not only sagittal knee motion (hyperextension) but also coronal knee motion (valgus), which can strain the ACL and be related to increased risk in athletes [8].

17.3 ACL Tear

The most common mechanism of ACL injury is a noncontact pivoting motion on a fixed foot or a trauma with the knee in hyperextension or rotation. If a hemarthrosis develops within a few hours after the trauma in the absence of a bony injury, there is a 70 % chance of ACL injury [9]. The examiner should assess gait and alignment, range of motion, and the affected joint and compare it with the contralateral joint, taking into account that most children may have hyperlaxity which decreases with maturity. Radiographs should be examined for bony injuries. Magnetic resonance imaging (MRI) can be useful but may not lead to better results than accurate clinical examination. In a pediatric athlete with an acute traumatic knee effusion, the Lachman test, anterior drawer test, and pivot shift test are clinical examinations that aid in making the diagnosis of an ACL tear. The Lachman test is considered the most accurate of the three commonly performed clinical tests for an acute ACL tear, showing a pooled sensitivity of 85 % (95 % confidence interval CI) and a pooled specificity of 94 % (95 % CI 92–95). The pivot shift test is very specific, namely, 98 % (95 % CI), but has a poor sensitivity of 24 % (95 % CI 21–27). Lastly, the knee arthrometer is an objective, accurate, and validated tool that measures, in millimeters, the amount of tibial translation relative to the femur while performing a Lachman test and, thus, augments the clinical examination when examining a patient with an ACL tear [10].

17.4 Management of ACL Tear

The management of ACL deficiency in skeletally mature children is still controversial, especially in terms of operative timing and surgical technique. Conservative management is not recommended, as it is accompanied by marked reduction in activity, decline in functional performance, and development of early osteoarthritis. Historically, delayed anatomic ACL reconstructions were preferred [11] recommending extensive rehabilitation and return to activities with a brace to skeletal maturity and growth plate closure, to allow an anatomical adult-like reconstruction. The present trend favors early reconstruction, using either extraphyseal techniques in very young athletes or anatomical reconstruction techniques placing the tibial and femoral tunnels close to the center on the growth plate of the tibia and femur in young athletes closer to skeletal maturity [12]. An ACL tear in a child is not a surgical emergency. Multiple timely discussions with parents and child about the appropriate management options and understanding of goals and expectations are very important. The general indications for surgery are the patient's inability to participate in his or her chosen sport, instability that affects activities of daily living, and an associated repairable meniscal tear or a knee injury with multiple torn ligaments. Treatment of ACL injuries in the skeletally immature patient remains controversial, because standard ACL reconstructions involve the use of drill holes that cross the open physes and may potentially cause growth disturbance, such as shortening or angulation of the child's leg. A meta-analysis of 55 studies suggested that the risk of leg length difference or angular leg deviations was approximately 2 % after ACL reconstruction in children and adolescents. The authors recommended randomized controlled trials to clarify this risk more accurately [13]. But ACL surgery is about 90 % successful in restoring knee stability and patient satisfaction. Ideally, surgical treatment of an ACL tear in a skeletally immature athlete would be postponed until skeletal maturity, and the athlete would not develop meniscal tears during that waiting time. Most recent literature now supports early surgery for pediatric athletes with an ACL-deficient knee and recurrent episodes of instability [14]. No consensus exists on the best method to treat an ACL tear in a pediatric athlete. Safe and effective surgical techniques continue to evolve. However, the current literature suggests reasonable, evidenced-based management options that minimize the risks of iatrogenic growth plate injury [15, 16]. The two principal ACL surgery techniques performed on a pediatric athlete are physeal spearing or transphyseal and all-inside.

17.4.1 Physeal Sparing Technique (Both Tibia and Femur)

Various physeal-sparing techniques have been described for primary repair of ACL. They were designed to avoid placing drill holes across both the tibial and the femoral growth physes because primary repair of ACL injury is associated with high rate of instability and failure. However, Brief [17] and recently Kocher et al. [18] have described a technique that avoids placing the tunnels across both the femoral and the tibial physes. This technique utilizes the distally attached semitendinosus and gracilis tendons or the iliotibial band graft by passing them under the anterior horn of the medial meniscus, through the intercondylar notch, passing over the top and attaching with staples above the physes of the lateral distal femoral condyle. There were no reports of growth disturbances in these patients at 36-month follow-up. Eight of the nine patients in the study said they had no instability and were satisfied with the result. Micheli et al. [19] also described the use of the iliotibial band as a femoral and tibial physeal-sparing technique in 17 prepubescent children. However, the validity of these techniques was limited by the small size of the number of patients and a relatively short-term follow-up.

17.4.2 Transphyseal and "All-Inside" Technique

This involves the transphyseal tibial and femoral passage of the graft. Athletes who were close to skeletal maturity were treated with standard techniques as in adults. Aichroth et al. [20] reported results of a prospective study of 45 adolescent patients treated for ACL injuries, whose average chronological age was 12.5 years. They used the four-strand hamstring technique. The drill holes originated from the anatomical footprint of the ACL and were oriented to cross the physes as perpendicular as possible. The mean follow-up period was 49 months. There were neither any leg length discrepancies nor any physeal arrest during the follow-up of these patients [14]. This study documented that placement of transphyseal tunnels may not cause clinically significant growth plate arrest when anatomy and choice of fixation devices are carefully planned and considered. The young average age of the patients studied (12.5 years) indicates that these patients had remaining growth potential which was not affected by ACL reconstruction.

Different surgeons have recently described [21, 22] an "all-inside" technique for ACL reconstruction using a second generation of retrodrill to create two small sockets in the tibia and femur, as perpendicular as possible to the physes, using only a quadruple semitendinosus with good results.

An accurate understanding of the athlete's physical maturity by determining skeletal age and Tanner stage helps to identify which treatment is best for a specific patient. The most common method of measuring the patient's skeletal age is to compare an anteroposterior radiograph of the patient's left hand and wrist to an age-specific radiograph in the Greulich and Pyle atlas. Tanner stage can be determined by self-assessment, which has been shown to be valid and reliable. [23]. Patients with open physes at Tanner stage III and skeletal age of less than 14 in girls and less than 16 in boys can be offered the option of activity modification, functional bracing, rehabilitation, and careful follow-up. Surgery is indicated in skeletally immature patients with a torn ACL and an additional repairable meniscal injury and in patients who failed conservative care. Rehabilitation after ACL surgery may need to be modified for the individual patient and the particular surgical procedure. In general, a graduated rehabilitation program emphasizing full extension, immediate weight-bearing, active range of motion, and strengthening of the quadriceps, hamstrings, hip, and core can be started in the first few weeks after surgery. Progressive rehabilitation during the first 3 months after surgery includes range-of-motion exercises, patellar mobilization, proprioceptive exercises, endurance training, and closed-chain strengthening exercises. Straight-line jogging, plyometric exercises, and sport-specific exercises are added after 4–6 months. Returning to play typically occurs 7–9 months after surgery [24].

In our experience, between the years 2002 to 2011, 71 patients aged 12–15 have undergone arthroscopic ACLR with ST-G using arthroscopy and then retrospectively reviewed.

The inclusion criteria were:

- Patients with Tanner scale of 3 and 4
- Patients with primary ACL lesion with or without associated meniscal injury
- Informed consent for the surgery signed by both parents of the patient

The exclusion criteria were:

- Difference of 5° angle or more in the coronal plane (in varus or in valgus) between the two lower limbs
- The presence of knee chondropathy requiring surgical intervention
- Rheumatic pathology and/or systemic inflammation at the time of surgical intervention
- Previous surgical interventions on the limb which is to be operated on

All patients were evaluated clinically using the visual analog scale (VAS), the Lysholm score, and the Tegner activity score [25] at the time of surgery (T0). In addition, an MRI of the knee was performed (to confirm the ACL injury and to assess for possible preexisting injury of the menisci or any associated chondropathies) and weight-bearing radiography in order to evaluate both the stage and the age of the bone and possible axial varus-valgus deviations in comparison with the contralateral limb.

All patients were reevaluated after a follow-up period of at least 2 years (T1) with a weight-bearing hip-knee-ankle alignment radiograph. On the obtained radiograph, a straight line was drawn from the center of the femoral head to the center of the knee. The straight line was then projected beyond the knee downward. We used the angle formed by the portion of the line, which was drawn from the center of femoral head to the center of the knee and further projected beyond the knee downward, to measure the tibial shaft axis (images were acquired by a digital system and measured with a software).

Patients were further evaluated using the visual analog scale (VAS), the Lysholm score, and the Tegner activity score in order to evaluate the operated limb at follow-up.

A difference of up to 2° in the knee axis in varus-valgus, measured by radiograph, between the operated limb and the healthy control limb, was considered acceptable [26].

Both pre- and postoperative evaluations were performed by the same blind expert observer (not the surgeon).

All reconstructions have been done using hamstrings tendon, the size of the graft was at least 7 mm and maximum 8 mm of diameter (ST-G doubled), and when possible, a meniscal repair had been performed.

The postoperative program was the same for all patients; they have been discharged from the ward on the 2 day and were allowed partial weight-bearing with the use of two crutches for 15 days with the goal of achieving a range 0–90° of motion by the end of the 2nd week and perform isometric contraction of the quadriceps; the use of a functional brace was not prescribed.

From the 15th day, weight-bearing as tolerated was allowed with the assistance of a crutch on the opposite side to the operated knee, achieving complete range of motion (ROM) by the 30th day of the surgical intervention. For patients in whom a meniscal suture was performed, touch-down weight-bearing of the operated limb was advised for 21 days, followed by progressive weight-bearing for 7 days.

During the second month, patients had stopped using the crutch and started physiotherapy in pool, freestyle swimming, and stationary bike.

From the 60th day, patients started muscle strengthening using closed-kinetic chain exercises with a ROM 0–60° as well as proprioception training exercises with mono- and bipedal weight-bearing.

At the end of the 4th month, straight line running was advised along with dynamic weight-bearing exercises to allow a gradual return to the sport-specific performance. Full return to sports activity has been advised after 6 months, and not before obtaining adequate recovery of muscle strength and proprioceptive control.

With regard to the main objective of this study, only three patients resulted in a valgus difference exceeding 2° in the knee axis, between the operated limb and the healthy control limb (4.2 %: 95 % CI 0.88 %–11.86 %). The average difference was less than 1° (0.3°, 95 % CI 0.04–0.55).

17.5 Discussion

The most important finding of the present study was a good safety profile of the technique used. None of the three cases mentioned with the axial deviation greater than 2° exceeded 5° axial deviation. This result was slightly greater than other results described in the literature [27], with axial deviation greater than 2° reported in only 4.2 % of the population studied.

The results of the secondary objective have also shown excellent clinical outcome. In fact, excellent results in terms of functional recovery were in more than 94 % of the study population. Besides a significant pain reduction were similar to the date seen in literature [7].

As noted, the main risk in ACL reconstruction in a young patient is the potential iatrogenic damage to the growth plates, which can ensue during the tunnel drilling or as a result of compression or shear forces applied from the outside. An interesting letter recently written to the editor by Chotel and Seil has shown that "adolescent are at a higher risk of epiphysiodesis, but often with low clinical consequences in terms of growth disturbance, whereas young children are at a lower risk of epiphysiodesis but sometimes with dramatic clinical consequences" [28].

Several authors showed that a lesion of less 7–9 % of distal femoral physis does not cause growth damage [6], and considering that a drill hole of 8 mm of diameter damaged 3–4 % of physis in a young girl, we took into consideration an adequate safety margin, a tunnel diameter of 7–8 mm.

As regards the choice of graft, we have always preferred the use of hamstring grafts over those with bone ends such as the bone-patellar tendon-bone (BPTB) graft in order to avoid bone bridging within the growth cartilage [19]. Therefore, it is important to pay attention to the diameter of the tunnel, the choice of graft, the method of fixation, and the patient age.

Conclusions

ACL injuries in children of 10–15 years of age are encountered more frequently in clinical practice, as a result of the increased participation of this age group in contact sports and the intensity with which these patients practice it [29]. These types of injuries are among the most devastating injuries a young athlete can sustain, given the frequent need for surgical repair and extensive rehabilitation, as well as the potential for long-term health problems such as osteoarthritis.

Although, to date, there is still no consensus regarding the therapeutic approach that should be taken, the choice of early reconstructive surgery over conservative treatment seems to be well established now, thus reducing the risks of secondary injuries due to untreated anterior knee instability [30].

Several surgical techniques have been proposed for the reconstruction of the anterior cruciate ligament in adolescents. However, there is still no agreement as to which is more favorable [9–14].

Among the different techniques described in literature, ligament reconstruction that preserves the growth cartilages (physeal-sparing) reduces the risk to the cartilages as they are not crossed with the drilling of the tunnels. Of the physeal-sparing techniques, the over-the-top (OT) variant does not include drilling of bone tunnels. Rather, the ligament is passed over the top around the lateral femoral condyle, passing under the anterior transverse meniscal ligament and then at the anterior tibial plateau [7]. This technique, however, does not guarantee anatomic ACL reconstruction. The all-epiphyseal (AE) variant, on the other hand, entails preparing a bone tunnel within the epiphysis but, unlike the transtibial technique, avoids crossing the growth cartilages. In the AE technique, in order to place the tibial tunnel proximally and the femoral one distally from the growth plate, they are inevitably prepared more horizontal and therefore more tangent to the cartilages. This increases the risk of extensive iatrogenic damage to the growth cartilage when compared with the transphyseal technique that has been used and described in our retrospective study. The lack of a randomized control group which would allow comparison between the different techniques represents a limitation to our study. Any data about stability, patients ingrowth of stature, and Tanner stage at follow-up were not collected by the authors. We believe that those elements are potentially significant limits of our study. Therefore, to shed more light on the advantages and disadvantages of the different surgical techniques for ACL reconstruction in children and adolescents, randomized control clinical studies are warranted and necessary.

A certain endemic level of ACL injury will always be associated with sports, yet an increased commitment should be made to reduce the incidence and severity of ACL injuries sustained in younger athletes. Future investigators should focus on the modifiable sport-specific risk factors for ACL injuries in order to drive the development of effective, evidence-based, targeted ACL injury prevention efforts. Until such programs are developed, the incidence of ACL injuries should be expected to continue to rise with the growing number of young people participating in sports.

References

1. Waldén M, Hägglund M, Werner J, Ekstrand J (2011) The epidemiology of anterior cruciate ligament injury in football (soccer): a review of the literature from a gender-related perspective. Knee Surg Sports Traumatol Arthrosc 19(1):3–10
2. Hewett TE, Zazulak BT, Myer GD (2007) Effects of the menstrual cycle on anterior cruciate ligament injury risk: a systematic review. Am J Sports Med 35(4):659–668
3. Myer GD, Ford KR, Hewett TE (2005) The effects of gender on quadriceps muscle activation strategies dur-

ing a maneuver that mimics a high ACL injury risk position. Electromyogr Kinesiol 15(2):181–189
4. Nylan JA, Caborn DN, Shapiro R, Johnson DL (1997) Fatigue after eccentric quadriceps femoris work produces earlier gastrocnemius and delayed quadriceps femoris activation during crossover cutting among normal athletic women. KSSTA 5(3):162–167
5. Shelbourne KD, Davis TJ, Klootwyk TE (1998) The relationship between intercondylar notch width of the femur and the incidence of anterior cruciate ligament tears. A prospective study. Am J Sports Med 26(3):402–408
6. Lombardo S, Sethi PM, Starkey C (2005) Intercondylar notch stenosis is not a risk factor for anterior cruciate ligament tears in professional male basketball players: an 11-years prospective study. Am J Sports Med 33(1):29–34
7. Trimble MH, Bishop MD, Buckley BD, Fields LC, Rozea GD (2002) The relationship between clinical measurements of lower extremity posture and tibial translation. Clinical Biomech 17(4):286–290
8. Soderman K, Alfredson H, Pietila T, Werner S (2001) Risk factors for leg injuries in female soccer players: a prospective investigation during one out-door season. KSSTA 9(5):313–321
9. Boden BP, Dean GS, Feagin GA Jr, Garret WE Jr (2000) Mechanism of anterior cruciate ligament injury. Orthopedics 23:573–578
10. Kocher MS, Saxon HS, Hovis WD, Hawkins RJ (2002) Management and complications of anterior cruciate ligament injuries in skeletally immature patients: survey of herodicus society and the ACL study group. J Pediatric Orthop 22:452–457
11. Pressman AE, Letts RM, Jarvis JG (1997) Anterior cruciate ligament tears in children: an analysis of operative versus nonoperative treatment. J Pediat Orthop 17:505–511
12. Kaeding CC, Flanigan D, Donaldson C (2010) Surgical techniques and outcome after anterior cruciate ligament reconstruction in preadolescent patients. Arthroscopy 26:1530–1538
13. Frosch KH, Stengel D, Brodhun T (2010) Outcomes and risks of operative treatment of rupture of anterior cruciate ligament in children and adolescents. Arthroscopy 26(11):1539–1550
14. Kocher MS, Smith JT, Zoric BJ, Lee B, Micheli LJ (2007) Transphyseal anterior cruciate ligament reconstruction in skeletally immature pubescent adolescent. JBJS Am 89(12):2632–2639
15. Volpi P, Galli M, Bait C, Pozzoni R (2004) Surgical treatment of anterior cruciate ligament injuries in adolescents using double-looped semitendinosus and gracilis tendons: supraepiphysary femoral and tibial fixation. Arthroscopy 20(4):447–449
16. Anderson AF (2004) Transepiphyseal replacement of the anterior cruciate ligament using quadruple hamstring grafts in skeletally immature patients. JBJS Am 86(A(pt 2 suppl 1)):201–209
17. Brief LP (1991) Anterior cruciate ligament reconstruction without drill holes. Arthroscopy 7(4):350–357
18. Kocher MS, Garg S, Micheli LJ (2006) Physeal sparing reconstruction of the anterior cruciate ligament in skeletally immature prepubescent children and adolescent. Surgical technique. J Bone Joint Surg Am 88(Suppl 1 Pt 2):283–293
19. Micheli LJ, Rask B, Gerberg L (1999) Anterior cruciate ligament reconstruction in patients who are prepubescent. Clin Orthop Relat Res 364:40–47
20. Duri ZA, Patel DV, Aichroth PM (2002) The immature athlete. Clin Sports Med 21(3):461–482
21. McCarthy MM, Graziano J, Green DW, Cordasco FA (2012) All-epiphyseal, all-inside anterior cruciate ligament reconstruction technique for skeletally immature patients. Arthroscopy Tech 1(2):e231–e239
22. Lubowitz JH, Schwartzberg R, Smith P (2013) Randomized controlled trial comparing all-inside anterior cruciate ligament reconstruction technique with anterior cruciate ligament reconstruction with a full tibial tunnel. Arthroscopy 29(7):1195–1200
23. Tanner JM, Davies PS (1985) Clinical longitudinal standards for height and height velocity for North American children. J Pediatrics 107(3):317–329
24. Ardern CL, Webster KE, Taylor NF, Feller JA (2011) Return to sport following anterior cruciate ligament reconstruction surgery: a systematic review and meta-analysis of the state of play. Br J Sports Med 45(7):596–606
25. Granan LP, Forssblad M, Lind M, Engebretsen L (2009) The Scandinavian ACL registries 2004–2007: baseline epidemiology. Acta Othop 80(5):563–567
26. LaBella CR, Henrikus W, Hewett TE (2014) Anterior cruciate ligament injuries: diagnosis, treatment and prevention. Pediatrics 133, e1437
27. Hewett TE, Myer GD, Ford KR (2004) Decrease in neuromuscular control about the knee with maturation in female athletes. JBJS Am 86-A(8):1601–1608
28. Chotel F, Seil R (2013) Growth disturbances after transphyseal ACL reconstruction in skeletally immature patients: who is more at risk? Young child or adolescent? J Pediatr Orthop 33(5):585–586
29. Shea KG, Pfeiffer R, Wang JH, Curtin M, Apel PJ (2004) Anterior cruciate ligament injury in pediatric and adolescent soccer players: an analysis of insurance data. J Pediatr Orthop 24(6):623–628
30. Lohmander LS, Englund PM, Dahl LL, Roos EM (2007) The long term consequence of anterior cruciate ligament and meniscus injuries: osteoarthritis. Am J Sports Med 35(10):1756–1769

ACL Revision

18

Jonathan G. Robin, Elvire Servien,
and Philippe Neyret

18.1 Introduction and Epidemiology

Football (soccer) is the most popular sport played worldwide, with a recorded participation of approximately 240,000,000 in 2005 [1] and more recently estimated to be close to 300,000,000. Approximately 30 % of severe injuries in football occur around the knee [1]. The most serious and frequent of these are to the anterior cruciate ligament (ACL), the posterior cruciate ligament (PCL), and medial collateral ligament (MCL) [1]. In Sweden football is the most common cause of ACL injury in males and females [2]. ACL injuries in football players can have a devastating effect on their career in the short and long term and carry a significant socioeconomic importance.

The incidence of ACL injuries in football players is varied and is dependent on multiple factors. These include the level of professionalism, gender, age, and country of origin. ACL injuries occur most frequently in professional players compared with amateurs and the general population [3]. Male professional players have an annual incidence of up to 616 injuries per 100,000 population compared to up to 1,599 per 100,000 for professional female players [3, 4]. Male amateur players have an incidence of 224 per 100,000 compared to 610 per 100,000 in amateur female players. In both professional and amateur football players, ACL injuries occur approximately 4 years earlier in females compared to males, with average age in females being 19 years old [5]. In the general population, the incidence of ACL injuries is 28 per 100,000 in the USA, equating to approximately 90,000 ACL injuries per year [3]. In Denmark this figure is approximately 47 per 100,000 equating to 2,500 ACL injuries. As these figures include the whole population, they are an underestimate compared to the highly active age group between 15 and 40 years of age [3, 6].

With an increasing number of ACL injuries and ACL reconstructions, there is also an increasing prevalence of failed surgery and subsequent revision ACL surgery. Current literature suggests that revision surgery for failure of primary ACL reconstruction occurs between 3 % and 25 % of cases [7, 8]. The literature is scarce regarding revision surgery in football players in particular; however, one study has shown that further ACL surgery was required in 12 % of players. This included 9 % of players who had an ACL reconstruction on the contralateral knee and 3 % who had a revision ACL reconstruction on the ipsilateral knee [9]. A smaller study of football players recorded a revision rate of 5 %; however, this was only one patient in their entire cohort [10].

J.G. Robin (✉) • E. Servien • P. Neyret
Department of Orthopaedic Surgery,
Hôpital de la Croix-Rousse,
103 grand rue de la Croix Rousse,
Lyon 69317, France
e-mail: jonathan@oasisortho.com.au;
elvire.servien@chu-lyon.fr;
philippe.neyret@chu-lyon.fr

P. Volpi (ed.), *Football Traumatology: New Trends*, DOI 10.1007/978-3-319-18245-2_18

Revision ACL reconstruction is a challenging surgery, and it is a commonly held belief that clinical outcomes are not as satisfactory compared to primary ACL reconstruction [11]. The reason for this is multifactorial; however, it is imperative that the main reason for failure of the primary reconstruction is identified prior to and addressed during the revision surgery. It is also important that patients due to undergo a revision procedure are aware of the general results of revision surgery, and their expectations of returning to playing football at the same level are counseled appropriately.

18.2 Etiology of ACL Graft Failure and Revision Surgery

Failure of ACL reconstruction occurs due to either graft failure or other general complications of the primary surgery [11]. General complications of ACL surgery include loss of range of motion, pain, arthritis progression, and extensor mechanism dysfunction. Combinations of these problems may occur simultaneously, making diagnosis and decision-making difficult. ACL graft failure often requires revision surgery, and this will remain the focus of the chapter.

18.2.1 ACL Graft Failure

ACL graft failures can be considered to be either traumatic or atraumatic.

Traumatic graft failures relate to graft rupture in technically well-performed primary ACL reconstructions. They may occur in the early postoperative period prior to biological fixation of the graft, especially if there is a premature return to sport prior to completion of full rehabilitation and return of neuromuscular control. Once there has been full rehabilitation, graft ruptures may occur from similar traumatic mechanisms and force that caused the primary injury.

Recent literature suggests that this figure may be as high at 30 % in the general population and may account for the greatest reason for graft failure in elite athletes [11, 12]. These ruptures, like native ACL tears, tend to occur mostly through the mid-substance of the graft.

Atraumatic graft failures are caused by technical errors of the index ACL reconstruction, diagnostic errors (of associated laxities and malalignment), and failure of biological graft incorporation.

Errors of surgical technique during index ACL reconstruction are the most common reason for the failure of ACL grafts leading to revision in the general population. Technical errors in the general population account for between 77 % and 95 % of reasons for revision ACL reconstruction [13]. The most common technical mistakes include malpositioning of osseous tunnels leading to poor graft orientation and mechanics, graft impingement, inadequate graft fixation, and improper graft tension. There is little in the literature documenting causation of graft failure specifically in football players, with some believing it to be mostly atraumatic in nature [10]

18.2.1.1 Technical Errors

Poor Tunnel Position

Nonanatomic femoral and tibial tunnel position is a very important cause of atraumatic ACL graft failure and accounts for 36–50 % of graft failures [11, 14, 15]. Inaccurate tunnel positions and graft orientations lead to changes in graft length during range of motion, plastic deformation, and eventually graft loosening. Graft impingement may also occur and is discussed below.

Despite anterior femoral tunnel positioning being a well-known cause for graft failure, this continues to be the most common technical error, three times more common than tibial tunnel malpositioning [11]. One possible reason for an anterior femoral tunnel placement may be difficulty in visualizing the "over-the-top" position during an "all-inside" arthroscopic technique.

The biomechanical consequences of anterior femoral tunnel placement include increased graft tension during flexion resulting in reduced knee flexion, excessive tension on the graft fixation site, and plastic stretching of the graft. Graft failure is related to the short intra-articular component of the graft when the patient engages in rehabilitation or return to sport [11]. In addition, there are high femorotibial contact pressures in knee flexion, which may contribute to large osteochondral lesions and pain [16].

Posterior malposition of the femoral tunnel causes excessive tension on the graft in full knee extension and associated mild laxity in flexion. Femoral tunnel malposition close to the central axis of the femur leads to poor rotational control over the knee despite it having adequate control in the sagittal plane.

Inadequate placement of the tibial tunnel may also lead to graft failure. Anterior malpositioning of the tibial tunnel will cause impingement in the femoral notch and inability to fully extend the knee, leading to knee flexion contracture. In order to prevent impingement when there is constitutional recurvatum, a slightly more posterior position of the tibial tunnel may be chosen. A tibial tunnel that is positioned too posteriorly, however, may lead to laxity in flexion, poor rotational control due to the graft being too vertical and risks impingement on the PCL. A posteriorly placed tibial tunnel can never correct the problem of an anteriorly malpositioned femoral tunnel.

Graft Impingement

Impingement of the ACL graft in the femoral notch is most commonly found when there is malposition of the femoral tunnels. This may also occur when the femoral notch is narrow or the graft is excessively large for the notch [17]. The mechanism of failure relating to impingement relates to chronic abrasion of the graft on the medial aspect of the lateral femoral condyle or roof of the notch. Chronic synovitis occurs first, followed by gradual graft attrition and finally failure [18, 19].

Failure of Fixation

Failure of fixation occurs during the early postoperative period prior to biological graft incorporation when there is lower load to failure of the graft fixation sites compared to the graft itself [20]. Graft fixation must be strong enough to keep the graft fixed while biological integration occurs. Fixation with interference screws is thought to be stronger than suture fixation around a post or soft tissue washer and screw fixation [21, 22]. There does not appear to be a difference between interference screws used as an "all-inside" technique compared to "outside-in" technique femoral fixation [23]. Interference screw fixation may have issues relating to incorrect bone plug sizing and inaccurate screw trajectory [21–24].

Inappropriate Graft Tensioning

It is controversial as to whether tensioning of the ACL graft prior to fixation leads to better outcomes. It is also unclear how tensioning relates to the different types of grafts [25]. In animal models, over-tensioning of the graft leads to failure after initially causing reduced motion, delayed revascularization, and myxoid degeneration [26]. Tensioning and fixing the graft with the knee at approximately 30° flexion appears to play more of a role in increasing graft force compared to the actual tension applied to the graft itself [27, 28].

18.2.1.2 Diagnostic Errors (Associated Laxities/Malalignment)

ACL injuries commonly occur in conjunction with acute injuries to other stabilizing structures around the knee. Injuries to these structures must be identified and addressed during the treatment of the primary ACL injury in order to improve the longevity of the ACL reconstruction. The most commonly unrecognized injury is to the structures of the posterolateral corner of the knee [11]. This occurs in approximately 15–20 % of knees with chronic ACL deficiency [29]. Injury to the posterior cruciate ligament (PCL), the posterior capsule, the medial collateral ligament (MCL), and the acute tears of the menisci may all play a role in further destabilizing the knee and must be identified [11, 30].

Preexisting factors may also predispose to ACL graft failure. These include previous meniscectomy and varus mechanical lower limb alignment. It is now well known that the menisci provide a stabilizing effect in the knee and intact menisci aid to protect the ACL graft from further mechanical stresses. The cumulative incidence of meniscectomies during the course of treatment for ACL deficiency has been found to be as high as 70 % [11]. Repetitive stretching of the ACL graft may also occur with varus alignment associated with a lateral thrust. In this situation, a valgus high tibial osteotomy to correct this alignment should be performed [31, 32].

18.2.1.3 Failure of Biological Graft Incorporation

Biological incorporation follows a predictable sequence of events [30]. Many factors may contribute to poor or delayed biological integration. Graft over-tensioning, notch impingement, immobilization, and infection may lead to reduced vascularity of the graft and poor graft integration [33, 34]. Animal models have demonstrated that BTB tunnel incorporation is faster compared to soft tissue grafts [35]. The clinical significance of this is unclear.

18.3 Clinical and Diagnostic Examination

It is essential that a thorough clinical history (including past surgical records), examination, and appropriate medical imaging are obtained in order to successfully treat the failed ACL reconstruction.

18.3.1 Clinical History and Examination

A careful patient history and examination are essential. The aim is to diagnose if the ACL graft has failed and if so identify a possible reason (or reasons) that can be addressed surgically.

Details regarding the mechanism of the primary ACL injury are important as severe force may indicate that a concomitant ligament or meniscal injury had occurred. These untreated injuries may be a subsequent source of ACL graft failure. The patient's current symptoms are crucial, and there needs to be a distinction made between instability and pain. Other mechanical symptoms may indicate a large meniscal tear or possibly a cyclops lesion.

It is imperative to obtain the surgical records of the primary ACL reconstruction. This will not only detail the technical aspects of the procedure, but gain an insight to the status of the menisci and chondral surfaces.

A general knee examination must be performed. Surgical scars are critical to identify as they may give a clue to the primary graft used and also allow for planning the revision approach. Assessing mechanical alignment is imperative as a varus alignment with a thrust may be an important mechanism for ACL graft failure. A careful assessment of gait in ACL-deficient knees may exhibit increased internal knee rotation during the initial swing phase [36, 37]. A more focused knee examination is required to diagnose ACL graft failure and identify other ligament injuries, which may have contributed to increased joint laxity. A close assessment of the posterolateral corner is crucial. The Lachman test and the pivot shift test must be performed to assess ACL graft status. The latter has been well correlated with patients' symptoms of instability and been shown to be a reliable test [38, 39].

18.3.2 Medical Imaging

Medical imaging plays the final crucial factor in diagnosing ACL graft rupture and planning a revision procedure. Plain radiographs and CT and MRI scans are utilized.

Plain radiographs can demonstrate graft rupture as well as the reason for failure. Poor tunnel position (in particular the femoral tunnel) is the most common reason for failure (Fig. 18.1). Plain x-rays also may identify hardware that has been used previously for fixation and its position as well as tunnel osteolysis. Long-limb alignment films will allow evaluation of mechanical alignment.

Stress radiographs are useful for diagnostic and planning purposes. Telos x-rays allow for an assessment of sagittal plane translation. Anterior tibial translation greater than 6 mm is indicative of gross laxity, which is important to consider during revision surgery. Likewise, stress radiographs may confirm collateral ligament injury in

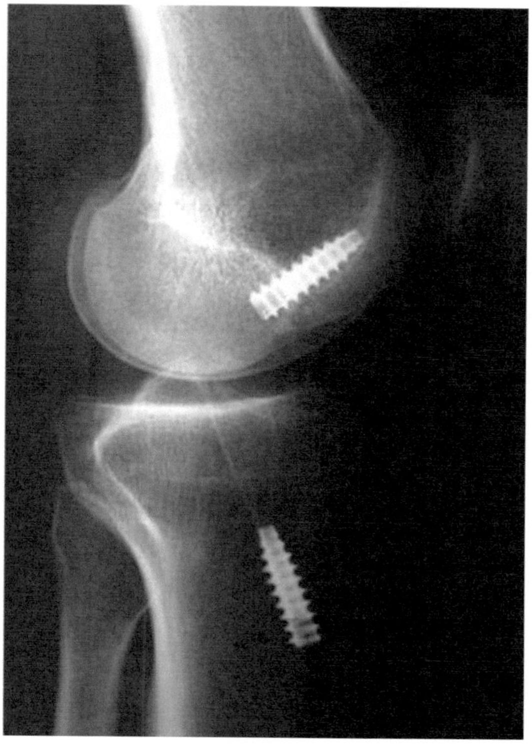

Fig. 18.1 Plain lateral radiograph demonstrating a malpositioned anterior femoral tunnel

the coronal plane, which may also need to be treated simultaneous to ACL revision reconstruction (Fig. 18.2). Finally, plain x-rays give an accurate assessment of joint arthrosis, which plays an important factor when considering reconstructive options.

CT is a very useful modality in assessing tunnel position and planning for revision surgery. It has been shown to be more accurate than plain radiographs [40]. Two main factors can be assessed: (1) tunnel position and orientation and (2) tunnel size (tunnel widening). Three-dimensional reformatting of CT scans can now produce an accurate representation of tunnel position and orientation [41] (Fig. 18.3). This technology is very helpful in determining whether the previous tunnel positions are beneficial or detrimental to revision ACL reconstruction. Tunnel size can be measured using all three planes possible with CT and allows for an assessment as to whether revision reconstruction may be performed as a single-stage or two-stage procedure and also as to which graft type may be suitable [41].

MRI scans are useful in determining the extent of soft tissue injury. Commonly, however, the

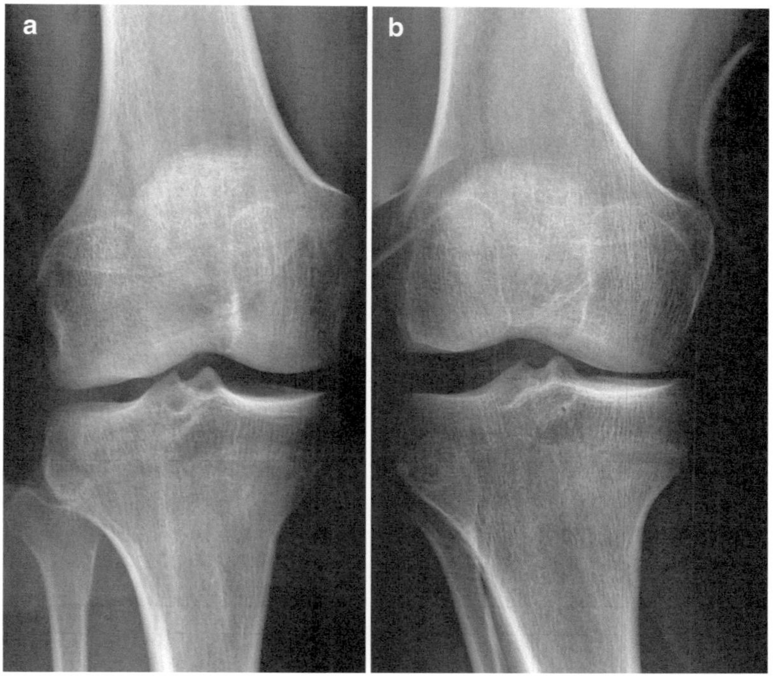

Fig. 18.2 (**a**) Plain anteroposterior radiograph and (**b**) stress view demonstrating lateral ligament insufficiency in the setting of chronic ACL deficiency

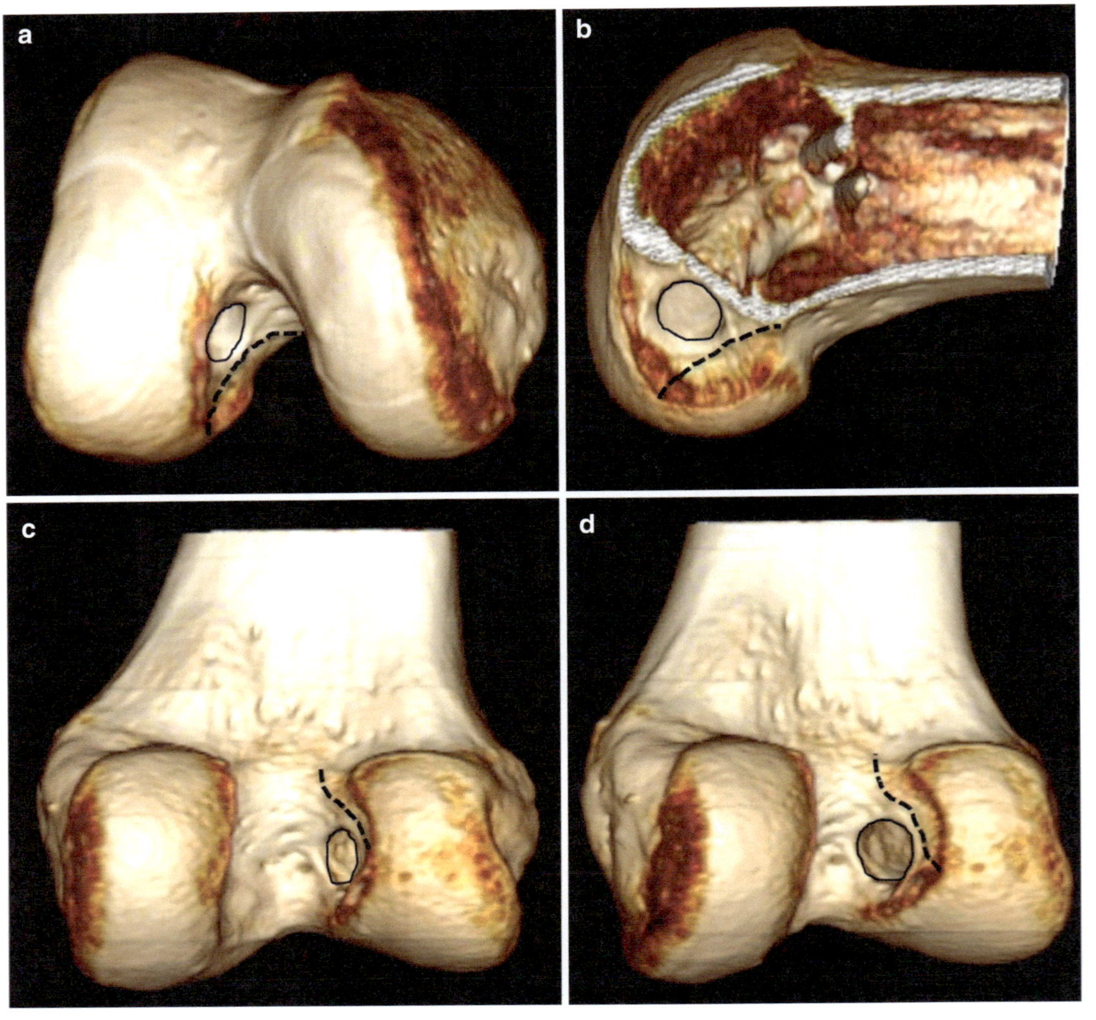

Fig. 18.3 (**a–d**) Three-dimensional CT reconstruction demonstrating malpositioned anterior femoral tunnel placement

diagnosis of ACL graft rupture is made prior to obtaining an MRI. Injury to other stabilizing structures such as the posterolateral corner ligaments and menisci is important to identify prior to and treat during revision ACL reconstruction.

18.4 Treatment Strategy

Prior to planning a revision ACL reconstruction, the patient must be seen as a person as well as a professional athlete. The considerations of further surgery vary for football players depending on which stage of their career they are in, their level of competition, the general state of their injured knee, what symptoms they are currently experiencing, and what stage of the football season it is. For a professional football player, there is a great deal of pressure to return to sport in the shortest possible time. These outside influences must be taken into account; however, the player's overall well-being is paramount. It is also very important to differentiate between symptoms of instability and pain. Revision ACL reconstruction should be performed to address recurrent symptoms of instability.

For a young elite player, who otherwise has a knee that is in good condition, the decision to perform a revision ACL reconstruction may well be appropriate. However, in an older player who is nearing the end of their career, or when there is already severe damage to the rest of the knee, revision surgery such that they can continue to play (and possibly further injure their knee) may not be the best option. It has been shown that return to sports after revision ACL reconstruction is associated with a higher risk of osteoarthritis [12]. In this setting there needs to be an open and frank discussion with the player who may need to consider retirement from high-level competition. This may also be the case for amateur athletes who will often have another profession or source of income.

When revision ACL reconstruction is going to be performed, the goal is to return stability, range of motion, and function of the patient's knee. In order to achieve this, contributing factors that lead to failure of the primary ACL reconstruction must be treated during the revision surgery. Each revision procedure must therefore be tailored to each individual patient. At all times, the patient's expectations from the surgery must be taken into account, and they must be counseled appropriately.

Specific technical considerations during revision ACL reconstruction include graft choice, management of osseous tunnels and graft fixation, choice of single- versus two-stage revision, correction of mechanical malalignment, and repair/reconstruction of other soft tissue stabilizers.

18.4.1 Graft Choice

There is no consensus as to the best graft to use in revision ACL reconstruction [42]. The choice of graft to be used during revision ACL reconstruction largely depends on the graft previously used, which graft is available, and surgeon preference.

Bone-patellar tendon-bone (BTB) autograft has been shown to have good results in revision ACL reconstruction [43]. If reinjury occurs less than 18 months from primary reconstruction, the contralateral BTB is used due to its robust bone plug in bone tunnel fixation [43] and the frequent use of autograft hamstring tendon as a graft in primary ACL reconstruction [44]. Ipsilateral BTB re-harvest is also possible; however, regeneration typically takes at least 18 months to 2 years [42]. Despite morphological analysis showing that the regenerated tendon has similar properties to the original BTB graft, clinical results using regenerated BTB have been disappointing [45, 46].

The use of hamstring tendons (semitendinosus and gracilis) for revision graft purposes can yield good results [47]; however, when there are large bone tunnels present, bone-bone fixation such as with BTB graft may be preferable [48]. It has also been shown that hamstring tendons may regenerate; however, their use as a graft has been controversial.

Little has been written in the literature regarding autograft quadriceps tendon, especially in ACL revision. One study has shown that good results can be achieved using this graft in 97 % of cases at a mean of 26 months after surgery [49]. The ipsilateral quadriceps tendon-bone block arrangement is particularly useful when BTB has been used primarily and a bone block is preferred when larger osseous tunnels are present [42].

The debate continues over the use of allograft versus autograft. Allograft avoids graft harvest site morbidity; however, allograft has limited availability in some countries and carries a potential risk of communicable diseases [42]. Allograft results in similar knee function compared to autograft; however, the latter has been shown to have greater biomechanical properties, produce superior stability, and have a lower risk of failure leading to re-revision [7, 42, 50, 51]. Synthetic graft choice is also available; however, its use is currently controversial.

18.4.2 Management of Bone Tunnels and Fixation

The bone tunnels on both the tibia and the femur may be well positioned, poorly positioned, or in an intermediate position. Femoral tunnels that have an intermediate position are the most difficult to deal with as they interfere with the positioning of new bone tunnels. In some of these cases, it may be more appropriate to perform a two-stage reconstruction by using bone graft to fill in tunnel defects [41].

18.4.2.1 Tunnels that Are Well Positioned

If the bony tunnels are well positioned, they may be reused during the revision surgery. Depending on the type of fixation used during the primary ACL reconstruction, it may be necessary to remove the fixation from within the tunnels. This may be simple if an interference screw is easily visualized at the aperture of the femoral and tibial tunnels. If, however, the screws have been well advanced into the tunnels, or overgrown with bone, removal of fixation may be very difficult. The surgeon must appreciate this preoperatively and be prepared with the correct screwdriver and materials for difficult hardware removal.

The tunnels should then be cleared of any graft material and then freshened up with a drill of increasing sizes over a guidewire in order to remove any sclerotic tunnel margins and to allow passage of the revision graft. This can be done on both femoral and tibial sides from an "all-inside" technique in the majority of cases.

An "outside-in" technique is very useful when metalware cannot be removed in well-positioned tunnels and in cases where the current tunnels may interfere with new tunnel placement. This technique uses a press-fit block in the femur away from the intra-articular space and origin of the original tunnel (Fig. 18.4).

Fixation depends on the graft being used, the tunnel sizes, and the surgeon's preference.

18.4.2.2 Tunnels That Are Poorly Positioned

Poorly positioned bone tunnels may be the technically "easiest" to deal with, and revision surgery for an anterior malpositioned femoral tunnel has been shown to provide statistically superior results than revision for any other cause [11].

It may not be necessary to remove metalware where the tunnels are well away from the desired new anatomical tunnel placement on the tibia or femur. After removing any remaining graft, new tunnels may be drilled in the desired positions and fixed according to graft size, type, and surgeon preference.

18.4.2.3 Tunnels That Are in Intermediate Position

Tunnels that are in an intermediate position are the most difficult to deal with as they often interfere with new tunnel placement. This may also be the case for other well-positioned tunnels that have expanded due to osteolysis and encroach on the potential position for an anatomical tunnel. In these situations, if an "all-inside" technique is used, careful attention must be paid to the direction of the new tunnel such that the femoral tunnel remains at a size that allows for adequate fixation. If this cannot be achieved, a two-stage procedure with initial bone grafting is indicated [52].

On the contrary, the "outside-in" technique is extremely useful in this situation, and using this technique, it is extremely rare to opt for a two-stage procedure. The main advantage of this technique is its proximal press-fit fixation on the femur, which avoids any large bone defects. It also allows for complete visualization of the intra-articular tunnel "entry" point in comparison with the old tunnel.

It may be possible to perform a single-stage revision in the presence of an interfering or enlarged tibial tunnel. This may be achieved by using an anterolateral starting point on the tibia, but an anatomical footprint intra-articularly. In this situation, the tunnel and graft position within the tibia is the inverse to the usual anteromedial tunnel, avoiding the pathological area [42].

18.4.2.4 Two-Stage Revision ACL Reconstruction

If it is not possible to perform a single-stage revision reconstruction due to tunnel misplacement or size, a two-stage procedure with initial bone grafting may be undertaken, followed by a delayed ACL reconstruction 3–6 months later [42]. The two most common reasons for requiring a two-stage revision are where the tibial tunnel is too far posterior and where a double-bundle primary ACL reconstruction has been performed.

There is no consensus on what defines the upper limit of tunnel size that will permit a

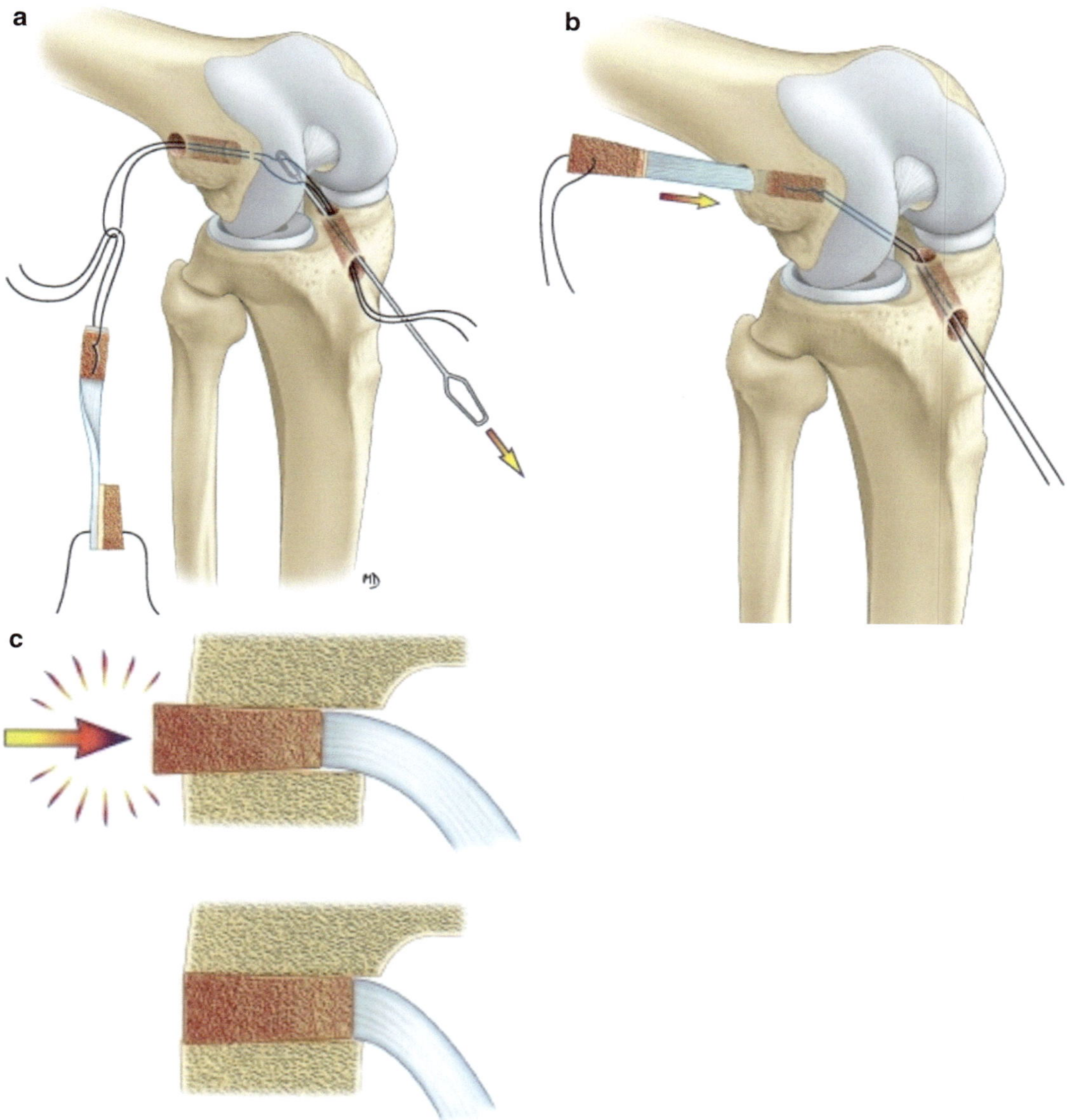

Fig. 18.4 (**a**, **b** and **c**) Schematic diagram of "outside-in" technique for ACL reconstruction

single-stage revision. Reports in the literature suggest that tunnels 16–17 mm in diameter are too large for a single-stage revision [53].

Multiple techniques have been described for the bone grafting process. All mandate that the old tunnels must be prepared meticulously to ensure that all remaining materials inside the tunnels are removed down to the bleeding cancellous bone. The size of the tunnels should be measured to allow for accurate procurement of the graft. The choice of graft is dependent on surgeon preference. Methods described include the use of autograft iliac crest or proximal tibia using a measured trephine as well as allograft femoral head bone dowels [54–56].

If there is significant knee stiffness preventing single-stage revision ACL reconstruction, this needs to be dealt with a priori, possibly necessitating a two-stage procedure.

18.4.3 Other Important Surgical Considerations

Primary ACL injury is frequently associated with a concomitant soft tissue injury to the lateral compartment of the knee and surrounding extra-articular envelope. In particular, the anterolateral and posteromedial soft tissues are affected with there being a resurgence in focus on the anterolateral ligament (ALL). The ALL is thought to provide significant rotational control to the knee in preventing internal tibial rotation and modest anterior translation. The combination of complete ACL rupture and ALL deficiency often leads to significant rotational instability symptoms often demonstrated clinically with an "explosive" pivot shift test. Telos x-rays will often demonstrate greater than 9 mm of tibial translation of the lateral compartment of the knee.

In this setting, and especially in young patients or those who wish to continue to play at a highly competitive level, reconstructing the ACL alone will often be insufficient. They may struggle to reach the same level of activity or may suffer a repeat injury leading to graft failure. In this light, the ALL should be considered as important as the other knee stabilizers and reconstructed to further stabilize the knee as well as protect the ACL graft during primary ACL reconstruction.

Where a lateral tenodesis is not performed initially, it is advocated that this be performed during revision ACL reconstruction [57]. Typically, in this situation there is no mechanical reason for the graft rupture, and the tunnel positions are good. There is some evidence that in revision ACL surgery a lateral tenodesis in association with the revision ACL graft improves stability compared to just using an intra-articular graft by itself [57]. This is irrespective of whether the revision ACL graft used is BTB or hamstring tendons. An extra-articular lateral tenodesis (or in fact and intra-articular augmentation) may also be considered where there is residual rotational laxity after primary ACL reconstruction. This may be the case when there is a vertically positioned graft from the primary ACL reconstruction.

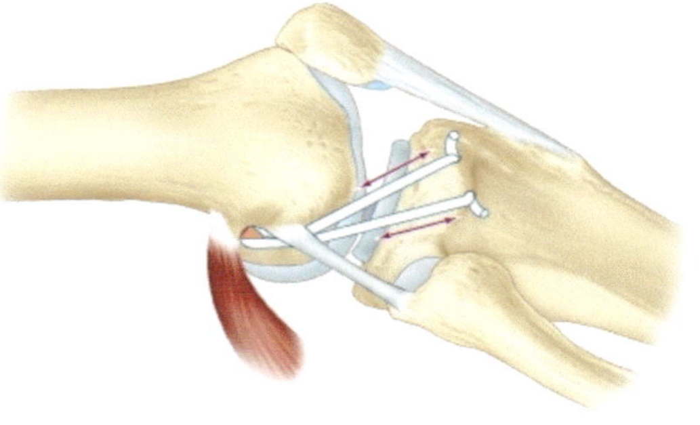

Fig. 18.5 Schematic diagram of lateral tenodesis in association with BTB ACL reconstruction

Many techniques have been described for the lateral tenodesis. One such technique is very useful in the revision setting as well as in primary ACL reconstruction. This technique uses an "outside-in" femoral tunnel with a press-fit BTB graft and a linked two-strand gracilis autograft (Fig. 18.5). This "outside-in" technique avoids fixation problems in the femur with interfering previous femoral tunnels, and linking the gracilis tendon avoids the need for individual fixation of the gracilis in the femur. This technique has been studied and shown to have very good results [57].

It is also recommended to correct concomitant ligamentous injuries or proximal tibial deformities (tibia vara and excessive posterior tibial slope) as a combined single-stage procedure with revision ACL reconstruction. These procedures are thought to protect the graft from undergoing excess stress and improve long-term outcomes [42]. Other soft tissue stabilizers such as the menisci must also be repaired where possible.

18.5 Results of Revision ACL Reconstruction

18.5.1 Literature Results

Most of the literature regarding results of revision ACL reconstruction consists of small case-control studies comparing the technical aspects of revision surgery techniques. More recently, population-based studies have shed some more light on the longer-term outcomes of revision ACL reconstruction, especially in comparison to primary ACL reconstruction.

Despite the fact that objective knee stability can be returned to the patient following revision ACL reconstruction, the clinical results are often inferior to that of primary ACL reconstruction [7, 58–60]. In particular, following revision ACL surgery, clinical outcome scores have been shown to improve from their preoperative levels; however, at 12-month follow-up, these scores are worse when compared to primary ACL reconstruction scores [61].

Only four studies in the literature have had large enough patient cohorts to reliably report on reinjury rates and failure of revision ACL reconstruction. None of these studies specifically address football players; however, it is noted that football players are included in some of the cohorts reported.

Two of these studies are population based and show quite different results. The Danish ACL registry reports an incidence of revision ACL reconstruction failure and re-revision in 5.4 % of cases at 5-year follow-up [7]. Even more recently, the Swedish ACL registry reports a failure rate of only 0.1 % leading to re-revision reconstruction. The authors concluded that this low value may be because the revisions did not re-tear to the same extent as the primary failures or that patients did not wish to undergo a second revision surgery [2].

Two large cohort studies have also reported their results. After an average of 6 years, Lind et al. reported a 6 % failure rate leading to re-revisions in a cohort of 126 patients [60]. Shelbourne et al. prospectively studied 3 cohorts of athletes of varying level of activity who had undergone a revision ACL reconstruction with BTB autograft. Failure of their revision ACL reconstruction grafts with a re-tear occurred in 2.3 % of a high school level cohort, 5.1 % of a college group, and 3.4 % of a recreational group. Of these, the majority of re-tears occurred in female basketball players and male American football players with only one re-tear in a football player belonging to the recreational group [62].

18.5.2 Rehabilitation and Return to Play

Rehabilitation following revision ACL reconstruction generally follows either an accelerated or delayed program. The rehabilitation technique depends on whether other soft tissue structures have been repaired or if a corrective osteotomy has been performed and is tailored to the individual patient. In the setting of single-stage revision procedures, a delayed program is often undertaken [63]. During the first 6–8 weeks, the patient is expected to have reduced swelling and increased range of motion and quadriceps strength [63]. Strengthening exercises for the quadriceps and hamstrings consist of closed-chain and isometric exercises. Straight line running could be considered at 6 months following which plyometric exercises, cutting maneuvers, may be considered between 9 and 12 months. The clinical indicators that a patient is ready to return to sport are controversial. Most advocate that when there is no effusion and the patient can reliably perform a controlled single-leg forward hop, then they will be able to return to sport. A change in MRI signal back to normal may also be another indicator.

Return to high-level sport is possible in many athletes following revision ACL reconstruction. In adults, the literature suggests that this is possible for between 50 % and 60 % of patients, while this figure can be as high at 72 % in high school and university/college students [62]. Reinjury rates within the first 5 years following revision surgery are varied, but are approximately between 2 % and 5 % of patients [7, 62]. This information is important when counseling patients prior to revision ACL surgery.

Conclusion

Football is one of the most popular sports worldwide and participation continues to grow. Knee injuries in football, in particular ACL injuries, are common. With an increase in ACL reconstructions being performed, graft failure and revision ACL reconstruction is becoming an increasingly performed procedure. The most common reasons for graft failure in general are technical errors (especially poor tunnel position) in the primary ACL reconstruction and reinjury. These factors are not well documented in football players.

As there are many different technical factors and anatomical situations to consider in revision ACL reconstructions, the surgeons must be prepared to deal with these and adapt their surgical technique as necessary. The literature shows that, in general, the outcomes of revision ACL reconstructions are inferior to that of primary ACL surgery. There is, however, a lack of literature regarding the results of revision surgery in football players, and this is an area that needs more research in the future. There is also a lack of consensus regarding rehabilitation following revision ACL reconstruction. Ultimately this must be tailored according to the surgery performed and the patients' postoperative progress.

References

1. Wong P, Hong Y (2005) Football injury in the lower extremities. Br J Sports Med 39:473–482
2. Kvist J, Kartus J, Karlsson J et al (2014) Results from the Swedish national anterior cruciate ligament register. Arthroscopy 30:803–810
3. Moses B, Orchard J, Orchard J (2012) Systematic review: annual incidence of ACL injury and surgery in various populations. Res Sports Med 20:157–179
4. Ekstrand J, Hägglund M, Waldèn M (2011) Injury incidence and injury patterns in professional football: the UEFA injury study. Br J Sports Med 45:553–558
5. Waldèn M, Hägglund M, Werner J et al (2011) The epidemiology of anterior cruciate ligament injury in football (football): a review of the literature from a gender-related perspective. Knee Surg Sports Traumatol Arthrosc 19:3–10
6. Gianotti S, Marshall S, Hume P et al (2009) Incidence of anterior cruciate ligament injury and other knee ligament injuries: a national population-based study. J Sci Med Sport 12:622–627
7. Lind M, Menhert F, Pedersen AB (2012) Incidence and outcome after revision anterior cruciate ligament reconstruction: results from the danish registry for knee ligament reconstructions. Am J Sports Med 40:1551–1557
8. Carson EW, Anisko EM, Restrepo C et al (2004) Revision anterior cruciate ligament reconstruction: etiology of failures and clinical results. J Knee Surg 17:127–132
9. Brophy R, Schmitz L, Wright R et al (2012) Return to play and future ACL injury risk after ACL reconstruction in football athletes from the multicenter orthopaedic outcomes network (MOON) group. Am J Sports Med 40:2517–2522
10. Zaffagnini S, Grassi A, Marcheggiani Muccioli G et al (2014) Return to sport after anterior cruciate ligament reconstruction in professional football players. Knee 21:731–735
11. Trojani C, Sbihi A, Djian P et al (2011) Causes for failure of ACL reconstruction and influence of meniscectomies after revision. Knee Surg Sports Traumatol Arthrosc 19:196–201
12. Lind M (2014) One stage revision: Danish approach. In: Siebold R, Dejour D, Zaffagnini S (eds) Anterior cruciate ligament reconstruction: a practical surgical guide. Springer, Heidelberg, pp p387–p403
13. Wolf RS, Lemak LJ (2002) Revision anterior cruciate ligament reconstruction surgery. J South Orthop Assoc 11:25–32
14. Allen CR, Giffin JR, Harner CD (2003) Revision anterior cruciate ligament reconstruction. Orthop Clin North Am 34:79–98
15. Getelman MH, Friedman MJ (1999) Revision anterior cruciate ligament reconstruction surgery. J Am Acad Orthop Surg 7:189–198
16. Weiler A, Wagner M (2008) Revision anterior cruciate ligament reconstruction using autologous hamstring tendons. In: The anterior cruciate ligament: reconstruction and basic science. Saunders, Philadelphia, pp 427–442
17. Tanzer M, Lenczner E (1990) The relationship of intercondylar notch size and content to notchplasty requirement in anterior cruciate ligament surgery. Arthroscopy 6:89–93
18. Howell SM, Clark JA (1992) Tibial tunnel placement in anterior cruciate ligament reconstructions and graft impingement. Clin Orthop 283:187–195
19. Howell SM, Taylor MA (1993) Failure of reconstruction of the anterior cruciate ligament due to impingement by the intercondylar roof. J Bone Joint Surg Am 75:1044–1055
20. George MS, Dunn WR, Spindler KP (2006) Current concepts review: revision anterior cruciate ligament reconstruction. Am J Sports Med 34:2026–2037
21. Kurosaka M, Yoshiya S, Andrish JT (1987) A biomechanical comparison of different surgical techniques of graft fixation in anterior cruciate ligament reconstruction. Am J Sports Med 15:225–229
22. Steiner ME, Hecker AT, Brown CH et al (1994) Anterior cruciate ligament graft fixation: comparison of hamstring and patellar tendon grafts. Am J Sports Med 22:240–246
23. Brown CH Jr, Hecker AT, Hipp JA et al (1993) The biomechanics of interference screw fixation of patellar tendon anterior cruciate ligament grafts. Am J Sports Med 21:880–886
24. Doerr AL Jr, Cohn BT, Ruoff MJ et al (1990) A complication of interference screw fixation in anterior cruciate ligament reconstruction. Orthop Rev 19:997–1000

25. Burks RT, Leland R (1988) Determination of graft tension before fixation in anterior cruciate ligament reconstruction. Arthroscopy 4:260–266
26. Yoshiya S, Andrish JT, Manley MT et al (1987) Graft tension in anterior cruciate ligament reconstruction: an in vivo study in dogs. Am J Sports Med 15:464–470
27. Bylski-Austrow DI, Grood ES, Hefzy MS et al (1990) Anterior cruciate ligament replacements: a mechanical study of femoral attachment location, flexion angle at tensioning, and initial tension. J Orthop Res 8:522–531
28. Gertel TH, Lew WD, Lewis JL et al (1993) Effect of anterior cruciate ligament graft tensioning direction, magnitude, and flexion angle on knee biomechanics. Am J Sports Med 21:572–581
29. Gersoff WK, Clancy WG Jr (1988) Diagnosis of acute and chronic anterior cruciate ligament tears. Clin Sports Med 7:727–738
30. Harner CD, Giffin JR, Dunteman RC et al (2001) Evaluation and treatment of recurrent instability after anterior cruciate ligament reconstruction. Instr Course Lect 50:463–474
31. Noyes FR, Barber SD, Simon R (1993) High tibial osteotomy and ligament reconstruction in varus angulated, anterior cruciate ligament-deficient knees. A two- to seven-year follow-up study. Am J Sports Med 21:2–12
32. Noyes FR, Barber-Westin SD, Hewett TE (2000) High tibial osteotomy and ligament reconstruction for varus angulated anterior cruciate ligament-deficient knees. Am J Sports Med 28:282–296
33. Arnoczky SP (1996) Biology of ACL reconstructions: what happens to the graft? Instr Course Lect 45:229–233
34. Muneta T, Yamamoto H, Takakuda K et al (1993) Effects of postoperative immobilization on the reconstructed anterior cruciate ligament. An experimental study in rabbits. Am J Sports Med 21:305–313
35. Rodeo SA, Arnoczky SP, Torzilli PA et al (1993) Tendon-healing in a bone tunnel: a biomechanical and histological study in the dog. J Bone Joint Surg Am 75:1795–1803
36. Georgoulis AD, Papadonikolakis A, Papageorgiou CD et al (2003) Three-dimensional tibiofemoral kinematics of the anterior cruciate ligament-deficient and reconstructed knee during walking. Am J Sports Med 31:75–79
37. Tashman S, Collon D, Anderson K et al (2004) Abnormal rotational knee motion during running after anterior cruciate ligament reconstruction. Am J Sports Med 32:975–983
38. Lucie RS, Wiedel JD, Messner DG et al (1984) The acute pivot shift: clinical correlation. Am J Sports Med 12:189–191
39. Kocher MS, Steadman JR, Briggs K et al (2002) Determinants of patient satisfaction with outcome after anterior cruciate ligament reconstruction. J Bone Joint Surg Am 84:1560–1572
40. Hoser C, Tecklenburg K, Kuenzel KH et al (2005) Postoperative evaluation of femoral tunnel position in ACL reconstruction: plain radiography versus computed tomography. Knee Surg Sports Traumatol Arthrosc 13:256–262
41. Magnussen RA, Debieux P, Benjamin B et al (2012) A CT-based classification of prior ACL femoral tunnel location for planning revision ACL surgery. Knee Surg Sports Traumatol Arthrosc 20:1298–1306
42. Servien E., Lustig S., Neyret P (2010) Chirurgie itérative dans la rupture du ligament croisé antérieur. EMC (Elseveier Masson SAS, Paris), Techniques chirurgicales – Orthopédie – Traumatologie, 44–783
43. Noyes F, Barber-Westin SD (2001) Revision ACL surgery with the use of bone patellar tendon bone autogenous grafts. J Bone Joint Surg Am 83:1131–1143
44. Middleton KK, Hamilton T, Ittgang JJ et al (2014) Anatomic anterior cruciate ligament (ACL) reconstruction: a global perspective. Part 1. Knee Surg Sports Traumatol Arthrosc 22:1467–1482
45. O'Shea JJ, Shelbourne KD (2002) Anterior cruciate ligament reconstruction using reharvested bone-patella tendon-bone graft. Am J Sports Med 30:208–213
46. Colosimo AJ, Heidt RS Jr, Taub JA et al (2001) Revision anterior cruciate ligament reconstruction with a reharvested ipsilateral patellar tendon. Am J Sports Med 29:746–750
47. Salmon LJ, Pinczewski LA, Russell VJ, Refshauge K (2006) Revision anterior cruciate ligament reconstruction with hamstring tendon autograft: 5- to 9-year follow-up. Am J Sports Med 34:1604–1614
48. Brown CH Jr, Carson EW (1999) Revision anterior cruciate ligament surgery. Clin Sports Med 18:109–171
49. Garofalo R, Djahangiri A, Siegrist O (2006) Revision anterior cruciate ligament reconstruction with quadriceps tendon-patellar bone autograft. Arthroscopy 22:205–214
50. Grossman M, ElAttrache N, Shields C et al (2005) Revision anterior cruciate ligament reconstruction: three- to nine-year follow-up. Arthroscopy 21:418–423
51. Fox J, Pierce M, Bojchuk J et al (2004) Revision anterior cruciate ligament reconstruction with nonirradiated fresh-frozen patellar tendon allograft. Arthroscopy 20:787–794
52. Tomas NP, Kankate R, Wandless F et al (2005) Revision anterior cruciate ligament reconstruction using a 2-stage technique with bone grafting of the tibial tunnel. Am J Sports Med 33:1701–1709
53. Kamath GV, Redfern JC, Greis PE et al (2011) Revision anterior cruciate ligament reconstruction. Am J Sports Med 39:199–217
54. Said HG, Baloch K, Green M (2006) A new technique for femoral and tibial tunnel bone grafting using the OATS harvesters in revision anterior cruciate ligament reconstruction. Arthroscopy 22(796):e1–e3
55. Franceschi F, Papalia R, Del Buono A et al (2013) Two-stage procedure in anterior cruciate ligament revision surgery: a five-year follow-up prospective study. Int Orthop 37:1369–1374
56. Coats AC, Johnson DL (2012) Two-stage revision anterior cruciate ligament reconstruction: indications, review, and technique demonstration. Orthopedics 35:958–960

57. Trojani C, Beaufils P, Burdin G (2012) Revision ACL reconstruction: influence of a lateral tenodesis. Knee Surg Sports Traumatol Arthrosc 20:1565–1570
58. Weiler A, Schmeling A, Stohr I et al (2007) Primary versus single-stage anterior cruciate ligament reconstruction using autologous hamstring tendon grafts: a prospective matched-group analysis. Am J Sports Med 35:1643–1652
59. Johnson D, Swenson T, Irrgang J et al (1996) Revision anterior cruciate ligament surgery: experience from Pittsburgh. Clin Orthop Relat Res 325: 100–109
60. Lind M, Lund B, Fauno P et al (2012) Medium to long-term follow-up after ACL revision. Knee Surg Sports Traumatol Arthrosc 20:166–172
61. Lind M, Menhert F, Pedersen A (2009) The first results from the Danish ACL reconstruction registry: epidemiologic and 2 year follow-up results from 5,818 knee ligament reconstructions. Knee Surg Sports Traumatol Arthrosc 17:117–124
62. Shelbourne D, Benner RW, Gray T (2014) Return to sports and subsequent injury rates after revision anterior cruciate ligament reconstruction with patellar tendon autograft. Am J Sports Med 42:1395–1400 [published online]
63. Heckmann TP, Noyes FR, Barber-Westin SD (2010) Rehabilitation of primary and revision anterior cruciate ligament reconstructions. In: Noyes FR (ed) Noyes' knee disorders: surgery, rehabilitation, clinical outcomes, 1st edn. Saunders, Philadelphia, pp p306–p336

PCL Lesion

19

Philippe Landreau and Jaleleddine Belhaj Ahmed

19.1 Introduction

Posterior cruciate ligament (PCL) injuries are less common in sport than anterior cruciate ligament (ACL) ruptures. Therefore, clinical studies and the experience of most physicians are more limited than for ACL injuries. In the last decade new anatomical, biomechanical and clinical studies have provided some novel insight concerning this ligament and renewed interest on this topic.

Football-related PCL ruptures are frequently associated with other pathologies, most commonly involving the posterolateral corner. It is critical to accurately diagnose PCL ruptures and their associated injuries because this will affect treatment and prognosis.

Injuries of the PCL can be classified according to the severity, timing (acute vs. chronic) and associated injuries (isolated vs. combined). The treatment options (conservative or surgical) are still a topic of debate.

P. Landreau, MD (✉)
Surgery Department,
Aspetar, Orthopaedic and Sports Medicine Hospital,
Doha, PO Box 29222, Qatar
e-mail: landreau@mac.com

J. Belhaj Ahmed, PT
Physiotherapy Department,
Aspetar, Orthopaedic and Sports Medicine Hospital,
Doha, PO Box 29222, Qatar
e-mail: jaleleddine.ahmed@aspetar.com

19.2 Anatomy

The PCL is a large ligament extending from the lateral surface of the medial femoral condyle to the posterior aspect of the tibia. Anatomically, it is closely related to other structures such as the joint capsule, the ACL, the menisci, the ligaments of Humphrey and Wrisberg, and the posterior neurovascular structures [1–5]. It consists of longitudinal collagen fibres narrower in their middle portion, extending largely at its femoral insertion and on a smaller surface area on the tibia. The PCL averages between 35 and 38 mm in length, and its width is 11 and 13 mm.

The ligament consists of two distinct but inseparable bundles with distinct footprints at both the femoral and tibial side. These are the anterolateral (AL) and the posteromedial (PM) bundles. The anterolateral bundle is twice as large as the posteromedial. It is the primary stabiliser of the knee when a posterior drawer test is applied.

The tibial insertion of the PCL is located 1.5 cm below the posterior joint line, in a trapezoidal fovea localised between the two tibial plateaus and slightly lateral (Fig. 19.1). The AL bundle is inserted on the superolateral portion and the PM bundle on the inferomedial portion of fossa. The more posterior and distal fibres are close to the posterior capsule (1–2 mm only). In order to understand the potential risk of perioperative vascular complication, it is important to mention that the anterior wall of the popliteal

P. Volpi (ed.), *Football Traumatology: New Trends*, DOI 10.1007/978-3-319-18245-2_19

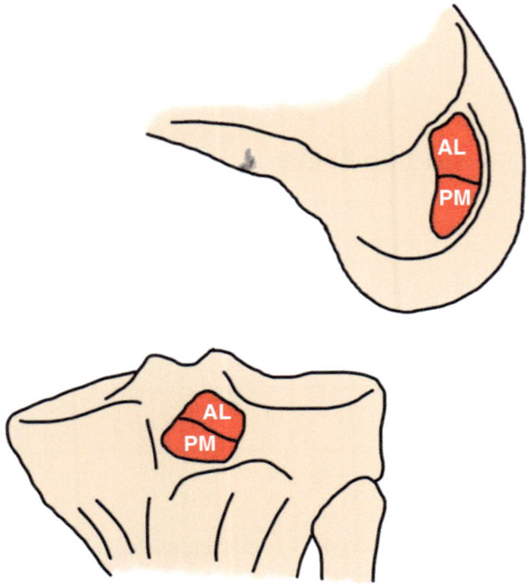

Fig. 19.1 The tibial and femoral insertions of the PCL

artery is located at a distance ranging from 7 to 10 mm from the posterior edge of the PCL [6, 7].

The femoral insertion of the PCL on the medial femoral condyle has a semicircular appearance (Fig. 19.1). Its distal portion follows the cartilage of the medial condyle at a distance of 1–2 mm. This insertion is spread in the coronal plane from 4 to 12 o'clock for the right knee and from 8 to 12 o'clock for the left knee. The surface of the insertion for the AL and PM bundles is distinct. During arthroscopy, the AL bundle is the more easily located bundle.

The PCL is sandwiched by the two meniscofemoral (MFL) ligaments. They are two distinct structures that connect the lateral meniscus to the medial intercondylar surface. The ligament of Humphrey passes in front of the PCL, and the ligament of Wrisberg is behind it. Recent anatomical dissections identified at least one MFL in 94–100 % of cases [1]. It can represent up to 25 % of the size of the PCL. They are secondary restraints of posterior tibial translation. Their presence probably explains the potential of the PCL to heal, when compared with the ACL, by acting as a splint to keep a torn PCL in position while it heals. If the MFL ligaments are not injured, they should be protected during PCL reconstructive surgery.

19.3 Biomechanics

The primary function of the PCL is to control posterior tibial displacement. Its secondary function is to assist with posterolateral stability and varus-valgus stress.

The tensile strength of the PCL ranges from 739 to 1,627 N, depending on the knee angle. The AL bundle has a 43 mm^2 cross-sectional area and a mean strength of 1,620 N, in comparison with 10 mm^2 and 258 N, respectively, for the PL bundle. Therefore, the AL bundle is clearly the stronger bundle of the PCL. A single bundle reconstruction must reconstruct this bundle. Note that the mean strength of the MFL averages 300 N (close to that of the PL bundle).

The tension of the two PCL bundles varies depending on the degree of knee flexion. In extension, the AL bundle is slack (appearing curved on the MRI), while the PL bundle is taut [3, 8]. With the knee in flexion, the AL bundle is taut. This knowledge indicates to the surgeon that the AL bundle graft must be fixed in a flexed position during PCL reconstruction and to the physiotherapist that extension is a protective position.

The posterolateral structures (PLS), which consist of the lateral collateral ligament, popliteofibular ligament and popliteus tendon, have an important synergistic relationship with the PCL to control posterior translation and external rotation. Biomechanical studies have shown that only the combined section of both PCL and PLS results in important laxity compared with an isolated section of structure alone. This means that severe posterior laxity on clinical examination should raise suspicions of a combined PLS lesion [9, 10].

19.4 Epidemiology and Mechanisms of Sports-related PCL Injury

The reported incidence of PCL ruptures in the literature ranges between 1 % and 44 % of all acute knee ligament injuries [11–13]. The variability is probably due to differences in the patient populations studied, as PCL injury rates are likely to vary when comparing trauma patients to an athletic population. In the general population, Miyasaka and Daniel [13] reported the incidence to be 3 %. The incidence in trauma or sporting activity is much higher. Fanelli [11] reported the incidence to be 37 % of all cases with acute haemarthrosis. In a large series, Schulz et al. [12] reported that of 494 complete PCL injuries, 45% of the injuries were related to traffic accidents and 40 % to a sports injury. These types of injuries are also reported in other publications [11, 13]. In the same series, motorcycle accidents were responsible for 28 % of PCL ruptures, in comparison with 14 % in car accidents. Football represented 25 % of the injuries usually as a result of falling on a flexed knee with the foot in plantar flexion, and it is notable that 18 % of all soccer-related PCL injuries involved the goalkeeper. Other sports such as rugby, American football and skiing are frequently associated with PCL injury (incidence range from 1 % to 4 %). Males are more frequently involved than females, probably due to the type of injuries and sports performed.

When comparing acute and chronic ruptures, the literature reports that sports injuries represented 70 % of acute PCL injuries in contrast to chronic ruptures, where motor vehicle accidents caused 60 % of injuries. Patients injured in high-energy motor vehicle accidents suffer a higher incidence of additional life-threatening injuries, and therefore ligamentous knee injuries can be easily overlooked. A combined injury (PCL and PLS) is frequent, particularly in traffic accidents, but can also occur in 50 % of athletic injuries [14].

Two main mechanisms can cause a PCL rupture [11, 12]. The most common is the 'dashboard injury' (40 %). Since the PCL is the primary restraint to posterior translation of the tibia relative to the femur, it is the first ligament to be injured in these dashboard injuries. In this setting, the knee is in a flexed position, and a posteriorly directed force is applied to the proximal tibia as the joint strikes the dashboard. With the knee in external rotation, the traumatic forces are directed toward the posterolateral and lateral structures of the joint. In football or rugby, falls on the flexed knee with the foot in plantar flexion are a common mechanism of injury. In this setting, the site of the impact is the tibial tubercle, and the proximal tibia is driven posteriorly relative to the femur. If the foot is in dorsiflexion, the force is transmitted more through the patella and distal femur, protecting the PCL from injury. Hyperextension is typically reported to be a cause of PCL rupture and may result in disruption of the posterior capsule (12 % in Schulz series), but a forced valgus or varus movement can result in a PCL rupture as well.

19.5 Clinical Examination

PCL ruptures as well as combined PCL and posterolateral structure lesions are frequently misdiagnosed. In many cases, the PCL rupture is missed despite typical injury mechanisms and symptoms. It is crucial to distinguish between PCL lesions that are isolated and those combined with other ligament injuries. A systematic clinical knee examination following trauma should always include PCL tests. It is essential to detect posterolateral laxity as the prognosis, and treatment will differ vastly if this is present [15, 16].

Begin the knee evaluation by obtaining a detailed history of the injury and attempting to delineate the mechanism. In contrast to ACL ruptures, the patient rarely reports hearing or feeling a 'pop' and does not relate a sense of instability if the PCL rupture is isolated. Patients with combined injuries, e.g. PCL and PLS, complain of pain, swelling and instability. The physical examination begins by exposing both lower extremities and observing the patient's gait pattern if he/she is able to walk. A varus thrust in combination with a hyperextended knee gait may indicate a chronic combined PCL and posterolateral corner injury.

19.5.1 Posterior Sag Test

In the posterior sag test, the knees are flexed to 90° and the feet placed on the table. A PCL injury can be suspected when observing and palpating the anterior joint line. Normally, the anterior

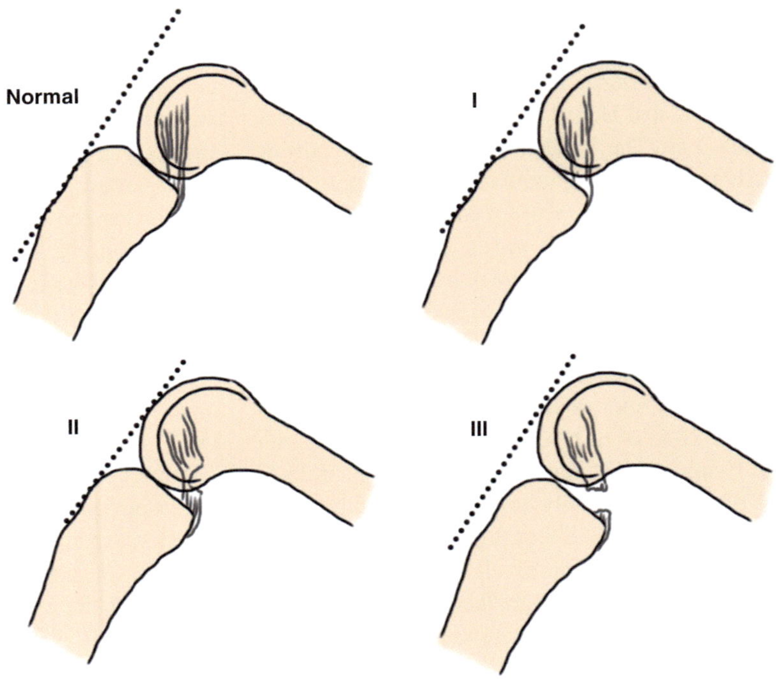

Fig. 19.2 Classification of PCL injuries, according to the posterior subluxation of the tibial plateau relative to the femoral condyle

border of the medial tibial plateau sits about 1 cm anterior to the medial femoral condyle. The normal step is easily palpable and compared with the contralateral side. In a PCL-deficient knee, gravity causes the tibia to rest in a posteriorly subluxed position compared with the intact knee. This test can be performed with the hip and the knee flexed to 90°, the examiner supporting the weight of the limb by the foot (Godfrey's test).

19.5.2 Posterior Drawer Test

The posterior drawer test is the most accurate clinical test for the assessment of PCL rupture. It is performed with the knee at 90° with the patient in supine position. The normal starting position is with the anterior border of the lateral tibial plateau 1 cm anterior to the lateral femoral condyle. Without a proper starting position, the examiner may elicit a false-negative posterior drawer and a false-positive anterior drawer test leading to an incorrect diagnosis. Isolated PCL injuries are usually classified by the degree of posterior subluxation of the tibial plateau relative to the femoral condyle. With a grade I injury, the tibial plateau remains anterior to the condyle, maintaining an anterior step-off. A grade II injury is likely when the anterior border of the tibia sits flush with the femoral condyle (5–10 mm translation). Grades I and II are usually partial tears. When the anterior border of the tibial plateau rests posterior to the femoral condyle (more than 10 mm of translation), a complete tear (grade III) is present, and associated posterolateral structure damage should also be suspected (Fig. 19.2).

19.5.3 The Quadriceps Active Test

In this test, the knee is placed at 60° of flexion and the examiner holds pressure on the foot. The patient is asked to contract the quadriceps isometrically. In the case of a complete rupture of the PCL, the quadriceps contraction achieves a dynamic reduction of the posterior displacement of the tibia.

19.5.4 Other Tests

As the treatment and the prognosis of combined laxities may differ from an isolated PCL injury, a complete ligament assessment of the joint must be performed, including particularly the tests for posterolateral, anterior and collateral laxities.

19.6 Imaging

The standard knee series must include bilateral standing anteroposterior and lateral views in flexion weight bearing ('Schuss views'). Look for subtle posterior tibial subluxation and avulsion fractures. Bony tibial avulsions, when recognised acutely, may be repaired primarily. In addition, long-leg cassette views allow an assessment of the lower limb alignment, particularly in chronic cases.

Stress radiographs (Telos), when available, can help the diagnosis and contribute to classifying the grade of the lesion.

MRI is the imaging study of choice for PCL ruptures [17]. Not only will it detect acute ruptures, it will determine the precise location of the lesion and assess the menisci and other supporting ligaments of the knee and articular surfaces.

19.7 Natural History of PCL Rupture and Conservative Treatment

The treatment of the PCL-injured knee is a controversial issue. Treatment should be based on the natural history of the PCL-deficient knee because this provides the baseline against which any interventions can be compared. Unfortunately, there are very few true natural history studies on the PCL-injured knee; most published studies are retrospective and include a mixture of patients and injuries. The retrospective studies generally report both acute and chronic injuries with various follow-up times, variable assessment criteria, small patient groups and even different PCL injury.

In a series of 45 patients, Dejour [18] described in 1988 the natural history of the isolated PCL injury as occurring in three phases:

1. Functional adaptation lasting 3–18 months, with return to sport
2. Functional tolerance continuing for 15–20 years
3. Osteoarthritic deterioration (medial tibiofemoral, femoropatellar or generalised) that does not become disabling until 25 years have passed

In a prospective study of the outcome of conservative treatment, Shelbourne [19] reported the outcomes of 271 athletes with acute, isolated, nonoperatively treated PCL injuries. 76 % were able to return to sport or activity at a similar level. Several series have described the intrinsic healing potential of the PCL, return to competitive sport, lack of symptomatic instability and good outcomes at midterm follow-up.

Conservative treatment, based on a physiotherapy protocol, gives good results if the PCL rupture occurs as an isolated injury, with return to sport which can, in some cases, be in less than 2 months. The current consensus is that grade 1 and grade 2 should be treated conservatively.

This PCL rehabilitation protocol is divided into an early (maximum protection), intermediate (moderate protection) and advanced (minimum protection) phase. Progression from one phase to the next is criteria based, not timeline based. The timelines provided are only approximate, and more importance should be placed on the criteria for progression when taking decisions. The protocol will require adaptation to each patient individually, depending on the specific treatment goals, the grade of the PCL injury and the level of sports activity.

The protocol may require adaptation for individuals with other associated injuries, and in these cases recommendations of the treating physician should be followed and accounted for when applying the protocol (Table 19.1).

19.8 Surgical Treatment

A combined acute lesion of the posterolateral structure must be diagnosed as the repair must be done within the first 3 weeks after the injury [20, 21]. The surgical management of displaced avulsion fractures will usually result in a favourable outcome. Suture or screw fixations are an appropriate method with a posterior surgical approach for cases where there is a large bony fragment. Some surgeons argue

Table 19.1 Aspetar PCL conservative rehabilitation protocol

General guidelines:	
Because the PCL has some potential of healing [19, 32], the early phase of rehabilitation is crucial in acute PCL injuries for the final outcomes by providing a maximum protection to the ligament and avoiding any stressful activity	
A statistical correlation exists between lower isokinetic quadriceps scores and lower function. Quadriceps isokinetic values in patients who fully returned to sport were greater than 100 % of the isokinetic values from the uninvolved side [19, 33, 34]. The quadriceps is the main agonist to the PCL by pulling the proximal tibia anteriorly between 0° and 60° of knee flexion, while the gastrocnemius is a secondary agonist muscle. Hamstrings act at antagonists to the PCL by pulling the proximal tibia posteriorly, and this action increases as the knee flexion angle increases. Open kinetic chain (OKC) hamstring strengthening should be postponed until the advanced phase of rehabilitation. All closed kinetic chain (CKC) exercises result in a posterior glide of the tibia that increases as the angle of knee flexion increases [35, 36]	
Proprioception and neuromuscular control of the knee are compromised after PCL injury [37–39]. Therefore, a regular strengthening and neuromuscular training programme should be continued after return to sport to maintain the knee performance	
Early phase (0–4 weeks)	
Goals	Protection of the healing PCL
	Decrease pain and swelling
	Maintain a minimum ROM
	Good quadriceps control and strengthening initiation
	Prepare for normal gait
General recommendations	Weight bearing as tolerated (WBAT) with crutches
	Brace: worn at all times including sleeping and rehabilitation (dynamic PCL brace ideally). If not available, use a hinged brace with a posterior tibial foam locked at 0° for 2 weeks, and add 20° every week: 4 weeks for grade 1, 6 weeks for grade 2 and 8 weeks for grade 3 [40–42]
	Avoid knee hyperextension
	RICE (avoid posterior sag with elevation: place a pillow below the proximal tibia)
	Start at phase 2 for patients with chronic PCL deficiency
Range of motion (ROM)	Gentle passive ROM exercises (0–60°) starting in prone to avoid the posterior sag
Strengthening	*Quadriceps*
	Quadriceps sets (may be done with ice application in the presence of a quadriceps inhibition) with a pillow below the proximal tibia
	Electrical muscle stimulation
	Straight leg raise (SLR): ensure good quadriceps control to avoid posterior sag
	Quadriceps bench/isometric quadriceps: 20°–40°–60°
	Terminal knee extension (progressively add weight or theraband resistance)
	Hip/gluteals
	SLR flexion/abduction/adduction
	Progress with a theraband resistance over the knee/progress from a plinth to standing position
	Multi-hip machine: flexion/abduction/adduction
	Gastrocnemius
	Calf press with extended knee
	Theraband-resisted ankle PF with the knee extended
	Bilateral heel raises as tolerated and progress to unilateral
Proprioception	Static single leg stance when tolerated
	Forward, backward and lateral steps as tolerated
	STAR excursion exercise
	Strengthening uninvolved leg
	Cardiovascular training
	Hydrotherapy: deep water walking

Table 19.1 (continued)

Progression criteria to move to next phase	Minimal or no swelling
	Normal gait without aid or brace
	Completed early exercise programme
	No quadriceps lag
	Less than 30 % deficit of uninvolved leg in isometric quadriceps strength
	Pain-free single leg squat to 60°
Intermediate phase (week 4–8)	
Goals	Normal gait
	Full pain-free ROM
	Less than 20 % deficit in isokinetic quadriceps test at 60°/s
	Improve balance and neuromuscular control
ROM	Passive ROM exercises as tolerated, start in prone
	Passive ROM in supine as physiotherapist pulls the tibia anteriorly (mobilisation with movement/MWM)
	Bike when more than 115 knee flexion/remove the clips to minimise the hamstrings activity
	Rowing machine/remove the foot clips and use mainly the upper arms
	Elliptical bike
	Stair master/retro climbing induces more quadriceps activity
Strengthening and endurance	Quadriceps/gastrocnemius/hip muscles
	Concentric and eccentric leg press (0–60°)
	Isotonic quadriceps (0–60°)
	Isokinetic quadriceps eccentric/concentric (0–60°) start with low speed and progress
	Bilateral mini squats: start at 45° and progress by adding depth and weights
	We may use the MWM/anterior glide with CKC exercises
	Wall slides/stable to unstable surface
	CKC (closed kinetic chain) terminal knee extension against theraband resistance (placed on the posterior aspect of the proximal tibia)
	Dead lifts
	Mini lunges: static, progress to dynamic and add weights
	Step ups: forward, backward and lateral. Progress by increasing step height and adding weight
	Total gym: bilateral/unilateral/mini-jump
	Multi-hip machine: flexion/abduction/adduction
	Multi-hip with theraband
Core stability	Prone plank
	Lateral plank
	Prone ball bridge
Calves	Calf press with extended knee
	Heel raises: bilateral/unilateral/add weights progressively
Maintenance strengthening of the uninvolved leg	CKC/OKC hip and knee muscle strengthening
	Isotonic/isokinetic strengthening
Proprioception	Double leg to single leg stance on foam/BOSU/trampoline
	Internal/external perturbations on varying surfaces (e.g. addition of squat/lunge/upper body exercise/catching/kicking)
	STAR excursion
	Biodex balance machine
	Ladder drills

(continued)

Table 19.1 (continued)

Cardiovascular	Continue as for early phase: increase intensity and time
Progression criteria to move to next phase	No swelling or pain
	No increase in laxity
	Full pain-free ROM
	Less than 20% deficit in isokinetic test
	Completed intermediate exercise programme
	No feeling of instability
Advanced phase (8–12 weeks)	
Goals	Less than 10% deficit in isokinetic test for both hamstrings and quadriceps
	Achievement of the running and sports-specific progression without problems
	Good stability and self-confidence with the exercises
	Continue the moderate phase programme
	Focus on power and endurance
Strengthening	Add hip extension resistance placed over the knee
	Single leg CKC
	Add hamstrings OKC strengthening if the deficit persists on isokinetic testing: heel digs, supine bridge, theraband, weights
	Single dead lifts with weights
	We may associate hamstrings retraining with an anterior tibial glide (MWM)
Proprioception	Balance squat
	Internal/external perturbations
	Star excursion exercises/add perturbation (e.g. ball tasks tubing resistance on waist)
	Biodex balance (increase complexity)
Running progression	Straight line running
	Progress in speed, acceleration, deceleration
	Changing direction, cutting, figure-8 running
Jumping progression	Bilateral to unilateral hops: anterior-posterior and lateral hop, triple hop, cross-over hop
	Step up/step down
	Bilateral jumps and progress to unilateral
Functional/sports-specific training	Single planar agility to multi-planar agility exercises
	Direction changes: low intensity, slow speed, anterior, posterior, lateral, progress speed and complexity in movements
	Acceleration/deceleration: gradual increase in intensity and progress to abrupt acceleration/deceleration
	Vertimax exercises: basic sports-specific progress to sports-specific rehabilitation on field
	Noncontact game situation
	Progress to contact situations
Cardiovascular	Continue intermediate phase training with increasing intensity/duration
Discharge criteria to return to play	Biodex <10 % difference compared to the uninvolved side (ideally no deficit for quadriceps)
	Hop testing <10 % difference compared to the uninvolved side with a good landing alignment
	Completed the sports-specific programme
	Good stability
	Self-reported confidence and no fear of reinjury

for the repair of some ligament avulsions without any bone avulsions, but in the majority of cases, a PCL reconstruction is carried out.

The general principles of the ligament reconstruction are based on the anatomical placement of the tunnels, use of a strong and large graft, graft tunnels avoiding sharp angulations, knowledge of the proximity of the popliteal vessels, tension and fixation of the anterolateral bundle between 70° and 90° of flexion, solid fixation of the transplant, as well as a suitable rehabilitation programme.

During PCL reconstruction, an autograft (patellar tendon, quadriceps tendon or hamstrings) can be used. However, an allograft, if available, is a suitable alternative. The Achilles tendon is often the allograft of choice [22, 23]. Several methods exist for reconstruction of the PCL.

19.8.1 The Single Bundle Transtibial Technique

The transtibial technique was the first developed technique. Initially using an open procedure, now performed arthroscopically [4, 22, 24, 25], it remains a technique of reference. Using an arthroscopic posteromedial approach and a specific tibial guide, a tibial tunnel is performed. The femoral tunnel is then made using an out-in or an in-out technique. The optimal tunnel positioning should take into consideration that the aim of the surgery is to recreate the anteromedial bundle of the native PCL. One of the key concerns with the transtibial technique is the so-called killer turn. This describes the sharp angulation of the graft at the posterior end of the tibial tunnel which can generate progressive damage and failure of the graft. The inlay technique was proposed in response to this concern.

19.8.2 The Inlay Technique [26]

Once the arthroscopic procedure has been achieved, including drilling of the femoral tunnel, the patient is repositioned for an open posterior approach. After protection of the neurovascular structures, the posterior tibial plateau is exposed and prepared for placement of the bone block. The graft is inlayed flush and fixed with screws. Then, the proximal part of the graft is passed through the femoral tunnel for a standard fixation. So far this modified technique does not show any superior clinical results when compared with the transtibial technique [24, 27].

19.8.3 The Double Bundle Reconstruction

In order to better reconstruct the anatomy of the native PCL, the double bundle reconstruction was developed [28]. The majority of the supporters of this surgical procedure perform two femoral tunnels. The tibial technique can be either single or double. Therefore, this technique can be carried out combining an inlay technique. Despite some cadaveric and biomechanical studies, no clinical difference has been found between single and double bundle reconstructions as of today [11, 21, 29].

19.8.4 Complications

Residual laxity is a common complication after PCL reconstruction, whatever the technique [30]. The most serious risk of surgery is a neurovascular complication, given the close proximity of the popliteal artery to the PCL [6]. Other postoperative complications include fractures, medial femoral condyle necrosis and arthrofibrosis [7].

19.8.5 Rehabilitation

Physiotherapy is crucial after PCL reconstruction. In contrast to ACL reconstruction, gravity tends to stretch the PCL graft. Therefore, some specific techniques of physiotherapy (immobilisation in extension, exercise in prone position) and a slower pace [31], compared to the accelerated rehabilitation of ACL injury, have been supported to allow complete healing of the PCL graft. Return to sport is rarely achieved before 8 months. The guidelines are comparable to those exposed for the conservative treatment in Table 19.1, with a different timeline.

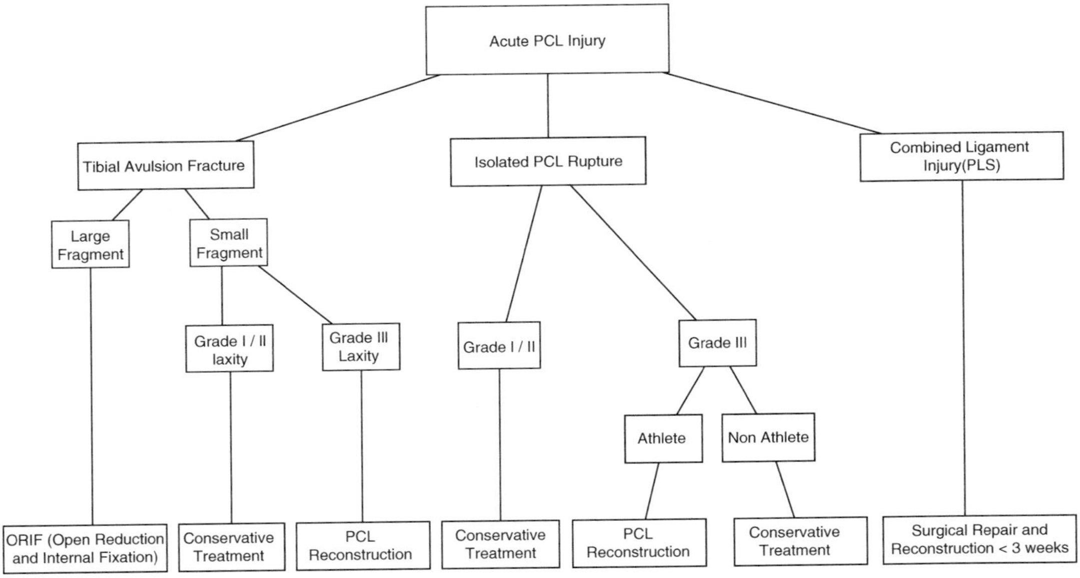

Fig. 19.3 Treatment algorithm for acute PCL injury

19.8.6 Clinical Outcomes After Surgical Reconstruction [20, 30]

The early results of surgical treatments reported in the literature were somewhat biased in that there was a mixture of acute, chronic, isolated and combined injuries. There are very few long-term results published. The conclusions of the 2004 symposium organised during the French Society of Arthroscopy Congress on isolated PCL ruptures were that PCL surgery can improve knee function and sports activity significantly, but that the graft cannot fully control posterior laxity, with the average gain being 6 mm [30]. Hammoud et al. [20] reported a systematic review of the evidence in 2010. Twenty-one papers in the literature reported the results after surgical treatment of isolated PCL injury. The percentage of return to same sports level activity ranges from 50 % to 82 % in comparison with the 19 % to 68% range in case of combined ligament injuries treated surgically (ten studies in the literature).

Based on our experience and the current literature, a treatment algorithm for acute PCL injury is proposed (Fig. 19.3).

Conclusion

The majority of isolated PCL ruptures can be treated conservatively with good results and return to sport in a few weeks. In the athletic population, grade I and II injuries are usually treated conservatively with success, and we recommend performing a PCL reconstruction in the case of grade III injuries. The combined injuries, particularly PCL and PLS lesions, must be treated surgically within the first 3 weeks following the injury as the treatment of the chronic posterolateral laxity is challenging.

References

1. Amis AA, Gupte CM, Bull AM, Edwards A (2006) Anatomy of the posterior cruciate ligament and the meniscofemoral ligaments. Knee Surg Sports Traumatol Arthrosc 14(3):257–263
2. Harner CD, Baek GH, Vogrin TM, Carlin GJ, Kashiwaguchi S, Woo SL (1999) Quantitative analysis of human cruciate ligament insertions. Arthroscopy 15(7):741–749
3. Girgis FG, Marshall JL, Monajem A (1975) The cruciate ligaments of the knee joint. Anatomical, functional and experimental analysis. Clin Orthop Relat Res 106:216–231

4. Forsythe B, Harner C, Martins CA, Shen W, Lopes OV Jr, Fu FH (2009) Topography of the femoral attachment of the posterior cruciate ligament. Surgical technique. J Bone Joint Surg Am 91(Suppl 2 Pt 1):89–100
5. Tajima G, Nozaki M, Iriuchishima T, Ingham SJ, Shen W, Smolinski P, Fu FH (2009) Morphology of the tibial insertion of the posterior cruciate ligament. J Bone Joint Surg Am 91(4):859–866
6. Cosgarea AJ, Kramer DE, Bahk MS, Totty WG, Matava MJ (2006) Proximity of the popliteal artery to the PCL during simulated knee arthroscopy: implications for establishing the posterior trans-septal portal. J Knee Surg 19(3):181–185
7. Zawodny SR, Miller MD (2010) Complications of posterior cruciate ligament surgery. Sports Med Arthrosc 18(4):269–274
8. Van Dommelen BA, Fowler PJ (1989) Anatomy of the posterior cruciate ligament. A Review. Am J Sports Med 17(1):24–29
9. Schulz MS, Steenlage ES, Russe K, Strobel MJ (2007) Distribution of posterior tibial displacement in knees with posterior cruciate ligament tears. J Bone Joint Surg Am 89(2):332–338
10. Sekiya JK, Whiddon DR, Zehms CT, Miller MD (2008) A clinically relevant assessment of posterior cruciate ligament and posterolateral corner injuries. Evaluation of isolated and combined deficiency. J Bone Joint Surg Am 90(8):1621–1627
11. Fanelli GC, Edson CJ, Reinheimer KN (2008) Arthroscopic single bundle versus double bundle posterior cruciate ligament reconstruction. Arthroscopy 24(Suppl):e26
12. Schulz MS, Russe K, Weiler A, Eichhorn HJ, Strobel MJ (2003) Epidemiology of posterior cruciate ligament injuries. Arch Orthop Trauma Surg 123(4):186–191
13. Miyasaka KC, Daniel DM (1991) The incidence of knee ligament injuries in the general population. Am J Knee Surg 4:3–8
14. Hochstein P, Schmickal T, Grützner PA, Wentzensen A (1999) Diagnostic and incidence of the rupture of the posterior cruciate ligament. Unfallchirurg 102(10): 753–762
15. Petrie RS, Harner CD (1999) Evaluation and management of the posterior cruciate ligament injured knee. Oper Tech Sports Med 7:93–103
16. Fanelli GC, Giannotti BF, Edson CJ (1994) The posterior cruciate ligament arthroscopic evaluation and treatment. Review. Arthrosc 10(6):673–688
17. Covey CD, Sapega AA (1993) Injuries of the posterior cruciate ligament. Review. J Bone Joint Surg Am 75(9):1376–1386
18. Dejour H, Walch G, Peyrot J, Eberhard P (1988) The natural history of rupture of the posterior cruciate ligament. Rev Chir Orthop Reparatrice Appar Mot 74(1):35–43
19. Shelbourne KD, Davis TJ, Patel DV (1999) The natural history of acute, isolated, nonoperatively treated posterior cruciate ligament injuries. A prospective study. Am J Sports Med 27(3):276–283
20. Hammoud S, Reinhardt KR, Marx RG (2010) Outcomes of posterior cruciate ligament treatment: a review of the evidence. Sports Med Arthrosc 18(4): 280–291
21. Wang CJ, Weng LH, Hsu CC, Chan YS (2004) Arthroscopic single- versus double-bundle posterior cruciate ligament reconstructions using hamstring autograft. Injury 35(12):1293–1299
22. Fanelli GC, Boyd J (2009) How I manage PCL injuries. Oper Tech Sports Med 17:175–183
23. Ahn JH, Yoo JC, Wang JH (2005) Posterior cruciate ligament reconstruction: double-loop hamstring tendon autograft versus Achilles tendon allograft—clinical results of a minimum 2-year follow-up. Arthroscopy 21(8):965–969
24. Bergfeld JA, McAllister DR, Parker RD, Valdevit AD, Kambic HE (2001) A biomechanical comparison of posterior cruciate ligament reconstruction techniques. Am J Sports Med 29(2):129–136
25. Mariani PP, Adriani E, Santori N, Maresca G (1997) Arthroscopic posterior cruciate ligament reconstruction with bone-tendon-bone patellar graft. Knee Surg Sports Traumatol Arthrosc 5(4):239–244
26. Berg EE (1995) Posterior cruciate ligament tibial inlay reconstruction. Arthroscopy 11:69–76
27. Markolf KL, Zemanovic JR, McAllister DR (2002) Cyclic loading of posterior cruciate ligament replacements fixed with tibial tunnel and tibial inlay methods. J Bone Joint Surg Am 84-A(4):518–524
28. Clancy WG, Bisson LJ (1999) Double tunnel technique for reconstruction of the posterior cruciate ligament. Oper Tech Sports Med 7:110–117
29. Harner CD, Janaushek MA, Kanamori A, Yagi M, Vogrin TM, Woo SL (2000) Biomechanical analysis of a double-bundle posterior cruciate ligament reconstruction. Am J Sports Med 28(2):144–151
30. Badet R, Chambat P, Boussaton M, Bousquet V, Chassaing V, Cucurulo T, Djian P, Franceschi JP, Potel JF, Siegrist O, Sbihi A, Cerciello S; et la Société Française d'Arthroscopie (2005) "Isolated" injury of the posterior cruciate ligament. Surgical treatment of isolated posterior cruciate ligament tears: a multicentric retrospective study of 103 patients. Rev Chir Orthop Reparatrice Appar Mot 91(S8):43–54
31. Fanelli GC (2008) Posterior cruciate ligament rehabilitation: how slow should we go? Arthroscopy 24(2):234–235
32. Tewes DP, Fritts HM, Fields RD, Quick DC, Buss DD (1997) Chronically injured posterior cruciate ligament: magnetic resonance imaging. Clin Orthop Relat Res 335:224–232
33. Markolf KL, O'Neill G, Jackson SR, McAllister DR (2004) Effects of applied quadriceps and hamstrings muscle loads on forces in the anterior and posterior cruciate ligaments. Am J Sports Med 32(5):1144–1149
34. Parolie JM, Bergfeld JA (1986) Long-term results of nonoperative treatment of isolated posterior cruciate ligament injuries in the athlete. Am J Sports Med 14(1):35–38

35. Escamilla RF, Fleisig GS, Zheng N, Barrentine SW, Wilk KE, Andrews JR (1998) Biomechanics of the knee during closed kinetic chain and open kinetic chain exercises. Med Sci Sports Exerc 30(4): 556–569
36. Wilk KE, Escamilla RF, Fleisig GS, Barrentine SW, Andrews JR, Boyd ML (1996) A comparison of tibiofemoral joint forces and electromyographic activity during open and closed kinetic chain exercises. Am J Sports Med 24(4):518–527
37. Clark P, MacDonald PB, Sutherland K (1996) Analysis of proprioception in the posterior cruciate ligament-deficient knee. Knee Surg Sports Traumatol Arthrosc 4(4):225–227
38. Grassmayr MJ, Parker DA, Coolican MR, Vanwanseele B (2008) Posterior cruciate ligament deficiency: biomechanical and biological consequences and the outcomes of conservative treatment. A systematic review. J Sci Med Sport 11(5): 433–443
39. Hewett TE, Paterno MV, Myer GD (2002) Strategies for enhancing proprioception and neuromuscular control of the knee. Clin Orthop Relat Res 402:76–94
40. Jacobi M, Reischl N, Wahl P, Gautier E, Jakob RP (2010) Acute isolated injury of the posterior cruciate ligament treated by a dynamic anterior drawer brace: a preliminary report. J Bone Joint Surg Br 92(10):1381–1384
41. Jansson KS, Costello KE, O'Brien L, Wijdicks CA, Laprade RF (2013) A historical perspective of PCL bracing. Knee Surg Sports Traumatol Arthrosc 21(5): 1064–1070
42. LaPrade RF, Smith SD, Wilson KJ, Wijdicks CA (2014) Quantification of functional brace forces for posterior cruciate ligament injuries on the knee joint: an in vivo investigation. Knee Surg Sports Traumatol Arthrosc 22(8):1–7 (Epub ahead of print)

Knee: Multiligament Injuries

20

Francesco M. Benazzo, Giacomo Zanon, and Loris Perticarini

20.1 Etiology

Knee ligament injuries are very common due to increased participation in sports, extreme events, and road traffic accidents. Multiligament knee injuries result in the disruption of at least two of the major ligaments of the knee and lead to significant functional instability. The anatomical classification system developed by Schenck and modified by Wascher [1, 2] to classify the knee dislocation is useful to guide the management of knee multiligament injury (Table 20.1).

It is important to remember that more than two-thirds of all knee dislocations will be spontaneously reduced by the time the patient presents for evaluation by the orthopedic surgeon.

Because of the close proximity of the neurovascular structures to the posterior part of the knee joint, peroneal nerve and popliteal artery injuries are not uncommon, and neurovascular status must be evaluated upon initial presentation.

Historically, treatment was primarily limited to closed reduction and casting or cast-bracing immobilization. However, with the improvement of instrumentation and technique, combined anterior and posterior cruciate ligament (ACL–PCL) tears associated with medial and/or lateral collateral ligament (MCL/FCL) disruption is typically managed surgically, with some allowed flexibility to adjust for patient-specific factors [3]. Proper comprehensive physical examination skills and a good understanding of the complex anatomy of the knee are necessary to accurately diagnose these frequently missed injuries [4]. Careful and thorough clinical evaluation is critical as is timely, appropriate treatment.

20.2 Injury Mechanism

20.2.1 Central Pivot and Posterolateral Corner (PLC)

Isolated tears of the posterior cruciate ligament (PCL) can be caused by a fall on the flexed knee (the upper tibia driven posteriorly with the knee flexed). These tears are relatively rare as well as

Table 20.1 Schenck modified classification of knee dislocation [1, 2]

KD I	Multiligamentous injury with intact cruciate ligament
KD II	ACL and PCL torn, collateral ligaments intact
KD IIIM	Both cruciate ligaments torn, PMC torn
KD IIIL	Both cruciate ligaments torn, PLC torn, medial side intact
KD IV	ACL, PCL, PLC, and PMC disrupted
KD V	Periarticular fracture/dislocation of the knee

F.M. Benazzo (✉) • G. Zanon • L. Perticarini
Fondazione IRCCS Policlinico San Matteo Pavia, Viale Golgi, 19, 27100 Pavia, Italy
e-mail: fbenazzo@unipv.it; zanon.g@libero.it; loris.perticarini@gmail.com

P. Volpi (ed.), *Football Traumatology: New Trends*, DOI 10.1007/978-3-319-18245-2_20

isolated injuries of posterolateral complex (PLC) that often occurs in association with other ligament disruptions.

Mechanisms resulting in PLC injuries include a posterolateral-directed force to the anteromedial tibia, knee hyperextension and varus injury [5], and/or severe tibial external rotation while the knee is partially flexed.

A different injury mechanism can lead to a different pattern of lesion: in knee hyperextension injuries, the posterior capsule is primarily involved, followed by the PLC and finally the PCL injury; in external rotation injuries, the knee partially flexed could have tears to the popliteus tendon, popliteofibular ligament, FCL, and the ACL.

20.2.2 MCL and Posteromedial Corner (PMC)

Higher-grade MCL disruptions almost always involve a direct blow to the lateral leg producing significant valgus and external rotation stresses. Pure valgus forces often produce isolated MCL injuries, but as external rotation is added to the proximal tibia, tears of the posterior oblique ligament and anterior cruciate ligament are often seen [6].

20.3 Clinical and Diagnostic Examination

Initial evaluation of a knee with multiple ligament injuries begins with a thorough and complete neurovascular examination, an assessment of the soft tissue, and determination of the instability pattern. Failure to recognize a vascular injury can lead to catastrophic. A knee dislocation with subsequent reduction should always be considered a multiligament injured knee and should be evaluated as such. If possible, the examination of the knee must be performed with the patient in the standing, sitting, and supine positions. The observation of the patient's gait is also important.

20.3.1 Clinical Evaluation: Medial Compartment

Comprehensive physical examination is necessary to differentiate between isolated MCL injuries and those involving the PMC. The entire course of the MCL should be palpated from proximal to distal. When examining medial-side knee injuries, it is important to distinguish between localized soft tissue swelling and an intra-articular effusion. The former is commonly seen with an isolated MCL injury; the latter is often associated with intra-articular pathology such as an ACL or meniscal tear [7].

The tests that should be used to evaluate medial side are:

- *Valgus stress test:* the examination is conducted at both 0° and 30° of knee flexion, and the amount of "opening" at the medial joint line is evaluated. A 30° test isolates the MCL and is typically performed first. It may be helpful placing a slight rotary stress on the foot and observing for any anteromedial rotation of the tibial plateau on the medial femoral condyle. A positive finding of rotary instability may suggest damage to the PMC of the knee. This finding may represent a subset of patients in whom the medial-side injury requires surgical repair, especially in the case of a concomitant ACL rupture.

Valgus stress testing positive n is the second part of this evaluation. Opening in full extension indicates a complete MCL rupture (grade III) and PMC damage. It may also be associated with ACL or posterior cruciate ligament (PCL) injury [7].

- *Anterior drawer test:* to assess the amount of anterior translation of the tibia with the knee flexed at 80° and the tibia externally rotated at 15°. If the test is positive, there was a tear of the meniscotibial ligaments that allows the meniscus to move freely.

20.3.2 Clinical Evaluation: Lateral Compartment

The tests that should be used to evaluate PLC are:

- *Posterolateral drawer test:* patient in supine, with the knee flexed to 80–90° and the foot externally rotated 15°. While the clinician stabilizes the patient's foot, a posterolateral drawer force is applied. It is useful to evaluate the popliteus tendon, popliteofibular ligament, and FCL.
- *Dial test:* patient positioned either supine or prone, the clinician rotates the tibia through the foot and observes the amount of tibial external rotation present at 30° and 90° of knee flexion. An increase of greater than or equal to 15°, as compared to the contralateral side, is considered positive [8]. A dial test that is positive at 30° of knee flexion but normal at 90° of knee flexion is indicative of a potential injury to the PLC (the popliteus complex) [8]. A positive test at both 30° and 90° of knee flexion indicates both a PCL and PLC injury [8].
- *Varus stress test*: patient supine, the examiner stabilizes the tibia from unwanted rotation and applies a varus stress to the knee through the foot/ankle, first with the knee at 30° of flexion and repeated with the knee extended to 0°. The injury of FCL is classified according to the amount of subjective translation (or joint opening) and the perceived quality of resistance at the endpoint (grade I, II, or III if it shows gapping without an endpoint). A positive varus stress test at 30° is indicative of a complete tear of the FCL, and if positive at 0° of knee extension, it indicates a more severe injury, which may include the PCL, FCL, meniscotibial ligament, popliteus tendon, and the superficial layer of the ITB.
- *External rotation recurvatum test*: is performed by lifting a supine patient's great toe, while gently stabilizing the distal thigh and observing the relative amount of genu recurvatum present. The test is used to detect a concomitant ACL–PLC injury. It has a high incidence of false-negative results, and it is rarely positive in PCL–PLC or isolated PLC injuries.
- *Reverse pivot shift:* the knee is flexed to 45°, and the foot is externally rotated with a valgus stress applied. It is positive if the tibia posterolaterally subluxes with injury of the PLC.
- *Standing apprehension test:* the patient stands with his/her weight on the injured knee and slightly flexes it, while the clinician applies a medially directed force on the anterolateral portion of the lateral femoral condyle [9]. Rotation of the condyle relative to the tibia, in addition to the patient feeling a giving-way sensation, indicates a positive test [10] to assess injury to the PLC.

20.3.3 X-Ray

A standard radiographic knee series is indicated in all cases of suspected multiligament injuries. As with all injuries, a complete "knee" series which includes anterior–posterior (AP) views, 45° flexion (tunnel) views, and a lateral and axial view is recommended. High-grade peripherical sprains, especially when combined with a cruciate injury, may show medial or lateral joint space widening on a supine AP view. Fractures, avulsions, or osteochondral fragments seen on x-ray could significantly affect the treatment plan. Every young player with increased laxity in varus or valgus stress and open physes should have stress views to rule out a fracture through the growth plate [7].

In chronic cases with instability, long-standing cassette radiographs of both lower extremities should be obtained to assess limb alignment. Moreover, in patients with chronic pain from a previous multiligament injury with MCL involved, radiographs may demonstrate crescent-shaped calcification along the MCL, known as a Pellegrini–Stieda lesion [11].

Fluoroscopic or radiographic stress examination is often helpful to assess for chronic ligament injuries, but difficult to perform in the acute injured knee. In chronic cases, at the stress examinations for posterior–anterior and varus–valgus laxity, a

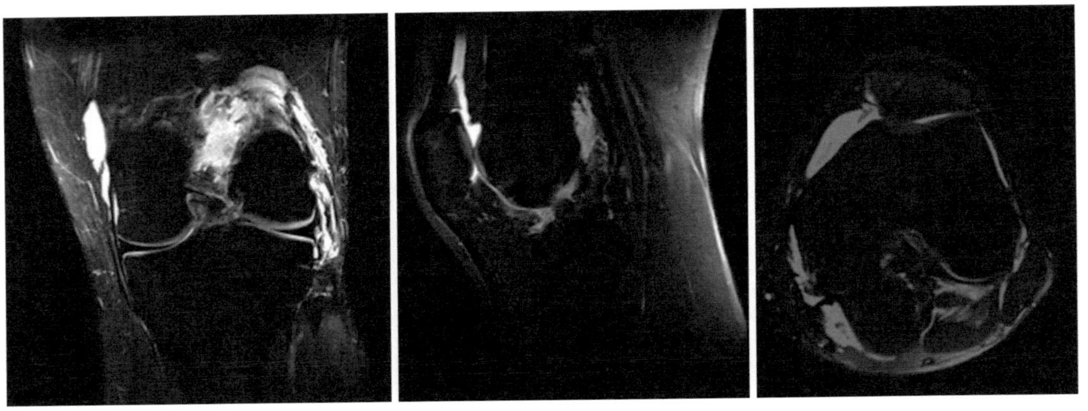

Fig. 20.1 ACL, FCL, PLC injury in elite football player

difference between the two knees of ≥3 mm can be considered pathologic using TELOS [12].

20.3.4 MRI

Magnetic resonance imaging (MRI) is important in assessing patients with complex multiligament knee injuries, though it should be used to supplement and support, rather than replace, physical examination findings. It is also important to stress that if an MRI is to be obtained, this should be done before operative fixation of any associated periarticular fractures, as metal susceptibility artifact will impede the quality of the scan. MRI scanning tends to overestimate injury to the ligamentous structures and should not be used as the only diagnostic tool for surgical planning. Physical examination under anesthesia (EUA) continues to be the most accurate for determining injury to the ligaments of the knee. MRI, however, may be more beneficial for detection of meniscus injury, or injury to the osteochondral surface, and it can also be very useful in determining avulsion versus midsubstance injuries (Fig. 20.1).

Surrounding edema is often observed in any acute ligament injuries, although it is nonspecific and can also be present in other knee problems, such as meniscal tears or osteoarthritis [13]. In the setting of a severe PLC injury, the adjacent peroneal nerve should be assessed for the presence of traumatic neuritis or disruption of nerve fascicles [14]. Halinen et al [15] demonstrated that MRI (1.5 T) ability to detect lateral meniscal tears was less than hoped, but medial meniscal tears, ligamentous injuries, and bone bruises were seen more precisely in 44 cases of multiligament knee injury. However, both MRI and EUA should be used in concert to appreciate the extent of injury to the knee following a high-energy injury.

20.4 Treatment Strategy

Decision-making often is based on each individual's pre-injury function and the extent of the ligament damage. Several studies have suggested patients receiving operative treatment have improved functional outcomes when compared with nonoperative treatment [16]. The timing of surgery is critical with evidence that shows if surgery is done immediately following the injury, an individual may experience increased postoperative stiffness and scarring. It is well demonstrated that outcomes of multiligament reconstruction have better outcomes when surgery is performed within 3 weeks from injury, after swelling from the initial injury is reduced [17–19]. The benefits of early surgery must be balanced against the risks of arthrofibrosis.

20.4.1 Central Pivot and Medial Side

Successful outcomes of complex multiligament injuries require that the surgeon differentiate between injuries to the medial collateral ligament (MCL) and those to the PMC, as this will be critical to the development of the surgical plan.

The high reparative potential of the MCL with conservative treatment and the complications (primarily knee stiffness) associated with surgical repair/reconstruction are at the base of the controversies regarding the treatment of medial/posteromedial ligamentous injuries.

If isolated MCL injury is present, nonoperative treatment can be the best choice, whereas outcomes with anteromedial rotatory instability (AMRI) typically improve with surgical reconstruction [20].

In case of combined MCL-ACL injury, should be considered the grade of MCL tear and the level of athlete; in grade I, the treatment is always conservative; in grade II, the tear could be treated conservatively, and the ACL reconstruction in low-level athletes is staged, while MCL and ACL should be repaired in one stage in elite athletes, especially if the collateral is detached from the tibia; in grade III, the surgical indication is mandatory whatever the level of participation.

In case of associated ACL, PCL, and PMC injuries, reconstruction of PMC and PCL should be performed first, while the second stage involves reconstruction of the anterior cruciate ligament 6 weeks following the initial operation [4]. By performing staged procedures with the PCL being addressed first, rehabilitation can follow a typical PCL protocol without stretching the ACL. Likewise, once the ACL has been reconstructed, the therapy program can switch to a pure ACL protocol, therefore maximizing the benefit for both cruciate ligaments [4].

20.4.1.1 Surgical Technique

In ACL–PCL and medial-side tears, the progression of the treatment in two stage (PCL and PMC on the first stage, ACL later) is a diagnostic arthroscopy to address meniscus pathology with repair or resection as indicated, perform reconstruction of PCL without tensioning and femoral fixation, and then reconstruct PMC. Graft tensioning and fixation of the PCL is then performed after the PMC reconstruction. The choice of the graft depends on the numbers and the structures involved: in multiligament injury, it is useful to consider one or more allograft (patellar tendon, Achilles tendon, tibialis anterior or posterior, semitendinosus). Fanelli et al. [21] prefer an Achilles tendon allograft for single-bundle posterior cruciate ligament reconstructions and the Achilles tendon and tibialis anterior allografts for double-bundle posterior cruciate ligament reconstructions. Either a tibialis anterior or a patellar tendon allograft is preferred for anterior cruciate ligament reconstructions, in case of one-stage reconstruction of all ligaments injured.

After 6 weeks, the anterior cruciate ligament reconstruction should be performed. The treating surgeon should choose a reconstruction technique, and the graft which he/she feels comfortable and confident in performing will provide good outcomes.

20.4.2 Central Pivot and Lateral Side

The lateral side of the knee is commonly injured as part of a multiligament knee dislocation complex. The modified Schenck classification [1, 2] of knee dislocations includes KD IIIL (injuries involving the anterior and posterior cruciate ligaments as well as the lateral complex). KD IV is less common and more severe because this injury involves both the medial and lateral sides as well as both cruciate ligaments. The lateral side of the knee is complex anatomically and therefore difficult to replicate with reconstructive techniques [21].

Surgical treatment is indicated by complete injuries or avulsions of the FCL; rotatory instabilities of the FCL and arcuate ligament, popliteus tendon, and fabellofibular ligament; and combined instability patterns of the FCL/posterolateral corner and ACL or PCL [22].

A controversial issue is whether to repair or reconstruct the posterolateral corner. Stannard et al. [23] and Levy et al. [24] indicate that reconstruction is probably better than repair. When surgery is performed within the first 3 weeks after the injury, a combination of repair and reconstruction can be done and should provide the best chance of producing a stable posterolateral corner [21].

20.4.2.1 Surgical Technique

Numerous surgical techniques to treat posterolateral corner injury have been described: Stannard et al. [23] used a modified two-tailed technique that reconstructs the popliteofibular ligament and fibular collateral ligament through transtibial and transfibular bone tunnels and around a single screw on the lateral femoral condyle; Levy et al. [24] reconstruct the posterolateral corner with a graft passed through the proximal part of the fibula, with both graft limbs inserting at an isometric point on the femur; the LaPrade technique use a two-tailed graft to reconstruct the fibular collateral ligament, the popliteofibular ligament, and the popliteus tendon with four tunnels: two in the femur (for the insertion of the fibular collateral ligament and the popliteus tendon), one in the fibula, and one in the proximal part of the tibia [25].

Geeslin and LaPrade [26] assert that the treatment of grade III PLC injuries with acute repair of avulsed structures, reconstruction of midsubstance tears, and concurrent reconstruction of any cruciate ligament tears resulted in significantly improved objective stability. The initial assessment addressed whether a damaged posterolateral corner structure was avulsed from its attachment and could be repaired or was torn in the midsubstance and required a reconstruction with use of an autogenous hamstring graft or an allograft [26].

Reconstruction of ACL must be performed, and the graft must be secured in the femoral tunnel. Fixation of the graft in the tibial tunnel must be performed later on, when repair and/or reconstruction of the posterolateral corner structures has already been done (Figs. 20.2 and 20.3).

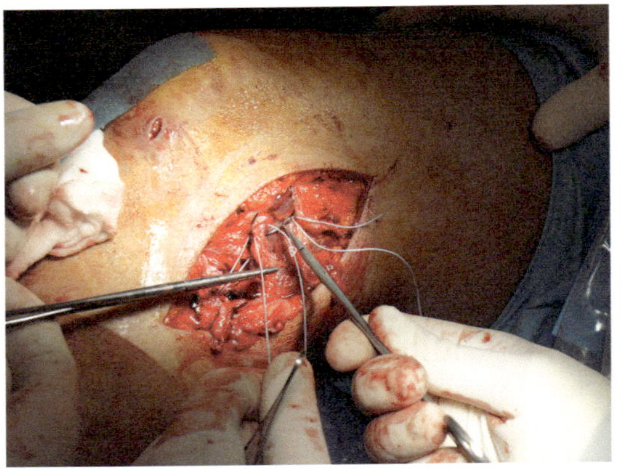

Fig. 20.2 Lateral side repair

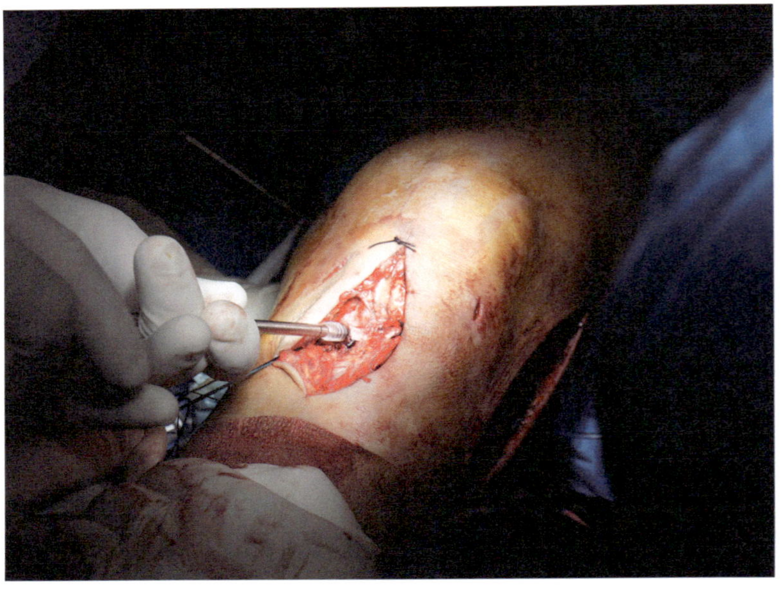

Fig. 20.3 ACL tibial fixation with interference screw

20.5 Rehabilitation and Return to Play

20.5.1 Rehabilitation

Following multiligament reconstruction is essential to regain motion, strength, and function. Initially after surgery the knee can be braced, and the use of crutches and weight bearing depend on the repaired/reconstructed ligaments. Gradually weight bearing and mobility is allowed to prevent stiffness postoperatively. The rehabilitation will slowly progress into strengthening, gait, and balancing activities. However, individual patients will progress at different rates depending on their age, associated injuries, pre-injury health status, rehab compliance, tissue quality, and injury severity.

20.5.1.1 Phase I

The goals of first phase are to protect the postsurgical knee, restore normal knee extension, improve scar and patellar mobility, eliminate effusion (swelling) and restore leg control. Usually the brace is locked for 15 days to protect the peripherical repair as well as the non-weight-bearing period. Thereafter passive range of motion is recovered, but the ROM is restricted until at least 4 weeks after surgery. Electric stimulation is necessary to stimulate quad control and straight leg raise (SLR) with brace locked.

20.5.1.2 Phase II

Phase II begins after meeting the Phase I criteria. The goals are normalized gait, single leg stand control, and quad control. The ROM must be greater then 125° in flexion and full in extension. Bike is allowed. No open-chain hamstring strengthening, isolated hamstring exercises, or hamstring stretching if PCL reconstruction was done. Quad, hip, and core strengthening are the key points in this phase (Fig. 20.4).

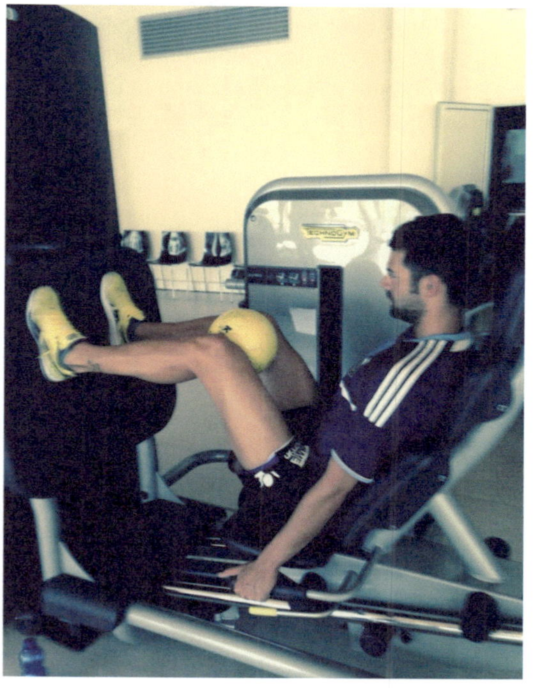

Fig. 20.4 Closed kinetic chain exercise for quadriceps

20.5.1.3 Phase III

Phase III starts after the Phase II goals are accomplished. The objectives are the single leg control (open and closed chain) and the good control and no pain with functional movements, including step ups/downs and squats. In addition, it is important to perform gait and balance drills.

20.5.1.4 Phase IV

In the last phase, the goals are to obtain a good dynamic neuromuscular control, no pain with multi-planar impact activities, and functional sports-specific progression. It is important to avoid post-activity swelling. The initiation of impact may occur if the involved leg has at least 80 % of the strength of the uninvolved leg when measured using a single leg press test.

The footballer must perform sports-specific balance and proprioceptive drills, progress impact control exercises to reactive strengthening and plyometrics, initiate a running program as appropriate, and continue quad strengthening. Movement control exercise begins with low-velocity, single-plane activities and progresses to higher-velocity, multi-plane activities from 1 foot to the other and then 1 foot to the same foot.

Rehabilitation of acute repair/reconstruction is much harder than rehabilitation following surgery for chronic cases. The reason is the amount of inflammation due to the massive soft tissue injury. Another important principle is that the PCL surgery dominates the rehabilitation. Note that the PCL is tensioned with flexion angles above 60° and stressed by gravity tending to produce a posterior tibial translation. The PCL is also tensed by open-chain hamstring activity. Not surprisingly, it is prone to stretching [22].

Early patellar mobilization is important to prevent a fat pad contracture. Full active and passive extension should be encouraged as soon as possible. Although collateral ligaments are tensioned in terminal extension, surgical technique should be good enough to allow for this [22].

In acute cases, the patient undergoes partial weight bearing for 4 weeks followed by full weight bearing. In chronic cases, if there is any significant varus/valgus that would compromise repair/reconstruction, osteotomy would be undertaken. The post-operative period after osteotomy requires that the patient remains touch weight bearing for 4 weeks and partial weight bearing for 2 weeks.

The reason for the slow recovery following surgery for these kinds of injuries is largely due to the slowness in restoration of proprioception. Structures other than those reconstructed have to upregulate their proprioceptive function [22].

20.5.2 Return to Play

Multiligament injury contains as seen a wide spectrum of injury. Many footballers have combined ACL and MCL injury, but only the cases previously described require surgery to the MCL. The majority of two ligament injuries will return to sport even at the highest level. Several athletes with three-ligament injuries return to sport at the highest level but only a few athletes with four-ligament involvement return to the pre-injury level of sport.

The footballer can return to play if he/she has dynamic neuromuscular control with multi-plane activities, without instability, pain, or swelling. Furthermore, he/she should be able to land from a sagittal, frontal, and transverse plane and leap and jump with good control and balance. Isokinetic and functional test should be done before the player returns to play.

References

1. Wascher DC, Dvirnak PC, DeCoster TA (1997) Knee dislocation: initial assessment and implications for treatment. J Orthop Trauma 11(7):525–529
2. Schenck R. (2003) Classification of knee dislocations. Oper Tech Sports Med 11(3):193–198
3. Levy BA, Fanelli GC, Whelan DB, Stannard JP, MacDonald PA, Boyd JL, Marx RG, Stuart MJ (2009) Controversies in the treatment of knee dislocations and multiligament reconstruction. J Am Acad Orthop Surg 17(4):197–206
4. Stannard JP, Bauer KL (2012) Current concepts in knee dislocations: PCL, ACL, and medial sided injuries. J Knee Surg 25(4):287–294
5. Fornalski S, McGarry MH, Csintalan RP, Fithian DC, Lee TQ (2008) Biomechanical and anatomical assessment after knee hyperextension injury. Am J Sports Med 36(1):80–84
6. Fanelli GC, Harris JD (2006) Surgical treatment of acute medial collateral ligament and posteromedial corner injuries of the knee. Sports Med Arthrosc 14(2):78–83
7. Kurzweil PR, Kelley ST (2006) Physical examination and imaging of the medial collateral ligament and posteromedial corner of the knee. Sports Med Arthrosc 14(2):67–73
8. Bae JH, Choi IC, Suh SW, Lim HC, Bae TS, Nha KW, Wang JH (2008) Evaluation of the reliability of the dial test for posterolateral rotatory instability: a cadaveric study using an isotonic rotation machine. Arthroscopy 24(5):593–598. doi:10.1016/j.arthro.2007.12.003
9. Ferrari DA, Ferrari JD, Coumas J (1994) Posterolateral instability of the knee. J Bone Joint Surg (Br) 76(2):187–192
10. Covey DC (2001) Injuries of the posterolateral corner of the knee. J Bone Joint Surg Am 83-A(1):106–118 ah. Stannard JP, Black BS, Azbell C, Volgas DA (2012) Posteromedial corner injury in knee dislocations. J KneeSurg25(5):429–434.doi:10.1055/s-0032-1322605
11. Duffy PS, Miyamoto RG (2010) Management of medial collateral ligament injuries in the knee: an update and review. Phys Sportsmed 38(2):48–54. doi:10.3810/psm.2010.06.1782
12. Larsen E, Jensen PK, Jensen PR (1999) Long-term outcome of knee and ankle injuries in elite football. Scand J Med Sci Sports 9(5):285–289
13. Wen DY, Propeck T, Kane SM, Godbee MT, Rall KL (2007) MRI description of knee medial collateral ligament abnormalities in the absence of trauma: edema

related to osteoarthritis and medial meniscal tears. Magn Reson Imaging 25(2):209–214
14. Farshad-Amacker NA, Potter HG (2013) MRI of knee ligament injury and reconstruction. J Magn Reson Imaging 38(4):757–773. doi:10.1002/jmri.24311
15. Halinen J, Koivikko M, Lindahl J, Hirvensalo E (2009) The efficacy of magnetic resonance imaging in acute multi-ligament injuries. Int Orthop 33(6):1733–1738. doi:10.1007/s00264-008-0689-6
16. Levy BA, Dajani KA, Whelan DB, Stannard JP, Fanelli GC, Stuart MJ, Boyd JL, MacDonald PA, Marx RG (2009) Decision making in the multiligament-injured knee: an evidence-based systematic review. Arthroscopy 25(4):430–438. doi:10.1016/j.arthro.2009.01.008
17. Liow RY, McNicholas MJ, Keating JF, Nutton RW (2003) Ligament repair and reconstruction in traumatic dislocation of the knee. J Bone Joint Surg (Br) 85(6):845–851
18. Harner CD, Waltrip RL, Bennett CH, Francis KA, Cole B, Irrgang JJ (2004) Surgical management of knee dislocations. J Bone Joint Surg Am 86-A(2):262–273
19. Tzurbakis M, Diamantopoulos A, Xenakis T, Georgoulis A (2006) Surgical treatment of multiple knee ligament injuries in 44 patients: 2–8 years follow-up results. Knee Surg Sports Traumatol Arthrosc 14(8):739–749
20. Stannard JP, Black BS, Azbell C, Volgas DA (2012) Posteromedial corner injury in knee dislocations. J Knee Surg 25(5):429–434. doi:10.1055/s-0032-1322605
21. Fanelli GC, Stannard JP, Stuart MJ, Macdonald PB, Marx RG, Whelan DB, Boyd JL, Levy BA (2011) Management of complex knee ligament injuries. Instr Course Lect 60:523–535
22. Adravanti P, Jakobsen BW, Marx RG, Santone DJ, Whelan DB, Williams A (2014) How to address multi-ligament injuries? In: Zaffagnini S et al (eds) ESSKA instructional course lecture book. Springer, Heidelberg, pp 79–96
23. Stannard JP, Brown SL, Farris RC, McGwin G Jr, Volgas DA (2005) The posterolateral corner of the knee: repair versus reconstruction. Am J Sports Med 33(6):881–888
24. Levy BA, Dajani KA, Morgan JA, Shah JP, Dahm DL, Stuart MJ (2010) Repair versus reconstruction of the fibular collateral ligament and posterolateral corner in the multiligament-injured knee. Am J Sports Med 38(4):804–809. doi:10.1177/0363546509352459
25. LaPrade RF, Johansen S, Wentorf FA, Engebretsen L, Esterberg JL, Tso A (2004) An analysis of an anatomical posterolateral knee reconstruction: an in vitro biomechanical study and development of a surgical technique. Am J Sports Med 32(6):1405–1414
26. Geeslin AG, LaPrade RF (2011) Outcomes of treatment of acute grade-III isolated and combined posterolateral knee injuries: a prospective case series and surgical technique. J Bone Joint Surg Am 93(18):1672–1683. doi:10.2106/JBJS.J.01639

Lateral Meniscus Injuries

21

Rene Verdonk

21.1 Introduction

The microscopic anatomy of the lateral meniscus is a cartilaginous construct containing 70 % of water, the rest being collagen fibers for 75 %, organized in order to sustain compressive and shearing forces. Like in the medial meniscus, the collagen fibers are circumferentially oriented including oblique and radial fibers.

The macroscopic anatomy is semicircular and is positioned between the lateral femoral condyle and the lateral tibial plateau, covering 70 % of its surface. It is tightly fixed, having two fixation horns. The anterior horn is rather flat and inserts just below the tibial anterior cruciate ligament fixation [1]. The posterior lateral meniscal horn is extremely strong and hits the tibial tubercle anterior to the posterior medial meniscal horn fixation.

Extra fixation is illustrated in anatomy with two meniscofemoral ligaments posteriorly [2]. The posterior fixation through the ligament of Wrisberg presents in 76 % of cases [2]. Finally there is most often also a transverse ligament uniting both medial and lateral menisci in the anterior part of the knee. In addition, the lateral meniscus is not fixed to the popliteal tendon (hiatus popliteus) [3]. Because there is no fixation to the lateral collateral ligament of the knee, the lateral meniscus is much more mobile versus the medial meniscus. This nicely fits the mobile expectations in normal knee function.

Vascular penetration of the lateral meniscus is decreasing after birth [4]. In the adult knee vascularization originates from the lateral genicular artery progressing to a capillary plexus on the outside of the meniscus [5]. Like in the medial meniscus, vascular penetration is only present in the periphery of this cartilaginous body.

Regarding innervation, most mechanoreceptors are located in the meniscal horns [6].

Biomechanically the lateral meniscus increases joint congruency and improves knee stability. Because of its specific fixation toward the musculus popliteus and the femur, the lateral meniscus is less subject to rotational trauma.

21.2 Etiology and Injury Mechanism

21.2.1 Stable Knee

Most of lateral meniscal lesions can be distinguished between:

– Vertical traumatic lesions [7]
– Lateral meniscal degenerative lesions [8]
– Degenerative meniscal lesions associated with arthritis which will not be discussed here [9]

R. Verdonk
Gent State University,
St Pietersnieuwstraat, 9000 Ghent, Belgium
e-mail: Rene.verdonk@ugent.be

P. Volpi (ed.), *Football Traumatology: New Trends*, DOI 10.1007/978-3-319-18245-2_21

The injured mechanism is mostly due to locking of the posterior horn in the maximum flexion of the knee joint, without specific rotational injury.

This injury leads to a more aggressive therapeutic approach, using arthroscopic surgery because of extension loss of the knee.

21.2.2 Unstable Knee

The natural history of anterior cruciate ligament injury retains a very high incidence of meniscal injury. This lesion, sometimes ab initio, always evolves dramatically, and if required, lateral meniscectomy will lead to major degenerative arthritis in the lateral compartment of the knee.

Today, up to 65 % of ACL rupture includes meniscal rupture, essentially in the lateral compartment. The clinical incidence presents more than 1/3 of lateral meniscal injury in case of acute anterior cruciate ligament rupture. This can be explained by the shearing force exerted on the posterior horn of the lateral meniscus during internal rotation on the lateral tibial plateau. Very often it shows a horizontal lesion at the posterior horn of the lateral meniscus and closely related to the hiatus popliteus, sometimes associated with an increase in length of this particular structure. Because of the vascularity of the location, healing is most often spontaneous. Indeed, in the late ACL repair, at 3–6 months, these vascularized shearing lesions at the edge of the meniscus have healed.

21.3 Clinical Diagnosis and Imaging

21.3.1 Stable Knee

As mentioned earlier in the etiology and injury mechanism, the clinical findings in the acute setting present with a locked knee with frank and painful extension deficit. No imaging is required in the experienced surgeon's hand.

When confronted with a chronic lateral meniscal lesion, the clinical picture is less clear. Imaging is required. Unless presenting with the degenerative knee complaints (in which case standing X-rays and Rosenberg's incidences are required), an MRI or possibly an arthro-CT scan must be requested. Van De Berg [10] has shown high sensibility and specificity using arthro-CT scan in meniscal injuries. MRI shows less sensibility according to Oei et al. [11] with good specificity in lateral meniscal lesions.

21.3.2 Unstable Knee

In the ACL injured knee joint, the laxity induces excessive forces on the menisci. More often in the medial compartment vs. the lateral compartment. Indeed, because of its mobility, the lateral meniscus stands these shearing forces better because of its excessive translation availability.

This evolves soon to become a chronic lateral meniscal tear because of episodes of new traumatic moments, onto unstable central pivot shift findings. Progressive mechanical joint line pain is mentioned by the patient, presenting with repeated hydrops. McMurray sign becomes more obvious. Sometimes, parrot beak lesions occur, presenting with locking symptoms. Today, however, since ACL repair is more readily done after injury, the frequency of these lateral meniscal lesions is decreasing in daily practice. These findings suggest again obvious ligament and meniscal cooperation in stabilizing the injured knee joint.

21.4 Treatment Strategy and Results

The purpose of meniscal repair is cartilage protection [12, 13].

Isolated partial (if possible) meniscectomy is only indicated in the more aged and sedentary individuals presenting without instability complaints.

On the other hand, adequate lateral meniscectomy in case of associated ACL ligament repair is only indicated if the symptomatic lesion is unrepairable. Masterly neglect of the lateral meniscal tear is probably the most appropriate approach as these lesions present a high frequency but only minimal extent [14–16]. When reviewing lateral meniscal repair, we found no secondary lateral meniscal

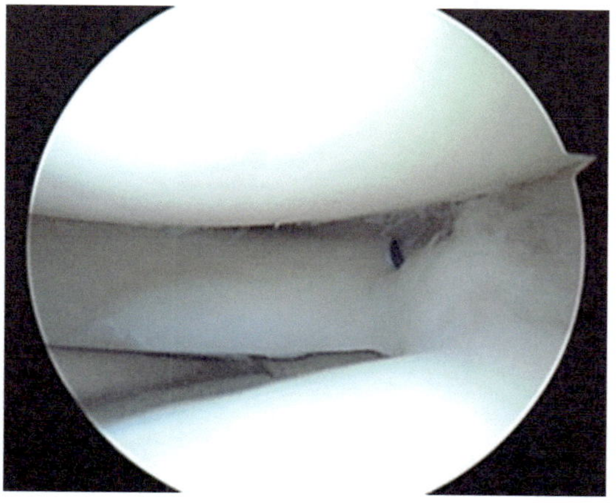

Fig. 21.1 After lateral meniscal bucket handle tear and arthroscopic reduction of the dislocation, a first vertical meniscal suture is positioned to reduce and hold the lateral meniscus in place (Courtesy dr J Hoher ESSKA meniscus presentation)

resection to be required on clinical grounds. Indeed, meniscal repair in the lateral meniscus is only indicated in unstable unrepairable lesions. Hybrid meniscal sutures using an all-inside technique are indicated around the popliteal hiatus (Fig. 21.1). These can be augmented in the medial and possibly anterior horn with an inside-out suture approach, increasing overall stability. Excellent results are expected and referred in literature [17, 18].

Hulet et al. [19] have investigated long-term results in lateral meniscectomies at plus 20 years of follow-up. The prevalence of OA was 56 % in the affected knee, and the difference of prevalence between the operated and healthy knees was 44 %. In those patients presenting with OA of the operated knee and a normal contralateral knee, the incidence of OA was 53 %. In their conclusions, the authors mention that in the long term arthroscopic lateral meniscectomy in stable knees without initial cartilage lesions might lead from good to excellent results in a young patient. Patients are at higher risk to the development of symptomatic OA if they are over 40, having a high BMI (more than 30), valgus malalignment, and cartilage lesions at the time of surgery. It is to be noted that in the younger patients, the lateral meniscus, presenting with a traumatic lesion and intact cartilage, clean minimal resection does not lead to further degeneration in well-aligned knees with stable and intact ligaments.

In the unstable, unrepaired ACL injured knee, lateral meniscectomy will lead to OA in 100 % of the cases.

After lateral meniscectomy short-term results may be complicated by swelling and prolonged joint line pain in the lateral compartment. Tabib et al. [20] have shown in young patients the swelling to be prolonged in time in 1/3 of the cases. Even in the presence of some weight-bearing cartilage degeneration, a conservative treatment is indicated, sometimes requiring cortisone intra-articular injections. It is suggested only to refer to a new arthroscopy at 6 months at the earliest. Chatain et al. [21] have found that re-arthroscopy for lateral resection in these cases is as high as 12 % as compared to less than 5 % in case of medial partial meniscectomy.

Charrois et al. [22] have illustrated that rapid chondrolysis is present in a limited number of patients. These findings require very careful approach in return to sports activities. A close follow-up is required sometimes using cortisone injections at the early stage [23].

Long-term complications arise, possibly including lateral compartmental OA [24]. In case of malalignment femoral corrective osteotomy is suggested [25]. Marti et al. [26] suggest tibial corrective osteotomy. None of these approaches are fully satisfactory. Indeed, varus femoral osteotomy is only effective in extension, not below 90° of flexion [13].

In light of these findings, recent investigations have suggested lateral meniscal replacement. Today's experience suggests two separate clinical situations:

- A chronic symptomatic joint line pain after partial lateral meniscectomy.
- A chronic symptomatic joint line pain after total lateral meniscectomy.

21.4.1 Partial Lateral Meniscal Replacement

Bouyarmane et al. [25] and Verdonk [27] have investigated prospectively in a single-arm multicenter study the safety and efficacy of the lateral

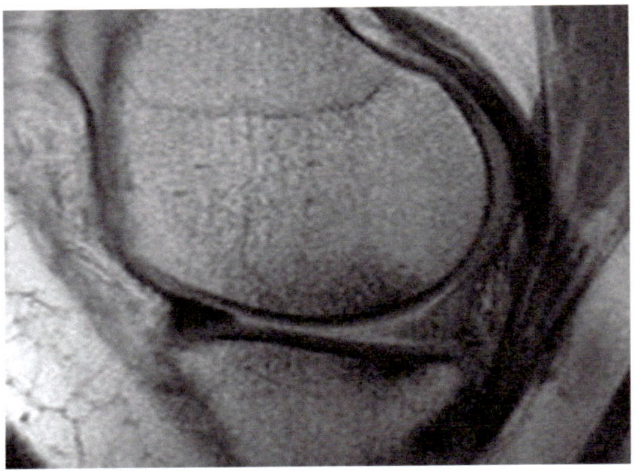

Fig. 21.2 This meniscal scaffold has been in place for 48 m. It is well fixed and well tolerated by the weight-bearing cartilage. This picture shows no scaffold regression however still with different contrast aspects vs. normal meniscal tissue

polyurethane meniscal scaffold (Actifit, Orteq Ltd, London, UK) for the treatment of post-meniscectomy syndrome. Fifty-four patients, aged between 16 and 50 years, who were treated between 2007 and 2011 with a polyurethane scaffold, presented with a non-repairable lateral meniscal tear or partial meniscal loss with intact rim. The knees were stable or had been stabilized within 12 weeks of the index procedure. The lateral defects were primarily localized in the posterior and middle segments of the lateral meniscus. Malaligned patients underwent distal femoral osteotomy. At 6 months clinical findings were improved from baseline. At 24 months, the clinical and KOOS continued to improve significantly (Fig. 21.2).

In case of chronic symptomatic medial joint line pain after partial medial meniscectomy, other alternatives are available using the CMI (collagen meniscal implant) [28]. Partial lateral meniscal replacement has been performed with similar effective results (personal communication).

21.4.2 Total Lateral Meniscal Replacement

According to current recommendations, meniscal allograft transplantation in the lateral compartment is indicated in three specific clinical settings:

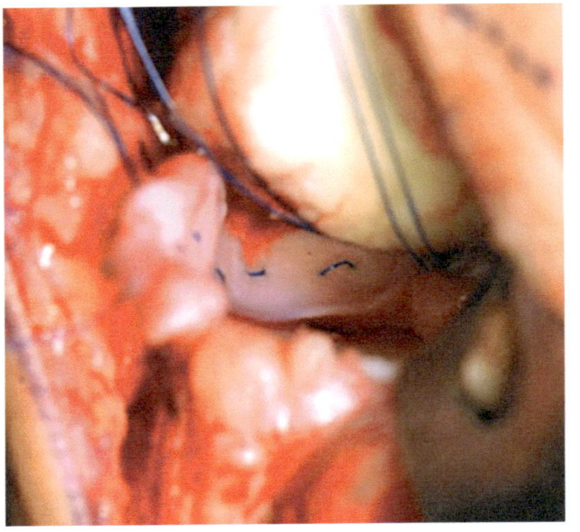

Fig. 21.3 In open surgery the lateral compartment of this right knee is opened through an osteotomy of the lateral collateral ligament insertion on the femoral condyle allowing for proper spacing and stable insertion of the lateral meniscal allograft using vertical/horizontal meniscal sutures

1. Young patients with a history of lateral meniscectomy with a localized joint line pain in a stable knee joint without malalignment and preferably with minor evidence of articular cartilage degeneration
2. Anterior cruciate ligament-deficient knees having sustained lateral meniscectomy requiring increased stability, supported by a new lateral meniscus
3. In an effort to avert early joint degeneration in the lateral compartment, young patients, most of them females, having sustained lateral total meniscectomy as a result of lateral discoid meniscus pathology

Both open (Fig. 21.3) and now routinely arthroscopically, this surgery results in a good satisfactory outcome [29].

In the majority of studies, these outcomes [30–42] suggest a clinical success rate of 70 % (Fig. 21.4). Overtime at the 10th to the 15th year, this rate tends to decrease. A higher failure rate is present in case of ligament instability or axial malalignment or pronounced cartilage degeneration at the index surgery.

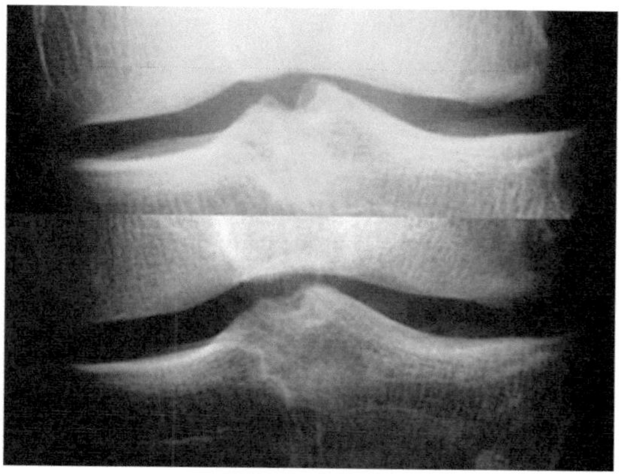

Fig. 21.4 Top and bottom: standing X-rays after lateral meniscal transplantation 10 years after the index surgery. No lateral joint narrowing is seen 10 years after lateral MAT

21.5 Rehabilitation and Return to Play

Supervised rehabilitation after partial meniscectomy can generally progress, as tolerated by the patient, with no substantial contraindications or limitations. The main goals are to control pain and swelling associated with surgery, more specifically in the lateral compartment, also to restore range of motion and to maintain muscle function, as well as optimizing lower extremity neuromuscular coordination and muscle strength [43].

In the early postoperative rehabilitation phase, weight bearing is allowed as tolerated by the patients. Ice packing is helpful in the first few days as treatment should focus in the reduction of pain and swelling. Reflex inhibition needs to be resolved rapidly because strengthening of muscles surrounding the knee cannot be initiated with this inhibition still being present.

Ice and the activity reduction in association with frequent low resistance active and passive movements stimulate joint recovery [44]. Progressive, active, and passive range of motion exercises of the knee need to be started immediately post surgery within the pain limits. Deep squats are not allowed until the 6th week following the surgery in order to avoid excessive load on the healing meniscus, more specifically in the lateral compartment. Progressively proprioceptive exercises are initiated to improve functional stability [43].

In the second phase, optimizing quadriceps strength is important as it adds to functional joint stability and protects knee function, being a shock absorber and dampening load during activity [45].

In combination, open kinetic chain and closed kinetic chain exercises can be used to improve upper leg muscle strength, but the latter becomes more important with time because these are more functional for the lower limb.

As soon as patients can tolerate weight bearing on the involved knee, closed kinetic chain exercises with a patient's own body weight can be started. The intensity of exercises can be increased by increasing the load enhancing muscle endurance.

In the third phase patients are generally able to go to work. In case of partial meniscectomy, careful sports activities can be resumed at 6–8 weeks. One should be more careful than in the partial medial meniscectomy.

Rehabilitation after stable meniscal repair in the lateral meniscus requires a similar approach as partial meniscal resection. However, partial weight bearing is required to be done carefully, as tolerated by the patients. Swelling has to subside as deep squatting is contraindicated, at least 3 months from the index surgery [46, 47].

In case of partial lateral meniscal replacement using the polyurethane implant, rehabilitation takes 16–24 weeks. Non-weight bearing is mandatory for the first 3 weeks, followed by progressive full weight bearing and a 100 % load at 9 weeks postimplantation. Flexion is progressively increased from 30° during 2 weeks, followed by 60° and progressively 90° at week 5–6. Light exercises including isometric quadriceps exercises, mobilization of the patella, heel slides, quadriceps and anti-equinus foot exercises, and Achilles tendon stretching are advised from week 1 [25].

Rehabilitation after lateral meniscal transplantation is comparable to extensive meniscal repair and fixation. In lateral meniscal transplantation, care has to be taken in regard with soft tissue or bony reinsertion of the anterior and posterior horn of the lateral meniscus. Today's techniques allow stable fixation of the allograft implant. Strict immobilization is to be avoided and progressive exercises initiated [29, 48].

Mobilization is started as tolerated through the first 60° of flexion in the first weeks. At 6 weeks weight bearing is allowed as no limitation of active flexion is instituted. Squatting is to be avoided for the first 3 months after the index surgery. Competitive sports may be considered at 6 months after proper regaining of function.

21.5.1 Particular Findings

21.5.1.1 Meniscal Cysts in Adults and Football

Introduction

Pathological meniscal cysts are essentially present in the lateral compartment. They are rare. Many issues on the lateral meniscal cysts are controversial: their true etiology is both degenerative and microtraumatic. The treatment approach has evolved over time because of more recent diagnostic tools and arthroscopic therapy.

Etiology

The etiology of the lateral meniscal cysts is controversial: initially, one considers a microcyst in the meniscal body to be created, consisting of synovial fluid, evolving toward the periphery [49–51]. Because of this weaker consistency, this interbody meniscal lesion develops toward a horizontal cleavage [49] with progressive clinical impact, this being caused possibly by collagen bundle rupture and influenced by shearing forces during sports activities like football. Hulet et al. [52, 53] find around 25 % of microtraumatic influence. Because of these traumatic incidents, the cyst becomes clinically symptomatic.

Reagan [54] has described further deterioration of the lesion being the development as a horizontal cleavage tear, progression of the lesion toward the peripheral wall of the meniscus, most often around the popliteal hiatus and then, because of weaker collagen structure developing toward the joint obviously, becoming symptomatic, more specifically with the active, mostly male, sportive individual.

Diagnostic Approach

Most often these patients are active sportsmen and, as they are middle aged, present with long-term symptomatology [52]. They present with complaints on the lateral joint line with intermittent swelling at the level of the popliteal hiatus. Pressure pain is present, while the McMurray sign becomes manifest. In most instances the meniscal cyst is relatively limited on the inside and also, sometimes, bilateral being symptomatic only unilaterally. Joint effusion is rarely associated with the presence of a lateral meniscal cyst. Obviously standing X-rays are required to evaluate possible evolving joint line width in the lateral compartment. Hulet [16] and Pedowitz [55] suggest the major role of MRI. Very often, it allows for finer diagnostics, whether or not the flap tear is present or there is a full connection from within the joint toward the periphery. This potential finding will lead to appropriate surgery, possibly suggesting partial meniscal resection associated with meniscal rim stabilization suture.

Arthroscopic and Associated Open Treatment

The final diagnosis is confirmed, and treatment suggestions are defined during arthroscopy. Being symptomatic, lateral meniscal cysts present usually with full horizontal cleavage [52]. They are obviously different from acute traumatic appearance. They are sometimes associated with smaller parrot beak meniscal lesions being the reason of their clinical symptoms. They very often present at the level of the popliteal hiatus [56, 57]. Probing allows for evaluating the entire lateral meniscal cyst, presenting outside the weight-bearing zone. Outside-in needling of the cyst allows for localizing the connecting canal [16].

Flap tear presence and the extensive degeneration of the meniscal body require adequate meniscectomies preserving the lateral meniscal wall if at all possible. It is possible then to use a mechanical shaver to address the intrameniscal cyst tissue, manipulating the shaver through the connecting canal into the cyst. If required then, after removing the degenerative tissue, an attempt can be made to suture the horizontal cleavage tear, being left after the partial meniscectomy, thus allowing for stabilization for both the femoral and the tibial parts of the meniscus. This being a somewhat degenerated tissue as well, it may require, in case of extensive meniscal cyst, an open approach on the lateral side of the knee by separate incision, allowing for an open resection of the meniscal cyst, associated with an all-outside meniscal stabilization suture.

These both inside and outside approaches will enhance chances of healing of the remnant meniscal wall with better care of the weight-bearing cartilage. As this is performed in an older and aged tissue, rehabilitation is slow, and immediate weight bearing needs to be avoided for 4–6 weeks and active contact sports avoided for 3–6 months.

Results

Objective results are satisfactory in almost 90 % of cases [52]. These results are comparable to lateral meniscal adequate resection [58–60]. This suggests the importance of preserving the continuity of the lateral meniscal wall, more specifically at the level of the hiatus popliteus if at all possible.

Lateral meniscal cyst recurrence is not a rare event, and 10–15 % is referred by Maffuli [61] and Reagan [54]. These authors are confronted with a more extensive degenerative tissue in redo surgery. This finding suggests a meniscal disease to be the reason of this type of pathology.

These findings are also in correlation with redo surgery in lateral meniscectomy [56]. At 5 years, these results also suggest further cartilage degeneration in the weight-bearing lateral compartment. This is also related to the age of the patient. Indeed, in the older-aged patient above 50 years, lateral meniscal cyst degeneration and surgery may originate toward further cartilage degeneration. These patients are different from the younger sportive individual with intact weight-bearing cartilage.

All these findings suggest the lateral meniscal cyst to be a degenerative pathology most possibly based on defective collagen material. This may be potentially initiated by local anatomy influenced by the presence of the hiatus popliteus, leading to higher stress and less peripheral vascularity. In the sportive individual this may lead to initiating mechanical pathology, even with minor and sometimes repetitive trauma as in football. Consequently the lateral meniscal cyst in the sportive individual may not be overlooked. It needs clinical diagnosis also confirmed by imaging, preferably MRI. This then may initiate an indication for arthroscopic surgery in extensive cases, associated with open meniscal cyst removal and meniscal wall suture in an all-outside fashion [62].

Conclusion

This not so frequent pathology of the lateral meniscus requires optimal clinical investigation and MRI to illustrate this degenerative pathology. Leading to operative arthroscopic surgery, it may require additional open approach to stabilize the meniscal wall, more specifically at the weak hiatus popliteus anatomy. Rehabilitation is suggested to be very progressive, and weight bearing may need to be delayed depending on the extent of the lesion. Prognosis is good and can be compared to adequate lateral meniscectomy with equal good follow-up at 15–20 years [53].

21.5.1.2 The Discoid Lateral Meniscus and Football

The lateral discoid meniscus is a congenital anatomic abnormality, quite rare, varying in gender and race [63, 64]. Major differences occur, while Caucasians have an incidence of about 5 % [65, 66] in contrast with the Japanese [64]. Watanabe et al. [67] suggest classification according to the covered surface of the lateral tibial plateau. Sometimes the posterior horn is not fixed on the tibial plateau in its posterior attachment but rather on the ligament of Wrisberg, inducing hypermobility with an O-shaped open discus.

Diagnosis and Clinical Findings

Discoid lateral menisci are very often associated with pathology in 70–80 % of cases [68, 69]. Clinical findings are highly variable because of individual anatomy. Wrisberg-type lateral discoid menisci are almost invariably symptomatic with lateral joint line pain and the presence of the snapping knee syndrome. However, less frequent versus pediatric occurrence. In the adult, knee locking [69], joint swelling, and instability are primarily present. Flexion to extension movement may cause clunk syndrome in 25 % of the cases. Imaging using MRI illustrates central cystic degeneration of the meniscal tissue inducing horizontal cleavage tears [70]. On regular basis, these clinical findings and symptoms are bilateral. According to Aichroth [71] and Matsumoto [72], the lateral discoid meniscus is associated with osteochondritis dissecans (OCD).

Arthro-CT scan and arthro-MRI may help in the precision diagnostics whether or not the discoid meniscus covers the entire lateral tibial plateau and presents with possible degenerative horizontal cleavage pathology.

Treatment

Once symptomatic the lateral discoid meniscus requires aggressive surgery.

Adequate meniscectomy is the rule. It allows for retaining the lateral meniscal wall, more specifically across the hiatus popliteus as suggested by Kaplan [73]. Technically and at arthroscopy, en bloc resection of the central part of the lateral discoid meniscus is difficult. Most often, arthroscopy allows for progressive resection using mechanical and sometimes thermal instrumentation [70, 74]. Partial meniscectomy sometimes referred to as "meniscoplasty" as described by Dickhaut [75] addresses most often degenerative central and horizontal cleavage tears. Meniscal repair is regularly performed in association with meniscal resection [64]. This approach is suggested in order to retain a maximum of meniscal tissue more specifically in the periphery and especially at the level of the hiatus popliteus [76]. This approach induces favorable results in many cases [77, 78].

Earlier literature retains potential arthrogenicity after extensive lateral meniscectomy [79]. In conclusion it appears that arthroscopic partial lateral meniscectomy in case of discoid malformation remains a difficult approach, requiring extensive experience in arthroscopic surgery in order to fully consider retaining maximal meniscal tissue [80].

Conclusion

In case of lateral meniscal tear, care must be taken to save meniscal tissues at all costs. In the young individual the repair needs to be pushed, and as in the older-aged patient, adequate limited resection becomes the rule.

In case of stable knees, long-term results suggest the partial lateral meniscus resection to be well tolerated. In the ACL-deficient knee, ligament repair has become the rule in the young patient as in these instances ab initio, the lateral meniscus is rarely involved.

In case of chronic symptomatic lateral meniscectomy, partial replacement presents with clear functional improvement.

In case of total meniscectomy and chronic symptomatic joint line pain – as may be the case after discoid meniscal resection – lateral meniscal allograft transplantation is an optimal indication to avoid inevitable joint line degeneration, even in the well-aligned knee joint [81].

Acknowledgment This chapter is based on the long personal clinical and surgical experience of the author but also on the SOFCOT 2005 round table on the lateral meniscus, coordinated by P. Beaufils and P. Hardy.

References

1. Messner K, Gao J (1998) The menisci of the knee joint. Anatomical and functional characteristics and a rationale for clinical treatment. J Anat 193:161–178
2. Kohn D, Moreno B (1995) Meniscus insertion anatomy as a basis for meniscus replacement: a morphological cadaveric study. Arthroscopy 11:96–103
3. Kim Y, Chung I, Yoo W et al (1997) Anatomy and magnetic resonance imaging of the posterolateral structures of the knee. Clin Anat 10:397–404
4. Petersen W, Tillmann B (1995) Age-related blood and lymph supply of the knee menisci. A cadaver study. Acta Orthop Scand 66:308–312
5. Arnoczky S, Warren R (1982) Microvasculature of the human meniscus. Am J Sports Med 10:90–95
6. Day B, Mackenzie W, Shim S et al (1985) The vascular and nerve supply of the human meniscus. Arthroscopy 1:58–62

7. Locker B, Hulet C, Vielpeau C (1992) Lésions traumatiques des ménisques du genou. Editions Techniques Encycl Med Chir (Paris) Appareil Locomoteur, 14084, A10, 12p
8. Dorfmann H, Juan LH, Bonvarlet JP et al (1987) Lésions dégénératives du ménisque interne en arthroscopie. Rev Rhum 54:4
9. Chatain F, Robinson AH, Adeleine P et al (2001) The natural history of the knee following arthroscopic medial meniscectomy. Knee Surg Sports Traumatol Arthrosc 9:15–18
10. Van De Berg BC, Lecouvet FE, Poilvache P et al (2000) Dual-detector spiral CT arthrography of the knee: accuracy for detection of meniscal abnormalities and unstable meniscal tears. Radiology 216:851–857
11. Oei EH, Nikken JJ, Verstijnen AC et al (2003) MR imaging of the menisci and cruciate ligaments: a systematic review. Radiology 226:837–848
12. De Haven KE, Black KP, Griffiths HJ (1989) Open meniscus repair. Technique and two to nine year results. Am J Sports Med 6:788
13. Chambat P, Aït S, Selmi T et al (2000) Varus tibial osteotomy. Oper Tech Sports Med 8:44–47
14. Cannon WD, Vittori JM (1992) The incidence of healing in arthroscopic meniscal repairs in anterior cruciate ligament reconstructed knees versus stable knees. Am J Sports Med 20:176–181
15. Daniel DM, Stone ML, Bobson BE (1994) Fate of the anterior cruciate ligament injured patients
16. Hulet C, Souquet D, Pierre A (2004) Arthroscopic treatment of 105 lateral meniscal cysts. Arthroscopy 20:831–836
17. Billot N (2004) Résultats des réparations méniscales des lésions verticales longitudinales sur genou stable. Symposium de la SFA 2003 sous la direction de P Beaufils et X Cassard. Rev Chir Orthop 90(S8): 3S67–3S69)
18. Beaufils P, Bamberg A, Pujol N (2004) Clivage horizontal sur genou stable chez le jeune athlète. Symposium de la SFA 2003 sous la direction de P Beaufils et X. Cassard. Rev Chir Orthop 90(S8):3S69–3S72
19. Hulet et al (2014) (ref: Christophe Hulet, Jacques Minnetrait, Philippe Beaufils, Pierre Chamba, Patrick Giant, Philippe Hardi, Jean-Francois Botelle, Elvire Servien, Romain Zail, SFA, Clinical and radiographic results of 89 arthroscopic lateral meniscectomies in stable knees with a minimum follow-up of 20 years – ASFT-D-14-00240)
20. Tabib W, Beaufils P, Prudhon JL (1993) Ménisectomies externes arthroscopiques sur genou avec ligament croisé antérieur sain. J Traumatol Sport 10:19–26
21. Chatain F, Adeleine P, Chambat P et al (2003) A comparative study of medial versus lateral arthroscopic partial meniscectomy on stable knee: 10 year minimum follow-up. Arthroscopy 10:842–849
22. Charrois O, Ayral X, Beaufils P (1998) Chondrolyse rapide après méniscectomie externe arthroscopique. Rev Chir Orthop 84:88–92
23. Beauvis P et al (2006) Le ménisque latéral de l'adulte. Rev Chir Orthop 92(5):2S 169–2S 194
24. Aglietti P, Menchetti PP (2000) Distal femoral varus osteotomy in the valgus osteoarthritis knee. Am J Knee Surg 13:89–95
25. Bouyarmane H, Beaufils P, Pujol N et al (2014) Polyurethane scaffold in lateral meniscus segmental defects: clinical outcomes at 24 months follow-up. Orthop Traumatol Surg Res 100(1):153–157
26. Marti R, Verhagen R, Kerkhoffs G et al (2001) Proximal tibial varus osteotomy: indications, techniques and five to twenty-one-year result. J Bone Joint Surg Am 83:164–170
27. Verdonk R, Verdonk P, Heinrichs EL (2010) Polyurethane meniscus implant. In: Beaufils F, Verdonk R (eds) The meniscus. Springer, Heidelberg, pp 389–394
28. Zaffagnini S, Muccioli GMM, Lopomp N et al (2011) Prospective long-term outcome of the medial collagen meniscus implant versus partial medial meniscectomy. Am J Sports Med 39:977–985
29. Verdonk P, Van Laer M, Atar ML et al (2010) titel verwijzing?? In: Beaufils F, Verdonk R (eds) The meniscus. Springer, Heidelberg, pp 349–363
30. Verdonk P, Demurie A, Almqvist KF et al (2005) Transplantation of viable meniscal allograft: survivorship analysis and clinical outcome of one hundred cases. J Bone Joint Surg Am 87:715–724
31. Stone KR, Walgenbach AW, Turek TJ et al (2006) Meniscus allograft survival in patients with moderate to severe unicompartmental arthritis: a 2 to 7-year follow-up. Arthroscopy 22:469–478
32. Rodeo SA (2001) Meniscal allografts – where do we stand? Am J Sports Med 29:246–261
33. Verdonk P, Demurie A, Almqvist KF et al (2006) Transplantation of viable meniscal allograft. J Bone Joint Surg Am 88(S1):109–118
34. Goble EM, Verdonk R, Kohn D (1999) Arthroscopic and open surgical techniques for meniscus replacement – meniscal allograft transplantation and tendon autograft transplantation. Scan J Med Sci Sports 9:168–176
35. Wirth CJ, Peters G, Milachowski KA et al (2002) Long-term results of meniscal allograft transplantation. Am J Sports Med 30:174–181
36. Noyes FR, Barber-Westin SD, Rankin M (2004) Meniscal transplantation in symptomatic patients less than fifty years old. J Bone Joint Surg 86A:1392–1404
37. van Arkel ER, Goei R, de Ploeg I et al (2000) Meniscal allografts: evaluation with magnetic resonance imaging and correlation with arthroscopy. Arthroscopy 16:517–521
38. van Arkel ER, de Boer HH (2002) Survival analysis of human meniscal transplantation. J Bone Joint Surg 84B:227–231
39. Sekiya JK, West RV, Groff YJ et al (2006) Clinical outcomes following isolated lateral meniscal allograft transplantation. Arthroscopy 22:771–780
40. von Lewinski G, Milachowski KA, Weismeier K et al (2007) Twenty-years results of combined meniscal allograft transplantation, anterior cruciate ligament reconstruction and advancement of the medial

collateral ligament. Knee Surg Sports Traumatol Arthrosc 15:1072–1082
41. Milachowski KA, Weismeier K, Wirth CJ (1989) Homologous meniscus transplantation. Experimental and clinical results. Int Orthop 13:1–11
42. Dienst M, Kohn D (2006) Die allogene Meniskustransplantation – allogenic meniscus transplantation. Oper Orthop Traumatol 5:463–480
43. Wittvrouw E, Thys Y (2010) Rehabilitation after meniscectomy. In: Beaufils F, Verdonk R (eds) The meniscus. Springer, Heidelberg, pp 147–154
44. Lederman E (2002) Harmonic techniques. Churchill Living-Stone, Edingburgh
45. Palmieri-Smith RM, Kreinbrink J, Ashton-Miller JA et al (2007) Quadriceps inhibition induced by an experimental knee joint effusion affects knee joint mechanics during a single-legged drop landing. Am J Sports Med 35:1269–1275
46. Becker R, Brettschneider O, Grobel KH (1995) Distraction forces on repaired bucket-handle lesions in the medial meniscus. Am J Sports Med 34:1941–1947
47. Richards DP, Barber FA, Herbert MA (2005) Compressive loads in longitudinal lateral meniscus tears: a biomechanical study in porcine knees. Arthroscopy 21:1452–1456
48. Boisrenoult P, Pujol N (2010) Arthroscopic techniques with bald plugs. In: Beaufils F, Verdonk R (eds) The meniscus. Springer-Verlag, Heidelberg, pp 343–347
49. Barrie HJ (1979) The pathogenesis and significance of meniscal cysts. J Bone Joint Surg (Br) 61:184–189
50. Ferrer-Rocca O, Vilalta C (1980) Lesions of the meniscus. Part 1: macroscopic and histologic findings. Clin Orthop 146:289–300
51. Ferrer-Rocca O, Vilalta C (1980) Lesions of the meniscus. Part 2: horizontal cleavages and lateral cysts. Clin Orthop 146:301–307
52. Hulet C, Schiltz D, Locker B, Beguin J et al (1998) Les kystes du ménisque latéral: étude rétrospective de 105 kystes traits par arthroscopie avec 5 ans de recul. Rev Chir Orthop 84:531–538
53. Hulet C, Menetrey J, Beaufils et al (2014) Clinical and radiographic results of arthroscopic partial lateral meniscectomies in stable knees with a minimum follow up of 20 years. Knee Surg Sports Traumatol Arthrosc (Epub ahead of print)
54. Reagan WD, Mcconkey JP, Loomer RL et al (1989) Cysts of the lateral meniscus: arthroscopy versus arthroscopy plus open cystectomy. Arthroscopy 5:274–281
55. Pedowitz EA, Feagin JA, Rajagopalan S (1996) A surgical algorithm for treatment of cystic degeneration of the meniscus. Arthroscopy 12:209–216
56. Chambat P, Neyret P, la SFA (1997) Résultats à 10 ans des méniscectomies arthroscopiques sur genou stable. Ann Soc Fr Arthroscop 95–154
57. Ramadier JO, Beaufils P, Dupont JY et al (1983) Ménisectomies arthroscopiques. Résultats à court et à moyen terme. Rev Chir Orthop 69:581–590
58. Tabib W, Beaufils P, Prudhon JL et al (1993) Ménisectomies externs arthroscopiques. Résultats à court et à moyen terme de 95 ans. J Trauma Sport 10:19–26
59. Jaureguito JW, Elliot JS, Lietner T et al (1995) The effects of partial lateral meniscectomy in an otherwise normal knee: a retrospective review of functional, clinical and radiographic results. Arthroscopy 11: 29–36
60. Chassaing V, Parier J, Artigala P (1985) L'arthroscopie opératoire dans le traitement du kyste du ménisque externe. J Med Lyon 66:449–453
61. Maffuli N, Petricciuolo F, Pintore E (1991) Lateral meniscal cyst: arthroscopic management. Med Sci Sports Exerc 23:779–782
62. Beaufils P, Frank A (1995) L'arthroscopie dans les lesions méniscales dégéneratives et dans l'arthrose fémoro-tibiale avérée. Ann Orthop Ouest 27:19–21
63. Barthel T, Pesch R, Lippert M et al (1995) Arthroskopische Behandlung des lateralen Scheibemeniskus. Arthroskopie 8:12–18
64. Ikeuchi H (1982) Arthroscopic treatment of the discoid lateral meniscus. Clin Orthop Relat Res 167: 19–28
65. Monleau J, Leon A, Cugat R et al (1998) Ring-shaped lateral meniscus. Arthroscopy 14:502–504
66. Smillie I (1948) The congenital discoid meniscus. J Bone Joint Surg (Br) 30:671–682
67. Watanabe M, Takeda S, Ikeuchi H (1979) Atlas of arthroscopy. Springer, Berlin
68. Rao PS, Rao SK, Paul R (2001) Clinical radiologic, and arthroscopic assessment of discoid lateral meniscus. Arhtroscopy 17:275–277
69. Pellacci F, Montanari G, Prosperi P et al (1992) Lateral discoid meniscus: treatment and results. Arthroscopy 8:526–530
70. Hayashi LK, Yamaga H, Ida K et al (1988) Arthroscopic meniscectomy for discoid lateral meniscus in children. J Bone Joint Surg Am 70:1945–1500
71. Aichroth PM, Patel DV, Marx CL (1991) Congenital discoid lateral meniscus in children. A follow-up study and evolution of management. J Bone Joint Surg (Br) 73:932–936
72. Matsumoto H, Suda Y, Otani T et al (2000) Meniscoplasty for osteochondritis dissecans of bilateral lateral femoral condyle combined with discoid meniscus: case report. J Trauma 49:964–966
73. Kaplan EB (1957) Discoid lateral meniscus of the knee joint; nature, mechanism, and operative treatment. J Bone Joint Surg Am 39:77–87
74. Kim SJ, Yoo JH, Kim HK (1996) Arthroscopic one-piece excision technique for the treatment of symptomatic lateral discoid meniscus. Arthroscopy 12:752–755
75. Dickhaut SC, Delee JC (1982) The discoid lateral-meniscus syndrome. J Bone Joint Surg Am 64: 1068–1073
76. Rosenberg TD, Paulus LE, Parkter RD et al (1987) Discoid lateral meniscus: case report of arthroscopic attachment of a symptomatic Wrisberg-ligament type. Arthroscopy 3:277–282
77. Bellier G, Dupont J, Larrain M et al (1989) Lateral discoid menisci in children. Arthroscopy 5:52–56
78. Vandermeer RD, Cunningham FK (1989) Arthroscopic treatment of the discoid lateral meniscus:

results of long-term follow-up. Arthroscopy 5: 101–109
79. Chambat P, Neyret P (1996) Résults à long terme des méniscectomies arthroscopiques. Annales du congrès de la Société Française d'Arthroscopie
80. Youm T, Chen AL (2004) Discoid lateral evaluation and treatment. Am J Orthop 33:234–238
81. Adachi N, Ochi M, Uchio Y et al (2004) Torn discoid lateral meniscus treated using partial central meniscectomy and suture of the peripheral tear. Arthroscopy 20:536–542

Medial Meniscus Injuries

22

Giancarlo Coari, Francesco Miele,
Alessandro Emanuele Tripodo, and Filippo Troiani

22.1 Introduction

Over the years, the concept of the meniscus has greatly evolved from being just a useless vestigial structure to a multifunctional and essential part of the knee. Currently, menisci are considered to be responsible for load transmission, joint lubrication, shock absorption, and joint stability [1, 2]. Since they are essential to normal functioning of the knee, it is not surprising that meniscus repair has become a common procedure. With increasing attention to meniscus repair, the need to devise a reliable and reproducible classification of meniscus tears has also arisen.

The menisci occupy 60 % of the contact area between the tibial and the femoral cartilage surfaces and transmit greater than 50 % of joint compression forces. After meniscectomy, the tibiofemoral contact area decreases by approximately 50 % and the contact forces increase two- to threefold [3–7]. Meniscectomy frequently leads to irreparable joint damage, including articular cartilage degeneration, flattening of articular surfaces, and subchondral bone sclerosis. Poor long-term clinical results have been reported by many investigators after partial and total meniscectomy, with Fairbank's signs of radiographic deterioration [8], and authors noted a 50 % rate of radiographic osteoarthritis in patients who underwent meniscectomy with a mean of 13 years postoperatively [9].

Problems do exist in many meniscectomy natural history studies such as including both partial and total meniscectomy in the same cohort; still, preservation of meniscal tissue and function remains paramount for long-term joint function.

G. Coari, MD (✉) • F. Miele, MD
A.E. Tripodo, MD • F. Troiani
Unità Funzionale di Ortopedia, Casa di Cura "San Camilo", Forte dei Marmi (LU), Milan, Italy
e-mail: francesco.miele@yahoo.it, francescomiele007@gmail.com

22.2 Etiology and Classification

Trauma is one of the most common etiologies of meniscus tears, and meniscus tears occur in 40–60 % of patients with anterior cruciate ligament (ACL) ruptures [10].The majority of these tears extend into the middle third avascular region. Magnetic resonance imaging (MRI) provides important information regarding the type of meniscus tear and potential for repair to preserve function [11]. Occasionally, MRI will indicate that a repair may be possible, such as in cases of large horizontal tears.

Degenerative meniscus tears are much less frequently repaired, because the meniscal tissue is poor in quality and often fragmented into multiple pieces. Frequently, the symptoms of tibiofemoral pain will diminish over 6–12 weeks in degenerative tears in older patients, allowing a conservative approach.

P. Volpi (ed.), *Football Traumatology: New Trends*, DOI 10.1007/978-3-319-18245-2_22

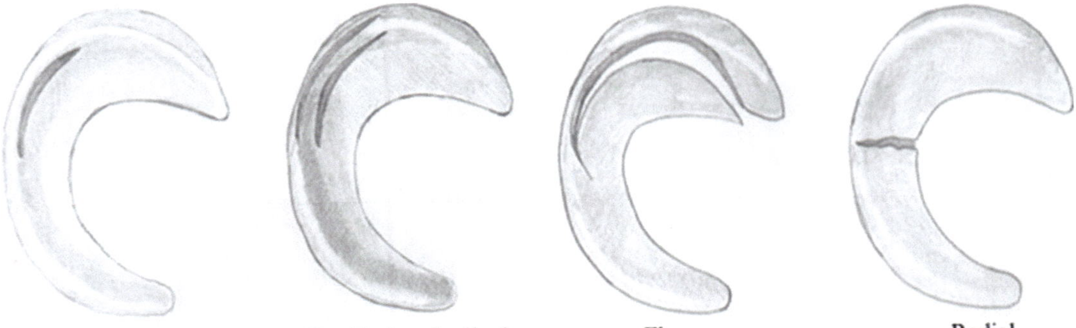

Fig. 22.1 Illustrations of the common complex and avascular meniscus tear patterns. Note the single-plane configuration of the single longitudinal and radial tears and the multiplane (complex) configuration of the double longitudinal and flap tears

Meniscus repair is frequently performed with concurrent operative procedures such as knee ligament reconstruction. Patients with lower extremity varus or valgus malalignment and associated meniscus tears are especially considered for meniscus repair. The malalignment produces high medial or lateral tibiofemoral compartment loads, and a functional meniscus is required to prevent articular cartilage deterioration.

Meniscus tears are classified according to location, type of tear, and integrity and damage to meniscal tissue and the meniscus attachment sites [12]. This classification, along with meticulous arthroscopic inspection of the tear site, allows the surgeon to determine whether a tear is reparable.

The meniscus body is divided into thirds: inner, middle, and outer. Tears located at the peripheral attachment sites (meniscofemoral and meniscotibial) are referred to as outer third tears. Single longitudinal tears are usually located in the outer third region or at the peripheral attachments (Fig. 22.1).

These tears are classified as red–red because both portions have an internal blood supply and are repaired in all cases with high success rates expected. Tears located in the middle third region are classified as either red–white or white–white (Fig. 22.2).

Red–white tears occur at the junction between the outer and the middle third regions where the vascular supply is present in the outer third portion of the tear. White–white meniscus tears are located in the inner third region where no blood supply is presumed to exist to either portion of the tear. When a repair is performed for these tears, the sutures may provide access to the vascular supply. In addition, the synovial migration of cells on the surface of the meniscus

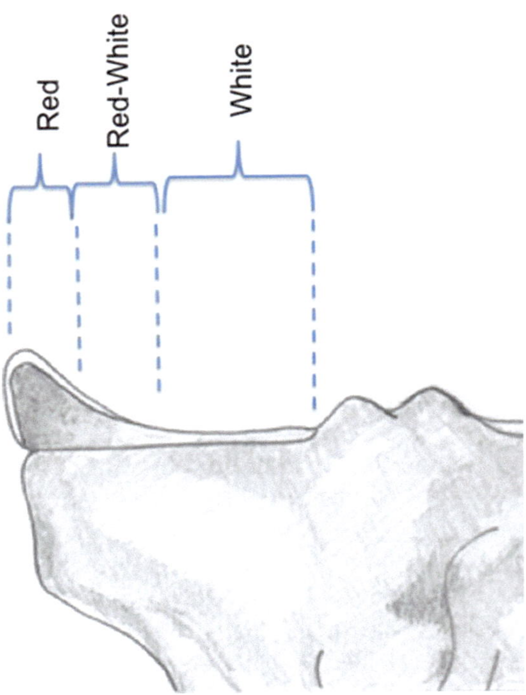

Fig. 22.2 Illustration of the different Zones of the meniscus

may occur after rasping of the meniscus–synovium border, providing a vascular supply to the repair site.

Repairs of complex tears and tears that extend into the middle third region are evaluated on an individual basis. Tear patterns in this region include single longitudinal, double longitudinal, triple longitudinal, horizontal, radial, and flap. The rationale for repair of these tears is that removal results in essentially a total meniscectomy because a substantial amount of meniscal tissue is resected. This is especially concerning in younger patients in their second to fourth decades of life and in all athletically active individuals. These tears are often reparable with reasonable success rates.

Single meniscus tears occur in a single plane, regardless of location. These include longitudinal, radial, and horizontal tears. These tears are most commonly found in the posterior horn and are usually reparable. Complex tears occur in more than one plane or direction. These include tears in the vertical plane (double or triple longitudinal), in the vertical and horizontal planes, or in the vertical and radial planes (flap tears). Each component of the tear is identified and may or may not be reparable.

The decision for repair includes the evaluation of the meniscal tissue regarding its integrity and absence of traumatic or degenerative changes. The meniscal tissue should appear nearly normal, with no secondary tears or fragmentation that would affect its projected function. This is a qualitative assessment regarding the quality of the tissue being repaired. The meniscal rim should be trimmed of tear fragments. A horizontal tear into the meniscal rim is a negative variable because it is difficult with sutures to fully restore the tear site owing to inner gaps between the horizontal tear arms. This is one indication in which a fibrin clot may provide a benefit. A meniscus that has been displaced in the notch may shorten and contract within 3–4 weeks, preventing reduction, and accordingly, early arthroscopy and repair are indicated. More specific recommendations of repair indications and techniques for specific tears are provided later in this chapter.

22.3 Injury Mechanism

22.3.1 Longitudinal Tears

Most meniscus tears are longitudinal, usually affecting the posterior segment of the meniscus. The lateral and medial menisci are equally affected, and complete and partial tears are seen with equal frequency. Because of structural differences, bucket-handle tears are more common in the medial meniscus [13].

The key element in the tearing of the medial meniscus is a rotational force on the partially flexed knee. Internal rotation of the femur pushes the medial meniscus to the center of the knee and posteriorly. With a strong posterior peripheral attachment of the meniscus, this movement is prohibited. Failure of this attachment, however, causes the posterior part of the medial meniscus to get caught between femur and tibia. In this situation, sudden extension of the knee will cause a longitudinal tear of the medial meniscus. With sufficient length, the central part of the tear can be locked behind the intercondylar notch and unable to return to its original position, resulting in a bucket-handle tear and causing acute locking of the knee [13].

22.3.2 Transverse, Radial, or Oblique Tears

Transverse, radial, or oblique tears can occur in either meniscus but more commonly involve the lateral meniscus. Transverse tears occur when the meniscus is stretched anteroposteriorly, separating the anterior from the posterior horn. A transverse tear results from the high amount of longitudinal stress on the middle part of the meniscus. The shorter radius of the lateral meniscus makes it more sensitive to this stress and thus to transverse tears. Any cause of reduction of meniscal mobility also adds to this stress.

The posterior horn of the lateral meniscus is stabilized by both the Wrisberg and the Humphrey ligament. Combined with the attachment to the popliteal tendon, this part of the meniscus is well connected to the lateral femoral condyle, reducing the risk of it getting caught in the center of the joint. Therefore, tears rarely start from the posterior horn of the lateral meniscus.

A radial tear greatly reduces the functional ability of the meniscus, more so than does a longitudinal tear, which can be explained by the longitudinal orientation of its fibers. As a consequence, radial tears result in massive loss of force transmission, which in turn results in higher pressures on the center of the medial femoral condyle and medial tibial plateau, eventually leading to degenerative changes in these areas.

22.4 Clinical and Diagnostic Examination

22.4.1 Clinical Examination

Before surgery, a presumptive diagnosis and a differential diagnosis should be established clinically by history taking, physical examination, and plain radiographs to provide the basis for informed consent discussions with patients and to determine if special studies, such as MRI or arthro-CT, are required for further evaluation. The physical examination should be preceded by careful history taking. A history of sudden pain on hyperflexion of the knee, catching, mechanical locking, and recurrent effusions requires a thorough investigation.

Examination of the tibiofemoral joint should note the presence of any cystic mass (ganglion) along the joint line, localized tenderness, crepitation, snapping, or clicking.

Meniscus tears occur as a result of injury to or degeneration of fibrocartilage. Physical examination of a knee with a torn meniscus reveals joint line tenderness with a palpable click or snap and occasionally the presence of an effusion. Range of motion may be limited secondary to a displaced meniscus tear. A block to full extension may be indicative of a locked knee with a large displaced tear.

22.4.1.1 Tests Commonly Used to Assess Meniscal Lesions

McMurray Test [14]

The McMurray test is performed with the patient supine. The examiner stands on the side of the affected knee and places one hand on the heel and the other along the medial aspect of the knee, providing a valgus force. The knee is extended from a fully flexed position while internally rotating the tibia. The test is repeated while externally rotating the tibia. Popping and tenderness along the joint line indicate a positive sign (Fig. 22.3).

Apley Test [15]

The Apley compression test is performed with the patient in prone position with the knee flexed to 90°. The tibia is compressed into the distal femur and rotated externally to assess the medial meniscus and internally to assess the lateral meniscus. The test is considered positive if it produces pain, which is less severe or relieved when the maneuver is repeated with distraction of the tibia.

Joint Line Palpation

Pain or discomfort is reproduced by palpation of the joint line.

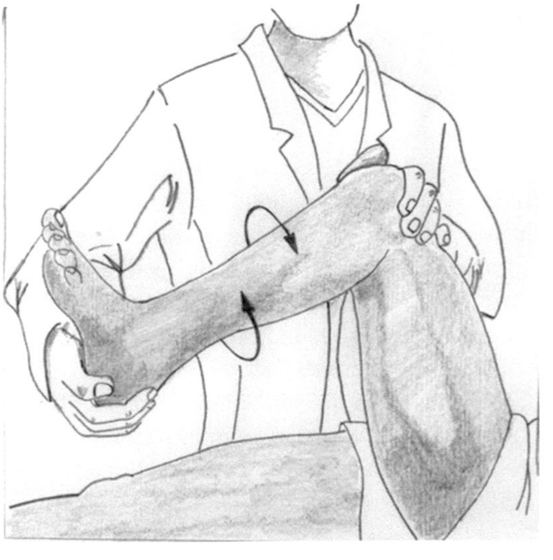

Fig. 22.3 McMurray test

Bragard Test
The Bragard test describes that external tibial rotation and knee extension increases tenderness along the medial joint line in the presence of a medial meniscus tear. This maneuver brings the medial meniscus more anterior and closer to the examining finger, therefore eliciting more pain. Internal rotation and flexion cause less tenderness by bringing the meniscus farther from the area of palpation. In the presence of a lateral meniscus tear, internal rotation of the tibia and extension will increase tenderness along the lateral joint line, while flexion and external rotation will reduce tenderness. If an articular surface irregularity of the femur or the tibia leads to tenderness, no difference between the two positions will be noted.

Steinman Second Test
The Steinmann second test demonstrates joint line tenderness that moves posteriorly with knee flexion and anteriorly with knee extension. This finding is consistent with a meniscus tear that moves with range of motion of the knee. On the other hand, with a fixed joint line disorder, tenderness should remain stationary throughout the range of motion.

The remaining tests for meniscal pathology depend on pain with rotation. The Apley grind forces the tibiofemoral surfaces together to elicit pain. A positive finding is believed to confirm a meniscus tear. On the other hand, the Apley test is performed with the knee surfaces distracted. If Apley test (distraction) elicits less discomfort than the Apley grind (compression), the finding of a meniscus tear is favored over a fixed joint line disorder. If the distraction test and compression are equally painful, an articular surface disorder is favored (such as an irregular surface secondary to osteoarthritic erosion).

If a medial meniscus tear is expected, the Bohler test can be performed by applying a varus stress to the knee. With a medial tear, a varus stress will result in increased pain caused by compression. Duck walking increases the compressive force on the posterior horns of the menisci, thus causing pain in the presence of a posterior meniscus tear.

A single clinical test is not sufficient to establish a correct diagnosis. Diagnostic accuracy is improved if the results of the three tests are combined. Generally, all clinical tests tend to be less reliable in the presence of concomitant ligamentous injury. Furthermore, physical examination is less accurate in patients with degenerative tears than in young patients with acute injuries [16].

22.4.2 Diagnostic Examination

Accurate imaging of the meniscus is essential to evaluate the damaged area and to select the most appropriate treatment. Similarly, in the postoperative meniscus, imaging is important for treatment, follow-up, and identification of any further injury. A number of factors have to be considered when selecting the most appropriate imaging technique.

Although the meniscus is not visible on *standard radiographs*, full-leg radiographs taken in a standing position are useful for the evaluation of knee alignment. Varus or valgus deviation results in abnormal pressure on the medial or lateral meniscus, which can lead to early degeneration and subsequent tearing of the meniscus. In a preoperative setting, meniscal transplantation is not indicated in knees with significant malalignment because the articular cartilage is usually completely degraded. Plain radiographs can also detect other indicators of meniscal lesions, including joint space narrowing and generalized degenerative changes of the femorotibial joint. Radiographic images taken before contrast injection can help distinguish between a tear and chondrocalcinosis, a pitfall on both CT and MR imaging.

A *CT* scan without a previous intra-articular iodinated contrast injection is no longer considered a good practice. CT arthrography and MR imaging have a similar level of accuracy when used for the detection of meniscus tears [17, 18]. CT arthrography is used less frequently than *MR* imaging because the technique is more invasive and involves the use of ionizing radiation. CT arthrography is, nonetheless, a valuable alternative

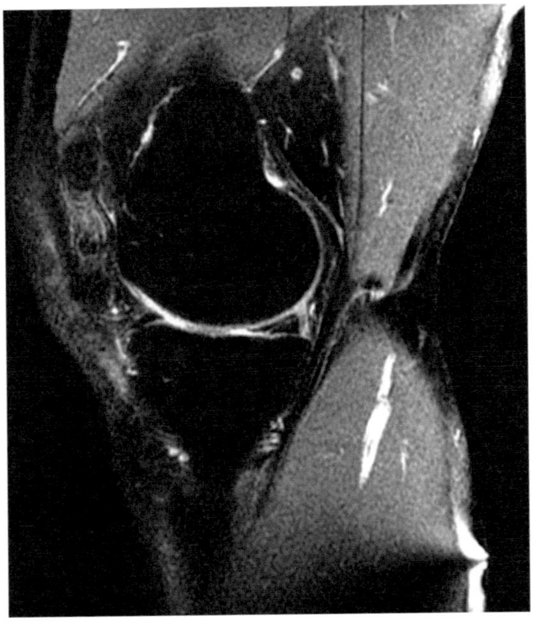

Fig. 22.4 Sagittal MRI image shows meniscus tear

when MR imaging is not available, in the presence of orthopedic hardware or in patients with contraindications for MR imaging. It is also indicated for the evaluation of repaired menisci, for largely the same reasons as MR arthrography.

MR imaging of the meniscus is highly effective and is the primary technique for evaluating internal derangements of the knee [19]. The technique is noninvasive and has a high level of accuracy in the detection of meniscal lesions (Fig. 22.4).

The sensitivity and specificity for the detection of medial meniscus tears are both estimated to be approximately 90 %. The same applies to the specificity for lateral meniscus tears, but here the sensitivity is lower (approximately 80 %).

The accuracy of detecting meniscal lesions in a nonoperated or postoperative knee is not significantly improved by using direct or indirect MR arthrography [20]. However, direct MR arthrography is useful after meniscus repair.

22.4.3 Arthroscopy

Arthroscopy is not part of the diagnostic methods, but allows to confirm or adjust a diagnosis based on history, physical examination, and imaging techniques. It permits the surgeon to define the exact size of the lesion and to identify other lesions. Arthroscopy has entirely replaced open surgery for the treatment of meniscus tears.

22.5 Treatment Strategy

The first goal always is to preserve as much viable tissue as possible. Other factors are location, length, tear pattern, stability of the tear, and any damage to the integrity of the meniscus body [21].

When conservative management is not feasible, arthroscopy is the method of choice for the treatment of a traumatic meniscus tear. It is essential to inform the patient about the postoperative consequences of the chosen treatment, with the rehabilitation period being short for meniscectomy, but much longer after repair. The final decision is always based on the intraoperative findings at arthroscopy, taking into account all of the previous parameters [22].

22.5.1 Conservative Treatment: Masterly Neglect

After diagnosing a meniscus tear, the first decision the surgeon has to make is whether it should be treated surgically or left alone.

Cascells [23] showed that not all meniscus tears cause clinical symptoms.

Tears that surgeons should consider leaving alone are partial-thickness split tears and full-thickness but short (5 mm or less) vertical or oblique tears, if the inner portion of the meniscus is stable with probing. This also applies to short (5 mm or less) radial tears. Some smaller lesions can be treated conservatively, especially when the patient does not perform strenuous physical activities [22].

Short inner radial tears (<5 mm) usually do not heal, but can be left alone because they may be asymptomatic [23]. Stable tears, defined as tears in which the central portion cannot be displaced more than 3 mm [23], can be left alone if they are less than 1 cm in length. Stable

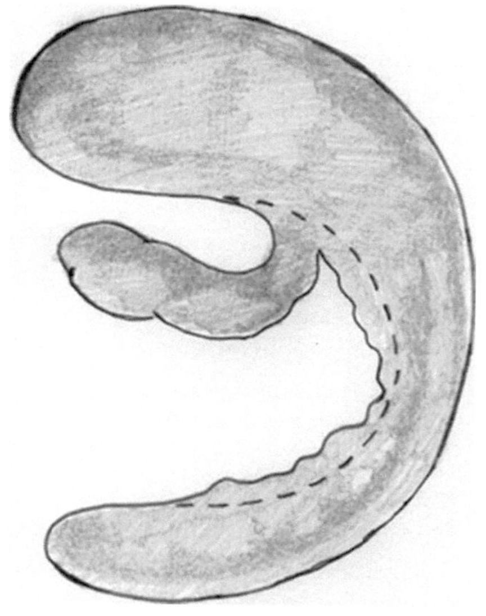

Fig. 22.5 Partial meniscectomy: tear in meniscus and area of resection

longitudinal tears in the peripheral two-thirds often can be left alone, particularly if they are less than 5 mm in length. The same applies to less than 5 mm long partial-thickness tears of various types (especially longitudinal) [22].

Therefore, it is essential that the surgery be performed by the same surgeon who has diagnosed the lesion and has suggested the indication for surgery [22].

22.5.2 Surgical Treatment

Symptomatic lesions in the avascular zone of the meniscus should be treated with meniscectomy (Fig. 22.5) [24].

22.5.2.1 (Sub)Total or Partial Meniscectomy

In the early days of meniscal surgery, little attention was paid to the preservation of healthy meniscal tissue. A tear in the meniscus was generally treated by total or subtotal meniscectomy. In 1948, Fairbank was the first to describe radiological changes in the knee following total meniscectomy, now known as Fairbank's changes (flattening of the femoral condyles, formation of peripheral ridges, and joint space narrowing) [24].

Roos et al. [25] compared knees of 123 patients who had undergone open total meniscectomy 21 years earlier, with normal knees of matched controls. They concluded that meniscectomy represented a significant risk factor for radiographic osteoarthritis of the knee, with the later appearance of degenerative changes being 14 times more likely in meniscectomized knees than in uninjured knees.

Literature reports had already shown the superiority of adequate partial resection of the meniscus to total meniscectomy [26, 27]. These findings initiated a mentality change, and surgeons, nowadays, always try to preserve as much meniscal tissue as possible [28].

When faced with a torn meniscus, the question arises whether the damaged tissue can be repaired. In the last two decades, different techniques have been developed to repair some, not all, meniscus tears. In the early days, meniscus tears were repaired during an open procedure. Currently, arthroscopy is generally accepted to be the method of choice for repairing a meniscal lesion. The arthroscopic management strategies can be divided into three groups: the inside–out technique, the outside–in technique, and the all-inside technique

22.6 Suitability and Indications for Repair

A thorough knowledge of the meniscus tear is necessary to determine its suitability for repair.

Besides the physical examination and the presence of associated lesions, the location is a critical factor. Only the peripheral third of the meniscus is sufficiently vascularized. DeHaven [21] considered tears within the peripheral third (3 mm) as vascular, 5 mm from the periphery as avascular, and between 3 and 5 mm as variable in vascularity. Current techniques allow some tears of the central and middle third to be repaired.

A more than 1 cm long tear in the vascular zone of the meniscus is an excellent indication for repair by suture [29].

The pattern, length, and stability of the tear are also important. With intact circumferential hoop fibers, the chance of healing is greater. In general, radial tears are less amenable to repair. Complex bucket-handle tears with radial components, often seen in chronic cases, have more difficulty healing with repair than simple bucket-handle tears. The same applies to oblique and horizontal tears. Longitudinal (vertical) tears in the periphery are most amenable to repair [30].

Any significant injury to the meniscus body, such as a complex tear, multiple cleavage tears, or change in the body contour, may compromise repair. Often, the structural integrity of the meniscus is damaged and vascularity may be impaired [21].

Some authors have reported better healing of acute vs. chronic tears [31].

22.7 Meniscal Grafts and Substitutes

When a symptomatic meniscal lesion can neither be repaired nor left untreated, the possibility of its replacement with either a graft or a synthetic substitute can be considered in association with ligament reconstruction.

The use of cryopreserved [32, 33] or viable [34] allografts has already been proposed with encouraging results. However, the results of these retrospective studies do not allow to confirm that meniscal substitution compensates the negative effects of meniscectomy associated with ACL reconstruction on the evolution of the joint.

Meniscus repair was first reported by Annandale [35], but it was not widely performed and sank into oblivion. Like other procedures in knee surgery, meniscus repair has benefited from advances in arthroscopy.

Arthroscopic techniques include inside–out, outside–in, and all-inside repairs [32, 36]. The first two techniques require the passage of suture through the skin, which exposes the patient to neurovascular complications. In the 1990s, various implants were introduced and these procedures became technically less demanding.

When meniscus repair is carried out under arthroscopic visualization, some common steps, which are independent of the technique, have to be followed.

Access to the posterior part of the medial meniscus is achieved by holding the knee in slight flexion and applying valgus stress.

Although imaging techniques can be helpful, the characteristics of a tear are best assessed arthroscopically. The final treatment decision is made at the time of arthroscopy. The type (vertical longitudinal, horizontal, radial, complex) and length of the tear are determined, and the distance from the meniscosynovial junction is measured using a probe. A short tear of 1–2 cm has a better chance of healing.

The peripheral 20–30 % of the medial meniscus is vascularized.

The location of the tear has been classified into zones, according to Arnoczky and Warren [37]. Zone 0 represents the peripheral meniscosynovial junction, zone 1 the red–red zone, zone 2 the red–white zone, and zone 3 the white–white zone. De Haven considered meniscus tears within 3 mm of the periphery as vascular, those 5 mm or more from the periphery as avascular, and between 3 and 5 mm as variably vascular [61]. Tears in the red–red and the red–white zone are amenable to repair. Meniscus repair for tears in the white–white zone has poor healing potential.

The macroscopic aspect of the meniscal tissue is assessed (normal or degenerative).

Finally, the meniscus is prepared. If a dislocated bucket-handle tear is present, it is reduced into its anatomic position.

In summary, the ideal candidate for meniscus repair is a young patient with a recent vertical tear within 3–4 mm of the peripheral rim and 1–2 cm in length, in a stable or stabilized knee.

22.8 Debridement

In case of a bucket-handle tear, the reducibility has to be assessed. An old bucket-handle tear can develop plastic shrinkage, leading to redislocation after reduction. The tensile forces are so important that they may compromise the fixation, regardless of the device implanted, and decrease the chance of healing.

For large bucket-handle tears, passing the probe through a transtendinous Gillquist portal permits to hold the inner segment in the proper position. Then, the tear can be fixed with the devices.

22.9 Technique

22.9.1 First Generation: Open Technique

The first-generation repairs involve an open procedure [35]. Open meniscus repair has been well described by DeHaven et al. [38] and requires an arthrotomy using a retroligamentous approach. The capsule is incised posterior to the collateral ligament, and the synovium is opened to give direct access to the posterior segment of the meniscus and the tear, provided that it is a vertical peripheral longitudinal tear. In case of a horizontal tear, the meniscosynovial rim needs to be dissected in order to expose the peripheral meniscal rim and the horizontal cleavage.

The repair is performed with vertically oriented, absorbable 4–0 sutures, incorporating the entire height of the meniscal rim and the capsular bed in an anatomic fashion. The individual sutures are placed 2–3 mm apart, beginning with the deepest or more centrally located suture. The repair sutures are tied inside the joint to reapproximate the capsular bed to the meniscal rim. Then, the knee is tested in full extension.

Variations of this technique involve vertically oriented sutures placed through the capsule and tied outside the joint, horizontally oriented sutures placed through the capsule and tied outside the joint, and the use of absorbable or nonabsorbable suture material.

This approach gives good access to the posterior and middle meniscal segments, but is much more difficult on the lateral side, due to the presence of the popliteus tendon. Open repair of the anterior segment (especially on the lateral side) requires an anterior approach.

The ability to achieve a strong fixation is the main advantage of this technique, which is suitable for lesions within 3 mm from the peripheral rim.

To remove the fibrous tissue, the walls of the tear are debrided using a basket punch, a rasp, or a shaver. Freshening must essentially be done on the outer part of the meniscus in order to promote the healing response and to preserve meniscal tissue in the inner part. In some cases, multiple perforations can be made with a needle in the meniscal rim to stimulate the bleeding through vascular channels. Debridement of the medial posterior segment can be difficult. The use of a posterior portal improves the accuracy of the abrasion, as proposed by Pujol et al. [39].

22.9.2 Fixation

Whatever the device and location of the meniscus tear (medial or lateral), the implants or the sutures are routinely inserted through the ipsilateral portal for the posterior segment and the contralateral portal for the middle segment. Sufficient sutures or devices need to be placed to avoid gaps of more than 3–5 mm. When using sutures, these should be nonabsorbable (such as Ethibond) or slowly absorbable (such as PDS).

Vertical longitudinal tears in the red–white zone (3–5 mm from the peripheral rim) are difficult to access through the posterior approach. In our opinion, this is the only suitable technique to repair horizontal cleavage tears.

The main disadvantage is the risk of neural damage to the saphenous nerve or its branches.

22.9.3 Second Generation: Arthroscopically Assisted Inside–Out or Outside–In Technique

The second-generation repairs are based on an arthroscopically assisted inside–out or outside–in technique. The goal is to reduce the morbidity associated with the posterior approach and to be able to repair meniscal lesions located in the red–white zone.

22.9.3.1 Inside–Out Meniscus Repair

Several systems have been developed using long curved single- or double-barrel cannulas.

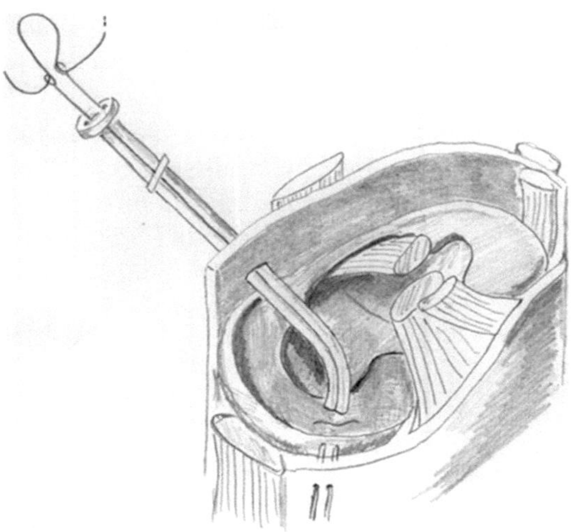

Fig. 22.6 Meniscus repair using the inside–out technique with a double-barrel cannula

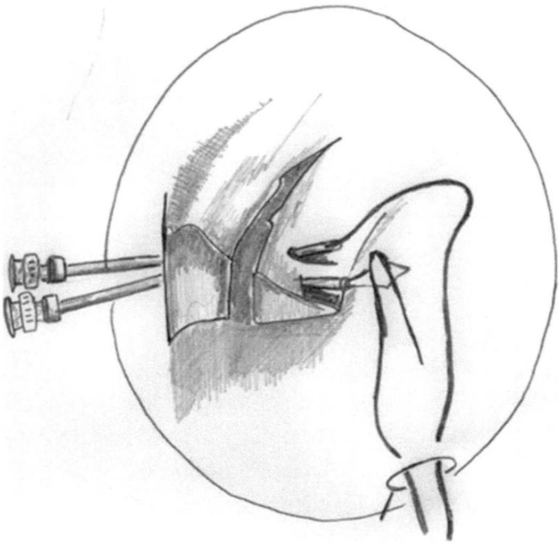

Fig. 22.7 Outside–in meniscus repair. The suture is passed through the needle and retrieved inside the joint

Absorbable or nonabsorbable 2-0 or 0 sutures are passed from inside to outside, using long flexible needles. Either horizontal or vertical mattress stitches can be done. The sutures are retrieved through an extra-articular posteromedial incision. The posterior neurovascular structures are protected with a large retractor. The knots are tied outside the joint over the capsule (Fig. 22.6).

As with the open technique, the main disadvantage is the risk of neurovascular complications. The saphenous nerve and vein are at risk on the medial side. The incision must be made behind the medial collateral ligament.

22.9.3.2 Outside–In Meniscus Repair

In 1985, Warren [40] introduced an outside–in technique that was initially designed to decrease the risk of peroneal nerve entrapment on the lateral side. A cannulated 18-gauge spinal needle is passed across the tear from the outside–in. Once the sharp tip of the needle is in view, the suture (monofilament absorbable 0-gauge PDS) is passed through the lumen of the needle and pulled through the arthroscopic ipsilateral portal. An interference knot is tied in the end of the suture and the suture is pulled back. The process is repeated and the free ends are tied two by two over the capsule through an accessory skin incision until the tear is stabilized. Sutures may be placed alternately on the femoral and tibial surface of the meniscus in order to balance the repair (Fig. 22.7).

The interference knot inside the joint can be avoided by passing the first suture through the second one tied as a lasso loop. The second suture is pulled back. The two ends of the first suture are retrieved outside the joint and tied over the capsule.

The inside–out and outside–in techniques are complementary. The first one is mainly indicated for posterior and middle segment repairs, while the second allows satisfactory access to the anterior segment of the meniscus.

Both techniques can be associated to repair extended longitudinal lesions.

22.9.4 Third Generation: Devices

Specific implants have been designed to replace the use of sutures and to allow all-inside meniscus repairs without the need for accessory skin incisions [41]. Staples, tacks, anchors, screws, etc. have been proposed. Most of the devices are bioabsorbable and composed of rigid poly-l-lactic acid (PLLA).

Albrecht-Olsen et al. were the first to present an all-inside procedure using a bioabsorbable tack, the Biofix meniscal arrow (Bioscience Ltd.,

Tampere, Finland). The implant consists of a T-shaped arrow with barbs on the stem, resembling a fishing hook. The barbed stem penetrates the meniscus, and its distal part is fixed in the peripheral part of the meniscus, while the T-head of the arrow is applied to the axial part of the meniscus, usually the upper surface.

An accessory incision being not needed and a lower risk of neurovascular complications are the advantages of this technique. Moreover, this technique is fast and easily performed.

The disadvantages are the lower strength of the arrows compared to vertical sutures [6, 19] and the risk of loose bodies, synovitis, cysts, and cartilage abrasion due to the head of the device at the surface of the meniscus [3, 11, 20, 42]. Low-profile heads have been proposed to decrease this risk.

22.9.5 Fourth Generation: All-Inside Technique with Sutures

The newest devices are self-adjusting suture devices, combining the advantages of all-inside meniscus repair (no accessory incision, lower neural complication rate) with those of suture (better strength). They are based on the same principles: an anchor is positioned behind the capsule, and a suture compresses and holds the axial meniscal part by using a sliding knot. These implants share the potential ability to deform and move with the meniscus during weight bearing and carry a lower risk of chondral abrasion. The three devices in this category are the RapidLoc (DePuy Mitek Products, Westwood, MA), the FasT-Fix (Smith and Nephew Endoscopy, Andover, MA) and, more recently, the Meniscal Cinch (Arthrex, Naples, FL) (Fig. 22.8).

22.10 Rehabilitation and Return to Play

22.10.1 Rehabilitation After Meniscectomy

Supervised rehabilitation after partial arthroscopic meniscectomy is frequently considered as nonessential because, usually, patients rapidly regain functional autonomy without specific postoperative treatment. However, quantitative evaluations of knee function after arthroscopic meniscectomy have shown recovery to be still incomplete 4–8 weeks after surgery, when the majority of patients already have resumed work and sports-related or other functional activities [42, 43]. Abnormalities in leg movements and muscle activations during submaximal locomotor activities such as gait and stairs ascent and descent have been observed up to 4 weeks postsurgery. At 8 weeks, patients often still walk and descend stairs at a slower pace, suggesting that complete locomotor recovery has not been attained [44]. In addition, strength evaluations have revealed residual deficits of 20–40 % in the knee extensor muscles and of up to 20 % in the knee flexor muscles, 3 weeks after partial arthroscopic meniscectomy [42].

Since a 10 % residual strength deficit of the extensor and flexor muscles has been associated to a higher frequency of knee (re)injury, it can be stated that progressive neuromuscular reeducation and strengthening of the knee after partial meniscectomy are warranted. Moffet et al. have demonstrated that an early, intensive, supervised physiotherapy program, applied in the first 3 weeks after arthroscopic meniscectomy, accelerates knee extensor strength recovery.

22.10.1.1 Rehabilitation Protocol

Supervised rehabilitation after partial meniscectomy can generally progress as tolerated by the patient with no substantial contraindications or limitations. The main goals of rehabilitation are to control the pain and swelling associated with surgery, restore the range of motion (ROM), restore or maintain isolated muscle function, and optimize lower extremity neuromuscular coordination and muscle strength [45].

22.10.1.2 Early Postoperative Rehabilitation Phase

Immediate weight-bearing is allowed as tolerated by the patient. Crutches are advised during the first few days after surgery and can be abandoned when the patient is able to place full weight on the involved leg without pain and has good control over the quadriceps muscle.

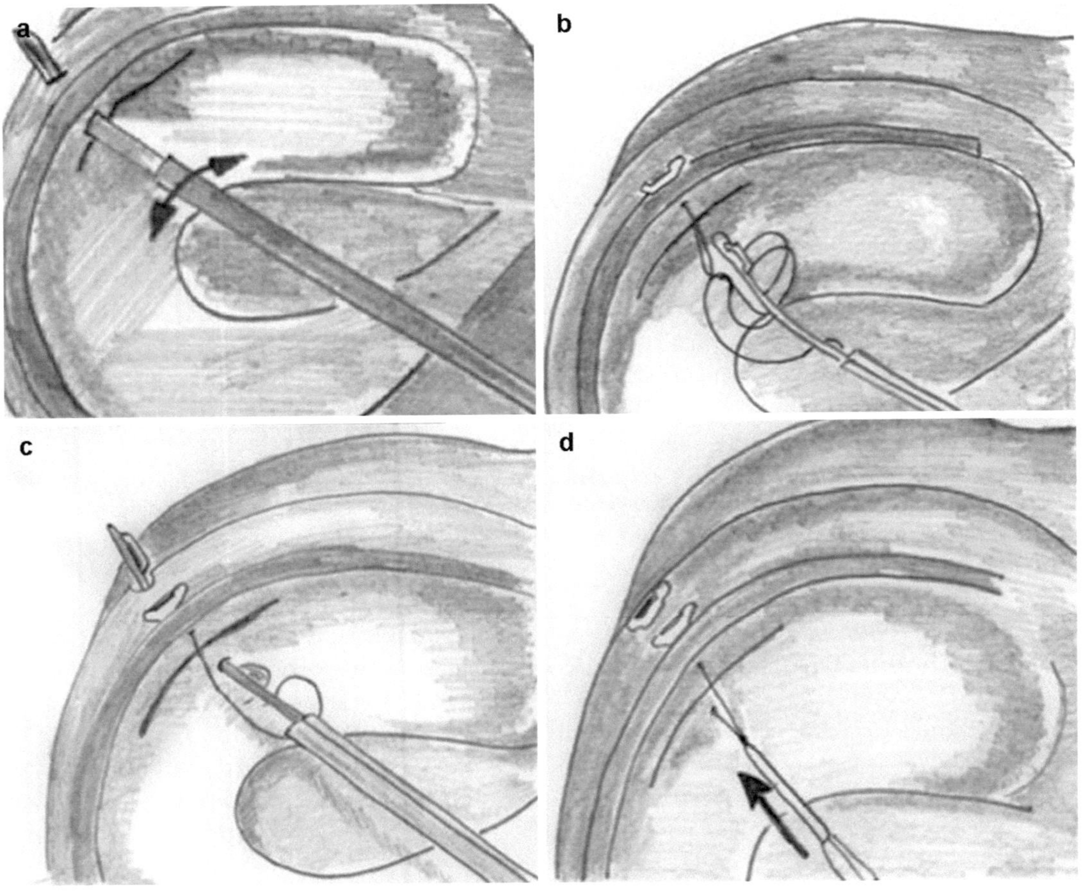

Fig. 22.8 FasT-Fix meniscus repair. (**a**) Insertion of the first implant with the needle. (**b**) The needle is positioned in front of the inner part of the meniscus. (**c**) The second implant is passed through the capsule. (**d**) Tensioning of the suture using the knot pusher

Postoperative treatment should initially focus on the reduction of pain and swelling, which may be present to a greater or lesser degree at the operated knee and are normal reactions of the affected tissue to the operation.

Reduction of pain and swelling is imperative for reducing "reflex inhibition," which may be present at the operated knee. "Reflex inhibition" represents a signal which is sent from an injured joint to the surrounding muscles in response to pain and joint effusion and which results in the inhibition of these muscles. This inhibition prevents the injured, weakened joint from being more damaged by excessive pressure in the joint caused by a strong contraction of the surrounding muscles. Hence, reflex inhibition acts as a natural protective mechanism of the body. As a result of reflex inhibition, however, the muscles surrounding the affected joint rapidly lose their strength, especially those that have their insertion closest to the joint, such as the vastus medialis muscle. In addition, the inhibition of the muscles limits their response to strengthening exercises [46].

Rapid reduction of pain and swelling is, therefore, an essential goal during the first postoperative week because strengthening of the muscles surrounding the knee cannot be initiated until reflex inhibition is resolved.

Initially, pain and swelling can be reduced by frequent application of ice (every 2 h for 30 min) and activity reduction. In addition, frequent (high repetitions) low-resistance active and passive movements (e.g., pendulum motions) within the pain-free ROM of the knee enhance the nutrition of the joint cartilage, and thus, stimulate joint recovery.

Progressive active and passive ROM exercises of the knee can be started immediately postsurgery within the pain limits. Examples of such exercises are heel slides, flexion–extension exercises while standing with the involved leg on a chair or bench, stationary cycling, and manual ranging of the knee joint. Deep squats are not allowed in the first 4 weeks following the operation to avoid excessive load on the healing meniscus.

The presence of reflex inhibition also causes a disruption of the neuromuscular coordination at the knee [47]. Because of the effects of reflex inhibition, the initial primary focus of muscle rehabilitation is not strengthening of the musculature surrounding the knee but improving the neuromuscular control of the muscles and the proprioception of the knee.

The neuromuscular coordination of the quadriceps muscle can initially be improved by performing muscle-setting exercises. The patient, lying in a supine position, is asked to perform an isolated isometric contraction of the quadriceps muscle in various knee angle positions. Setting exercises of the quadriceps muscle are, however, not recommended with the knee in full extension because this might cause impingement of the knee capsule. Eventually, the patient should be capable to maintain the isometric muscle contraction for 10 s. Patients are advised to daily perform ten series of ten repetitions until they regain full control of the quadriceps muscle in supine position, after which they can perform the setting exercises in more functional, weight-bearing positions such as sitting and standing.

Co-contractions of the quadriceps and hamstring muscles in different positions (lying, sitting, and standing) at various knee angles are also essential components of the rehabilitation program, because they play an important role in anterior–posterior stability of the knee.

Proprioceptive exercises are essential to improve the functional stability of the knee joint. They can be started immediately after the operation, proceeding from exercises in a lesser weight-bearing position (e.g., repositioning exercises, exercises in lying position) to exercises in more weight-bearing positions (e.g., unilateral balance exercises on a stable/unstable surface) to optimally facilitate the proprioceptive receptors.

22.10.1.3 Second Phase

Once the patient has regained good control of the muscles surrounding the knee, muscle strengthening exercises can be initiated. Optimizing quadriceps strength is especially important since, in addition to providing functional joint stability, the quadriceps musculature also has a protective function, serving as shock absorber capable of dampening loads during activity. Poor quadriceps strength decreases this shock-absorbing function and results in increased loading of the meniscus [47].

A combination of open kinetic chain (OKC) and closed kinetic chain (CKC) exercises can be used to improve upper leg muscle strength, but the latter become more important with time because they are more functional for the lower limb.

Depending on how much weight the patient can tolerate on the involved knee, CKC exercises are initially carried out with partial weight-bearing and then progressively with full weight-bearing. The progression in exercise intensity is guided by the amount of pain and effusion the patient experiences at the knee during or after the exercise and can be increased when there is no marked reaction of the knee to the exercise. The intensity of the exercises has to be modified so that they can be performed within the pain limits. Examples of CKC exercises that can be performed are leg press exercises, squats, forward and sideways lunges, and step exercises.

As soon as patients can tolerate full weight-bearing on the involved knee, CKC exercises with the patients' own body weight as load can be started at a frequency of three series of 10–12 repetitions. When these can comfortably be performed, the number of repetitions can progressively be increased to four series of 30 repetitions to enhance muscle endurance.

Subsequently, the intensity of the exercises can be increased by increasing the load. The number of repetitions is then initially reduced to three series of 15 repetitions and can progressively be increased again to four series of 20 repetitions. When there is no negative reaction (pain or effusion) of the knee joint to the intensity of the exercises, loading can be increased to 60–70 % of one repetition maximum (1RM) at a frequency of three series of 15 repetitions and eventually to 80 % of 1RM in a series of 8–12 repetitions.

22.10.1.4 Third Phase

Functional activities, rotational activities, jumps, running, and sport-specific exercises can be integrated in the rehabilitation program 3–4 weeks after surgery.

Patients are generally able to return to work after 1–2 weeks and to resume sports activities and training by 3–4 weeks following the operation [48].

22.10.2 Rehabilitation After Meniscus Repair

In the treatment of meniscus injuries, preservation of the meniscus has become a major priority. Consequently, contemporary meniscal surgery is aimed at retaining the structure and function of the meniscus whenever possible. The shift in focus from meniscectomy to meniscus repair noted in the last decade has entailed a change in the rehabilitation protocol because the finest surgical technique can be fraught with frustration if rehabilitation is inadequate or incomplete.

In an attempt to protect the repaired meniscus, a significantly less aggressive approach should be used in the postoperative management and rehabilitation than when meniscectomy has been performed. In one of the first landmark papers concerning postoperative care after meniscus repair, authors advocated immobilization of the knee in 30° of flexion and no weight-bearing during the first two postoperative months. In the following years, other rehabilitation protocols were described, and it is probably the poorly understood healing rate of meniscus repair that has led surgeons to suggest various restrictions. Full weight-bearing is postponed for various amounts of time (from 8 to 3 weeks) or is allowed immediately. A similar disagreement is found with regard to the ROM and the return to sports activities.

Despite the conflicting reports in the literature, clinicians and researchers all agree about the time-honored principles of aftercare for meniscus repair. These include a period of maximum protection to provide the best opportunity for healing to occur, followed by a period of continuing restriction from potentially harmful stresses while the healing process undergoes maturation and becomes sufficiently strong to resist re-rupture under heavy stress.

Simply stated, the rehabilitation program after meniscus repair needs to consider when to allow motion, weight-bearing and resumption of activities. In order to answer these questions, we need to know how these activities influence the healing meniscus.

22.10.2.1 Healing of the Meniscus

Healing Rate After Meniscus Repair

The key question is how long it takes for a meniscus to heal and how strong the healed tissue is. Roeddecker et al. [49] showed in rabbits that 12 weeks post-repair, the energy required to tear the suture-repaired meniscus was 23 % of the energy required to tear a normal meniscus. This suggests that even after 12 weeks, a repaired meniscus is still significantly weaker than a healthy meniscus. In contrast to this, other experimental studies showed that lesions of the vascular portion of the meniscus heal completely after 10 weeks and that it takes several months for fibrocartilage to regain a normal appearance [50]. Four to five weeks are usually required for early histological evidence of meniscus repair.

Extrinsic Factors Influencing Meniscus Healing After Meniscus Repair

Immobilization

Studies have shown decreased collagen content in meniscus repairs subjected to prolonged immobilization [51]. These findings encourage early ROM exercises after meniscus repair. In addition, it has been demonstrated that a rehabilitation program implementing immediate knee motion from the first postoperative day after meniscus repair (with or without anterior cruciate ligament (ACL) reconstruction) is not deleterious to the healing meniscal tissue [52]. As a result, most postoperative rehabilitation protocols now allow immediate mobilization.

Weight-bearing

Restricted weight-bearing and limited ROM are common in an attempt to avoid undue forces which could impair meniscal healing. However, Staerke et al. [53] showed that compression of the meniscus can substantially increase the pull-out resistance of meniscus repair implants and, thus, does not seem to negatively influence the stability of the repair. On the basis of their results, these authors rather support early weight-bearing, although some caution is warranted while drawing clinical implications from ex vivo studies. Moreover, these results are in agreement with the fact that the hoop stresses caused by weight-bearing are primarily absorbed at the periphery of the meniscus. In addition, it was shown that immobilization and non-weight-bearing did not improve meniscal healing in sheep and rabbits after suture repair in the avascular and vascular zone [54].

In conclusion, there is very little evidence showing that weight-bearing alone causes significant distension forces on a meniscal lesion. However, scientific evidence proving the opposite is also rather scarce. As a result, it is not very surprising that no consensus has yet been reached in this respect. Many authors do not allow immediate postoperative weight-bearing, while others do.

Intrinsic Factors Influencing Meniscus Healing After Meniscus Repair

Intrinsic key factors in meniscus repair include (a) vascular supply (determined by age and localization of the tear); (b) suture fixation, which can lead to early failure if too vigorous a program is initiated; (c) anatomical site of the tear (anterior, posterior, medial, or lateral); (d) tear size and type; and, finally, (e) other intra-articular disorders.

Therefore, it seems evident that a rehabilitation protocol after meniscus repair should take these intrinsic factors into account and, accordingly, provide for some variations. For example, peripheral repairs heal rapidly, whereas complex tears extending into the central avascular region heal more slowly and require greater caution. Radial repairs must be especially protected, as excessive weight-bearing in an early postoperative stage can disrupt the repair site. A higher rate of failure of tears has been observed in the medial versus the lateral meniscus (30–45 vs. 16–20 %). Tears longer than 4 cm had a 59 % failure rate, which dropped to 15 % for tears smaller than 2 cm [55]. In addition, modifications may be required if significant articular cartilage deterioration is present. Obviously, this might affect the design of an exercise program.

22.10.3 Protocol

22.10.3.1 Conventional Rehabilitation Protocol

In most of today's conventional protocols, weight-bearing is not allowed the first 3–4 weeks. A 4-week period of restricted ROM (until 90°) is recommended. Controlled knee extensor–flexor strengthening exercises in an OKC are initiated after 2–3 weeks and in a CKC after 4–5 weeks. Stationary cycling is allowed at 2 months. Since backward pedalling offers lower tibiofemoral compressive loads compared to normal forward pedalling, we suggest that backward pedalling be started 2 weeks earlier. Return to light work and running are allowed at 5–6 months. Full participation in pivoting sports is deferred until 9–12 months postoperatively [56, 57].

22.10.3.2 Accelerated Rehabilitation Protocol

An accelerated rehabilitation program after meniscus repair includes immediate full weight-bearing as tolerated. Patients are allowed to actively move their knees within the pain-free ROM immediately after surgery. Progressive early motion is permitted as the swelling decreases. Forced knee flexion should be avoided, especially if effusion or soft-tissue swelling is present. Loaded knee flexion should not exceed 90° for the first 6 weeks. Unloaded ROM from 0° to 90° is allowed from the first postoperative day, with flexion advanced to 120° by the third to fourth week. Full knee flexion is permitted after 6 weeks. Caution is used to avoid hyperextension in individuals who have had anterior-horn meniscus repairs.

OKC strengthening exercises are allowed after the first postoperative week and CKC strengthening exercises from the fifth postoperative week. Low-resistance stationary cycling and swimming are allowed at 6 weeks. When effusion is absent, full extension, full flexion, and straight-ahead jogging are permitted 4–5 months postsurgery. Patients are allowed to return to pivoting sports when there is no pain, swelling, or reduced motion despite running and agility training (5–7 months postsurgery) [58].

Based on clinical, MRI, and arthroscopic evaluations, several authors reported an 80 % success rate after an aggressive rehabilitation program [59]. These results are consistent with those reported after nonaggressive rehabilitation. Although these studies have documented an equal success rate, no randomized control trials have been performed to compare these two rehabilitation protocols.

22.10.3.3 Individualized Rehabilitation Protocol

We suggest, together with other authors [60], to avoid using a "cookbook" (conventional or accelerated) protocol but rather recommend an individualized program based on the patient's intrinsic key factors influencing the healing of the meniscus (vascular supply, suture fixation, anatomical site of the tear, tear size and type, and other intra-articular disorders).

The therapist needs to thoroughly evaluate the patient to implement the appropriate protocol. The individualized program will be a mixture of elements from the conventional program and the accelerated program, depending on the patient's intrinsic risk factors. If more than two risk factors are present (e.g., large tear of the medial meniscus), the individualized program will be similar to the conventional program. In contrast, if less than two risk factors are present, the individualized program will largely correspond to the accelerated program. The initial goal of this individualized program is to prevent excessive weight-bearing forces. The limitation is designed to control high compressive and shear forces that could disrupt the healing meniscus repair. The supervised physical therapy program is supplemented with home exercises performed on a daily basis. Patients are warned that an early return to strenuous activities, including impact loading, jogging, deep knee flexion, or pivoting, carries a definite risk of a repeat meniscus tear. This is particularly true in the first 4–6 months postoperatively, where full flexion or deep-squatting activities may disrupt the healing repair sites.

Conclusion

Saving the meniscus, especially in young patients, to decrease the risk of secondary osteoarthritis is challenging. Meniscus repair techniques are well established and allow surgeons to address tears of different complexity and location. There exists no universal technique, but rather several techniques which are adapted to different indications.

Even if all-inside fourth-generation devices are now the gold standard in the majority of cases, inside–out, outside–in, and even open techniques are still indicated in selected cases. The ultimate goal is to achieve a strong repair.

In the future, the next step will be biological meniscus repair by introducing factors such as stem cells, growth factors, or cytokines at the site of the repair to enhance healing. These can be regarded as biological mediators, which regulate key processes in tissue repair (cell proliferation, directed cell migration, cell differentiation, and extracellular matrix synthesis).

References

1. Arnoczky SP, McDevitt CA (2000) The meniscus: structure, function, repair and replacement. In: Buckwalter JA, Einhorn TA, Simon SR (eds) Orthopaedic basic science. American Academy of Orthopaedic Surgeons, Rosemont

2. Volesky M, Johnson DH (2006) The meniscus. In: Johnson DH, Pedowitz RA (eds) Practical orthopaedic sports medicine and arthroscopy. Lippincott Williams & Wilkins, Philadelphia
3. Ahmed AM, Burke DL (1983) In-vitro measurement of static pressure distribution in synovial joints—part I: tibial surface of the knee. J Biomech Eng 105:216–225
4. Fukubayashi T, Kurosawa H (1980) The contact area and pressure distribution pattern of the knee. A study of normal and osteoarthrotic knee joints. Acta Orthop Scand 51:871–879
5. Kettelkamp DB, Jacobs AW (1972) Tibiofemoral contact area—determination and implications. J Bone Joint Surg Am 54:349–356
6. Kurosawa H, Fukubayashi T, Nakajima H (1980) Load-bearing mode of the knee joint: physical behavior of the knee joint with or with- out menisci. Clin Orthop Relat Res 149:283–290
7. Verma NN, Kolb E, Cole BJ et al (2008) The effects of medial meniscal transplantation techniques on intra-articular contact pres- sures. J Knee Surg 21:20–26
8. Scheller G, Sobau C, Bulow JU (2001) Arthroscopic partial lateral meniscectomy in an otherwise normal knee: clinical, functional, and radiographic results of a long-term follow-up study. Arthroscopy 17:946–952
9. Rockborn P, Messner K (2000) Long-term results of meniscus repair and meniscectomy: a 13-year functional and radiographic follow- up study. Knee Surg Sports Traumatol Arthrosc 8:2–10
10. Noyes FR, Bassett RW, Grood ES, Butler DL (1980) Arthroscopy in acute traumatic hemarthrosis of the knee. Incidence of anterior cruciate tears and other injuries. J Bone Joint Surg Am 62:687–695, 757
11. Fox MG (2007) MR imaging of the meniscus: review, current trends, and clinical implications. Radiol Clin North Am 45:1033–1053, vii
12. Scott GA, Jolly BL, Henning CE (1986) Combined posterior incision and arthroscopic intra-articular repair of the meniscus: an examination of factors affecting healing. J Bone Joint Surg Am 68:847–861
13. Miller RH III (2003) Knee injuries. In: Canale ST (ed) Campbell's operative orthopaedics. Mosby Elsevier, St. Louis
14. McMurray T (1942) The semilunar cartilages. Br J Surg 29:407–414
15. Apley A (1947) The diagnosis of meniscus injuries. J Bone Joint Surg 29:78–84
16. Terry GC, Tagert BE, Young MJ (1995) Reliability of the clinical assessment in predicting the cause of internal derangements of the knee. Arthroscopy 11: 568–576
17. Manco LG, Berlow ME (1989) Meniscus tears–comparison of arthrography, CT, and MRI. Crit Rev Diagn Imaging 29:151–179
18. Manco LG, Kavanaugh JH, Fay JJ et al (1986) Meniscus tears of the knee: prospective evaluation with CT. Radiology 159:147–151
19. Vande Berg BC, Lecouvet FE, Poilvache P et al (2000) Dual- detector spiral CT arthrography of the knee: accuracy for detection of meniscal abnormalities and unstable meniscus tears. Radiology 216:851–857
20. White LM, Schweitzer ME, Weishaupt D et al (2002) Diagnosis of recurrent meniscus tears: prospective evaluation of conventional MR imaging, indirect MR arthrography, and direct MR arthrography. Radiology 222:421–429
21. DeHaven KE (1990) Decision-making factors in the treatment of meniscus lesions. Clin Orthop Relat Res 252:49–54
22. Verdonk R, Almqvist FA (2005) Lésions traumatiques des ménisques du genou. In: EMC appareil locomoteur. Elsevier, Paris 14-084-A-10, 1–16
23. Casscells SW (1980) The place of arthroscopy in the diagnosis and treatment of internal derangement of the knee: an analysis of 1000 cases. Clin Orthop Relat Res 151:135–142
24. Weiss CB, Lundberg M, Hamberg P et al (1989) Non-operative treatment of meniscus tears. J Bone Joint Surg 71A:811–822
25. Roos H, Lauren M, Adalberth T et al (1998) Knee osteoarthritis after meniscectomy: prevalence of radiographic changes after twenty-one years, compared with matched controls. Arthritis Rheum 41:687–693
26. Gillquist J, Hamberg P, Lysholm J (1982) Endoscopic partial and total meniscectomy. A comparative study with a short- term follow-up. Acta Orthop Scand 53:975–979
27. Northmore-Ball MD, Dandy DJ (1982) Long-term results of arthroscopic partial meniscectomy. Clin Orthop Relat Res 167:34–42
28. Howell JR, Handoll HH. Surgical treatment for meniscal injuries of the knee in adults. Cochrane Database Syst Rev. 2000;(2):CD001353
29. Tapper EM, Hoover NW (1969) Late results after meniscectomy. J Bone Joint Surg 51A:517–526
30. Newman AP, Anderson DR, Daniels AU et al (1989) Mechanics of the healed meniscus in a canine model. Am J Sports Med 17:164–175
31. Cannon WD Jr, Vittori JM (1992) The incidence of healing in arthroscopic meniscus repairs in anterior cruciate ligament-reconstructed knees versus stable knees. Am J Sports Med 20:176–181
32. Boyd KT, Myers PT (2003) Meniscus preservation; rationale, repair techniques and results. Knee 10:1–11
33. Kurosawa H, Fukubayashi T, Nakajima H (1980) Load- bearing mode of the knee joint: physical behavior of the knee joint with or without menisci. Clin Orthop 149:283–290
34. McDermott ID, Richards SW, Hallam P, Tavares S, Lavelle JR, Amis AA (2003) A biomechanical study of four different meniscus repair systems, comparing pull-out strengths and gapping under cyclic loading. Knee Surg Sports Traumatol Arthrosc 11:23–29
35. Annandale T (1885) An operation for displaced semilunar cartilage. Br Med J 1:779
36. Barber FA, McGarry JE (2007) Meniscus repair techniques. Sports Med Arthrosc 15:199–207
37. Arnoczky SP, Warren RF (1982) Microvasculature of the human meniscus. Am J Sports Med 10:90–95

38. DeHaven KE, Black K, Griffiths HJ (1989) Open meniscus repair. Technique and two to nine year results. Am J Sports Med 17:788–795
39. Pujol N, Panarella L, Selmi TAS, Neyret P, Fithian D, Beaufils P (2008) Meniscal healing after meniscus repair. A CT arthrography assessment. Am J Sports Med 36:1489–1495
40. Warren RF (1985) Arthroscopic meniscus repair. Arthroscopy 1:170–172
41. Barber FA, Herbert MA (2000) Meniscus repair devices. Arthroscopy 16:613–618
42. Durand A, Richards CL, Malouin F et al (1991) Strength recovery and muscle activation of the extensor and flexor muscles after arthroscopic meniscectomy. Clin Orthop Rel Res 262:210–226
43. Moffet H, Richards CL, Malouin F et al (1994) Early and intensive physiotherapy accelerates recovery post-arthroscopic meniscectomy: results of a randomized controlled study. Arch Phys Med Rehab 75:415–426
44. Durand A, Richards CL, Malouin F et al (1993) Motor recovery after arthroscopic partial meniscectomy: analysis of gait and the ascent and descent of stairs. J Bone Joint Surg 75:202–214
45. Brindle T, Nyland J, Johnson L (2001) The meniscus: review of basic principles with application to surgery and rehabilitation. J Athl Train 36(2):160–169
46. Stokes M, Young A (1984) The contribution of reflex inhibition to arthrogenous muscle weakness. Clin Sci 67:7–14
47. Palmieri-Smith RM, Kreinbrink J, Ashton-Miller JA et al (2007) Quadriceps inhibition induced by an experimental knee joint effusion affects knee joint mechanics during a single-legged drop landing. Am J Sports Med 35:1269–1275
48. Stpierre DMM (1995) Rehabilitation following arthroscopic meniscectomy. Sports Med 20(5):338–347
49. Roeddecker K, Muennisch U, Nagelschmidt M (1994) Arthroscopic meniscus repair evaluated by second-look arthroscopy. J Surg Res 56:20–27
50. Arnoczky SP, Warren RF (1983) The microvasculature of the meniscus and its response to injury. An experimental study in the dog. Am J Sports Med 11:131–141
51. Dowdy PA, Miniaci A, Arnoczky SP (1995) The effect of cast immobilization on meniscal healing. An experimental study in the dog. Am J Sports Med 23:721–728
52. Rubman MH, Noyes FR, Barber Westin SD (1998) Arthroscopic repair of meniscus tears that extend into the avascular zone. A review of 198 single and complex tears. Am J Sports Med 26:87–95
53. Staerke C, Bochwitz C, Groebel KH (2004) The effect of meniscus compression on the biomechanical properties of repaired meniscal lesions. Arch Orthop Trauma Surg 124:221–225
54. Guisasola I, Vaquero J, Forriol F (2002) Knee immobilization on meniscal healing after suture: an experimental study in sheep. Clin Orthop Relat Res 395: 227–233
55. Tuckman DV, Bravman JT, Lee SS et al (2006) Outcomes of meniscus repair. Minimum 2-year follow up. Bull Hosp Joint Dis 63(3–4):100–104
56. Horibe S, Shino K, Nakata K et al (1995) Second-look arthroscopy after meniscus repair. J Bone Joint Surg Br 77:245–249
57. Tenuta JJ, Arciero RA (1994) Arthroscopic evaluation of meniscus repairs factors that effect healing. Am J Sports Med 22:797–802
58. Mariani PP, Santori N, Adriani E et al (1996) Accelerated rehabilitation after arthroscopic meniscus repair: a clinical and magnetic resonance imaging evaluation. Arthroscopy 12:680–688
59. Barber FA, McGarry JE (2007) Meniscus repair techniques. Sports Med Arthrosc Rev 15:4
60. Heckmann TP, Barber-Westin SD, Noyes FR (2006) Meniscus repair and transplantation: indications, techniques, rehabilitation, and clinical outcome. J Orthop Sports Phys Ther 36(10):795–814
61. DeHaven KE (1990) Decision-making features in the treatment of meniscal lesions. Clin Orthop 252: 49–54

Anterior Knee Pain in Football

23

Paulo Renato Fernandes Saggin and David Dejour

23.1 Introduction

Anterior knee pain (AKP) is a common complaint of football players. Although many may still play while affected, it can pose significant disability and demand temporary withdrawal from sport. The complex interplay of factors involved in its genesis, the poorly understood mechanism of pain generation, and the heterogeneous literature regarding this disorder create several obstacles to the adequate management of this frequent and poorly known pathology. A pragmatic approach is therefore essential to manage patients with anterior knee pain. For the purpose this chapter, anterior knee pain and patellofemoral pain syndrome are considered synonyms, and alternative diagnosis creating pain around the anterior aspect of the knee are excluded (Table 23.1).

P.R.F. Saggin, MD (✉)
Instituto de Ortopedia e Traumatologia de Passo Fundo, Rua Uruguai 2050, 99010-111 Passo Fundo, RS, Brazil
e-mail: paulosaggin@yahoo.com.br, prsaggin@gmail.com

D. Dejour, MD
Lyon-Ortho-Clinic; Clinique de la Sauvegarde, 8 Avenue Ben Gourion, 69009 Lyon, France
e-mail: corolyon@wanadoo.fr

23.2 Etiology

The variable relationship between abnormality and pain originates most of the controversy regarding AKP. Patellofemoral chondral pathology

Table 23.1 Possible causes of anterior knee pain

Articular cartilage injury
Hoffa's disease
Neuromas
Patellar instability/subluxation
Patellofemoral arthritis
Plica synovialis
Quadriceps tendinopathy
Sinding-Larsen-Johansson syndrome
Bone tumors
Iliotibial (IT) band syndrome
Osgood-Schlatter disease
Patellar stress fracture
Patellofemoral pain syndrome
Prepatellar bursitis
Referred pain from lumbar spine or hip joint pathology
Symptomatic bipartite patella
Chondromalacia patellae
Loose bodies
Osteochondritis dissecans
Patellar tendinopathy
Pes anserine bursitis
Previous surgery
Saphenous neuritis

Several are the pathologies that can present with anterior knee pain (Adapted from: Waryasz and McDermott [1])

P. Volpi (ed.), *Football Traumatology: New Trends*, DOI 10.1007/978-3-319-18245-2_23

(chondromalacia or chondropathy) and malalignment may cause pain, but asymptomatic individuals bearing these conditions are frequent. On the other side, individuals with a normal anatomy of their knees may complain of AKP. From this perspective it becomes clear that some individuals may suffer from pain that in fact does not originate from the evident abnormalities the orthopedic surgeon and the sports medicine specialist may diagnose on a first evaluation [2–4]. This is especially important because effective treatment must address the true causes of pain and not the confounding findings.

Pain may arise from several mechanisms. Recently, the soft tissues around the knee have gained popularity as possible causes of pain, since histological studies have demonstrated abnormalities that could possibly be the origin of pain. This is particularly true when considering the lateral retinaculum, where fibrosis, demyelination, and tissular neuromas have been found [5, 6]. Other soft tissue potential sources of pain are the medial retinaculum, the infrapatellar fat pad, and the synovium.

Cartilage damage alone cannot cause pain since cartilage is aneural [4]. Chondral pathology, however, may contribute to pain. Despite the evidence showing that advanced chondral damage may exist in asymptomatic individuals, the lack of cartilage and its protective effect over the bone favors the subchondral bone overload, which is richly innervated and thus a possible cause of pain. Also, synovitis may arise from the cartilage debris.

The patellofemoral articulation (as any other articulation) may be subjected to a variable range of load while keeping its homeostasis. Particularly in high-demand sports like football, excessive loading of the joint may alone be responsible for homeostasis loss, generating inflammation and nociceptive output (pain). These overuse/overload injuries are common when increasing frequency or intensity of sports. Most of the time, the history is clear, and so the overuse diagnosis is straightforward. Other times, however, the training abuses are not elicited, and the diagnosis becomes cloudy.

Skeletal anatomy and muscular balance determine patellar tracking and joint mechanics. From this standpoint, it becomes clear that the interplay of a lot of factors can potentially lead to abnormal loading of the patellofemoral joint even in the absence of excessive exercise practice. Most of the time, these *small abnormalities* do not reach a pathological threshold to be diagnosed on clinical examination and imaging or even to be considered significantly different from the population average. This is particularly true when we consider the wide range of anatomical patterns that are considered normal regarding osseous anatomy and becomes even more complicated when we add to this formula the multitude of muscular imbalance possibilities (and considering that there is still a lot to discover). From a pragmatic standpoint, however, we must consider what has already been studied and so far established.

Recently, the dynamic valgus theory has gained popularity. It advocates that the cause for maltracking of the patella in some patients with AKP may not be part of a structural fault but rather a dynamic or functional malalignment. Potential risk factors involved in the genesis of dynamic valgus include hip weakness (abductors and external rotators), iliotibial band tightness, excessive quadriceps (Q) angle, abnormal *vastus medialis obliquus/vastus lateralis* reflex timing, and rear-foot eversion (causing compensatory tibial and femoral internal rotation). Other risk factors involved in the genesis of anterior knee pain include weakness in functional testing; gastrocnemius, hamstring, or quadriceps tightness; generalized ligamentous laxity; deficient hamstring or quadriceps strength; and patellar compression or tilting [1] (Fig. 23.1).

When we consider gross deviations from normal as pathological, we can refer to them as structural abnormalities. Structural abnormalities may contribute to the overload of the PF joint. Torsional abnormalities and elevated tibial tubercle – trochlear groove distance (TT-TG) – increase the lateralizing vector acting on the patella during flexion, increasing the PF reaction force on the lateral facet and allowing symptomatic overload to become apparent. Simultaneously, insufficient load of the medial facet may generate loss of homeostasis and equally provoke pain.

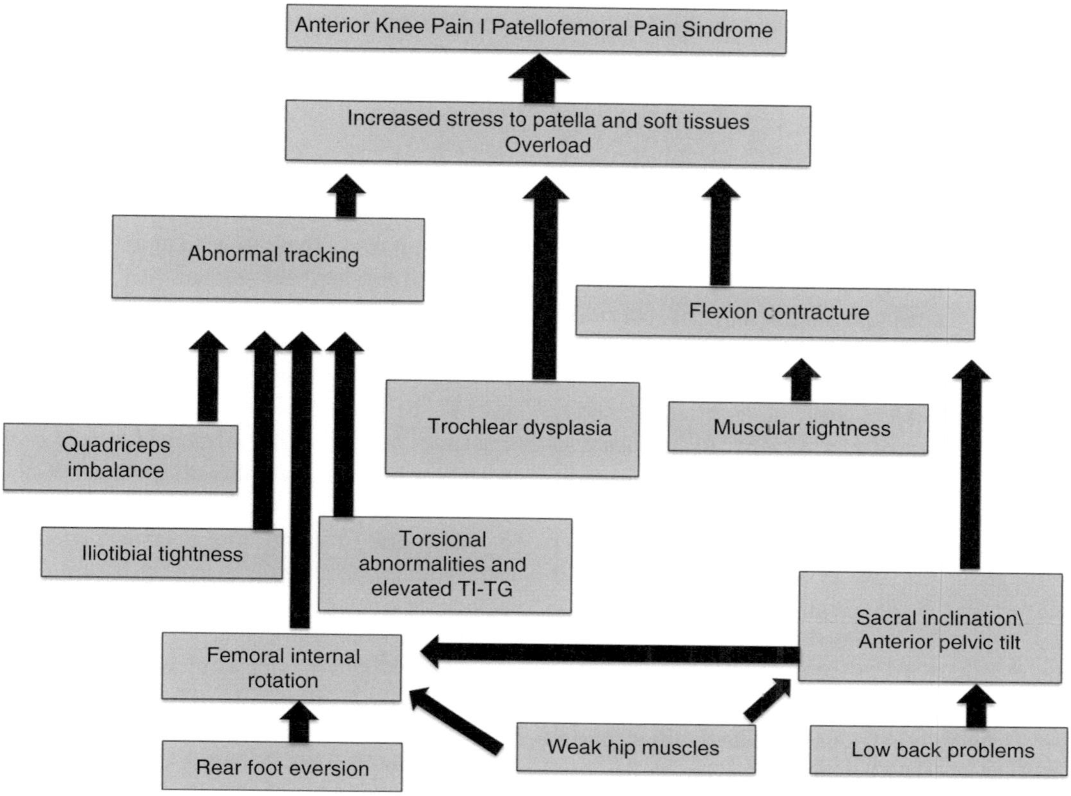

Fig. 23.1 Proposed mechanisms of anterior knee pain generation (Adapted from: Petersen et al. [7])

Trochlear dysplasia is another potential contributor to the genesis of anterior knee pain. Keser et al. [8] have demonstrated a considerable higher prevalence of trochlear dysplasia in AKP patients compared to controls (16.5 % vs. 2.7 %). In their study, trochlear dysplasia was assessed with the lateral trochlear inclination angle (LTI) on magnetic resonance. LTI was investigated by Carrilon et al. [9], calculated by means of a line tangential to the subchondral bone of the posterior aspect of the two femoral condyles crossed with a line tangential to the subchondral bone of the lateral trochlear facet. Choosing 11° as the threshold value for LTI, results were excellent in identifying trochlear dysplasia (considered present if LTI was equal or below 11°) with sensitivity of 93 %, specificity of 87 %, and accuracy of 90 %.

In trochlear dysplasia the position of the trochlear sulcus is prominent in relation to the anterior femoral cortex. In a study performed by Dejour et al. [10], the trochlear sulcus in normal knees was at a mean distance of 0.8 mm posterior to a line projected from the anterior femoral cortex, and in knees with dysplastic trochlea, its mean position was 3.2 mm forward this same line. This increases the contact force between the patella and the trochlea (anti-Maquet effect) possibly contributing to pain generation.

23.3 History and Clinical Examination

In AKP, pain is usually anterior, not well localized, and diffuse. It may also be referred to the medial retinaculum or to the lateral retinaculum. Sometimes the pain is located below the patella as a bar. Posterior knee pain, although rare, may also be possible, especially if an articular effusion is present. Usually, the pain is worse during or after activities that cause overload, such as those that demand jumping, running, or vigorous quadriceps contraction. Complaints of instability may occur due to quadriceps inhibition (reflex) as a result of pain but without loss of contact of the articulating surfaces.

Adequate interviewing of the athlete often brings to light the possible factors leading to the overload. Appearance of pain after training modifications is strongly suggestive of overload. Coach replacement and progression of category could indirectly suggest that overload is present. The time from the onset of pain and previous responses to exercise cessation also contribute to the overload diagnosis.

Clinical examination is often unspecific. Tenderness over the medial and lateral retinacula is frequent. Compression tests (e.g., grind test and patellar engagement sign, Zohlen test) lack specificity. Since most of the time structural abnormalities are absent, physical examination is unnoteworthy. Adequate examination must search for different causes of pain and potential contributors to pain generation.

Crepitation usually correlates with chondral pathology but is nonspecific. Effusion must be an alert signal for associated intra-articular pathology, but is similarly nonspecific. They must alert for possible chondral damage that usually correlates with overuse and structural abnormalities (in contrast to simple patellar pain in low-demand adolescents). Patellar tilt over 10°, when present, is clinically evident on palpation [11] and rarely is found alone, indicating that malalignment and trochlear dysplasia may be associated. Hypermobility is usually evaluated with the glide test. It can possibly lead to erratic tracking causing overload. Patellar and quadriceps tendon palpation is fairly reliable to exclude tendonitis (tendinopathy) and must be indispensable.

Abnormalities that increase the valgus vector acting on the patella, like increased Q angle and malalignment (increased femoral anteversion and increased tibial external rotation), may be evident already in the static inspection, becoming worse when the patient is asked to walk (dynamic inspection). The torsional "profile" of the patient estimated on the static clinical examination is clinically apparent during walking as the patient develops intoeing or the patellae point inward.

The feet must be assessed during walking and from behind the patient. Hyper-pronation can potentially cause excessive internal rotation of the tibia and femur, what is roughly equivalent to lateralizing the patella. The functional "malalignment" or dynamic valgus can be visualized clinically with one-legged squats (Fig. 23.2). Crossley et al. [12] have demonstrated that a valgus collapse of the knee joint during one-legged squat indicates weakness of the hip abductors.

Tightness of the posterior and anterior muscular chains must be assessed as it increases the patellofemoral reaction force. Hamstrings are tested with the patient supine and the opposite leg extended and flat over the table. The hip is flexed 90° and the knee is then extended as far as possible. The popliteal angle is observed and compared to the opposite side. The quadriceps is tested with the patient prone, and in most patients the heels should touch the buttocks. The iliotibial band is tested with the Ober test – with the patient in lateral decubitus position (the side to be tested up), the hip is extended and abducted, and the knee is extended. From this position, the thigh is released and allowed to adduct. Most patients will be able to touch the exam table with the medial aspect of the knee.

The spine and the pelvis (and therefore the sacroiliac articulation) must be assessed thoroughly. Stiffness of this "system" avoids adequate stretching of the quadriceps (remember the *rectus femoris* origins from the pelvis). Irreducible lordosis is an indicator of anterior pelvic tilt and its commonly associated features (weak abdominals, weak glutes and hamstrings, and tight hip flexors). Anterior pelvic tilt may cause femoral internal rotation (and relative lateralization of the patella) due to changes in acetabular orientation. Static inspection begins with the patient sited in front of the physician (thoracic abnormal kyphosis is already apparent) and continues when the patient is asked to stand up (pelvic anterior tilt and lumbar hyperlordosis can be evaluated from

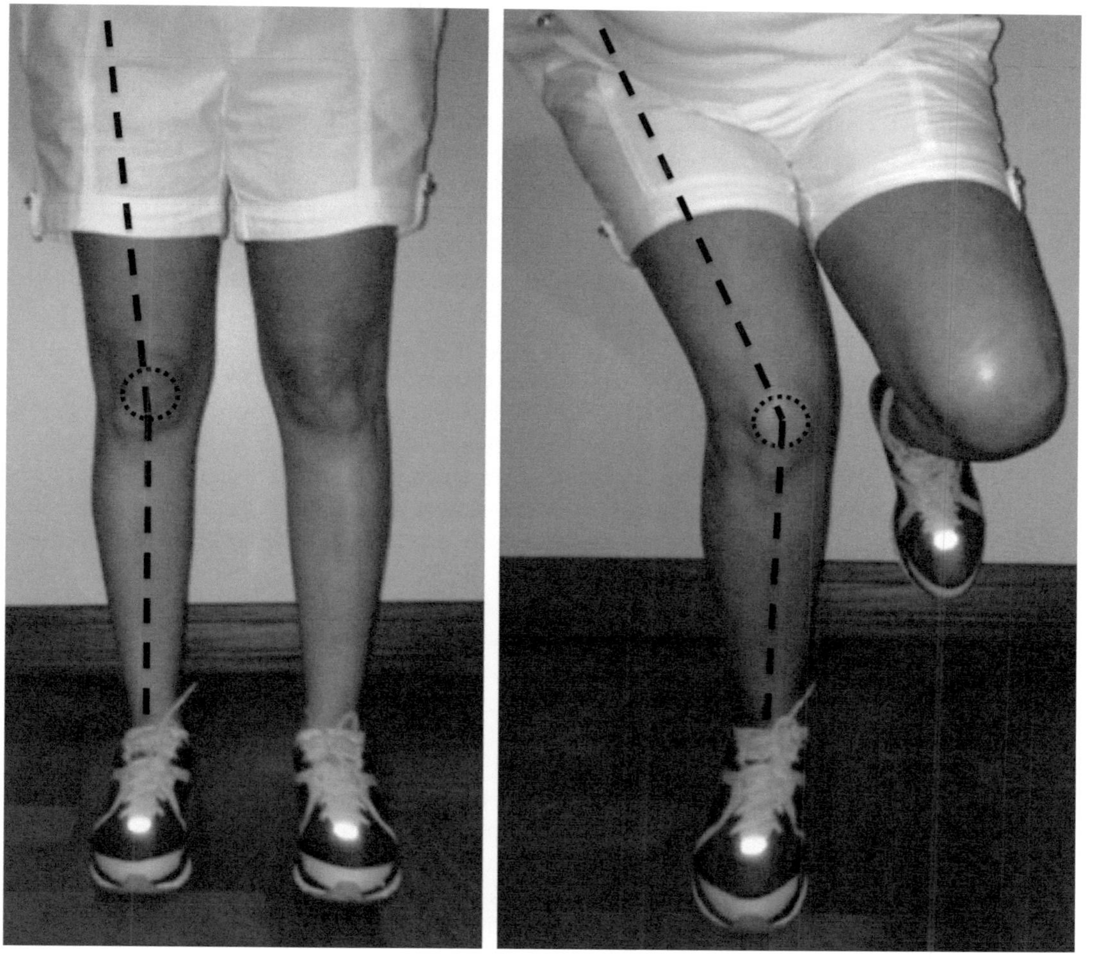

Fig. 23.2 Apparently well-aligned limbs can demonstrate dynamic valgus when the patient is asked to perform a single leg squat

the side of the patient). A simple test may be performed asking the patient to stand with the back against the wall. He/she must be able to touch the wall with his heels, the back of the knees, the buttocks, and his back (lumbar region) and shoulders. Inability to do so and stand flat against the wall reflects stiffness and muscular imbalance (Fig. 23.3).

In summary, knee biomechanics is complex and exceeds local anatomical relations. The patella is a sesamoid bone inserted in a biarticular muscle which function relies in the interplay of several factors. Failure to evaluate the individual thoroughly avoids an accurate diagnosis.

23.4 Imaging

Pain is subjective, but imaging modalities are fundamental for identifying the associated structural abnormalities and quantifying them and for excluding alternative causes of pain.

Ultrasound is commonly prescribed but is dependent on the observer experience, and its usefulness is limited to the superficial soft tissues evaluation (e.g., tendinopathy evaluation and differential diagnosis). CT, arthro-CT, and MRI have increasing abilities to image intra-articular structures and grow in importance to exclude alternative causes of pain.

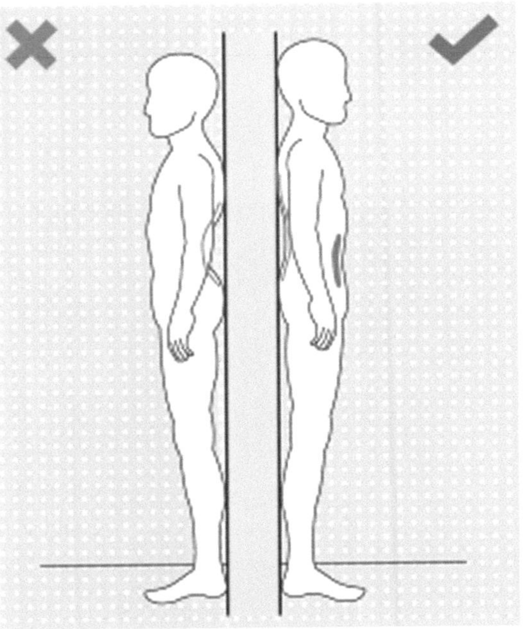

Fig. 23.3 Spine and pelvis flexibility can be evaluated with this simple test – the patient is asked to stand flat against the wall. Inability to do so reflects imbalance or stiffness of this "system"

Abnormal tilt, increased TA-GT, patella alta, and other abnormal tracking measurements may be present. Objective patellar instability (previous dislocations) must be ruled out.

X-ray lateral views are the key to the diagnosis of the patella alta. Several methods of measurement (and diagnosis) have been described. Patellar height can also be reliably measured on MRI. CT and MRI axial views provide a clue to patella alta diagnosis when the patella is not found facing the upper part of the trochlea.

TT-TG is a simple way to measure the valgus (lateralizing) forces acting on the patella. TT-TG is the distance from the bottom of the most proximal part of the trochlear groove to the proximal part of the tibial tubercle, measured with two CT superimposed cuts and expressed in millimeters.

Another important contribution of CT produced by the superimposition of images is the assessment of torsional deformities, such as femoral anteversion and external tibial torsion [10].

Patellar tilt and subluxation refer to the abnormal position of the patella in relation to the trochlear groove. While tilt means increased lateral inclination of the transverse diameter of the patella, subluxation refers primarily to abnormal mediolateral displacement of the patella in relation to the trochlea. Tilt seems to be the result of a complex interplay of factors, including trochlear and patellar shape and congruence, medial restraint insufficiency, and lateral retinacular tightness. Several methods of evaluating tilt and subluxation have been described for axial views, which are the gold standard for its evaluation.

Standard lateral x-ray films are the key to trochlear dysplasia diagnosis (strict lateral views, with perfect superimposition of the posterior medial and lateral femoral condyles). The crossing sign is typically found in this projection and represents the point where the trochlea becomes flat (the bottom of the groove reaches the height of the facets). Additional findings include the double-contour sign and the supratrochlear spur [13, 14]. Axial x-ray views performed in 45° of knee flexion allow the measurement of the sulcus angle [15]. CT and MRI have the ability to image the entire trochlea in sequential cuts, from its most proximal part until its distal end. This allows better visualization of the dysplastic upper part. Frequently, dysplasia found in these modalities is missed on x-ray axial views.

Despite the multitude of possible associated features, imaging is frequently normal. Several authors have shown that x-rays are not useful for AKP diagnosis, and the alignment parameters used for instability are within normal values in many AKP patients. MRI findings also are not useful in differentiating AKP patients from a control group [16]. Thus, imaging is complimentary to the physical examination but cannot predict the onset of pain neither can it quantify the contribution of the evidenced abnormality to the final pain status.

Bone scans may provide some functional information. Scintigraphy has the ability to demonstrate metabolic changes otherwise not visualized in other imaging modalities, but its contribution to treatment or diagnosis remains to be established. Dye and Boll [17] noted that about one-half of patients with patellofemoral pain demonstrated increased patellar uptake in technetium 99 m methylene diphosphonate scintigraphy, compared with only 4 % of the control subjects. The increased osseous metabolic activity of the patella, detected by the bone scan, was biopsy proven to represent increased remodeling activity of bone compared with controls. When these patients underwent follow-up imaging, it was noted that many who experienced resolution of painful symptoms also demonstrated resolution of the bone scan to normal activity, representing restoration of osseous homeostasis [18]. Bone SPECT/CT can similarly be employed and provide equivalent information [19]. These imaging modalities could be used to follow up patients after unloading procedures or devices.

23.5 Treatment Strategy

Conservative treatment is always the first line. In the short term, a period of rest and adequate pain control are usually sufficient to alleviate symptoms. The importance of rest or activity decrease in the initial phase cannot be overemphasized, because it reduces load and allows homeostasis to be reestablished. The absence of evident tissue damage on the imaging evaluation usually hinders the physician from prescribing sports suspension, delaying complete recovery and, at times, worsening the symptoms. Pain must not be withstood, but rather avoided. The strategy of *no pain, no gain* must be abandoned.

Pharmacological treatment is aimed to reduce pain. With this purpose, nonsteroidal anti-inflammatory drugs and weak analgesics can be employed. Ice may contribute to pain reduction during pain exacerbations.

Flexibility training or muscular tightness should always be part of a successful AKP treatment strategy. Stretching exercises can be initiated in the initial phase and must be maintained during the late and rehabilitation phases. Stretching exercises should aim loosening potentially tight anatomical structures that could predispose to AKP. Fully extending the knee against tight hamstrings, iliotibial band, or gastrocnemius muscles can increase the patellofemoral joint reaction force and precipitate pain [20]. Similarly tight quadriceps may lead to the same consequences in deep flexion. Patients must be informed that flexibility is a goal to be chased for lifetime.

After the pain subsides, and for the long term, physical therapy becomes the mainstay of treatment. Quadriceps and hip strengthening are the most important goals to be achieved, and exercises comprising them can be prescribed almost universally to patients, except for those who still suffer from pain.

Quadriceps weakness, selective *vastus medialis obliquus* (VMO) weakness and altered activation pattern of VMO relative to *vastus lateralis* have been associated with AKP development. Proximal musculature (core musculature) imbalance and weakness also have been associated with AKP. Hip weakness and adduction and greater femoral internal rotation have been shown in AKP patients [21, 22]. These could theoretically lead to overload of the lateral PF joint, since this time the trochlear sulcus is medialized under the patella. Hip extensors are responsible for at least 25 % of impact during landing [23]. Therefore, strengthening of hip external rotators and abductors could correct this and could be further enhanced with strengthening of hip flexors and extensors [21, 24].

The best way to achieve quadriceps strengthening nowadays is still subject of controversy. Both open and closed kinetic chain exercises apparently can be employed with success, but from a logical standpoint, these exercises must be performed in manners that do not impose excessive load to the patellofemoral joint. To achieve this purpose, closed kinetic chain exercises must be performed from knee extension to 45° of flexion, while open kinetic chain exercises must be performed from 90° to 45° of flexion [22, 23, 25]. Exercises must be performed without pain, and the patient must remain pain-free in the next hours (many times pain arises after the exercise cessation due to a cytokine flare). Preferential activation of the *vastus medialis obliquus* during quadriceps strengthening would be of particular importance to treatment, but its feasibility remains a topic of debate.

Hip strengthening is targeted preferentially to abductors and external rotators, but the addition of hip flexors and extensors must be considered. Most of the data concerning strengthening of the proximal musculature is still experimental and inconclusive, but it leads us toward an important direction. Roughly, it can be proposed that strengthening can restore more normal kinematics by avoiding non-physiological loading to occur as a result of abnormal kinematics or insufficient musculature. Although more conclusive data is missing, the prescription of strengthening exercises must not neglect the hip musculature.

Recently, more attention has been paid to the core musculature. Weakness of the abdominals, glutes, and back musculature can contribute to AKP, so these groups must not be neglected during rehabilitation. Patients with weakness in these muscles are grossly defined as having "bad posture." In this setting, some non-specialized works like *Pilates* could be beneficial.

Knee or patella orthotics may correct abnormal tracking and unload compromised areas, but interestingly, they may also provide alternative afferent stimuli, *competing* with the nociceptive information, thus alleviating pain and allowing an exercise program to be developed or initiated. Its efficacy is still controversial, but despite the lack of consensus, adverse events from its use are improbable, and short-term usage remains an option for pain control [26, 27].

Foot orthotics are another commonly suggested option for anterior knee pain control, but recommendations concerning football players and their specific footwear are difficult to make. Since the foot orthotics can generate adverse events like pain around the ankle, it is the authors' opinion that their use should be restricted to those with evidence of pathology/abnormality involving the feet or ankles. Again, the importance of proper physical examination cannot be overemphasized.

Failure of initial conservative management is common due to the lack of validated standardized treatment protocols and the multitude of possible approaches. The physician should be aware of the employed exercise regimens before the efficacy of treatment is questioned. Patient adherence is another crucial factor to treatment success. Periodical evaluations therefore are essential before complete pain relief is achieved. Persistence is an indispensable quality to the team assisting the patient, and several trials of conservative management are the rule before a failure can be defined.

Surgery indications for patients complaining exclusively of pain are exceptions and must be made for correctable (treatable at least) structural abnormalities which cause pain with a reasonable amount of probability. Surgical procedures employed for anterior knee pain usually are tibial tubercle transfers in patients with evidence of malalignment and cartilage procedures for those who suffer from chondral pathology. In the absence of clear indications, surgery may even aggravate the symptoms.

23.6 Return to Play

Anterior knee pain is normally treated conservatively, and sports can be resumed as soon as the pain subsides. Many patients continue to play despite the pain, but care should be taken to not aggravate the symptoms. It is logical to propose that sports return should be undertaken slowly and progressively and that when pain reappears during training, its intensity should be decreased.

References

1. Waryasz GR, McDermott AY (2008) Patellofemoral pain syndrome (PFPS): a systematic review of anatomy and potential risk factors. Dyn Med 7:9. doi:10.1186/1476-5918-7-9
2. Dye SF (2005) The pathophysiology of patellofemoral pain: a tissue homeostasis perspective. Clin Orthop 436:100–110
3. DeHaven KE, Collins HR (1975) Diagnosis of internal derangements of the knee. The role of arthroscopy. J Bone Joint Surg Am 57:802–810
4. Dye SF, Vaupel GL, Dye CC (1998) Conscious neurosensory mapping of the internal structures of the human knee without intraarticular anesthesia. Am J Sports Med 26:773–777
5. Sanchis-Alfonso V, Roselló-Sastre E (2003) Anterior knee pain in the young patient–what causes the pain? "Neural model". Acta Orthop Scand 74:697–703. doi:10.1080/00016470310018225
6. Fulkerson JP, Tennant R, Jaivin JS, Grunnet M (1985) Histologic evidence of retinacular nerve injury

associated with patellofemoral malalignment. Clin Orthop 197:196–205
7. Petersen W, Ellermann A, Gösele-Koppenburg A et al (2014) Patellofemoral pain syndrome. Knee Surg Sports Traumatol Arthrosc 22:2264–2274
8. Keser S, Savranlar A, Bayar A et al (2008) Is there a relationship between anterior knee pain and femoral trochlear dysplasia? Assessment of lateral trochlear inclination by magnetic resonance imaging. Knee Surg Sports Traumatol Arthrosc 16:911–915. doi:10.1007/s00167-008-0571-5
9. Carrillon Y, Abidi H, Dejour D et al (2000) Patellar instability: assessment on MR images by measuring the lateral trochlear inclination-initial experience. Radiology 216:582–585. doi:10.1148/radiology.216.2.r00au07582
10. Dejour H, Walch G, Nove-Josserand L, Guier C (1994) Factors of patellar instability: an anatomic radiographic study. Knee Surg Sports Traumatol Arthrosc Off J ESSKA 2:19–26
11. Grelsamer RP, Weinstein CH, Gould J, Dubey A (2008) Patellar tilt: the physical examination correlates with MR imaging. Knee 15:3–8. doi:10.1016/j.knee.2007.08.010
12. Crossley KM, Zhang W-J, Schache AG et al (2011) Performance on the single-leg squat task indicates hip abductor muscle function. Am J Sports Med 39:866–873. doi:10.1177/0363546510395456
13. Maldague B, Malghem J (1985) Significance of the radiograph of the knee profile in the detection of patellar instability. Preliminary report. Rev Chir Orthop Reparatrice Appar Mot 71(Suppl 2):5–13
14. Dejour D, Saggin P (2010) The sulcus deepening trochleoplasty-the Lyon's procedure. Int Orthop 34:311–316. doi:10.1007/s00264-009-0933-8
15. Merchant AC (1997) Femoral sulcus angle measurements. Am J Orthop Belle Mead NJ 26(820):822
16. MacIntyre NJ, Hill NA, Fellows RA et al (2006) Patellofemoral joint kinematics in individuals with and without patellofemoral pain syndrome. J Bone Joint Surg Am 88:2596–2605. doi:10.2106/JBJS.E.00674
17. Dye SF, Boll DA (1986) Radionuclide imaging of the patellofemoral joint in young adults with anterior knee pain. Orthop Clin North Am 17:249–262
18. Dye SF, Peartree PK (1989) Sequential radionuclide imaging of the patellofemoral joint in symptomatic young adults. Am J Sports Med 17:727–727. doi:10.1177/036354658901700598
19. Hirschmann MT, Schön S, Afifi FK et al (2013) Assessment of loading history of compartments in the knee using bone SPECT/CT: a study combining alignment and 99mTc-HDP tracer uptake/distribution patterns. J Orthop Res Off Publ Orthop Res Soc 31:268–274. doi:10.1002/jor.22206
20. Al-Hakim W, Jaiswal PK, Khan W, Johnstone D (2012) The non-operative treatment of anterior knee pain. Open OrthopJ6:320–326.doi:10.2174/1874325001206010320
21. Bolgla LA, Boling MC (2011) An update for the conservative management of patellofemoral pain syndrome: a systematic review of the literature from 2000 to 2010. Int J Sports Phys Ther 6:112–125
22. Werner S (2014) Anterior knee pain: an update of physical therapy. Knee Surg Sports Traumatol Arthrosc Off J ESSKA 22:2286–2294. doi:10.1007/s00167-014-3150-y
23. McCarthy MM, Strickland SM (2013) Patellofemoral pain: an update on diagnostic and treatment options. Curr Rev Musculoskelet Med 6:188–194. doi:10.1007/s12178-013-9159-x
24. Tyler TF, Nicholas SJ, Mullaney MJ, McHugh MP (2006) The role of hip muscle function in the treatment of patellofemoral pain syndrome. Am J Sports Med 34:630–636. doi:10.1177/0363546505281808
25. Witvrouw E, Werner S, Mikkelsen C et al (2005) Clinical classification of patellofemoral pain syndrome: guidelines for non-operative treatment. Knee Surg Sports Traumatol Arthrosc Off J ESSKA 13:122–130. doi:10.1007/s00167-004-0577-6
26. Barton C, Balachandar V, Lack S, Morrissey D (2014) Patellar taping for patellofemoral pain: a systematic review and meta-analysis to evaluate clinical outcomes and biomechanical mechanisms. Br J Sports Med 48:417–424. doi:10.1136/bjsports-2013-092437
27. Callaghan MJ, Selfe J (2012) Patellar taping for patellofemoral pain syndrome in adults. Cochrane Database Syst Rev 4, CD006717. doi:10.1002/14651858.CD006717.pub2

Patellar Instability in Football Players

24

Alexis Lion, Alexander Hoffmann, Caroline Mouton, Daniel Theisen, and Romain Seil

24.1 Injury Mechanism

Patellar instability, also known as patellofemoral or kneecap instability, is an abnormal movement of the patella in the patellofemoral groove of the femur [1]. It is characterized by patellar dislocation and subluxation [2] that mainly occur in the coronal plane [3]. The other types of patellar dislocation (i.e., the patella can dislocate superiorly and inferiorly or rotate about its longitudinal axis without vertical translation) are extremely rare [4].

Patellar dislocations can be induced by a direct contact on the medial side of the patella (contact between two players or with the ground) that knocks the patella out of the joint [5]. However, they are mainly caused by atraumatic events. In those cases, the injury is the consequence of the combination of intrinsic characteristics with an inciting event. Predisposing anatomical factors such as patella alta, abnormal bone morphology, increased Q-angle, genu valgum and/or genu recurvatum, ligament hypoplasia or hyperlaxity, muscular insufficiency, external tibial torsion, femoral anteversion, and subtalar joint pronation can indeed increase the risk for a patellar dislocation [6, 2]. Twisting or changing direction during sports, running on uneven surfaces, and walking on slippery or icy surfaces have been described as the most common inciting events [7]. Patellar dislocation is mainly induced by the internal rotation of the femur on the tibia combined with contraction of the quadriceps (acting as a lateralizing force), followed by a knee flexion movement combined with an external rotation of the femur (Fig. 24.1) [8–10]. This mechanism is comparable to the valgus collapse known to cause anterior cruciate ligament injuries. In football, this situation can be enhanced by the fixation of the foot on the field via the studs at the beginning of the injury mechanism.

A. Lion • C. Mouton • D. Theisen
Sports Medicine Research Laboratory,
Luxembourg Institute of Health,
76, Rue d'Eich, L-1460 Luxembourg, Luxembourg
e-mail: alexis.lion@lih.lu;
caroline.mouton@lih.lu;
daniel.theisen@lih.lu

A. Hoffmann
Department of Orthopaedic Surgery,
Centre Hospitalier de Luxembourg – Clinique d'Eich,
78, Rue d'Eich, L-1460 Luxembourg, Luxembourg
e-mail: hoffmann.alexander@chl.lu

R. Seil (✉)
Department of Orthopaedic Surgery,
Centre Hospitalier de Luxembourg – Clinique d'Eich
and Sports Medicine Research Laboratory,
Luxembourg Institute of Health,
78, Rue d'Eich, L-1460 Luxembourg, Luxembourg
e-mail: rseil@yahoo.com

24.2 Epidemiology/Etiology

Acute patellar dislocation represents 2–3 % of all knee injuries [11]. In the general population, the incidence rate represents up to 6.8 per 100,000

P. Volpi (ed.), *Football Traumatology: New Trends*, DOI 10.1007/978-3-319-18245-2_24

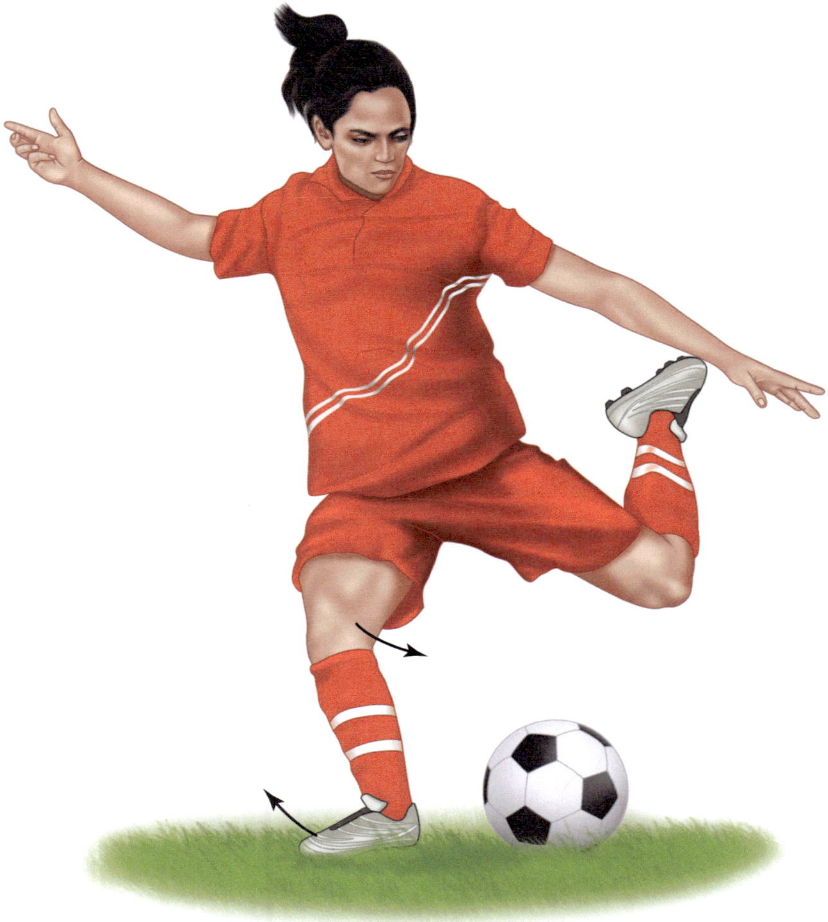

Fig. 24.1 Mechanism of noncontact injury

person-years [12–14] and varies from 2.3 to 242.0 per 100,000 person-years depending on the targeted population [12, 15–17, 13, 18, 14].

24.2.1 Influence of Exercise

The active population is more at risk to sustain a patellar dislocation (>69.0 per 100,000 person-years) [15, 18, 17]. Over half of the patellar dislocations indeed occur during athletic activities [12, 16, 17, 13, 14]. In football players, the incidence rate of patellar dislocation has not been specifically investigated. Football is however the most common sport with patellar dislocations (7.0 % of all patellar dislocations in Finland [19] and 6.9 % in the United States of America (USA) [13]) as it involves contacts and cutting situations.

24.2.2 Influence of Age

Patellar dislocations are more common in adolescents and young adults under 20 years old. Indeed, the incidence rate ranges from 11.2 to 107.0 per 100,000 person-years [12, 18, 16, 13, 15], highest incidence rate being observed between 9 and 15 years of age [16]. Between 15 and 19, the incidence rate is 25-fold higher compared to individuals aged between 50 and 54 years [13]. Patients with rare patellar dislocations, such as superior and inferior patellar dislocations, were more likely to be older than 38 and presented signs of knee arthritis [4], the degenerative knee being a risk factor for patellar dislocation [20].

24.2.3 Influence of Sex

The influence of sex in the occurrence of patellar dislocations is still being discussed. While Waterman et al. did not find any difference according to the sex [13], three other studies reported that females have a higher risk to sustain patellar dislocation than males [14, 12, 15], especially when they are under 20 years old. This sex-related difference is even more marked in teenagers with prior subluxation/dislocation (female: 18.0 per 100,000 person-years; male: 6.0 per 100,000 person-years) [12].

24.2.4 Influence of Ethnicity and Family History

Two studies conducted in the USA showed that black and white people were at higher risk than other racial category [15] or Hispanic people [13]. This observation is probably due to the differences of the anatomy of the lower extremities (including the knees) and the athletic exposure between racial categories. In nontraumatic patellar dislocation, the family history is important to take into account and should be systematically investigated [19, 21]. Indeed, 29 % of patients with nontraumatic patellar dislocation had a positive family history versus only 6 % of patients with traumatic patellar dislocation [19]. Moreover, family history plays a role in the recurrence of patellar dislocation [19, 22].

24.2.5 Influence of Prior Subluxation/Dislocation

The incidence rate of patellar dislocation is 206.0 per 100,000 person-years in individuals with a previous knee dislocation [17]. Patients with a prior history of patellar dislocation have seven times higher odds of subsequent instability episodes during follow-up than first-time dislocators [12]. Depending on predisposing risk factors for patellar instability, a patella redislocation rate from 25 % to 69 % is described in the literature [22–24].

24.2.6 Influence of Osseous Factors

Beside the aforementioned risk factors, trochlear dysplasia, patella alta, and a non-physiologic distance between the tibial tubercle and the trochlear groove have been reported to be related to recurrent patellar instability [2, 25, 1].

Trochlear dysplasia can be defined by a sulcus angle (defined as the angle formed between lines joining the highest points of the bony medial and lateral condyles and the lowest bony point of the intercondylar sulcus – Fig. 24.2a) greater than 145°, the trochlear groove being possibly flat or convex [26]. The sulcus angle is estimated to be abnormal in 14 % of first-time dislocators and 11 % of recurrent dislocators [12]. In average, it is higher in dislocators than in controls although both groups often have a sulcus angle greater than 145° [27, 28]. This difference was not confirmed in teenagers [29]. Trochlear dysplasia is also characterized by the measurement of the trochlear depth (abnormal if 4 mm or less), the presence of crossing sign, and the trochlear prominence (abnormal if 3 mm or more) [30, 26]. Trochlear dysplasia is present respectively in 85 % of patients with recurrent instability but not in controls (0 %) [25]. The 4-grade classification of Dejour (Fig. 24.2b) [26] also helps to discriminate low-grade (type A) and high-grade trochlear dysplasia (types B–D) [31]. Patients with high grade are 4.25-fold more at risk of recurrent dislocations [32].

Patellar height (or patella alta) can be measured with the Blackburne-Peel, the Insall-Salvati, or the Caton-Deschamps ratios (Fig. 24.2c) (patella alta is considered abnormal when the ratio is >1 according to Blackburne-Peel ratio, >1.20 according to Insall-Salvati, and ≥1.20 according to Caton-Deschamps ratio

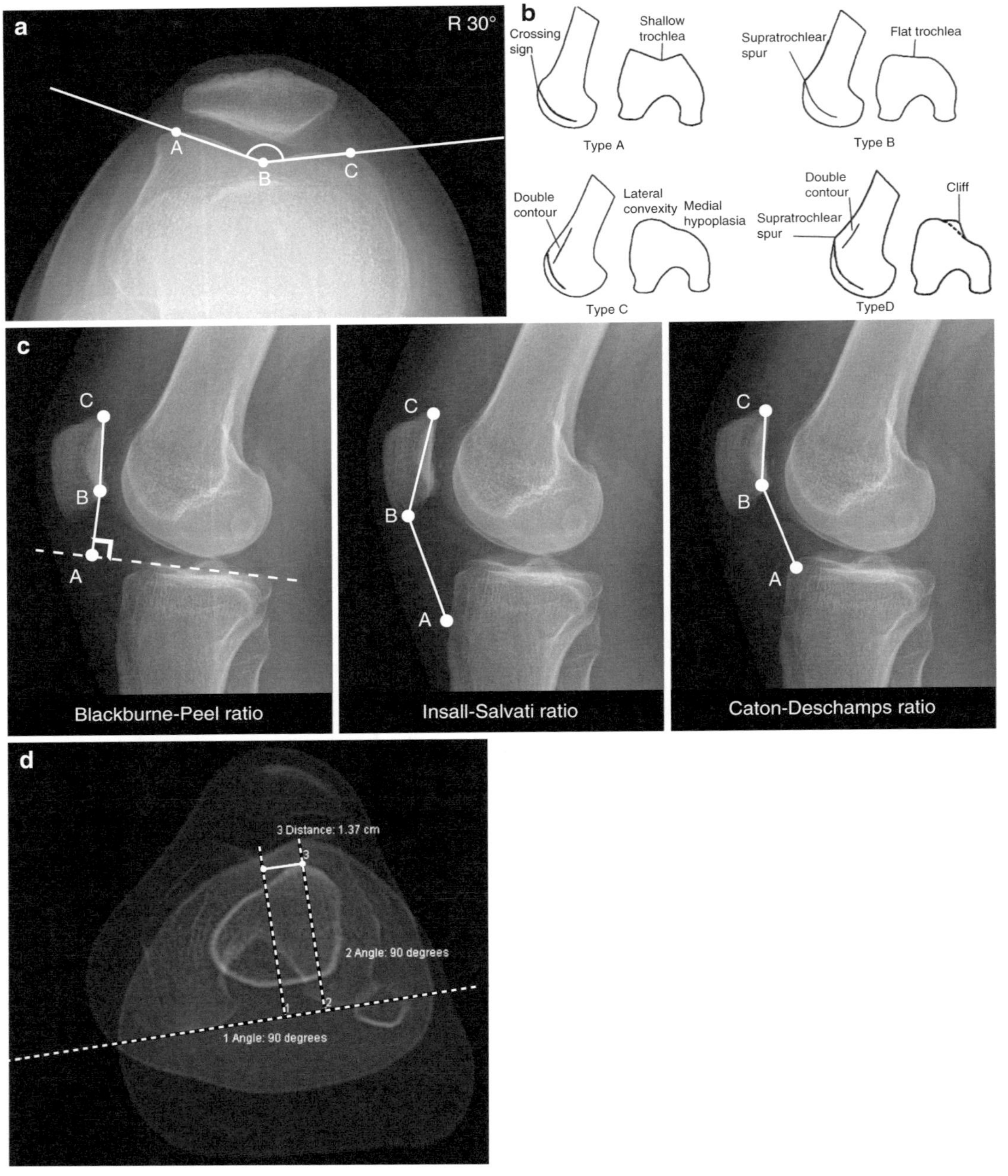

Fig. 24.2 *Panel a*: sulcus angle ($\widehat{ABC}$). *Panel b*: trochlear dysplasia classification (Dejour). Type A: crossing sign, trochlear morphology preserved (fairly shallow trochlea >145°). Type B: crossing sign, supratrochlear spur, flat or convex trochlea. Type C: crossing sign, double contour (projection on the lateral view of the hypoplastic medial facet). Type D: crossing sign, supratrochlear spur, double contour, asymmetry of trochlear facets, vertical link between medial and lateral facet (cliff pattern). With the kind permission of Wolters Kluwer and Dejour et al. [26]. *Panel c*: Blackburne-Peel, Insall-Salvati, and Caton-Deschamps ratios ($ratios = AB/BC$). *Panel d*: distance (straight line) between the trochlear groove (dotted line n°1) and the tibial tubercle (dotted line n°2) in the frontal plane (TT–TG distance)

[25, 33–35]). In the first degrees of knee flexion, an elevated patella induces an insufficient engagement into the proximal trochlea which is necessary to prevent lateralization of the patella [36]. Patella alta (Caton-Deschamps ratio ≥1.20) has been observed in dislocators (24 %) but not in controls [25]. Moreover, patella alta was also observed in recurrent dislocators [27, 37]. However, this finding was not consistent throughout the literature [12, 32].

The distance between the tibial tubercle and the trochlear groove in the frontal plane (TT–TG distance) characterizes the lateralization of the tibial tuberosity and the medialization of the trochlear groove (Fig. 24.2d). TT–TG distance has been shown to be longer in patients with patellar instability compared to controls [38, 39, 25]. The TT–TG distance was in average 20 mm in patients with instability and 13 mm in adults without history of patellar instability [25]. A similar trend has been observed in younger populations. The TT–TG distance ranged between 14.6 and 16.3 mm in young athletes with patellar instability and between 10.6 and 11.7 mm in matched controls [39, 38]. The TT–TG distance does not differ between first-time and recurrent dislocators [32] neither between the symptomatic (16.9 mm) and the healthy (15.6 mm) knee of patients with recurrent unilateral patellar instability [40].

24.2.7 Influence of Soft Tissue Factors

Patients with patellar instability can have associated lesions of the medial patellofemoral ligament (MPFL) and/or medial collateral ligament (MCL) [41, 2]. MCL and MPFL are anatomically close and a lesion of the MPFL could be associated with a lesion of the MCL, and vice versa.

The MPFL is a retinacular band of tissue stretched between the superior medial aspect of the patella and the medial femoral epicondylar region. This soft tissue structure, which is 38–60 mm long, keeps the patella within the trochlear groove and is the primary restraint to its lateral dislocation, especially between 0° and 30° of knee flexion [42, 43]. Patellar dislocation thus injures the MPFL, which is in average 13.5 mm longer in patients with patellar instability and patellar dislocation [44]. Patients with lateral patellar dislocation and the classic bone marrow bruise pattern on MRI are likely to present a rupture of the MPFL [45]. MPFL tears are indeed present in more than 98 % of patients with acute lateral patellar dislocation [46, 47]. In 80 % of the cases, its avulsion occurs at the femoral insertion site [48].

A previously nonrecognized feature was recently described by Quinlan et al. who observed that 50 % of the patients with transient patellar dislocation displayed signs of medial collateral ligament (MCL) injury [49]. The valgus laxity induced by MCL injury has indeed been demonstrated to be associated with patellar dislocations [41]. MCL insufficiency increases the Q-angle, the angle between the lines of action of the patella and the quadriceps tendon. Increased Q-angle has been considered as a risk factor for patellar dislocation, but its reliability remains discussed [50]. As a consequence, strengthening of vastus medialis obliquus (VMO) is targeted in rehabilitation. It appears however that there is no difference in the VMO parameters (i.e., VMO cross-sectional area, muscle-fiber angulation, and the craniocaudal extent of the muscle in relation to the patella) between first-time dislocators, recurrent dislocators, and controls [51].

24.2.8 Classification

According to the risks factors detailed above, a classification of patellar instability has been proposed [10]. Patients can be dichotomized in two groups: TONES and LAACS (Fig. 24.3). Patients of the TONES group display a unique unilateral traumatic injury that often induces osteochondral fractures. The anatomical architecture and function of the patellofemoral joint are normal. Conversely, the patients of the LAACS group display an atraumatic, recurrent, and often bilateral instability. The anatomical architecture of the patellofemoral joint and the ligamentous laxity are abnormal.

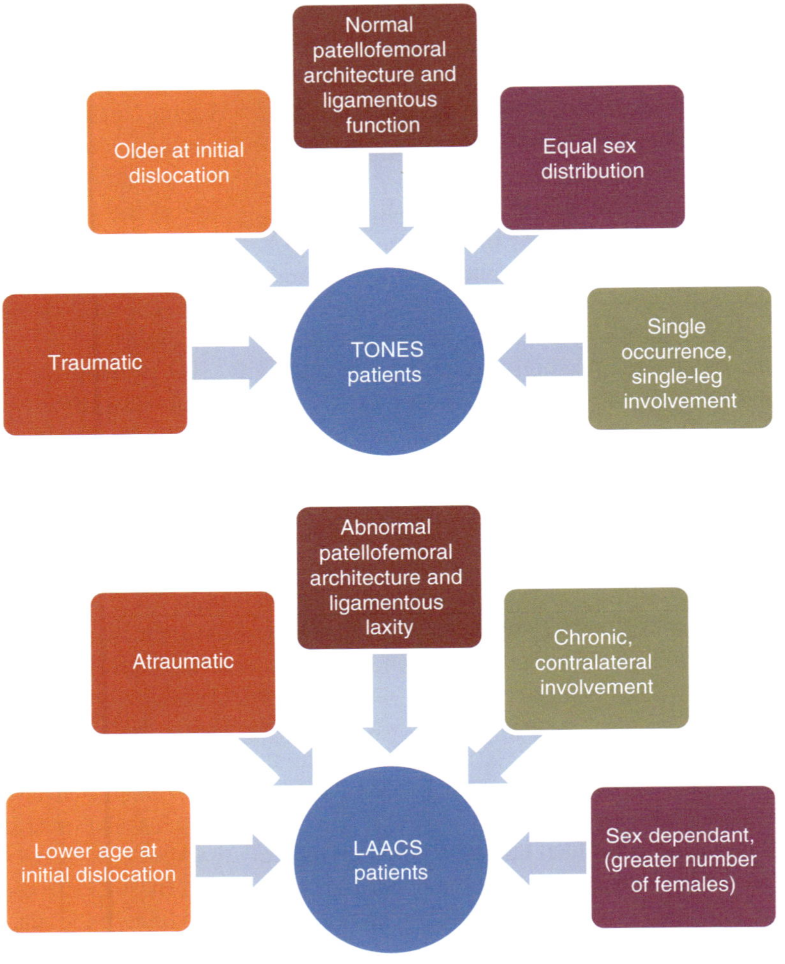

Fig. 24.3 Classification of patellar instability (adapted from Hinton and Fullick [10])

24.3 Clinical and Diagnostic Examination

A dislocated locked kneecap is an obvious sign for patellar dislocation. However, after spontaneous relocation, the diagnosis is far more difficult. The clinical pathway to detect a first patellar dislocation necessitates a detailed anamnesis, including the exact trauma mechanism and a possible family history of patellar dislocations or soft tissue hyperlaxity.

The physical examination of the injured joint may be inadequate on the day of the accident, due to the pain, stress, and discomfort of the patient. The limited examination options in the acute setting should be completed by a second examination some days later. Acute patellar dislocation is very often accompanied by a severe hemarthrosis. The aspiration of the intra-articular blood is, besides the pain relieve to the patient, a valuable diagnostic tool. The presence of fatty globules can be a sign of an osteochondral fracture or of an additional bony injury. Concomitant intra- and extra-articular injuries have to be excluded. The inspection prior to the physical examination can provide hints of predisposing factors leading to patellar dislocation such as valgus instability or the torsion of tibia and femur. Furthermore, the amount of effusion, subcutaneous hematoma, and prior skin incisions can give valuable hints for the diagnosis and treatment options.

The physical examination must include a palpation of all relevant soft tissue structures such as tendons, retinacula, and muscles. Clinical tests should include the patella apprehension test and the J sign/tracing test. For the patella apprehension test, the patella is pushed laterally with the leg in full extension. The apprehension test is to be noted positive by a verbal response of the patient or by an increasing quadriceps muscle contraction. For the J sign test, the patient is asked to move the knee slowly from flexion to extension. In patients with patellar instability, the patella will undergo a sudden lateral movement. Evaluation of the mediolateral mobility of the patella in the extended knee is mandatory. It should be semiquantified with the quadrant method [52]. A helpful diagnostic indicator is also the hypermobility of articular joints (elbow and knee hyperextension greater than 10°) [24].

To obtain a detailed description of the pathology, radiographs are essential. Anteroposterior and lateral radiographs of both knees as well as long-leg standing radiographs of the lower limbs are needed to evaluate patella height, degree of trochlea dysplasia, axial deformities, as well as the presence of osteochondral fragments. Since the CT scan has limitations in determining the location and extent of soft tissue defects or cartilaginous flake fractures, the MRI is currently the diagnostic tool of choice. Besides its ability to detect concomitant injuries, this imaging technique can also provide valuable information concerning the extent of trochlear morphology, status of the growth plates, and the TT–TG distance. A medial patella bone marrow edema in combination with a lateral femur condyle bone marrow edema on MRI is pathognomonic for a patellar dislocation.

24.4 Treatment Strategy

Persistent patellar instability leads to a decreased level of sporting activity due to evolving patellofemoral osteoarthritis, recurrent kneecap dislocations, and pain. For that reason, the treatment strategy is first to reestablish the patellofemoral joint stability, to ensure a normal development of the joint in the skeletally immature patients, and to diminish the risk of secondary osteoarthritis.

The management of patellar instability in the football player should take into account the intrinsic and extrinsic risk factors (Fig. 24.4). Patients with patellar instability are often complex cases, with a combination of bony and soft tissue abnormalities. It is fundamental to analyze all possible dislocation factors to develop an appropriate treatment strategy. A consensus for the management of first traumatic patellar dislocation does not exist [53]. A laterally first-time subluxated patella is generally treated nonoperatively in the absence of an osteochondral fracture, malalignment, or severe trochlear dysplasia. In the case of a patella redislocation or persistent patellar instability symptoms despite appropriate rehabilitation, a surgical treatment is recommended. Because of the heterogeneity of factors leading to patellar instability, an adequate surgery addressing the individual pathology needs to be performed. Numerous surgical interventions have been described and performed over the last century [54]. With further knowledge of the complexity of patellar instability, there has been a paradigm change in the treatment strategies over the last decades. Irrespective of trochlear morphology and the medial capsule/ligament complex, the "traditional surgical procedures" were addressing only the realignment of the quadriceps force vectors, in order to decrease lateralizing forces to the patella and hence increase its stability in the trochlea. Currently, surgical procedures focus on the reconstruction of the passive patella stabilizers such as bony geometry of the trochlea and the MPFL.

Since young adolescents are one of the main groups at risk for patellar dislocations, the presence of open growth plates must be taken into account in the debate of treatment options. Distal bony realignment procedures may compromise the growth plate on the tibial tuberosity and can lead to severe genu recurvatum [55]. Damaging the growth plate on the distal femur where 70 % of the length development takes place can lead to genu varum and valgum [56]. This is especially relevant if MPFL reconstructions with open growth plates are performed. It is mandatory to avoid an injury of the growth plate at the femoral

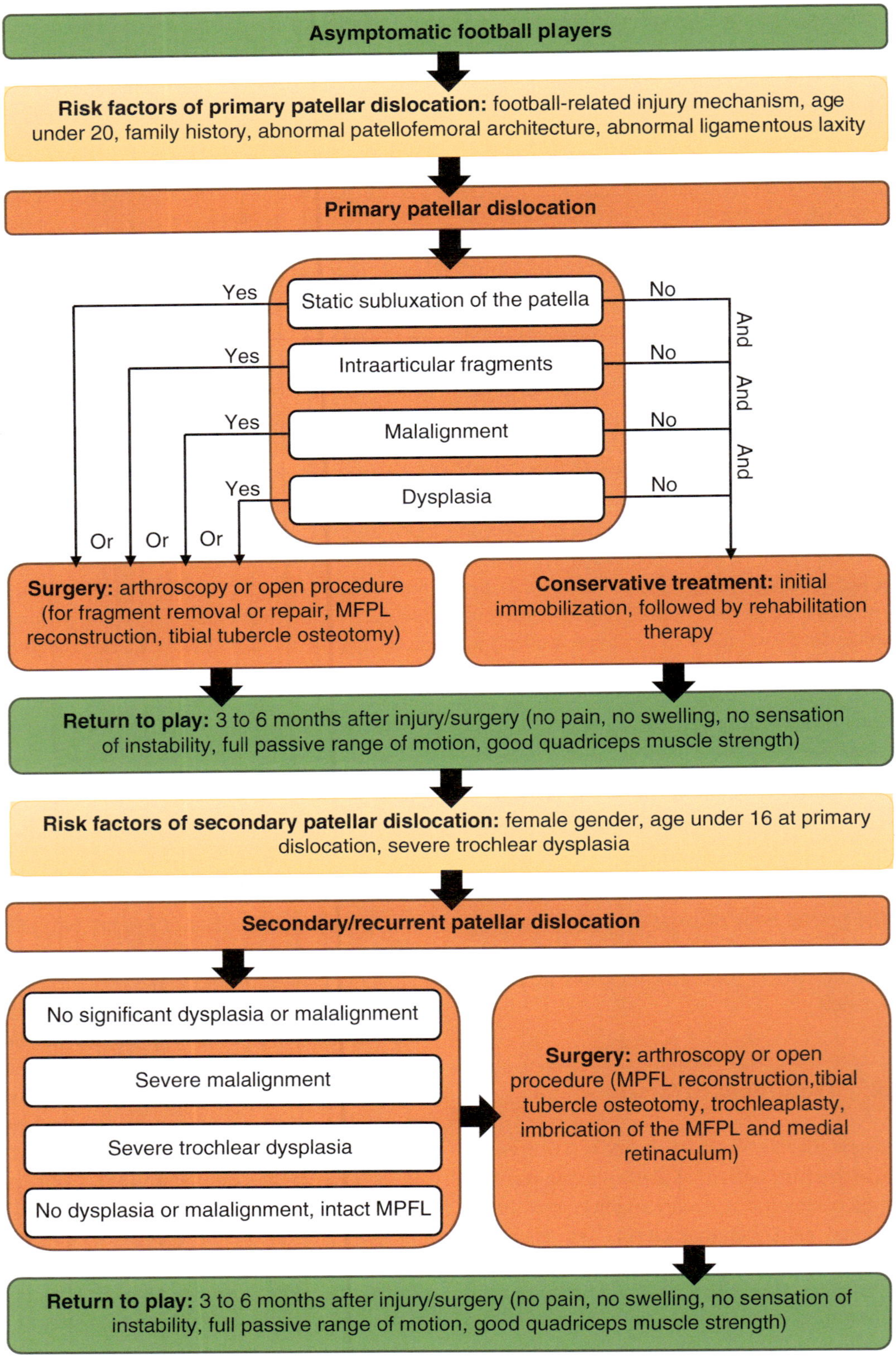

Fig. 24.4 Algorithm for the management of patellar instability in football players (adapted from Golant et al. [59])

insertion of the MPFL. This insertion is always located distally to the growth plate, on the epiphyseal side [57].

24.5 Rehabilitation and Return to Play

24.5.1 Rehabilitation

The current rehabilitation (conservative treatment or after surgery) aims to restore the strength of the quadriceps and the range of motion of the injured limb. Between 40 % and 60 % of the patients with first-time patellar dislocation have satisfactory results with a nonoperative treatment. This rehabilitation includes bracing and immobilization, electrotherapy, strengthening, and proprioception exercises [58]. For acute dislocation, brace or cast immobilization with the knee locked in extension is recommended for 2–6 weeks, depending on the patient's age and the lesion [59]. However, the immobilization should not be too long to avoid muscle atrophy and knee stiffness. In the acute inflammatory phase, rehabilitation aims to eliminate pain and swelling (3–4 first weeks) and to improve range of motion. Later on, it should focus on regaining muscle strength, stabilizing patellofemoral tracking, improving proprioception of the knee, and normalizing the gait pattern [59]. During rehabilitation, taping can be used to stabilize the patella. Strengthening the VMO is the muscular aim to target and closed-chain exercises may be more efficient [59].

For operated patients, the postoperative treatment should be adapted to the preoperative instability, the type of surgery, and the patient's risk factors. Weight bearing is typically limited for 4–6 weeks to prevent excessive traction on the patella tendon after osteotomies [59]. Conversely, partial weight bearing with the knee locked in extension is allowed immediately after MPFL reconstruction [60]. Full weight bearing without brace is generally recommended after 4–6 weeks. The rehabilitation aims also to regain full range of motion, passive and active range of motion being targeted at 0–3 weeks and 2–6 weeks, respectively. Isometric quadriceps strength and straight leg raise exercises should be performed immediately after surgery. Subsequently, specific exercises aiming to improve concentric muscular strength (quadriceps, hamstring) and proprioception are generally proposed 6–8 weeks after surgery. Running, cycling, and "mild" sports are allowed 2–4 months after surgery, whereas return to competitive sports can generally be considered after 6 months. The rehabilitation of the currently used minimally invasive MPFL reconstructions is by far easier and faster than the formerly used procedures.

24.5.2 Return to Play

Regardless of the treatment, patients are allowed to return to play after complete disappearance of pain and swelling, if there is no remaining sensation of instability, if they have reached a full passive range of knee motion, if they regained 85–90 % of quadriceps muscle strength compared with the noninjured limb, and if they had excellent dynamic stability [14, 61]. This may be expected at the earliest by 3 months from initial injury and surgery. At this time, patients should be able to run and jump on the injured leg without limping, apprehensions, or pain, but should wear a brace that stabilizes the patella during pivoting activities.

The time required to return to play depends on different factors, including the underlying anatomy and physiology, whether conservative or surgical treatment was used, and the type of surgical treatment performed. The delay for returning to sport is variable [60, 62–64] and can range from 3 to 6 months after MPFL surgery. In the literature, the percentage of patients able to return to play between 24 and 46 months after surgery (Fulkerson osteotomy or MPFL surgery) has been reported to be as high as 97–100 % [65, 63, 57]. However, only 32–82 % of patients return to their preoperative level of sport 16–38 months after MPFL surgery [66, 63, 67, 68, 62, 57]. The main factors described to limit the return to sport to a preoperative level are decreased knee function, fear of reinjury, and lack of interest. Athletes who do not return to their level reported that they avoid the high-pivot sports, such as football, associated with increased risk for reinjury [63].

References

1. Fithian DC, Neyret P, Servien E (2007) Patellar instability: the Lyon experience. Tech Knee Surg 6(2): 112–123
2. Colvin AC, West RV (2008) Patellar instability. J Bone Joint Surg Am 90(12):2751–2762
3. Boden BP, Pearsall AW, Garrett WE Jr, Feagin JA Jr (1997) Patellofemoral instability: evaluation and management. J Am Acad Orthop Surg 5(1):47–57
4. Ofluoglu O, Yasmin D, Donthineni R, Muzaffler Y (2006) Superior dislocation of the patella with early onset patellofemoral arthritis: a case report and literature review. Knee Surg Sports Traumatol Arthrosc 14:350–355
5. Varatojo R (2010) Clinical presentation of patellofemoral disorders. In: Zaffagnini S, Dejour D, Arendt EA (eds) Patellofemoral pain, instability, and arthritis. Springer, Berlin/Heidelberg, pp 35–39
6. Kantaras AT, Selby J, Johnson DL (2001) History and physical examination of the patellofemoral joint with patellar instability. Oper Tech Sports Med 9(3):129–133
7. Smith TO, Donell ST, Chester R, Clark A, Stephenson R (2011) What activities do patients with patellar instability perceive makes their patella unstable? Knee 18(5):333–339
8. Michels F, Pouliart N, Oosterlinck D (2008) Locked patellar dislocation: a case report. J Med Case Rep 2:371
9. Davis WL Jr, Fulkerson JP (1999) Initial evaluation of the athlete with anterior knee pain. Oper Tech Sports Med 7(2):55–58
10. Hinton RY, Fullick RK (2012) Patellar instability. In: Scott WN (ed) Insall & Scott surgery of the knee, 5th edn. Elsevier Churchill Livingstone, Philadelphia, pp 881–894
11. Casteleyn PP, Handelberg F (1989) Arthroscopy in the diagnosis of occult dislocation of the patella. Acta Orthop Belg 55(3):381–383
12. Fithian DC, Paxton EW, Stone ML, Silva P, Davis DK, Elias DA et al (2004) Epidemiology and natural history of acute patellar dislocation. Am J Sports Med 32(5):1114–1121
13. Waterman BR, Belmont PJ Jr, Owens BD (2012) Patellar dislocation in the United States: role of sex, age, race, and athletic participation. J Knee Surg 25(1): 51–57
14. Atkin DM, Fithian DC, Marangi KS, Stone ML, Dobson BE, Mendelsohn C (2000) Characteristics of patients with primary acute lateral patellar dislocation and their recovery within the first 6 months of injury. Am J Sports Med 28(4):472–479
15. Hsiao M, Owens BD, Burks R, Sturdivant RX, Cameron KL (2010) Incidence of acute traumatic patellar dislocation among active-duty United States military service members. Am J Sports Med 38(10): 1997–2004
16. Nietosvaara Y, Aalto K, Kallio PE (1994) Acute patellar dislocation in children: incidence and associated osteochondral fractures. J Pediatr Orthop 14(4): 513–515
17. Sillanpaa P, Mattila VM, Iivonen T, Visuri T, Pihlajamaki H (2008) Incidence and risk factors of acute traumatic primary patellar dislocation. Med Sci Sports Exerc 40(4):606–611
18. Kuikka PI, Pihlajamaki HK, Mattila VM (2013) Knee injuries related to sports in young adult males during military service – incidence and risk factors. Scand J Med Sci Sports 23(3):281–287
19. Maenpaa H, Lehto MU (1995) Surgery in acute patellar dislocation–evaluation of the effect of injury mechanism and family occurrence on the outcome of treatment. Br J Sports Med 29(4):239–241
20. Bankes MJ, Eastwood DM (2002) Inferior dislocation of the patella in the degenerate knee. Injury 33(6): 528–529
21. Carter C, Sweetnam R (1958) Familial joint laxity and recurrent dislocation of the patella. J Bone Joint Surg Br 40-(b)(4):664–667
22. Palmu S, Kallio PE, Donell ST, Helenius I, Nietosvaara Y (2008) Acute patellar dislocation in children and adolescents: a randomized clinical trial. J Bone Joint Surg Am 90(3):463–470
23. Schneider FJ, Thumfart A, Linhart WE (2009) Behandlung der Patellaluxation im Kindes- und Jugendalter. Arthroskopie 22(1):60–67
24. Stefancin JJ, Parker RD (2007) First-time traumatic patellar dislocation: a systematic review. Clin Orthop Relat Res 455:93–101
25. Dejour H, Walch G, Nove-Josserand L, Guier C (1994) Factors of patellar instability: an anatomic radiographic study. Knee Surg Sports Traumatol Arthrosc 2(1):19–26
26. Dejour D, Le Coultre B (2007) Osteotomies in patello-femoral instabilities. Sports Med Arthrosc 15(1):39–46
27. Charles MD, Haloman S, Chen L, Ward SR, Fithian D, Afra R (2013) Magnetic resonance imaging-based topographical differences between control and recurrent patellofemoral instability patients. Am J Sports Med 41(2):374–384
28. Balcarek P, Jung K, Ammon J, Walde TA, Frosch S, Schuttrumpf JP et al (2010) Anatomy of lateral patellar instability: trochlear dysplasia and tibial tubercle-trochlear groove distance is more pronounced in women who dislocate the patella. Am J Sports Med 38(11):2320–2327
29. Regalado G, Lintula H, Eskelinen M, Kokki H, Kroger H, Svedstrom E et al (2014) Dynamic KINE-MRI in patellofemoral instability in adolescents. Knee Surg Sports Traumatol Arthrosc. 22(11):2795–2802
30. Latt LD, Christopher M, Nicolini A, Burk DR, Dezfuli B, Serack BJ et al (2014) A validated cadaveric model of trochlear dysplasia. Knee Surg Sports Traumatol Arthrosc 22(10):2357–2363
31. Lippacher S, Dejour D, Elsharkawi M, Dornacher D, Ring C, Dreyhaupt J et al (2012) Observer agreement

on the Dejour trochlear dysplasia classification: a comparison of true lateral radiographs and axial magnetic resonance images. Am J Sports Med 40(4):837–843
32. Balcarek P, Oberthur S, Hopfensitz S, Frosch S, Walde TA, Wachowski MM et al (2014) Which patellae are likely to redislocate? Knee Surg Sports Traumatol Arthrosc 22(10):2308–2314
33. Hinton RY, Sharma KM (2003) Acute and recurrent patellar instability in the young athlete. Orthop Clin North Am 34(3):385–396
34. Insall J, Salvati E (1971) Patella position in the normal knee joint. Radiology 101(1):101–104
35. Seil R, Muller B, Georg T, Kohn D, Rupp S (2000) Reliability and interobserver variability in radiological patellar height ratios. Knee Surg Sports Traumatol Arthrosc 8(4):231–236
36. Ward SR, Terk MR, Powers CM (2007) Patella alta: association with patellofemoral alignment and changes in contact area during weight-bearing. J Bone Joint Surg Am 89(8):1749–1755
37. Escala JS, Mellado JM, Olona M, Gine J, Sauri A, Neyret P (2006) Objective patellar instability: MR-based quantitative assessment of potentially associated anatomical features. Knee Surg Sports Traumatol Arthrosc 14(3):264–272
38. Pennock AT, Alam M, Bastrom T (2014) Variation in tibial tubercle-trochlear groove measurement as a function of age, sex, size, and patellar instability. Am J Sports Med 42(2):389–393
39. Balcarek P, Jung K, Frosch KH, Sturmer KM (2011) Value of the tibial tuberosity-trochlear groove distance in patellar instability in the young athlete. Am J Sports Med 39(8):1756–1761
40. Caplan N, Lees D, Newby M, Ewen A, Jackson R, St Clair Gibson A et al (2014) Is tibial tuberosity-trochlear groove distance an appropriate measure for the identification of knees with patellar instability? Knee Surg Sports Traumatol Arthrosc 22(10):2377–2381
41. Hermans K, Claes S, Bellemans J (2013) Valgus instability as a cause for recurrent lateral patellar dislocation: a new mechanism for patellofemoral instability? Acta Orthop Belg 79(5):495–501
42. Amis AA, Firer P, Mountney J, Senavongse W, Thomas NP (2003) Anatomy and biomechanics of the medial patellofemoral ligament. Knee 10(3):215–220
43. Feller JA, Amis AA, Andrish JT, Arendt EA, Erasmus PJ, Powers CM (2007) Surgical biomechanics of the patellofemoral joint. Arthroscopy 23(5):542–553
44. de Oliveira V, de Souza V, Cury R, Camargo OP, Avanzi O, Severino N et al (2014) Medial patellofemoral ligament anatomy: is it a predisposing factor for lateral patellar dislocation? Int Orthop 38(8):1633–1639
45. Guerrero P, Li X, Patel K, Brown M, Busconi B (2009) Medial patellofemoral ligament injury patterns and associated pathology in lateral patella dislocation: an MRI study. Sports Med Arthrosc Rehabil Ther Technol 1(1):17
46. Nomura E (1999) Classification of lesions of the medial patello-femoral ligament in patellar dislocation. Int Orthop 23(5):260–263
47. Balcarek P, Ammon J, Frosch S, Walde TA, Schuttrumpf JP, Ferlemann KG et al (2010) Magnetic resonance imaging characteristics of the medial patellofemoral ligament lesion in acute lateral patellar dislocations considering trochlear dysplasia, patella alta, and tibial tuberosity-trochlear groove distance. Arthroscopy 26(7):926–935
48. Smirk C, Morris H (2003) The anatomy and reconstruction of the medial patellofemoral ligament. Knee 10(3):221–227
49. Quinlan JF, Farrelly C, Kelly G, Eustace S (2010) Co-existent medial collateral ligament injury seen following transient patellar dislocation: observations at magnetic resonance imaging. Br J Sports Med 44(6):411–414
50. Cooney AD, Kazi Z, Caplan N, Newby M, St Clair Gibson A, Kader DF (2012) The relationship between quadriceps angle and tibial tuberosity-trochlear groove distance in patients with patellar instability. Knee Surg Sports Traumatol Arthrosc 20(12):2399–2404
51. Balcarek P, Oberthur S, Frosch S, Schuttrumpf JP, Sturmer KM (2014) Vastus medialis obliquus muscle morphology in primary and recurrent lateral patellar instability. Biomed Res Int 2014:326586
52. Kolowich PA, Paulos LE, Rosenberg TD, Farnsworth S (1990) Lateral release of the patella: indications and contraindications. Am J Sports Med 18(4):359–365
53. Hing CB, Smith TO, Donell S, Song F (2011) Surgical versus non-surgical interventions for treating patellar dislocation. Cochrane Database Syst Rev. doi:10.1002/14651858, CD008106.pub2(11):Cd008106
54. Arendt EA, Dejour D (2013) Patella instability: building bridges across the ocean a historic review. Knee Surg Sports Traumatol Arthrosc 21(2):279–293
55. Pappas AM, Anas P, Toczylowski HM Jr (1984) Asymmetrical arrest of the proximal tibial physis and genu recurvatum deformity. J Bone Joint Surg Am 66(4):575–581
56. Seil R, Pape D, Kohn D (2008) The risk of growth changes during transphyseal drilling in sheep with open physes. Arthroscopy 24(7):824–833
57. Nelitz M, Dreyhaupt J, Reichel H, Woelfle J, Lippacher S (2013) Anatomic reconstruction of the medial patellofemoral ligament in children and adolescents with open growth plates: surgical technique and clinical outcome. Am J Sports Med 41(1): 58–63
58. McConnell J (2007) Rehabilitation and nonoperative treatment of patellar instability. Sports Med Arthrosc 15(2):95–104
59. Golant A, Quach T, Rosen J (2013) Patellofemoral instability: diagnosis and management. In: Hamlin M, Draper N, Kathiravel Y (eds) Current issues in sports and exercise medicine. InTech, Rijeka, pp 87–117
60. Fisher B, Nyland J, Brand E, Curtin B (2010) Medial patellofemoral ligament reconstruction for recurrent patellar dislocation: a systematic review including rehabilitation and return-to-sports efficacy. Arthroscopy 26(10):1384–1394
61. Menetrey J, Putman S, Gard S (2014) Return to sport after patellar dislocation or following surgery for

patellofemoral instability. Knee Surg Sports Traumatol Arthrosc 22(10):2320–2326
62. Ronga M, Oliva F, Longo UG, Testa V, Capasso G, Maffulli N (2009) Isolated medial patellofemoral ligament reconstruction for recurrent patellar dislocation. Am J Sports Med 37(9):1735–1742
63. Lippacher S, Dreyhaupt J, Williams SR, Reichel H, Nelitz M (2014) Reconstruction of the medial patellofemoral ligament: clinical outcomes and return to sports. Am J Sports Med 42(7):1661–1668
64. Smith TO, Chester R, Clark A, Donell ST, Stephenson R (2011) A national survey of the physiotherapy management of patients following first-time patellar dislocation. Physiotherapy 97(4):327–338
65. Tjoumakaris FP, Forsythe B, Bradley JP (2010) Patellofemoral instability in athletes: treatment via modified Fulkerson osteotomy and lateral release. Am J Sports Med 38(5):992–999
66. Howells NR, Barnett AJ, Ahearn N, Ansari A, Eldridge JD (2012) Medial patellofemoral ligament reconstruction: a prospective outcome assessment of a large single centre series. J Bone Joint Surg Br 94(9): 1202–1208
67. Mariani PP, Liguori L, Cerullo G, Iannella G, Floris L (2011) Arthroscopic patellar reinsertion of the MPFL in acute patellar dislocations. Knee Surg Sports Traumatol Arthrosc 19(4):628–633
68. Panni AS, Alam M, Cerciello S, Vasso M, Maffulli N (2011) Medial patellofemoral ligament reconstruction with a divergent patellar transverse 2-tunnel technique. Am J Sports Med 39(12):2647–2655

25 Knee Cartilage Repair

Lars G. Peterson and Haris S. Vasiliadis

25.1 Introduction

Football is one of the biggest global sports attracting boys and girls, men and women, professionals and amateurs and billions of spectators and fans. Around the world about 260 million male and female players are licensed within FIFA (Federation Internationale de Football Association). A problem following the popularity of football is the increasing speed, body contacts and competitions causing injuries.

25.1.1 Aetiology-Epidemiology

The incidence of the injuries of knee articular cartilage is found to be increasing among athletes [1]. In several football studies it has been shown that foul play is responsible for about 30 % of all injuries and that knee injuries are among the most common injuries and may be career ending. In acute and chronic ACL injuries, between 40 % and 70 % are combined with meniscus and articular cartilage injuries [2]. Isolated cartilage lesions (grade I–IV, ICRS classification) have been reported in about 61–63 % by Curl et al. and by Hjelle et al. at arthroscopy for knee pain [3, 4]. Any grade I–IV lesion can progress into posttraumatic osteoarthritis over time and may accelerate by continued sport activities. A cartilage lesion was reported in about half of the athletes treated with an ACL reconstruction, while these cases are already very common among recreational or high competitive athletes [5, 6]. A study in NFL (American football) reported 8 cartilage injuries annually for 14 consecutive years, whereas about half of them were treated surgically [7].

L.G. Peterson, MD, PhD (✉)
Department of Orthopaedics, Sahlgrenska Academy, Gothenburg University, S413 45 Gothenburg, Sweden
e-mail: peterson.lars@telia.com

H.S. Vasiliadis, MD, PhD (✉)
Department of Orthopaedics, University of Ioannina, Leoforos Panepistimiou, 45500 Ioannina, Greece
e-mail: vasiliadismd@gmail.com

25.1.2 Injury Mechanism

The increased repetitive forces applied to the knee joint during the demanding training programme and frequent games lead to an increased incidence of cartilage lesions in high-level football players, compared with the general population. Knee injuries can be caused by intrinsic forces (generated by the player him/herself, e.g. by landing on one leg and forcing the knee in a valgus rotation) and/or by extrinsic forces (generated from outside the individual, e.g. tackles from the opponent or foul play). This incidence is further increased in contact sports with frequent pivoting, like football, indoor handball or American football. One explanation may be the pivoting movements which substantially overload especially the medial compartment causing MCL and ACl ruptures and simultaneously subject the cartilage to shearing

P. Volpi (ed.), *Football Traumatology: New Trends*, DOI 10.1007/978-3-319-18245-2_25

forces. The alert position of the athletes followed by rapid "explosive" accelerations or decelerations applies severe and sudden forces to the knee ligaments and also to the patellofemoral joint leading to patella and/or trochlea lesions. Finally, the frequent injuries apparent in contact sports additionally increase the incidence of ligamentous instability, mainly due to ACL ruptures or deficiencies that secondarily contribute to meniscal and cartilage lesions. Noyes found articular cartilage injuries in 40–70 % of acute and chronic ACL injuries [2, 8]. Background factors must be identified and addressed such as varus–valgus malalignment, instability (ACL, PCL, MCL, LCL or MPFL rupture) meniscus deficiency and bone deficiency/pathology, as contributing to and accelerating articular cartilage injuries.

25.1.3 The Risks of Delayed Treatment and Special Considerations

Under the pressure of the running league and the players' contracts, the background lesions may frequently remain practically untreated until they severely interfere with the player's performance. At this point the treating physician usually faces severe, multiple neglected cartilage lesions demonstrating signs of posttraumatic osteoarthritis. Several studies have demonstrated a highly increased risk of knee OA in high demanding professional players, up to 12-fold, compared to the general population [9, 10].

The repair of cartilage defects in professional players is a great challenge, being a rather complicated issue. There are many factors that a treating surgeon may need to encounter in order to decide if a lesion requires early or late surgical intervention and, if yes, which is the best intervention for the specific player. Of course lesion characteristics like the size (e.g. contained or not), the location (medial or lateral femoral or tibial condyle, patella, trochlea) and the number (isolated or multiple) play a crucial role for the decision of the most appropriate treatment. Concomitant procedures to correct ligament instability (ACL, PCL, MCL, LCL, MPFL), meniscus lesions or insufficiency, varus or valgus malalignment, bone defect or pathology and patellar maltracking or instability have to be included in the analysis. When this is the situation for a professional player, the decision will need to be further individualised, based on the age and the level of the player, the time of the running league season, the anticipated time to return to play or the anticipated (or scheduled) time up to the retirement of the player or even the financial issues related with his running contract.

There are two very important factors that affect or even define the final success of a treatment: (1) the clinical outcome itself and (2) the time that it will take the player to achieve this outcome. There is also one third factor, the duration of the results, which however is usually underestimated and usually not taken as first priority when it comes to high-level active players.

The best repair treatment of cartilage lesions is still a controversial issue. A number of treatment options are currently used in clinical practice, with certain advantages and disadvantages that accompany any of these. The importance of fast return to play and the need for top performance, if possible from the first postoperative day, further complicates the final decision and final treatment approach.

The success of the treatment in professional players is mainly counted with the return to preinjury level. However, the rate of players that finally return to sports may be limited and many of them may have to cope with a lower level, never achieving their preinjury level, if the lesions are undertreated. In a systematic review that assessed 11 studies, 66 % of patients reached their preinjury level, which highly defers between treatment approaches [11]. However, the fact that this percentage is highly related to the treatment approach and substantially differs among different treatments stresses the necessity of a meticulous approach to these patients and of the conduction of the best possible treatment.

25.2 Clinical and Diagnostic Examination

The diagnostic approach is similar if not identical to that of the general population and the diagnosis of articular cartilage lesions based on an adequate history and a physical examination.

A thorough history of symptoms, acute trauma, or repetitive excessive loading related or not to the sports is important. Any history of previous cartilage treatment, meniscal repair, or meniscectomy may interfere with the condition of the cartilage. An ACL reconstruction or previous realignment of the patellofemoral joint may be associated with a "diseased" knee that already before the time of surgery sustained a cartilage injury, which may have remained untreated or undertreated. Clinical examination, including signs of local tenderness, swelling, range of motion and crepitation, is performed. Pain, swelling, locking, catching, giving-way sensation and crepitation along with signs of tenderness, effusion, muscle weakness and pain on weight-bearing movements may be indicative of coexisting cartilage lesions along with other potential injuries.

The clinical examination should additionally focus on the assessment of the ligament stability in order to detect any anteroposterior or lateral instability of the knee joint or any instability of the patella. Clinical assessment of the function and volume of the quadriceps and hamstrings should be included. A careful record of previous surgery is also of great importance.

Standing X-rays including both limbs (hip–knee–ankle) and comparison to contralateral knee are necessary. Varus and valgus deformities are assessed, and patella malalignment, maltracking or instability is further assessed if clinical signs exist. Further examinations include MRI to assess articular cartilage, meniscus and the subchondral bone and other pathology and also CT scan in full extension with and without Q-ceps contraction (in patellar–trochlear lesions and instability).

An arthroscopy may be performed to confirm the diagnosis and to evaluate the features of the lesion (location, size, containment, opposing surface, shouldering) along with the identification of potentially concomitant lesions (ACL, PCL rupture or insufficiency, meniscal lesions, etc.). High-level players usually aim for a fast diagnosis, fast repair and fast recovery in as less surgical steps as possible. In these cases a very careful preoperative planning is even more important. The surgeon should rely on clinical and radiological findings and be prepared for addressing in one step if possible all the concomitant lesions (cartilage, ACL, meniscal). It is most important to propose the optimal treatment in each individual case. The surgeon should also inform about and be prepared with alternative treatment plans according to the intraoperative findings.

A detailed discussion with the patient preoperatively and an analysis of the treatment approach is necessary. The patients should be fully informed of the situation, the treatment approach, the rehabilitation time, the anticipated final outcomes and the perspectives for return to the preinjury level of sports performance as well as the prognosis for short- and long-term results.

25.3 Treatment Strategy

The aim for football players is to minimise the symptoms with an as brief as possible rehabilitation and as long as possible duration of the results. Three different categories of players will be discussed in an algorithm.

First the teenage player in the beginning of his career, second the established player in his active career between 20 and 35 years and third the player in the end of his career or post career. These groups will be discussed in relation to available treatments.

In general, there are many different treatment options for cartilage lesions, such as debridement, coblation, drilling, abrasion, microfracturing, mosaicplasty (OATS), use of osteochondral allografts or ACI. The treatment strategy is usually individualised according to many factors, including the priorities of the patient-athlete. The currently available scientific evidence provides a background for the best possible approach.

25.3.1 Active Teenage Football Players

In this patient group osteochondritis dissecans (OCD) is a relatively frequent entity that has to be treated. An OCD lesion requires a different approach than a purely traumatic lesion and a "sandwich technique" is often necessary to address the bone pathology or defects involved.

Just removal of the fragment or loose body will give fast relief of symptoms but will increase the risk to almost 100 % for early posttraumatic osteoarthritis with continued sports like football.

Another differentiation is related with the younger age and the consequently increased anticipated time for participation in sports. The good quality of the repair tissue at the site of cartilage lesion and the high durability of the good treatment outcomes are mandatory for a durable successful career of the teenage player. Therefore, ACI is usually suggested as a treatment option in this patient group. The more prolonged rehabilitation time is not so important and has not much impact on the performance, as a progress of a cartilage injury would have.

Teenage players treated for cartilage lesions have a very high recovery rate, with a greater chance for returning to full sports activities. However, an unsuccessful treatment would lead to an early end of a career and an increased risk of developing posttraumatic osteoarthritis.

25.3.2 Active Adult Football Players

Microfractures are currently the most common intervention that is performed for the treatment of cartilage lesions in active athletes. In 14 consecutive years in NFL American football, in 118 cases half of each were operated, 43 % were treated with MF, and 31 % were treated with debridement [7]. In the majority of the studies assessing cartilage repair in athletes (8 of the 11 included), microfractures were assessed [11]. According to the systematic review of Harris et al., the return to preinjury level in athletes differs between treatments. MF patients have a lower possibility for full recovery (59 %, range 25–100 %, 8 studies), while ACI results in a higher possibility (78 %, range 27–100 %, 3 studies). OATS according to one study (57 patients) provides the best chance of full recovery to sports activities (93 %). Moreover, OATS offers also a relatively faster return followed by MF. ACI results in a more prolonged rehabilitation time [11]. Similar outcomes have been found by another systematic review reporting good and excellent results in 67 % after MF, in 82 % of ACI patients and in 93 % of patients treated with OATS. Return to sport was achieved 7 months after MF, 8 months after OAT and 18 months after ACI [5]. The size, location of the lesions are very important factors for the final outcome.

The only RCT available compares OATS with MF. According to this study in 57 high performance athletes, OATS provide a better rate of return to preinjury level (93 % vs. 52 %) with a clinical improvement between the 1st and 3rd postoperative year (86 % and 96 %, respectively). On the other hand, the MF athletes showed a significant deterioration (76 % and 52 % in 1 and 3 years, respectively) [12].

Continued sports participation at the preinjury level, thus a long-term durability of good clinical outcomes, was seen in 96 % of ACI-treated patients, in 52 % of MF and 52 % of OAT patients [5]. This clearly suggests a better repair tissue after treatment with ACI.

The rate of full recovery of MF-treated athletes differs among studies. Steadman reports a return to NFL in 76 % of 25 players, with a good postoperative performance [13]. Another study in 24 NBA basketball players showed that one third never returned to the league. Only 14 returned to NBA for more than a year, but had to deal with shorter length of play and less points scored per game, although no other performance indexes were affected [14]. Another similar study also reported 20 % of players treated with MF not returning to NBA and a significantly reduced performance at 1st and 2nd year for the rest. The mean time to return to an NBA game was 30 weeks [15].

One thing that needs to be considered is definitely the characteristics of the cartilage lesion. The algorithm that has been set for the common population may not be directly applied to high competitive athletes; however, some main guidelines and suggestions should be considered [16]. For small contained lesions of less than 1 or 2 cm^2, MF or OATS may definitely be efficient at least for short-term return, whereas double-stage or more demanding treatments like ACI should be selected for lesions larger than 2 cm^2 and/or more complex cases where a longer career is more important than a quick return for established players. However, ACI should be considered for young players early in their careers even for these small lesions.

For larger lesions or for multiple and/or kissing lesions, the ACI is the only reliable treatment with accepted results (good recovery rate, long-lasting good results). Although MF may be used as a palliative treatment, even if good results are initially provided, the possibilities of long-term good results are very low. This is probably related to the insufficient repair tissue (mainly fibrous tissue) in the lesion area after MF; this tissue subsequently fails to withstand the high forces of sports activities and in due time it leads to symptoms' relapse. Mosaicplasty (MP) gives good results but leads to high donor site morbidity due to the harvest of osteochondral plugs. Provided the usually large multiple defects in football players, there is a limited number of patients that may profit from the use of MP. Osteochondral allografts may be used in large defects. However, there is no evidence to support their use in athletes.

Another dilemma in the treatment approach of active athletes is usually related with the need of assessing the concomitant injuries or the need of correcting the limb axis or a patella malalignment. In regard to the ACL or meniscal ruptures, they should definitely be assessed and addressed along with the cartilage repair. Regarding though the need of osteotomies, there is a controversy. It is shown that osteotomies are accompanied by a further rehabilitation time, a higher complication incidence and a recovery that nearly never reaches the preinjury level of sports performance. There was a general rule that osteotomies should not be used for high-level football players and other athletes if they intend to continue participating at the same level. However, this rule is based on the old indications (unicompartmental osteoarthritis in older population) where old techniques with large overcorrections and insufficient fixation systems were prevailing. In the treatment of cartilage injuries, there is quite a different situation where you have to analyse the background factors of importance and correct them to create an optimal environment for the repair tissue to survive in the short and long term. The surgeon should fix a varus malalignment in medial compartment large unipolar or bipolar defect(s), by unloading with an osteotomy if necessary. The modern approach to osteotomies is to just overcorrect the mechanical axis by 2–4°, use open wedge osteotomy, correct the malalignment and use a stable internal fixation. If the malalignment is mainly due to abnormal biomechanics in the femur, the osteotomy should be performed in the distal femur. If the biomechanics are located in the proximal tibia, it should be corrected in the proximal tibia. Nagel et al. reported that 59 % returned to sports after high tibial osteotomy [17].

25.3.3 Retired or to Be Retired Football Players

The aim of the treatment of these patients is to eliminate the symptoms they experience and to delay or even to prevent the arthroplasty. This patient group resembles more the "normal" patients. A differentiation usually comes to the severity of lesions they suffer from. They are usually patients with severe and extended lesions despite the relatively low age. This is related to the prolonged period in high competitive sports and to the fact that these lesions have not been treated before or been undertreated. In many cases the knee fully resembles a severe osteoarthritic knee, with neglected cartilage lesions, resected meniscus lesions, instability and usually malalignment (mainly varus knees). The cartilage lesions are often multiple and kissing. The challenge is that the too young age is a contraindication for salvage procedures as the knee replacement. The "advantage" though is the fact that the short rehabilitation time is not so important as for the active players.

The different hierarchy of treatment goals sets a different hierarchy of treatment options to be followed. In this patient group, when large lesions occur (>3–4 cm^2), the ACI should be definitely preferred, aiming to a better repair tissue and to durable good clinical outcomes. A long-term follow-up study has shown that ACI was an effective and durable treatment even for neglected large cartilage lesions or multiple kissing lesions, for which a resurfacing of the knee joint with ACI was performed [18]. In this series none of the 224 cases followed had a knee arthroplasty 10–20 years after the chondrocyte implantation. ACI provides the ability to a biological resurfacing of the joint in order to repair the usually extended bare bone surfaces.

In many of these cases, the bony surface is completely exposed and rather sclerotic (providing a "polished" surface appearance). In these cases, the lesion area should be carefully abraded without causing bleeding. If the subchondral bone is sclerotic, often with cyst formations, bone marrow oedema and osteophytes (which are related to poor outcomes), a meticulous removal of this pathologic subchondral bone may be needed. Then the defect area should be filled with autograft cancellous bone using the "sandwich technique" [19].

In this patient group, of retired football players, more radical surgical treatments should be used, as the demand for very fast return to very high performance no longer exists. In this sense, a more sophisticated treatment approach involve unloading osteotomies, reconstructions of ACL or PCL as well as meniscus transplantation when needed in order to correct the functional anatomy of the joint and to unload the repaired cartilage. On the other side, in this patient group the surgeon usually deals with more extended, severe, multiple and usually chronic lesions, which all are considered as negative prognostic factors and add to the treatment challenge.

25.4 Rehabilitation and Return to Play

The importance of an adequate rehabilitation in cartilage repair techniques is as important as the surgical procedures themselves. The articular cartilage is dependent on diffusion of synovial fluid for the transportation of nutrition and oxygen to the chondrocytes. The cells are responsible for the production of matrix, mainly collagen type II and proteoglycans, responsible for the high water content in cartilage, necessary for the shock absorption capacity. This structure provides the mechanical strength and function of the articular cartilage throughout our life. During unloading of the joint, the negatively charged proteoglycans attract water, and during the weight bearing (WB) the synovial fluid is pressed back into the joint. This exchange of water is necessary for the survival and function of the chondrocytes and their maintenance of the cartilage matrix turnover. Irrespective of surgical repair techniques, the chondrocytes need the loading–unloading for their survival and regeneration of the tissue. Progressive increase of WB over time is necessary for the cell survival and for the new matrix to mature into functional cartilage.

After ACI the maturation process of the cartilage takes about 9 months to reach 80 % return of the normal concentration of proteoglycans, and for deeper and larger lesions, it takes 12–15 months to reach normal concentrations of proteoglycans and collagen II, a guarantee for long-term survival and function of the cartilage.

25.4.1 Rehabilitation Protocol

Intermittent continuous passive motion is started 6–8 h after surgery. Active knee extension–flexion movements are started the first postoperative day and increased as tolerated. The rehabilitation protocol is dependent on the characteristics of the cartilage lesion.

Lesions Up to 6–8 cm2 Contained: Weight bearing is limited to 20–30 kg for the first 3–6 weeks as tolerated by pain. Then progressive increase per 20 kg every 2 weeks, up to full weight bearing at 12 weeks. Stationary biking with low resistance when flexion allows. Outdoor biking at full weight bearing. Progressive increase walking distances. Water training freestyle swimming. Running at 6–9 months.

Lesions Over 8 cm2 or Multiple Lesions (Two or More in the Same Knee) and Uncontained Lesions: Weight bearing is limited to 20–30 kg for the first 6–8 weeks. Then progressive increase per 20 kg every 2 weeks, up to 12–16 weeks. Training protocol as above. Running at 6–12 months (individual decision).

Bipolar Lesions + Concomitant Procedures: Weight bearing is limited to 20–30 kg for the first 8 weeks. Then progressive increase per 20 kg every 2 weeks, up to full weight bearing at 16 weeks. Training protocol as above. Running 9–12 months(individual decision).

Return to football and other impact sports may be allowed in average 12–15 months, on an individual basis.

The rehabilitation following ACT is long and focuses mainly on functional training and motion training. Return to football is judged on an individual level. Clinical follow-up, including strength and endurance tests as well as arthroscopic evaluation and indentation testing of the stiffness of the repair tissue, is important before allowing the player to go back to football training. MRI enhanced with gadolinium contrast may be useful for assessing the healing. The player starts with individual training and then gradually goes back to individual football training and then to competitive training and matches [20, 21].

25.5 Prediction of Outcomes

It seems that the *age* is a very important prediction factor determining the capability of return to sports and return to preinjury level, in all the treatment options. Mithoefer et al. showed a more frequent return to sports in players younger than 40 years that were treated with MF, comparing with older players [1]. In another group of football/soccer players treated with ACI, 70 % of players younger than 25 years returned versus only 30 % of older players [22]. The return to sports was even much higher in adolescent athletes reaching the 95 %, while 60 % to an equal or higher level [23]. The higher age has been shown to negatively affect the outcome of a cartilage repair treatment also in the general population probably because of an inferior intrinsic repair capability of the lesion area [24, 25]. In the case of high-level professional athletes, a severe injury and surgery at higher age (35–40) followed by a prolonged rehabilitation programme obviously affects and probably stresses to a decision for earlier retirement.

Another important factor that has also been stressed by studies in general population is the *duration of symptoms prior to the treatment* [24–26]. It appears that it applies also for high competitive athletes. The shorter preoperative time seems to provide a higher success rate as has been shown by several studies [1, 22, 23, 27]. Athletes who were symptomatic for less than 12 months returned to sports in 66 % and 67 % of cases after MF and ACI, respectively. When symptomatic period exceeded the 12 months, these rates radically declined to 14 % and 15 %, respectively [5].

Finally, the higher *number of previous cartilage surgeries* has also been correlated to a higher failure or not sufficient outcomes both in the general population and competitive athletes [1, 23, 28]. Although this has not been confirmed, it is thought that the multiple previous cartilage surgeries and/or the long duration of cartilage lesions prior to surgery contributes to increased stiffness with worsening of repair capabilities of the subchondral bone and the overlying cartilage repair. It has been suggested that the subchondral bone in these cases is more sclerotic with increased stiffness and the knee joint has turned into a posttraumatic osteoarthritic knee. This probably results in an inferior environment usually deteriorated by a varus knee that has been gradually settled and the subsequent overloading of the diseased bone and cartilage.

Defect-specific features like the size of a lesion definitely also play a role. The general guidelines and the up-to-date algorithms determine that MF should not be used for large uncontained lesions due to inferior results with gradual recurrence of symptoms [16]. An inferior result in larger lesions has also been shown by Gudas et al. in athletes treated by MF, but not in his OATS group [12]. The upper border of 2 cm^2 for the MF has also been confirmed in athletes by Mithofer et al. They found a higher rate of return to sports in patients with lower than 2 cm^2 lesions compared with the larger ones (64 % vs. 22 %) [1]. A negative effect of large lesions has also been found in ACI-treated football/soccer players. The best outcomes were found in athletes with moderate lesions (5 cm^2) in contrary to the group with larger ones (8.5 cm^2) [22]. Other background anatomical factors when remain untreated play a negative role for the success of any cartilage treatment. For example, a repair of a cartilage lesion on the medial condyle of a varus knee has a very low chance for long-term good results if the medial compartment is not unloaded (e.g. with a valgus osteotomy).

Concomitant injuries like ACL or meniscal lesions play definitely an important role. The successful treatment along with the cartilage treatment substantially increases the chance for an uneventful, successful and durable recovery to preinjury sports activities. These concomitant lesions seemed not to affect the final outcome in medium and long term, if treated along with the treatment of cartilage lesions with ACI [18, 29, 30]. The results have been durable and at last follow-up, 82 % had good or excellent clinical result. No sagittal or rotational instability was reported and the macroscopic assessment of the cartilage repair tissue (according to ICRS evaluation) after simultaneous ACI and ACL surgery showed a very good filling, surface appearance and integration to the surrounding healthy cartilage (10.9 points out of 12). Biopsies taken revealed a "hyaline-like" microscopic appearance in 80 % of the cases. In summary ACI/ACL patients have been followed up repeatedly up to 20 years and over 80 % reported good/excellent results with objectively supported data. Ninety two percent reported that they would do the ACI/ ACL operation again [18].

Nevertheless, the good clinical result especially in this demanding patient group of high competitive athletes is highly dependent on the quality of the repair tissue at the cartilage lesion area. The systematic review of Harris et al. has shown that "ability to return to play and ability to perform on return are affected positively after ACI and negatively after microfracture" [11]. In large defects MF results in a lower rate of return to sports and in a lower performance of the athletes that finally return. Even in the successive cases there is a higher possibility of gradual deterioration of the clinical scores and performance over the first years [1, 31–33]. There is evidence to show that this deterioration is not found, at least not to this degree, in the ACI-treated patients.

25.6 Conclusion/Suggestions

It seems that there is not an optimal treatment for the cartilage defects in football players and other athletes. Although the algorithms set for the general population may be of great prognostic value, a lot of other factors may influence and determine our treatment protocol. These factors may have to do with the lesion and the medical situation itself, although sadly it is very often that other nonmedical factors related to the career perspectives of the athlete play the most critical role.

Therefore, a careful assessment of the patient-player is required along with a detailed discussion of the treatment options, the possibilities, the anticipated outcomes and all the parameters related to the anticipated rehabilitation time, the complication rate and the potential long-term impact on the knee joint.

The currently available evidence shows a superiority of ACI in terms of return to sports, return to preinjury levels and durability of good outcomes. However, the ACI is a two-stage operation, associated with a longer and more demanding rehabilitation protocol. On the other hand, although MF is associated with a less postoperative morbidity and a short-term good outcome may be observed, it is associated with a lower sports performance, higher rate of retirement and long-term deterioration of the clinical outcomes. Regarding MP-OATS, although good results have been reported, there is not much evidence to allow for safe conclusions. No evidence exists for other treatment options like osteochondral allografts or one-step procedures with the use of scaffolds.

Regarding concomitant lesions like ACL or meniscal injuries, they should definitely be assessed along with the cartilage treatment, if possible addressed in the same surgery. Osteotomies may be needed to correct the limb axis or patellofemoral alignment, although this should be made clear to the athlete that they are accompanied with an increased morbidity and the chances for full-performance sports participation may be reduced.

Overall, a general algorithm that could apply for high competitive players is provided in the algorithm (Figs. 25.1, 25.2, and 25.3).

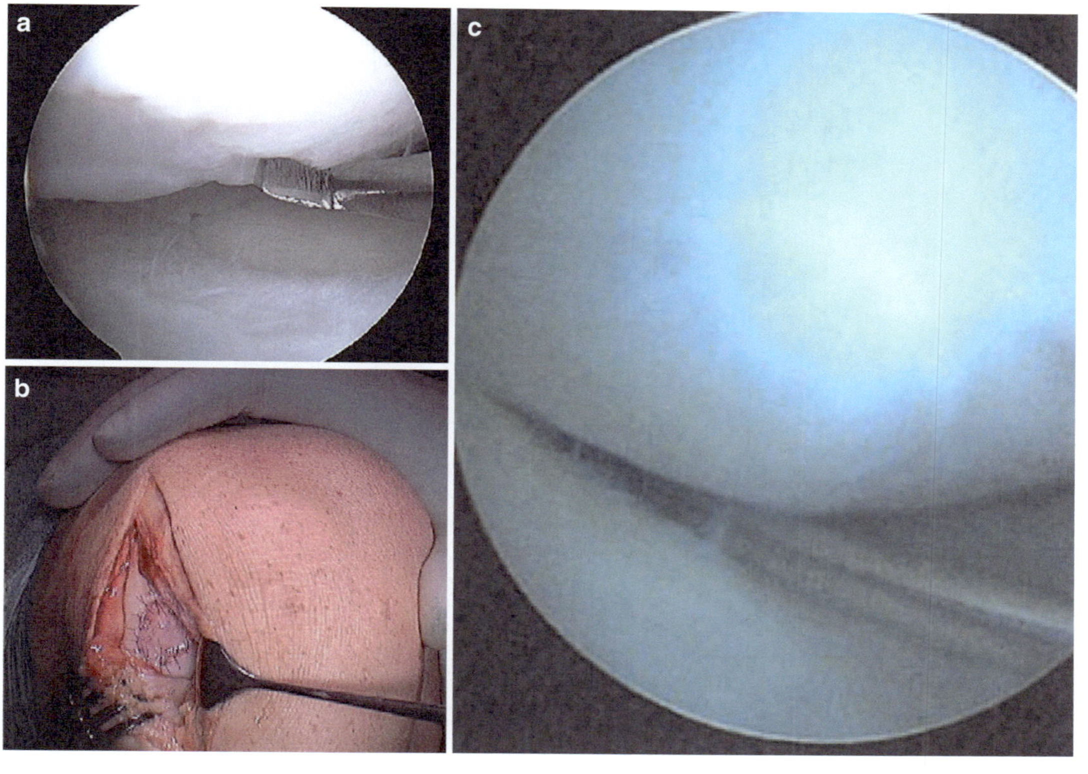

Fig. 25.1 (**a**) A 32-year-old professional football player in English Premier League. Arthroscopy 1 year after failed microfracture of lateral femoral condyle lesion. (**b**) ACI through lateral mini-arthrotomy. (**c**) Arthroscopy 12 months after ACI showing complete healing. Returned to football at 15 months

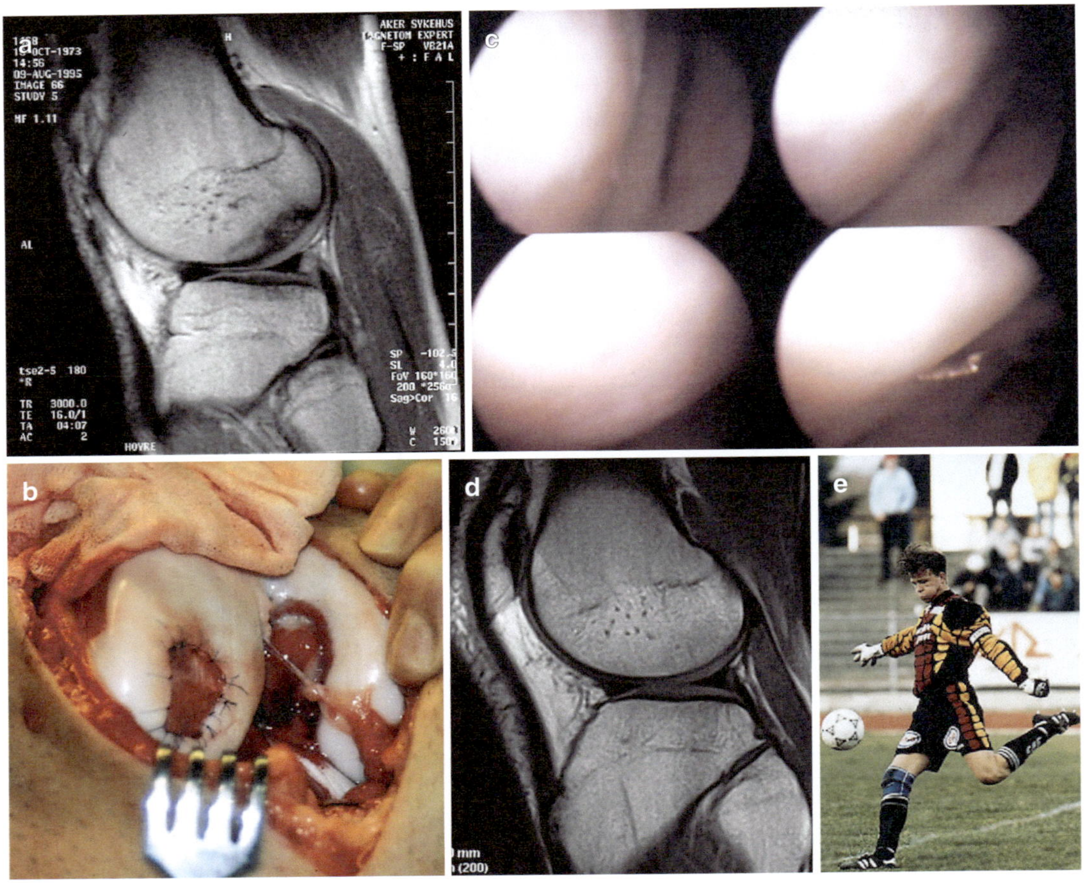

Fig. 25.2 (**a**) A 24-year-old football player in the English Premier League. Periodic knee pain and swelling since teenage. Recurring catching and the last year synovitis and massive hydrops making it impossible to play, a career-threatening situation. MRI showing osteochondritis dissecans on the lateral femoral condyle. (**b**) Arthrotomy with ACI in1995 with removal of the unstable fragment, diagnosed earlier by arthroscopy followed by debridement of the fibrous tissue in the bony bottom and cell implantation under a periosteal flap. (**c**) Arthroscopy 12 months later showing a complete healing, good stiffness, smooth surface and complete integration of the repair tissue on probing. Returned to football and first match 15 months postop. (**d**) Followed by repeated MRI and 9 years after surgery, MRI showed a complete healing of bone and overlying cartilage. Signed a new contract at that time. (**e**) Still playing in his national league 18 years after ACI

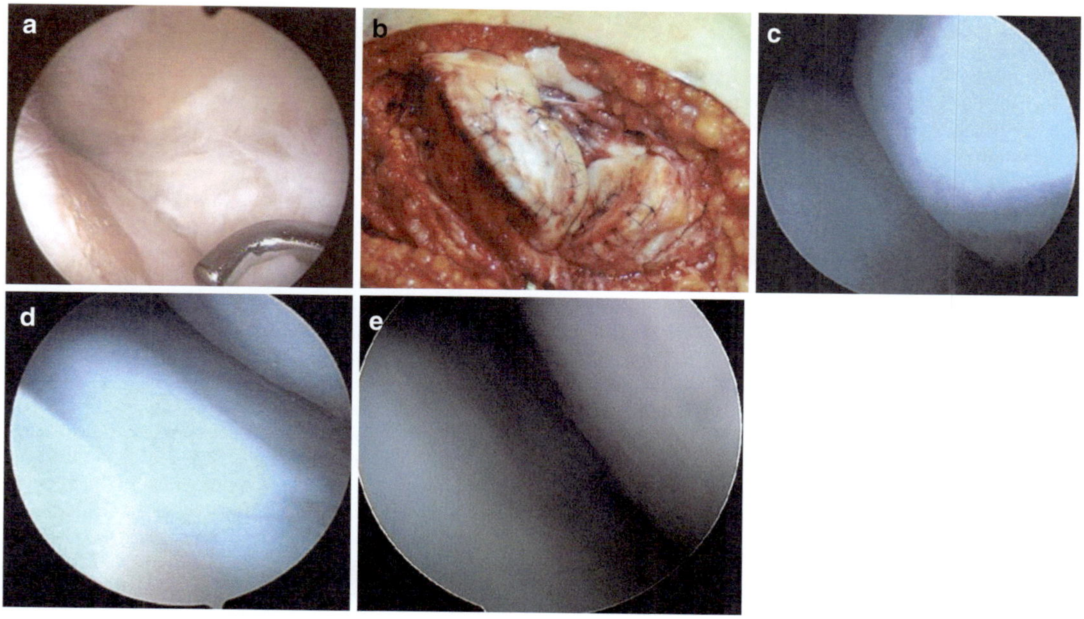

Fig. 25.3 (**a**) A 39-year-old ex-female football player, who injured her left knee and had a total medial meniscectomy at the age of 16 years. Arthroscopy 1995 and 1998 with shaving of articular cartilage legion medial femoral and tibial condyles. Arthroscopy 2000 showed bipolar lesions down to bone in medial compartment. (**b**) ACI performed on medial femoral condyle (size 32 × 17 mm) and medial tibial condyle(size 30 × 15 mm) and unloading HTO closing wedge. (**c**) Arthroscopy 16 months postop showed complete healing of femoral condyle lesion in medial compartment. (**d**) Same arthroscopy at 16 months showing tibial condyle lesion with complete healing. (**e**) Arthroscopy at 4 years showing durable healing medial compartment. At 14 years after ACI, the patient is completely free of symptoms, is working full time as an X-ray technician and is in regular physical training

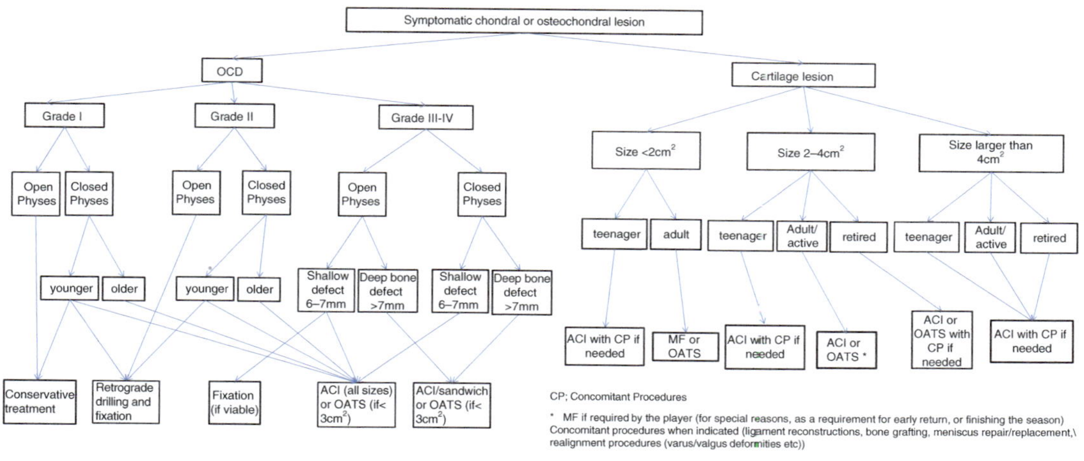

References

1. Mithoefer K, Williams RJ, Warren RF, Wickiewicz TL, Marx RG (2006) High-impact athletics after knee articular cartilage repair: a prospective evaluation of the microfracture technique. Am J Sports Med 34:1413–1418
2. Noyes FR, Bassett RW, Grood ES, Butler DL (1980) Arthroscopy in acute traumatic hemarthrosis of the knee. Incidence of anterior cruciate tears and other injuries. J Bone Joint Surg Am 62:687–695, 757
3. Curl WW, Krome J, Gordon ES, Rushing J, Smith BP, Poehling GG (1997) Cartilage injuries: a review of 31,516 knee arthroscopies. Arthrosc J Arthrosc Relat Surg Off Publ Arthrosc Assoc N Am Int Arthrosc Assoc 13:456–460
4. Hjelle K, Solheim E, Strand T, Muri R, Brittberg M (2002) Articular cartilage defects in 1,000 knee arthroscopies. Arthrosc J Arthrosc Relat Surg Off Publ Arthrosc Assoc N Am Int Arthrosc Assoc 18:730–734
5. Mithoefer K, Hambly K, Della Villa S, Silvers H, Mandelbaum BR (2009) Return to sports participation after articular cartilage repair in the knee: scientific evidence. Am J Sports Med 37(Suppl 1):167S–176S
6. Piasecki DP, Spindler KP, Warren TA, Andrish JT, Parker RD (2003) Intraarticular injuries associated with anterior cruciate ligament tear: findings at ligament reconstruction in high school and recreational athletes. An analysis of sex-based differences. Am J Sports Med 31:601–605
7. Brophy RH, Rodeo SA, Barnes RP, Powell JW, Warren RF (2009) Knee articular cartilage injuries in the National Football League: epidemiology and treatment approach by team physicians. J Knee Surg 22:331–338
8. Noyes FR, Mooar PA, Matthews DS, Butler DL (1983) The symptomatic anterior cruciate-deficient knee. Part I: the long-term functional disability in athletically active individuals. J Bone Joint Surg Am 65:154–162
9. Drawer S, Fuller CW (2001) Propensity for osteoarthritis and lower limb joint pain in retired professional soccer players. Br J Sports Med 35:402–408
10. Kujala UM, Kettunen J, Paananen H, Aalto T, Battié MC, Impivaara O, Videman T, Sarna S (1995) Knee osteoarthritis in former runners, soccer players, weight lifters, and shooters. Arthritis Rheum 38:539–546
11. Harris JD, Brophy RH, Siston RA, Flanigan DC (2010) Treatment of chondral defects in the athlete's knee. Arthrosc J Arthrosc Relat Surg Off Publ Arthrosc Assoc N Am Int Arthrosc Assoc 26:841–852
12. Gudas R, Stankevicius E, Monastyreckiene E, Pranys D, Kalesinskas RJ (2006) Osteochondral autologous transplantation versus microfracture for the treatment of articular cartilage defects in the knee joint in athletes. Knee Surg Sports Traumatol Arthrosc Off ESSKA 14:834–842
13. Steadman JR, Miller BS, Karas SG, Schlegel TF, Briggs KK, Hawkins RJ (2003) The microfracture technique in the treatment of full-thickness chondral lesions of the knee in National Football League players. J Knee Surg 16:83–86
14. Namdari S, Baldwin K, Anakwenze O, Park M-J, Huffman GR, Sennett BJ (2009) Results and performance after microfracture in National Basketball Association athletes. Am J Sports Med 37:943–948
15. Cerynik DL, Lewullis GE, Joves BC, Palmer MP, Tom JA (2009) Outcomes of microfracture in professional basketball players. Knee Surg Sports Traumatol Arthrosc Off J ESSKA 17:1135–1139
16. Cole BJ, Pascual-Garrido C, Grumet RC (2009) Surgical management of articular cartilage defects in the knee. J Bone Joint Surg Am 91:1778–1790
17. Nagel A, Insall JN, Scuderi GR (1996) Proximal tibial osteotomy. A subjective outcome study. J Bone Joint Surg Am 78:1353–1358
18. Peterson L, Vasiliadis HS, Brittberg M, Lindahl A (2010) Autologous chondrocyte implantation: a long-term follow-up. Am J Sports Med 38:1117–1124
19. Peterson L (2003) Autologous Chondrocyte Implantation, In; Master Techniques in Orthopaedic Surgery: Reconstructive Knee Surgery. Second Edition. Douglas W. Jackson (Ed). Lippincott Williams & Wilkins, Philadelphia, 2002; 353–373
20. Peterson L (2009) Autologous chondrocyte implantation. In: Noyes FR (ed) Noyes knee disord surg rehabil clin outcomes saunders https://books.google.gr/books?id=s-4cvT0c3E8C&dq=Peterson+L+%282009%29+Autologous+chondrocyte+implantation.+In:+Noyes+FR+%28ed%29+Noyes+knee+disord+surg+rehabil+clin+outcomes+saunders&lr=&source=gbs_navlinks_s
21. Peterson L (2003) Articular Cartilage lesions in football players. In; Football Traumatology: Current Concepts: from Prevention to Treatment. Piero Volpi (ed), Springer Milan, pp 255–261
22. Mithöfer K, Peterson L, Mandelbaum BR, Minas T (2005) Articular cartilage repair in soccer players with autologous chondrocyte transplantation: functional outcome and return to competition. Am J Sports Med 33:1639–1646
23. Mithöfer K, Minas T, Peterson L, Yeon H, Micheli LJ (2005) Functional outcome of knee articular cartilage repair in adolescent athletes. Am J Sports Med 33:1147–1153
24. Vanlauwe J, Saris DB, Victor J, Almqvist KF, Bellemans J, Luyten FP, TIG ACT (2011) Five-year outcome of characterized chondrocyte implantation versus microfracture for symptomatic cartilage defects of the knee: early treatment matters. Am J Sports Med 39:2566–2574
25. De Windt TS, Bekkers JEJ, Creemers LB, Dhert WJA, Saris DBF (2009) Patient profiling in cartilage regeneration: prognostic factors determining success of treatment for cartilage defects. Am J Sports Med 37(Suppl 1):58S–62S
26. Knutsen G, Drogset JO, Engebretsen L, Grøntvedt T, Isaksen V, Ludvigsen TC, Roberts S, Solheim E, Strand T, Johansen O (2007) A randomized trial comparing autologous chondrocyte implantation with microfracture. Findings at five years. J Bone Joint Surg Am 89:2105–2112

27. Riyami M, Rolf C (2009) Evaluation of microfracture of traumatic chondral injuries to the knee in professional football and rugby players. J Orthop Surg 4:13
28. Minas T, Gomoll AH, Rosenberger R, Royce RO, Bryant T (2009) Increased failure rate of autologous chondrocyte implantation after previous treatment with marrow stimulation techniques. Am J Sports Med 37:902–908
29. Peterson L, Brittberg M, Kiviranta I, Akerlund EL, Lindahl A (2002) Autologous chondrocyte transplantation. Biomechanics and long-term durability. Am J Sports Med 30:2–12
30. Peterson L, Minas T, Brittberg M, Nilsson A, Sjögren-Jansson E, Lindahl A (2000) Two – to 9-year outcome after autologous chondrocyte transplantation of the knee. Clin Orthop 374:212–234
31. Blevins FT, Steadman JR, Rodrigo JJ, Silliman J (1998) Treatment of articular cartilage defects in athletes: an analysis of functional outcome and lesion appearance. Orthopedics 21:761–767, discussion 767–768
32. Gobbi A, Nunag P, Malinowski K (2005) Treatment of full thickness chondral lesions of the knee with microfracture in a group of athletes. Knee Surg Sports Traumatol Arthrosc Off J ESSKA 13: 213–221
33. Kon E, Gobbi A, Filardo G, Delcogliano M, Zaffagnini S, Marcacci M (2009) Arthroscopic second-generation autologous chondrocyte implantation compared with microfracture for chondral lesions of the knee: prospective nonrandomized study at 5 years. Am J Sports Med 37:33–41

Patellar Tendon Lesions

26

E. Prospero, M. Denti, A. Quaglia, L. Pulici, L. Brambilla, and Piero Volpi

26.1 Introduction

Tendinopathy and patellar tendon ruptures are two different clinical entities representing an important problem in many sports. The former is a tendon degenerative pathology following a functional overload. Symptoms occur in 20 % of athletes. The clinical course of this disease can lasts for 32 months because of a high rate of recurrence of symptomatology [1, 2]. The latter is a rare and acute event which can be so severe to impair an athlete's career. It often occurs in tendons previously mechanically stressed and it has been considered as the last step of the degenerative evolution of the tendon structure. Rarely it can affect apparently healthy tendons. Basketball and volleyball are the sports more interested by these pathologies, respectively, with an incidence of 31.9 % and 44.6 % [3], mostly because of the mechanics of sport-specific gestures, characterized by high speed and power demand on the extensor apparatus. This disease was described in 1973 by Blazina as "jumper's knee" and this definition has been preserved until now [4].

The prevalence of tendinitis in football players ranges from 5 % to 32 % [5–7]. It is less than in the sports mentioned above, likely because the different sport-specific gestures imply less mechanical stress. Both diseases imply a difficult management of the athlete: : or because of the severe symptomatology and severe impairment of sport performance or because of the long period of stop in case of tendon rupture.

E. Prospero (✉) • M. Denti • A. Quaglia • L. Pulici
L. Brambilla
Knee Surgery and Sport Traumatology, Humanitas Research-IRCCS, 20089 Milan, Italy
e-mail: emanuele.prospero@humanitas.it

P. Volpi
Knee Orthopedics and Sport Traumatology Unit, Humanitas Clinical Institute IRCCS, Milan, Italy

Head of Medical Staff FC Internazionale Milan, Milan, Italy

26.2 Epidemiology and Risk Factors

Data on this topic show a variable prevalence of patellar tendinopathy ranging from 5 % to 32 % in football players with an incidence peak between 15 and 30 years: it is the period in which most patients practice sport activities. Going on with sport activities can lead to other cases in older ages. Hagglund et al., according to others, show that during an entire season, the 2. 4 % of football players investigated didn't take part to some training sessions or matches because of patellar tendinopathy. In most cases the absences lasted a maximum of 1 week, but there was a high rate of recurrence because of the chronic trend of this pathology [8]. The risk was related to the exposition, showing an incidence of 0, 12 injuries every 1,000 h played. There are no available data about the rupture of the patellar tendon: no cases

P. Volpi (ed.), *Football Traumatology: New Trends*, DOI 10.1007/978-3-319-18245-2_26

are reported in the study mentioned above. This confirms the rarity of the event, but anyway it is extremely feared for the possible complications for the career. In sportsmen the patellar tendon rupture can be considered as the final stage of the tendinopathy, so it can be supposed that, in the professional players investigated by Hagglund et al., an early diagnosis and an adequate treatment, including load reduction on the tendon during the symptomatic period, may have helped to prevent this complication. Different risk factors for the diseases are described and can be classified into intrinsic and extrinsic.

Intrinsic risk factors can't be modified and can give information about which groups of athletes have to be monitored:

- Gender: the incidence is double in male than females. This was due to different capacity in generating force and to the ability of the athletic movement [1].
- Age: the tendinopathy is considered to be linked to overload, so the greater the age, the greater the stress on the tendon at the same level of sport activity.
- Rheumatologic diseases and collagenopathies: these can change the structure of the tendon and decrease the mechanical resistance.
- Injury of the contralateral tendon: patients with a contralateral overload can be more susceptible for developing pathologies of the other tendon.
- Anatomy: there are different opinions about anatomical features predisposing to jumper's knee tendinopathy [9].

Extrinsic risk factors are the most interesting for the professional sportsman and are the once for whom it is possible to apply preventive measures.

Sport-specific gestures: it is impossible to modify them, but it is possible to improve the technique of execution to reduce the load and the frequency of execution in at-risk or symptomatic people.

- Environment and playground: in volleyball players it was shown that a harder ground increases the risk of developing the tendinopathy [1]. Concerning football players no differences were indicated between the incidence of the pathology in athletes playing on natural ground and the incidence in athletes playing on synthetic ground.
- Equipments: mechanical properties of footwear and cleats can change the friction coefficient and the mechanical load on the limb. It is important to choose the best footwear according to the features of the ground, in order to reduce microtrauma from impact with the ground. More often knee bandages are used to reduce the load on the tendon in athletes who have early symptoms, but their benefit is doubtful.
- Exposition level: many hours of training and sports are the most important risk factor for the development of patellar tendon pathology [2, 10]. Some authors have shown a relation between the risk of developing the jumper's knee and 12 h/week training or matches; the same link has been pointed out with 5 h/week training with weights [11, 12]. This is the risk factor more difficult to manage because of the growing agonistic demand and the difficulty of a simultaneous management of the needs of the athlete and those of the company and the team.

26.3 Biomechanics of the Extensor Apparatus

Patellar tendon is the terminal part of the thigh's extensor apparatus, responsible for leg extension, so the tendon supports the work of the muscles and endures a high mechanical stress, mostly at the level of its patellar origin and its tibial insertion. The extensor apparatus can perform both eccentric and concentric work. Patellar tendon is very durable to tensile force and it is proven that a very high strength is required to break a healthy tendon [13, 14]. However, the continuous stress, due to repetitive sport-specific gestures, can lead to an overload pathology. Patellar tendon is stressed in different ways according to the degree of knee flexion: between 45° and 60° the position of the patellae and the high forces exerted on the tendon result in a higher probability of having injuries, above during eccentric work [15]. The greatest muscle strength, produced in an eccentric way, is 1, 5–2 times higher than the greatest isometric force and the higher concentric force, above at high speeds [16]. The force transmitted from the ground varies according to different athletic feats and corresponds to 2.8 times the body weight during long-distance running, to six times the body weight during volleyball jumping, and to ten times the body weight during the takeoff of the long jump [17]. The highest forces of load transmission to the quadriceps occur during the ballistic reaction with the "drop jumps," during which the forces transmitted to the quadriceps are proportional to the reaction force of the ground. So it is reasonable to assume a link between the working model of the quadriceps and the prevalence of the jumper's knee. This assumption seems to be validated by the distribution of the prevalence reported in several studies. This is highest in basketball, volleyball, and athletics and low or negligible in other sports.

26.4 Pathogenesis

The features underlined by histopathological studies concerning patellar tendinopathy are the separation of the collagen fibers with eventual loss of the normal organization, a most fundamental mucoid substance, morphological changes of tenocytes, fibrocartilaginous metaplasia, and cell and capillary proliferation [18, 19]. The connection between the conditions of mechanical load and the pathophysiological response is unknown. It was suggested that the mechanical overload can produce partial ruptures in the tendon tissue and the histological results have been interpreted as partial tendon ruptures [6, 7, 12]. The hypoechoic lesions, observed in the proximal patellar tendon, associated to tendinopathy are usually described as a result of the failed healing or as partial tendon ruptures. Some classical theories suppose that the lack of traction promotes healing and adaptation of tension; a too high traction might prevent healing and promote the accumulation of degenerative tissue. Other authors suggest that an excessive mechanical stretching of the tenocytes may activate some signal pathways able to induce apoptosis. Histological findings, observed during tendinopathy, are compatible with an apoptotic process. It can be possible that when the mechanical load is higher than the adaptive response of tenocytes, apoptosis is induced [20].

26.5 Clinical Symptoms

Patellar tendinopathy is characterized by pain; it can manifest in an acute, subacute, or in an intermittent way, usually not following local trauma; it can be associated to a change in the type or in the frequency of training, to a work overload. Usually the pain is reported in specific sites, mostly located at the level of insertion near the lower apex of the patella; in the remaining cases the pain can be localized to the tendon or to the distal insertion of it. For a long time the clinical classification more followed was Blazina's that was improved and divided into six stages according to clinical symptoms (Table 26.1).

In the first Blazina's classification, the last step was related to the catastrophic rupture of the patellar tendon, a rare but possible eventuality. Usually the symptoms described above disappear with a break from sports activities, especially if it is the first episode, but symptoms can recur if the patient resumes physical training too early or with excessive workloads. More attention should be paid to the recovery time of patients with chronic tendinopathy. Concerning patellar tendon rupture, the physician should carefully evaluate the swelling and the hematoma in the patella that can be associated with a hemarthrosis. The more evident and limiting clinical sign is the inability to an active extension of the leg and to lift the extended limb; this makes the gait difficult also using some aids.

Table 26.1 Classification of patellar tendinopathy according to clinical symptoms

Stage 0	No pain
Stage I	Rare pain with normal performance
Stage II	Moderate pain during sports activities with normal performance
Stage III	Pain during sports activities with initial qualitative or quantitative limitation of performance
Stage IV	Pain during sports activities with an important decrement of performance
Stage V	Pain during daily life and impossibility in practice sport

26.6 Instrumental Diagnosis

Injuries of the patellar tendon can be investigated by using conventional radiology, echography, and MRI. It is possible to evaluate the presence of insertional or peritendinous calcifications by standard radiographies, mostly in case of chronic pathologies, bipartite patella, and outcomes of Osgood-Schlatter disease or Sinding-Larsen-Johansson. Performing X-ray, when the patellar tendon is broken, enables to investigate the possible ascent of the patella, with the lateral projections, and any bone avulsions, including those that are articular. The echography, using linear high-resolution probes, can point out the presence of hypoechoic areas in tendon, associated with the presence of an edematous perilesional variably extended. Ultrasound allows to make regular inspections to investigate the evolution of the patellar injury in a practical and noninvasive way. The execution of ultrasound also in patients with patellar ruptures is indicated for assessing the location and the extent of the lesion, the hemorrhage, and the involvement of the surrounding soft tissues. MRI is an exam very sensible for evaluating the patellar pathology, allowing to assess the morphology of the tendon and to delimit the location and the extent of damage of the tendon. Using MRI it is possible to highlight an area of high signal intensity on T1 and T2 (Fig. 26.1), and often the tendon with tendinopathy appears thickened and deformed [21, 22]. Performing MRI in patients affected by rupture of the patellar tendon allows also to assess the quality of the tendon and the type and the site of the lesion. In this group of patients, it can be useful also to identify associated joint injuries.

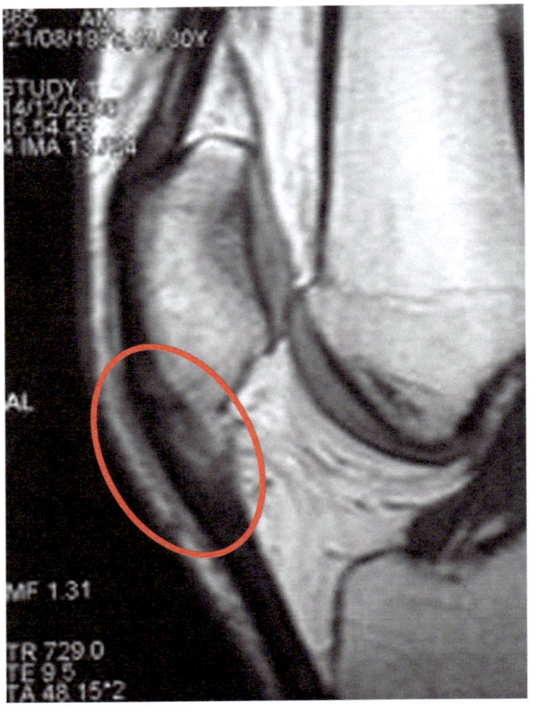

Fig. 26.1 Tendon with deformity and altered signal

26.7 Treatment

Usually the treatment for an athlete affected by patellar tendinopathy is conservative; surgery is often postponed. The treatment should be carefully planned and the physician should modulate and quantify the type, the load and the timing of exercise, the abstention from particular activities, and the rest period. The athlete needs to be informed about what happened and a protocol should be started for the reeducation, rehabilitation, and redistribution of the load and of the intensity of work. The sportsman, during the symptomatic period, should begin a training including all kinds of exercises but mostly eccentric ones and stretching. These are suggested to all patients with acute tendinopathy, working mainly on the phase of deceleration and on gradual recovery of elasticity; this treatment can be associated with hydrokinesitherapy and with manual massage to relax the quadriceps.

We can divide therapies into medical and physical. The medical ones help to solve the clinical symptoms; for this reason there are many drugs available, above FANS, with systemic and local action. There are different opinions about appropriateness of local injections of cortisone; these can be useful in reducing symptoms temporarily, but on the other hand, these can cause tendon ruptures. In order to improve the clinical symptoms, physical therapies can be performed. Cryotherapy, TENS, laser, ultrasound, Tecar Therapy, shockwave, and magnetic fields are the most used techniques on the tendon to relieve pain. Especially the shockwave seems to play an additional role in stimulating tendon tissue regeneration [23, 24]. Another kind of therapy that has spread in the last decade for the patellar tendinopathy is the injection with autologous platelet-rich plasma (PRP)[25]; the purpose is to try to stimulate healing of the tendon tissue using platelet growth factors. One or more injections can be performed in a few days. Comparing them with shockwave seems that the results of PRP injections are better from the biological point of view [26]. Anyway in the literature the results are controversial, mostly because of the different method of preparation and concentration of the substance to inject [27].

This approach in patients affected by patellar tendinopathy might allow the recovery of the sport activities in a period ranging from a few weeks up to 6 months; if symptoms persists or worsen, surgery should be considered. There are various surgical options, but all have as their main purpose the stimulation and facilitation of the tendon healing. Since in most cases the tendinitis is proximal, the most used surgical approach consists of some steps: slice longitudinally the tendon for a few centimeters, in correspondence with the injured area, previously evaluated with MRI; remove the part of possible degenerated tendon tissue (Fig. 26.2); and perform a cruentation of the patellar apex and some small perforations in the apex in order to facilitate the flow of blood in the interested area. It is possible to perform some tendon scarification if the injured area is extended. The same procedure can be used in case of distal tendinopathy, performing scarifications and perforations of the ATA, eventually associated with the removal of the degenerated tissue. During the execution of this surgical technique, it is possible to use PRP gel (Fig. 26.3).

In case of patellar tendon rupture, a discriminating factor able to condition a good outcome of the surgical treatment and of the function recovery is the time since the accident. The injuries treated in the acute phase seem to have a better complete functional recovery. The surgical treatment of the acute rupture of the proximal or distal insertion of the patellar tendon consists in the reinsertion of the tendon to the bone component. It can be made using transosseous sutures or suture anchors in order to restore the bone-tendon continuity. This first step has to be associated to a biological augmentation (Fig. 26.4) in a resorbable or nonresorbable material [15]. Some authors suggest also a transosseous wire augmentation.

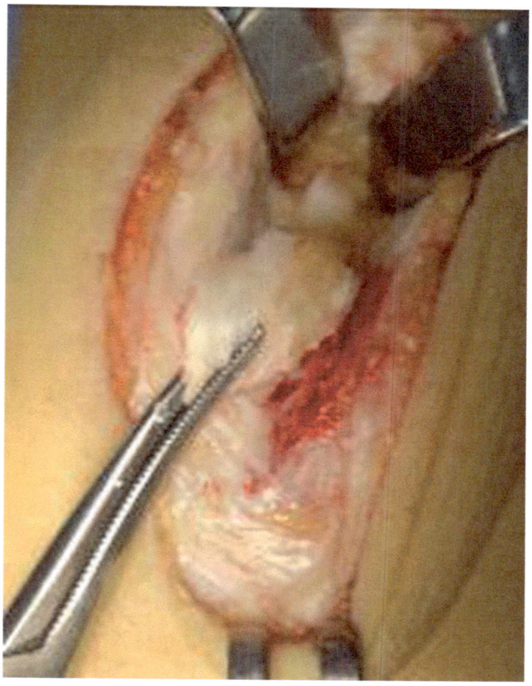

Fig. 26.2 Removal of degeneration tendon tissue

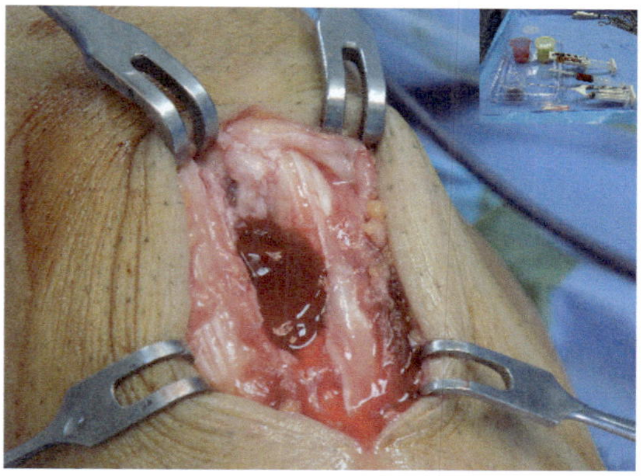

Fig. 26.3 Preparation and application of PRP

In case of ruptures of the central part of the tendon, the continuity of it has to be restored taking back the patella to its original site and eventually associating an augmentation, biological or in resorbable material. Also in this case there are

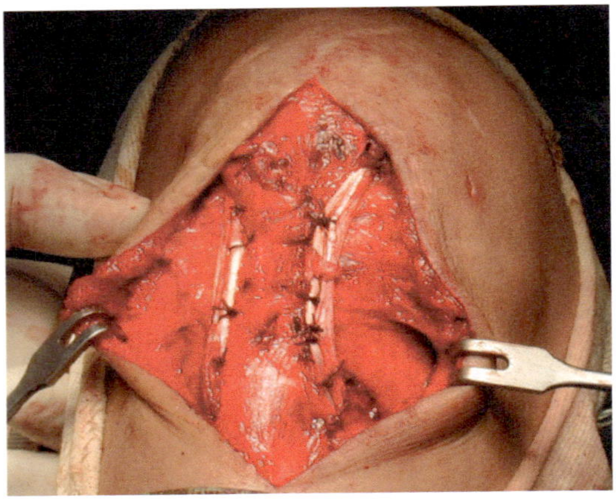

Fig. 26.4 Patellar tendon rupture treated with suture and biological autologous augmentation

authors who suggest a transosseous wire augmentation. Often if lesions are unrecognized or chronic, perilesional or calcific scar tissue is present associated to anatomical deformity of knee detectable at the physical examination. In these cases the surgical approach is more complex with the possible difficulty to recover the right position of the patella. The treatment consists in the initial removal of the scar tissue and calcifications and in the cruentation of the ends of the tendon. Sometimes the gap cannot be filled without a "zed" elongation of the patellar tendon. If the ruptures are inveterate with a considerable ascent of the patella, it is possible to use the technique suggested by Dejour, transplanting the distal part of the extensor apparatus of the contralateral knee [28]. Alternatively tendon allograft or autologous tendon transplantation (semitendinosus and gracilis tendons) can be used to minimize the iatrogenic lesions for the contralateral healthy knee.

References

1. Lian OB, Engebretsen L, Bahr R (2005) Prevalence of jumper's knee among elite athletes from different sports: a cross-sectional study. Am J Sports Med 33(4):561–567, Epub 2005 Feb 8
2. Hägglund M, Zwerver J, Ekstrand J (2011) Epidemiology of patellar tendinopathy in elite male soccer players. Am J Sports Med 39(9):1906–1911, Epub 2011 Jun 3
3. Ferretti A (1986) Epidemiology of jumper's knee. Sports Med 3(4):289–295
4. Blazina ME, Kerlan RK, Jobe FW, Carter VS, Carlson GJ (1973) Jumper's knee. Orthop Clin North Am 4(3):665–678
5. Raatikainen T, Karpakka J, Puranen J, Orava S (1994) Operative treatment of partial rupture of the patellar ligament. A study of 138 cases. Int J Sports Med 15(1):46–49
6. Martens M, Wouters P, Burssens A, Mulier JC (1982) Patellar tendinitis: pathology and results of treatment. Acta Orthop Scand 53(3):445–450
7. Karlsson J, Lundin O, Lossing IW, Peterson L (1991) Partial rupture of the patellar ligament. Results after operative treatment. Am J Sports Med 19(4):403–408
8. Fredberg U, Bolvig L, Andersen NT (2008) Prophylactic training in asymptomatic soccer players with ultrasonographic abnormalities in Achilles and patellar tendons: the Danish Super League Study. Am J Sports Med 36(3):451–460, Epub 2007 Dec 13
9. Khan KM, Cook JL, Maffulli N (2005) Patellar tendinopathy and patellar tendon rupture-Tendon Injuries. Springer 166–177
10. Gaida JE, Cook JL, Bass SL, Austen S, Kiss ZS (2004) Are unilateral and bilateral patellar tendinopathy distinguished by differences in anthropometry, body composition, or muscle strength in elite female basketball players? Br J Sports Med 38(5):581–585
11. Cook JL, Khan KM, Kiss ZS, Griffiths L (2000) Patellar tendinopathy in junior basketball players: a controlled clinical and ultrasonographic study of 268 patellar tendons in players aged 14–18 years. Scand J Med Sci Sports 10(4):216–220
12. Lian Ø, Refsnes PE, Engebretsen L, Bahr R (2003) Performance characteristics of volleyball players with patellar tendinopathy. Am J Sports Med 31(3):408–413
13. Rauh M, Parker R (2009) Patellar and quadriceps tendinopathies and ruptures. In: DeLee JC (ed) DeLee and Drez's orthopaedic sports medicine. Saunders, Philadelphia, pp 192–200
14. Zernicke RF, Garhammer J, Jobe FW (1977) Human patellar-tendon rupture. J Bone Joint Surg Am 59(2): 179–183
15. Lee D, Stinner D, Mir H (2013) Quadriceps and patellar tendon ruptures. J Knee Surg 26:301–308
16. Herzog W (2000) Muscle properties and coordination during voluntary movement. J Sports Sci 18(3): 141–152
17. McNitt-Gray JL (2000) Musculoskeletal loading during landing. In: Biomechanics in sport. Encyclopaedia of sports medicine, vol 9. Blackwell Science, Oxford
18. Cook JL, Khan KM, Harcourt PR, Grant M, Young DA, Bonar SF (1997) A cross sectional study of 100 athletes with jumper's knee managed conservatively and surgically. The Victorian Institute of Sport Tendon Study Group. Br J Sports Med 31(4): 332–336
19. Khan KM, Bonar F, Desmond PM, Cook JL, Young DA, Visentini PJ, Fehrmann MW, Kiss ZS, O'Brien PA, Harcourt PR, Dowling RJ, O'Sullivan RM, Crichton

KJ, Tress BM, Wark JD (1996) Patellar tendinosis (jumper's knee): findings at histopathologic examination, US, and MR imaging. Victorian Institute of Sport Tendon Study Group. Radiology 200(3):821–827
20. Lian Ø, Scott A, Engebretsen L, Bahr R, Duronio V, Khan K (2007) Excessive apoptosis in patellar tendinopathy in athletes. Am J Sports Med 35(4):605–611, Epub 2007 Jan 23
21. Yu JS, Popp JE, Kaeding CC, Lucas J (1995) Correlation of MR imaging and pathologic findings in athletes undergoing surgery for chronic patellar tendinitis. AJR Am J Roentgenol 165(1):115–118
22. El-Khoury GY, Wira RL, Berbaum KS, Pope TL Jr, Monu JU (1992) MR imaging of patellar tendinitis. Radiology 184(3):849–854
23. De Girolamo L, Stanco D, Galliera E, Viganò M, Lovati AB, Marazzi MG, Romeo P, Sansone V (2014) Soft-focused extracorporeal shock waves increase the expression of tendon-specific markers and the release of anti-inflammatory cytokines in an adherent culture model of primary human tendon cells. Ultrasound Med Biol 40(6):1
24. Furia JP, Rompe JD, Cacchio A, Del Buono A, Maffulli N (2013) A single application of low-energy radial extracorporeal shock wave therapy is effective for the management of chronic patellar tendinopathy. Knee Surg Sports Traumatol Arthrosc 21(2):346–350
25. Volpi P, Quaglia A, Schoenhuber H, Melegati G, Corsi MM, Banfi G, de Girolamo L (2010) Growth factors in the management of sport-induced tendinopathies: results after 24 months from treatment. A pilot study. J Sports Med Phys Fitness 50(4):494–500
26. Smith J, Sellon JL (2014) Comparing PRP injections with ESWT for athletes with chronic patellar tendinopathy. Clin J Sport Med 24(1):88–89
27. Moraes VY, Lenza M, Tamaoki MJ, Faloppa F, Belloti JC (2014) Platelet-rich therapies for musculoskeletal soft tissue injuries. Cochrane Database Syst Rev 29(4):CD010071
28. Dejour H, Denjean S, Neyret P (1992) Treatment of old or recurrent ruptures of the patellar ligament by contralateral autograft. Rev Chir Orthop Reparatrice Appar Mot 78(1):58–62

PRP in Football Players

27

Ramon Cugat, Xavier Cusco, Roberto Seijas, Pedro Alvarez, Gilbert Steinbacher, and Marta Rius

27.1 Introduction

Football is played by approximately 5 % of the Spanish population aged between 15 and 35 years old and regulated by the Spanish Football Federation. This high prevalence also carries a high rate of associated injuries. The Catalan Soccer Federation is a sports association in the autonomous region of Catalonia, Spain, with more than 140,000 members. Approximately

R. Cugat (✉) • P. Alvarez
Mutualidad de Futbolistas, Real Federacion Espanola de Futbol, Ronda de San Pedro 19, 08010 Barcelona, Spain

Chair of Medicine and Regenerative Surgery, Garcia Cugat Foundation and CEU Cardenal Herrera University, C/Tirant lo Blanc, 7, 46115, Alfara del Patriarca, Valencia, Spain

Department of Orthopaedic Surgery, Sports Medicine and Trauma, Hospital Quiron Barcelona, Artroscopia gc,S.L, Plaza Alfonso Comin, 5–7, 08023 Barcelona, Spain

Facultad de Medicina, Universitat Internacional de Catalunya, Carrer Inmaculada, 22, 08017 Barcelona, Spain
e-mail: ramon.cugat@sportrauma.com; drpedroalvarezdiaz@gmail.com, info@artroscopiagc.es, info@fundaciongarciacugat.org, www.fundaciongarciacugat.org, www.artroscopiagc.es

X. Cusco
Chair of Medicine and Regenerative Surgery, Garcia Cugat Foundation and CEU Cardenal Herrera University, C/Tirant lo Blanc, 7, 46115, Alfara del Patriarca, Valencia, Spain

Department of Orthopaedic Surgery, Sports Medicine and Trauma, Hospital Quiron Barcelona, Artroscopia gc,S.L., Plaza Alfonso Comin, 5–7, 08023 Barcelona, Spain
e-mail: info@fundaciongarciacugat.org, www.fundaciongarciacugat.org, info@artroscopiagc.es, www.artroscopiagc.es

R. Seijas
Chair of Medicine and Regenerative Surgery, Garcia Cugat Foundation & CEU Cardenal Herrera University, C/Tirant lo Blanc, 7, 46115, Alfara del Patriarca, Valencia, Spain

Department of Orthopaedic Surgery, Sports Medicine and Trauma, Hospital Quiron Barcelona, Artroscopia gc,S.L, Plaza Alfonso Comin, 5–7, 08023 Barcelona, Spain

Facultad de Medicina y Ciencias de la Salud, Universitat Internacional de Catalunya, Immaculada, 22, 08017 Barcelona, Spain
e-mail: roberto6jas@gmail.com, info@fundaciongarciacugat.org, info@artroscopiagc.es, www.fundaciongarciacugat.org, www.artroscopiagc.es, www.uic.es

G. Steinbacher • M. Rius
Mutualidad de Futbolistas, Real Federacion Espanola de Futbol, Ronda de San Pedro 19, 08010 Barcelona, Spain

Chair of Medicine and Regenerative Surgery, Garcia Cugat Foundation and CEU Cardenal Herrera University, C/Tirant lo Blanc, 7, 46115, Alfara del Patriarca, Valencia, Spain

Department of Orthopaedic Surgery, Sports Medicine and Trauma, Hospital Quiron Barcelona, Artroscopia gc,S.L, Plaza Alfonso Comin, 5–7, 08023 Barcelona, Spain
e-mail: gsteinbacher1@hotmail.com; martarius@hotmail.com, info@artroscopiagc.es, www.artroscopiagc.es, info@fundaciongarciacugat.org, www.fundaciongarciacugat.org

P. Volpi (ed.), *Football Traumatology: New Trends*, DOI 10.1007/978-3-319-18245-2_27

22,000 injuries occur annually among members of the Federation, most of which are muscle, ankle, and knee lesions. The *Mutualitat de Futbolistes* is an organization within the Catalan Soccer Federation that provides health insurance coverage for all soccer-related injuries sustained by federated soccer players in Catalonia. The idiosyncrasy of the patient in a sport like football involves diagnosis and management of the markedly different injuries when compared to the occasional athlete. The three most common injuries treated at the *Mutualitat de Futbolistes* are muscle, ankle, and knee injuries [109].

27.2 Plasma Rich in Growth Factors (PRGF-Endoret®) Preparation

PRGF-Endoret® is obtained from small volumes of the patients' blood (20 cc). It is not a platelet concentrate and is obtained after single-stage centrifugation. It does not contain leukocytes and is simply platelet-rich plasma. White cells, and especially leukocytes, contain proinflammatory cytokines and express metalloproteinases (MMP-8 and 9) capable of degrading the extracellular matrix. PRGF-Endoret® is 100 % autologous and biocompatible [6].

PRGF-Endoret® activation is performed with a standard dosage of calcium chloride, taking advantage of the patient's own thrombin and not using bovine thrombin; hence biosecurity risks are avoided. It obtains a platelet concentration of 2–3 times higher than the physiological, which is the optimum concentration; as lower doses would be subtherapeutic and superior concentrations do not induce superior effects, they can even exert inhibitory actions [6].

Culture studies with the use of PRGF-Endoret® have shown a cellular increase in tendon tissues and especially an increase in collagen levels [6, 31, 61, 137].

27.3 Knee Injuries

Knee injury is common in soccer. Anterior cruciate ligament (ACL) injury is one of the most frequent, reaching 70 % and typically with an indirect injury mechanism of deceleration-rotation without contact [51]. In the USA, 50,000 patients require ACL surgery annually [24, 58, 112]. The majority is sports related and affects patients between 15 and 45 years old with 47 % taking place in the 30–40-year-old age range [51]. It is estimated that one ACL tear occurs every 1,500 h of sports practice, including sports such as soccer, basketball, rugby, and skiing, which is equivalent to one injury for every 1,750 citizens of the USA [51]. The cost of an ACL reconstruction surgery in the USA is an estimated $ 17,000 to which one can add an additional $2,000 for the cost of the initial care of all ACL injuries and/or the conservative treatment of the patients who do not undergo ACL reconstruction. The annual cost of treating only ACL injuries is an estimated 1 billion dollars [51]. Overall costs of sports-related injuries in the USA in 2002 were estimated at about 15.8 billion dollars [122].

ACL reconstruction in a high number of cases is performed with BTB (patellar tendon) of which 4–60 % present anterior knee pain [15, 74, 87, 112]. Recovery from joint injuries in active athletes is increasingly faster due in part to the progress and improvement of surgical techniques and the application of biological elements that promote rapid tissue regeneration [40]. This improved ligamentization has been shown in ACL graft maturation (90, 97, 104, 110) and the patellar tendon donor site [23, 29, 72, 73, 112].

The assessment of tendon regeneration has led to the realization of various studies with both magnetic resonance imaging (MRI) and ultrasound, depending on the location and accessibility of the tissue [1, 36, 132]. In ligaments and tendons such as the ACL, MRI has been used most [57, 97, 110]. Seijas et al. performed a study on 100 football players that underwent BTB ACL ligament graft, and after randomly dividing them into two groups, at the end of the surgery, group A received a dose of PRGF-Endoret®, while the other was used as control. MRI was performed on all of the patients at 4, 6, and 12 months to assess the grade of graft maturation. The MRI classification system was based on the study by Howell [57] with certain variants added by Jordi Català, which lead to the creation of the Català

Classification [110]. In another study by the same group of authors [112], a clinical trial was performed comparing a group that received PRGF-Endoret® exclusively at the donor site and the rest served as control. A follow-up protocol was followed with ultrasound to assess the donor site at 4, 8, 16, 24, 48, and 96 weeks, comparing the grade of maturation [112]. Populations with complete ACL tear were included in both studies, all of them athletes, as described in papers [110, 112]. Surgical procedures were performed by the same surgical team that employed the same surgical technique with inclusion and exclusion criteria described in both papers. In the ultrasonographic assessment, a classification was created (Rius classification) based on a previous study on 10 patients, 50 measurements, and two sonographers with correlation higher than 95 % [67].

In the first study the MRI at 4 months showed statistically different maturation grade ($p=0.003$) between the two groups, as well as the assessment at 6 months ($p=0.0001$). Once they reached 1 year, no significant differences ($p=0.354$) between both groups were observed. In the second study, groups were composed of 23 and 19 patients who underwent ACL surgery with and without PRGF-Endoret® at the donor site. The PRGF group showed significantly increased maturation speed at 4th postoperative month ($p=0.0037$). The studies reviewed show that the application of PRGF-Endoret®, both at an articular level and at the donor site, favors a faster maturation process in the ligaments evaluated, which is in line with results published in previous studies [37, 90, 97].

In recent years the application of platelet-rich plasma (PRP) or plasma rich in growth factors (PRGF) has been linked to faster tissue regeneration in bone, cartilage, ligaments, and tendons, for studies in vitro, in vivo, and in humans [40, 66, 99, 102–104]. There are several ways to obtain and apply PRP, and it is therefore of utmost importance that the technique employed, the product obtained, and the subsequent designated treatment protocols are described in detail when research is published to avoid the unfortunate misinterpretation of data. The system for obtaining plasma rich in growth factors is not always uniform, with different techniques being followed by various authors, making the resultant products significantly different without reaching any conclusion about the degree of effectiveness from one to the other [131]. The PRGF-Endoret system (BTI) has European (European CE mark) and American (FDA Approval) health certifications, both for the different applications of the product and for each and every one of the elements necessary for their application [110, 112].

It is known that in order for the tissue repair-regeneration process to take place, a multitude of elements must interact, from various cellular components to proteins, metabolites, and electrolytes, all encompassed within an appropriate environment [122]. During this process, both in the acute inflammatory phase and in the cellular proliferation and remodeling phase [18, 19], platelets play an important role, not only based on hemostatic capacity but also on their chemotactic activity and on growth, morphogenesis, and cell differentiation [4–7]. Over the last 20 years, several studies have been published which aimed at taking advantage of the benefits offered by this cell type in tissue repair, stimulating research and development in the field of regenerative medicine [6, 70, 102, 103, 130, 136].

The tissue repair process is based on a complex cascade of biological events controlled by a long list of growth factors and proteins with biological activity. The environment in the spatio-temporal action of this group of mediators at the area of damaged tissue regulates the mechanisms and phases that govern tissue repair and regeneration. Throughout this process, another set of factors regulates the dynamic balance between stimulation and inhibition of cell proliferation, angiogenesis, and the formation of extracellular matrix [6]. The tissue repair process involves several phases including angiogenesis, tissue proliferation, and extracellular matrix deposition. The remodeling and maturation processes are combined with the mechanical stresses to which the tissue in question is subjected [103]. Growth factors are substances of polypeptide nature, soluble and diffusible regulating growth, differentiation, and phenotype of many cell types [128]. These provide the initial signals for the activation of the cells in surrounding tissue. In response to signals provided by these molecules, local cells and those infiltrated undergo changes in proliferation, differentiation, and protein synthesis with different biological functions. These proteins act in an autocrine and/or paracrine manner. They affect cell behavior, binding to specific receptors located in cell membranes. Not all cell phenotypes have the same receptors; therefore, the effect of the growth factors will not be the same in all tissues and in all situations [118]. All these phenomena, together, define the process known as cell activation [100].

Animal studies also show increases in cell density, neovascularization, and resistance force between 30 % and 65 % according to studies [3, 7, 9, 107] with an improvement within biomechanical properties in the medial collateral ligament in its early stages. Weiler showed how the application of autologous PDGF into the graft during surgery was able to alter natural maturation, improving tension and resistance, increasing the rate of maturation, and improving collagen quality [132]. The study by Xie et al. suggested a role of PRGF in promoting synthesis of extracellular matrix after ACL reconstruction, in a study performed with dogs [136]. Along the same lines, the study by Fernandez-Sarmiento et al. showed histological changes at 8 weeks, consistent with an accelerated early healing process in repaired Achilles tendons in sheep after surgical disruption and repair treated with PRGF-Endoret® [37]. The work by Xie et al. also states that the use of PRP alters the expression of some target genes at certain time points, especially during the early stages of graft remodeling, which might explain the enhancing effect of PRP on the ACL graft maturation process, which at a cellular level, could explain the result in both animals and human studies, including the two studies evaluated [37, 110, 112, 136].

Different studies show a series of stages in the revascularization of the patellar graft used as anterior cruciate ligament. After a phase of graft avascular necrosis, with hypocellularity and collagen fragmentation, revascularization is produced through a synovial cover which originates from both the distal and proximal insertions of the graft that starts covering it and promotes intratendinous vascular growth up to complete coverage and cellularization at 1 year postsurgery [8, 22]. With specific reference to the ACL graft, PDGF, FGF-1, and some TGF subtypes are responsible for the acceleration of tissue healing and increased graft tension [97]. PRGF was associated with histological changes consistent with an accelerated early healing process in repaired Achilles tendons in sheep after experimental surgical disruption. PRGF-treated tendons showed improvements in the morphometric features of fibroblast nuclei, suggesting a more advanced stage of healing. At 8 weeks, histological examination revealed more mature organization of collagen bundles, lower vascular densities, and decreased fibroblast densities in PRGF-treated tendons than in tendons infiltrated with saline solution. These findings were consistent with a more advanced stage of the healing process [37]. Kondo et al. also demonstrated that the application of growth factors in ACL elongations achieved improved tension compared with patients where growth factors were not applied [66].

Studies show maturation of patellar graft evolution in terms of vascularization, cellularity, collagen fiber, and pattern, and the presence of metaplasia with a high correlation [36] showed maturity with a peak at just after 1-year postsurgery but with vascularity and fiber pattern similar to normal in a period of 6–12 months. Aim [1] studied the patellar graft viability by microangiography and histology showing revascularization at 8 weeks with tissues rich in collagen and a similar structure to the original ligament at 4–5 months. In the first months the grafted plasty is in the process of maturation, a fact that has left ACL surgeons reluctant to carry out aggressive rehabilitation in the initial period for fear of plasty failure [101]. Rougraff in his study of graft biopsies in patellar ligamentoplasties showed that tissue obtained in the early postoperative period (3–8 weeks post-op) shows no more than 30 % tissue necrosis, in contrast to animal studies where the percentage is much higher. Therefore, he concluded that postoperative rehabilitation programs proposing an acceleration of physical therapy not only don't have detrimental outcomes but if not followed could lead to worse outcomes [101]. Even patellar tendon studies to evaluate the maturation process that takes place at the donor site show an enhanced maturation process in histological studies in animals in accordance with Sarmiento and the study by our team with ultrasound evaluation [37, 72, 73, 112].

From a clinical point of view, the published studies present conflicting results. On one hand studies like that by Orrego showed greater maturation for the patellar graft assessed by MRI at 6 months without an increased tibial tunnel diameter [90]. Studies like that by Magnussen [74] with 2 years clinical evaluation or that by Nin [86] show no significant differences with the application of plasma rich in growth factors in ligament grafts. The results obtained with the assessment carried out at 1 year postsurgery are concurrent with those obtained in our study showing equal numbers of completely mature ligaments in both groups with no differences between the two groups. The main difference between the author's study and previous studies is that the authors assessed the grade of maturity at earlier intervals, noting that although the two groups (PRP and control) reach maturity at 1 and 2 years at similar rates, the speed at which they do so is different. In 2010 Radice published graft maturation rates, assessed by MRI, which showed figures 48 % faster for grafts treated with growth factors with respect to the speed of maturity [97]. Sanchez for his part showed how the use of PRGF also accelerated the maturation process in hamstring grafts [104]. De Almeida showed that PRP had a positive effect on patellar tendon harvest site healing on MRI after 6 months and also reduced pain in the immediate postoperative period [29].

In another study by Seijas et al. [111] about football players with partial ACL ruptures, it demonstrated that the application of PRGF in the remnant ACL in arthroscopic surgery allowed patients to return to football in less than 4 months in 95 % of the players [111]. The study performed by Seijas [110, 112] showed enhanced maturation speed in both the donor site and the graft around 4–6 months. The results at 1 year show that there are no differences between the two groups and maturation is observed to be complete in both groups. These results are similar to those previously reported by Magnussen and Nin, wherein no significant differences were found at 1 and 2 years follow-up [74, 86]. The publications reviewed insist that the role PRGF plays in the maturation process of ligaments takes place in the early stages. Therefore, the changes that may be proposed at a clinical level should be based on these biological findings. The next lines of research should consider safe methods and protocols for speeding up the rehabilitation process and evaluating the biochemical and histological structural components of neoligaments, assessing the similarity to normal ligaments.

27.4 Hip Injuries

Regarding hip pathology within professional athletes, three specific lesions have received increased attention over recent years: adductor lesions, hernias, and femoroacetabular impingement (FAI) [78]. FAI has been identified as one of the main causes of hip pain in athletes, resulting in reduced range of motion (ROM) and decreased sports activity [44, 81]. The bony or mechanical abnormality that causes FAI has been associated with labral, joint, and cartilage damage in patients with hip pain, i.e., correcting FAI could delay or even avoid arthritic progression in the joint [16, 17, 20, 41, 125]. Reducing the acetabulum and femoral head surface that contact each other or impinge may prevent the continuous trauma that takes place in movements that combine flexion, adduction, and internal rotation of the hip. Studies of nonathletic asymptomatic volunteers demonstrated an incidence of cam-type deformity at 14 % [52], although this percentage varies in several studies, ranging between 36 % and 76 % [2, 10, 62, 68, 96, 116]. Alternatively, studies in asymptomatic athletes describe figures reaching up to 64 % of deformities, 31 % being cam type [116].

In the treatment of this pathology, after attempting the conservative route by physiotherapy with stretching and joint flexibility and the persistence of mechanical problems that involves femoroacetabular impingement, surgical options are indicated. The result of surgical treatment in athletes is satisfactory in more than 90 %, but the most limiting of these results is the status of the articular cartilage. If patients have grade 4 cartilage defects, satisfactory results with the patient's return to their usual sports can decrease up to 50 % in experienced hands [115]. An articular joint space greater than 2 mm radiologically is a prognostic factor that can help to calculate the outcome of treatment in higher-demand patients. The risk of having to perform total hip replacement after hip arthroscopy in patients with decreased femoroacetabular space below 2 mm is 38 times higher than in those that have more than 2 mm [115]. Therefore, the most significant joint survival predictor is the condition the cartilage is in [69, 95, 115]. It is widely known that the risk of prosthesis is greater in athletes than in the general population [49].

Surgical correction of a condition that creates a conflict and a mechanical disturbance in the normal functioning of the hip joint must be one of the steps for resolution and minimizing risk in athletes hips especially in rough contact sports like football that place extra stress on joints. Although the application of biological treatments certainly plays a vital role in the preservation of the joint as already demonstrated in other joints such as the ankle or knee in similar patient populations [65, 109, 127, 130]. The use of plasma rich in growth factors (PRGF) is reported as a good treatment to improve pain, stiffness, and functional capacity of articular surfaces [65, 130]. The use of PRP in hip arthroscopy has demonstrated improved postoperative pain, edema, and improved short-term outcomes compared to control patients treated arthroscopically for FAI [46, 76]. Not only in the context of surgery but the application of PRGF under ultrasound guidance in patients with FAI has shown favorable results with improvements in pain and stiffness in the short to medium term [14, 105]. In hips with femoroacetabular chondropathies in moderate stages of arthritis, different authors have reported to have performed arthroscopic debridement with 50 % good results at 2 years and reoperation in the other 50 % requiring hip prosthesis. In similar cases where PRGF was applied additionally, over 70 % of patients in moderate stages of arthritis were able to avoid prosthesis at 2 years with good functional results [69, 95, 115].

In the context of hip pathology in footballers, femoroacetabular impingement is undoubtedly the pathology to pay attention to for the biomechanical consequences it entails, and the professionals dealing with this patient population should recognize their requirements when considering treatment approaches. Correction of the conflict and mechanical disturbance has been the main objective to date, and it is the biological status of the cartilage which has demonstrated to be a deciding factor in the survival of the joint and therefore the application of biological therapies associated with mechanical treatments is the path to follow.

27.5 Ankle Injuries

Ankle injuries are extremely common in the majority of field sports, and sprains are the most common ankle injuries [39, 83]. It is thought that injury to the lateral aspect of the talus is associated with specific traumatic events. The anterolateral aspect of the talus dome collides with the fibula when the ankle is in forced inversion or dorsiflexion [11, 84].

In ankle injuries we have noted that the most commonly injured ligaments are the talofibular, the calcaneofibular, the posterior talofibular, and in many cases the distal tibiofibular syndesmosis with distal tibiofibular. This location can contribute to an increase in thickness by inflammation and scarring of the distal tibiofibular ligament and cause mild impingement in the anterior aspect of the ankle. Conservative treatment with immobilization techniques such as taping, proprioception exercises, and application of PRGF in injured ligaments accelerates recovery from these injuries. In addition, some works indicate that more than 50 % of acute ankle sprains and fractures develop some form of chondral injury [82]. Osteochondral lesion of the talus is a relatively broad term used to describe an injury or abnormality of the talar articular cartilage and adjacent bone [12]. Osteochondral lesions can lead to mechanical pain and swelling that precludes resumption of sports activity [126]. The ability to return to play at preinjury level is a good indication that the lesion has resolved satisfactorily [133]. As is true for most sports-related injuries, osteochondral lesions are usually managed conservatively. It is only after this approach has failed that alternative surgical strategies are contemplated.

27.6 Osteochondritis

Osteochondral lesions of the talus are uncommon injuries, occupying the third position in order of frequency following knee and elbow involvement, and represent 4 % of all the osteochondral lesions of the body [108]. The portion of the talar dome bearing the medial load is most often affected and less commonly the lateral load area [11, 89, 98]. There are two common patterns of osteochondral lesions of the talus. Anterolateral talar dome lesions result from inversion and dorsiflexion injuries of the ankle at the area impacting against the fibula. Posteromedial lesions result from inversion, plantar flexion, and external rotation injuries of the ankle at the area impacting against the tibial ceiling of the ankle joint [114]. Injuries involving the lateral aspect are usually more severe (grades III and IV) [106]. Recent studies suggest that after studying the location of injuries by MRI, it seems that most lesions are located medially and centrally on the talar dome [55].

Seijas et al. [109] presented a series from a group of soccer players with Tegner activity level 9 and 10, suffering from osteochondral injuries which after 3 months of conservative treatment, pain persisted and impeded sports activity [109]. In this series, 94 % were medial lesions, and in more than 60 % there was a traumatic causal relationship without injury to the lateral dome, in agreement with a previous study by Burns and Rosenbach [21]. In 70 % of cases, there were associated lesions, including soft tissue impingement in 50 %, rupture of the external lateral ligament (lateral collateral ligament) in 13 %, and fracture of the fibula in 6 %.

The clinical symptoms of osteochondral talar lesions include pain, recurrent synovitis, joint balance alterations, and obstruction due to the presence of loose bodies. The recurrent synovitis and balance alterations are the likely cause of tibiotalar arthritis [53]. The symptoms are not specific to this condition, and because these are uncommon lesions, they can be mistaken for acute or chronic ankle sprains. For this reason, when the symptoms persist and the initial X-ray shows normal findings, it is advisable to perform CT or MRI to investigate the injury [21]. MRI shows the osteocartilaginous lesion [79], with a high degree of correlation, and can detect lesions that may be missed on plain films [71, 119]. Prevention of ankle sprains by proprioceptive training exercises is necessary to reduce the susceptibility of the joint to osteocartilaginous lesions [60].

The initial treatment indicated is usually conservative [12]. The common treatment strategies of symptomatic osteochondral lesions include nonsurgical treatment, with rest, cast immobilization, and use of nonsteroidal anti-inflammatory drugs (NSAIDs) [12]. The mere presence of osteocartilaginous injuries on imaging studies does not imply that they will progress or lead to arthrotic degeneration. For this reason, treatment is only contemplated in symptomatic cases [84]. When the patient's condition fails to improve, arthroscopic surgery obtains results equal to or better than arthrotomy, with the associated advantages of lower morbidity and faster recovery [13, 84]. Some authors consider arthroscopy the treatment of choice, leaving the option of open surgery for cases in which the access is difficult and malleolar osteotomy is required [113]. In addition to enabling treatment of many types of injuries, ankle arthroscopy provides a more accurate assessment of the problem than imaging, thereby facilitating the decision as to the most appropriate therapeutic approach [106]. A meta-analysis of published studies using different treatments has shown success rates of 78 % in series in which excision and curettage were carried out and 86 % when microfracture was additionally performed [129]. Until randomized studies are conducted and more conclusive results can be obtained, these are the most effective treatments available. Conservative treatment has yielded a success rate of 45 % [120, 124, 129, 138]. The study of Seijas et al. shows excellent results in 81.75 % and good in 18.25 %, which are in accordance with the reported outcome of other studies [11]. Arthroscopic bone marrow stimulation techniques, such as microfracture and drilling, perforate the subchondral plate with multiple openings to recruit mesenchymal stem cells from the underlying bone marrow to stimulate the differentiation of fibrocartilaginous repair tissue in the defect site [82].

In a randomized study, Gobbi et al. reported similar findings with the use of microfractures or autografts with chondrocytes for osteocartilaginous talus lesions [48]. Hankemeier et al. obtained excellent or good outcome in 89 % of patients with osteochondral ankle lesions treated by debridement and abrasion of the subchondral space [54]. In a prospective study, Takao et al. found that the debridement of the osteochondral bed favored cartilaginous improvement at the site of the lesion in more than 90 % of cases [121]. Thermann and Becher reported a success rate of 93 %, 2 years after performing microfractures, and proved that age was not a criterion favoring a poor prognosis [123]. Giza presented a series of 10 patients, wherein after conservative treatment and arthroscopy with debridement/curettage without good results they then underwent matrix-induced autologous chondrocyte implantation (MACI) showing improvements in AOFAS and SF-36 scales [47].

Clinical improvements have been reported in different studies on cartilage lesions with the use of plasma rich in growth factors (PRGF) [127, 130]. When working with PRGF, the methodology described by its author should be followed with regard to its preparation and application to ensure traceability [4] and thus render the results comparable to the various studies published. As indicated by Taylor, when obtaining PRP, taking different paths leads to the preparation of different products, with the huge possibility of getting different results [122].

Giannini presents favorable results in a 4-year follow-up with improvements in AOFAS scores and objectified by MRI T2 mapping sequences. Patients were treated in one surgical procedure with bone marrow-derived cell transplantation [45]. The study with meta-analysis by Niemeyer evaluated 16 publications with autologous chondrocyte implantation wherein he concluded that although clinical outcome as described in the studies available seems promising (with regard to a lack of controlled studies) a superiority or inferiority to other techniques such as osteochondral transplantation or microfracturing cannot be estimated [85]. Paul et al. presented a series treated by talar osteochondral transplantation where they found that patients modify their postoperative sporting activities, and they noted a reduction of participation in high-impact and contact sports [91].

The series described here is composed of a highly homogeneous population of federated soccer players of similar age. Treatment by arthroscopy and debridement is not extremely aggressive and provides good results in terms of functional recovery. Based on the review of the literature, there are insufficient works with high levels of evidence that recommend a specific type of treatment in cases of osteochondritis of the talus. However, based on the accumulated experience gained at the Spanish Football Federations' Mutualitat de Futbolistes, ankle osteochondritis (if symptomatic) is initially treated conservatively by physiotherapy and with biological techniques such as the infiltration of plasma rich in growth factors. If conservative treatment fails, surgical techniques are indicated with ankle arthroscopy and curettage of the lesion down to the healthy bone and the application of articular PRGF-Endoret®.

27.7 Muscles Injuries

Inferior extremity or lower limb muscle injuries are excessively common in sports, especially in football [34]. It is estimated that muscle injuries represent 30 % of all injuries (1,8–2,2/1,000 h of exposure), meaning that a professional football team suffers about 12 muscle injuries per season, of them 92 % affecting the four groups in the lower limb, with the adductors in second place after the hamstrings [32, 34]. Hamstrings are the most frequently injured muscles representing 25 % of all muscle injuries in sports [30, 42]. In the hamstring group, the long head of the biceps femoris is injured the most, making it the most injured muscle in the body [94]. Clanton et al. described that hamstring injuries are the most common injuries in athletes and have the most re-injuries [25]. The high number of injuries in the hamstrings and rectus femoris musculature could be due to the considerable amount of muscle junctions and layers of aponeuroses. Depending on the anatomic location,

Table 27.1 Myotendinous junction (MTJ)

Classifications of muscle injuries	Hamstring injuries	Rectus femoris
	Proximal avulsion	Avulsions
	Disinsertion ruptures of the proximal myotendinous junction	MTJ proximal indirect or intermuscular septum
	Isolated avulsions of the semimembranosus	MTJ proximal direct or superficial
	High lesions of the common tendon	MTJ distal or deep fascia
	Lesions in the middle third affecting myotendinous junctions of the biceps femoris and the semitendinosus	
	Injuries to the distal third, medial, and lateral	

different types of hamstring and rectus femoris injury can be distinguished in Table 27.1. Violent stretching or fast contraction of the hamstrings leading to injury at the myotendinous junction usually causes hamstring injury. This typically occurs during acceleration, jump, and sprint or during the deceleration phase with the knee in extension, by the sudden or abrupt change from maximal eccentric to concentric contraction [134].

The diagnosis of muscle injury is important not only to confirm the clinical suspicion of the existence of an injury, but it allows us to give a prognosis and suggested treatment. For diagnosis, imaging techniques are helpful such as ultrasound and magnetic resonance imaging (MRI), allowing physicians to diagnose, quantify, and locate the lesion. Ultrasound has advantages over other diagnostic techniques, such as being a noninvasive technique, and allows for a dynamic assessment of the injury.

Although various treatment protocols have been used and described, there is no consensus on which method is the most effective in achieving the ultimate goal, which is the rapid return to competition. Currently few methods are guided by prospective randomized studies [59, 93, 135], and despite this, the length of time to return to sport hovers around 6 weeks depending on the extent of the injury [26]. The appearance of PRP has opened new avenues for the treatment of muscle injuries. Advances in basic science have focused attention on the application of autologous biologics in the treatment of muscle injuries. Muscle injury passes through an initial phase of destruction (inflammatory phase) which affects the muscle cells, blood vessels, connective tissue, and intramuscular nerves leading to necrosis [63]. This initial phase is followed by the repair and remodeling phase wherein undifferentiated cells, in response to various growth factors, proliferate and differentiate into mature myoblasts, trying to replace injured muscle fibers [5, 64, 77]. The inflammatory process that occurs after the muscle injury causes accumulation of inflammatory cells (neutrophils and macrophages). Also in this initial phase, platelet activation occurs. Platelet activation results in the degranulation of alpha granules and the release of various substances, among which are the growth factors. Also found in platelets are growth factors that are involved in the acceleration of the repair in tendons and muscles [27].

Animal studies showed shortened repair times with the application of PRP in tibialis anterior muscle injury from 21 to 14 days [75]. Wright-Carpenter et al. in 2004 conducted a study in which the injection of autologous conditioned serum (ACS) in muscle injury shortened the time to return to sports by 30 % [26]. Moreover Sanchez et al., at the second World Congress on Regenerative Medicine 2005, presented a work in which the ultrasound-guided application of growth factor (PRGF) reduced the expected recovery time of muscle injury by 50 %. Finally in 2010 the IOC concluded that there is little scientific evidence of the effectiveness of PRP in sports injuries, and in a recent systematic review, no randomized trials on the effectiveness of the application of PRP in muscle injury repair were found, and only four papers, evidence level 3–4,

Table 27.2 Diagnosis and treatment of muscle injury is assessed by ultrasound, and the protocol in this table can be followed, with reassessment by ultrasound in the weeks following the injury *RICE* rest, ice, compression, elevation, *NSAID* nonsteroidal anti-inflammatory drug, *US* ultrasound study, *PRP* platelet-rich plasma

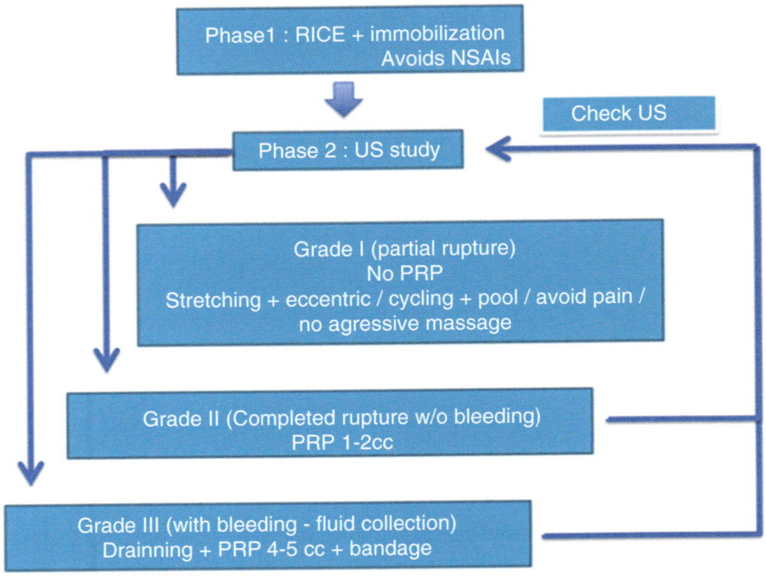

proposed conducting more scientific studies to assess the effectiveness of PRP [102, 35]. In the group to which the authors belong and based on the work of Sanchez and collaborators and the authors' experience in treating muscle injuries at the Catalan Football Federation in which more than 140,000 injuries are treated annually, with muscle injuries being the most common injuries, the following treatment protocol for professional football players is adhered to: Firstly, it is essential to identify the injury location and the extent of the damage. It is therefore essential to perform a clinical and ultrasound evaluation as explained in previous sections. Treatment depends on both the location and at which point in the healing process the injury is found to be in as described in Table 27.2.

Patients tend to present with chronic tendon injuries such as patellar tendon and Achilles tendon pathology and acute tendinitis. The work by De Mos et al. showed that PRP stimulated proliferation and collagen production in cultured human tenocytes [31]. Schnabel showed increased collagen types I and III in horse flexor tendons with the use of plasma rich in growth factors [107], corroborated in vivo in the study by Kajikawa et al. [61].

Animal studies showed that using PRGF® increased cell density and neovascularization without side effects or fibrosis [7]. The study on Achilles tendon ruptures in athletes showed that using PRGF® favored early mobility and return to sports [103].

In vivo animal studies have shown increased resistance of the Achilles tendon by 30 % in a series of 263 rats with 3 mm defects in the Achilles tendon treated with PRP at 6 h after surgery [9] as well as repair of the rotator cuff tendons [67].

Hildebrand showed the usefulness of growth factors (PDGF-BB) in a series of in vivo studies, improving the biomechanical properties of the medial collateral ligament at earlier stages of the ligament healing process [56].

Studies in chronic tendinopathy have also been treated with good results according to several studies with regard to pain reduction in more than 90 % [33, 40, 43, 50, 80, 92, 117].

Randelli published results using PRP in rotator cuff surgeries finding significant differences at 2 years follow-up in terms of pain and function [99]. Meanwhile Foster cites in his publication a series presented in 2009 by Cugat at ISAKOS [28] on the application of growth factors in the medial collateral ligament in football players with a 27 % reduction in recovery time [40].

In cases of patellar tendinopathy, Filardo published in 2010 that the use of PRP provided improved functional indices in athletes at 6 months follow-up [38].

Conclusions

Soccer is definitely a sport that generates a high rate of injury, especially in the lower extremities. If one also takes the level of sports activity into account, it becomes clear that this is a highly demanding sport with a patient population possessing a particular set of requirements for recovery and return to play.

PRGF treatment, in different injuries and over several years of use, has been shown to improve and facilitate standardized treatments. Healing, maturation, and tissue regeneration are shown to have been facilitated and improved with the use of PRGF. Shortening recovery times and ultimate return to play are of particular interest within this patient population; soccer players' can benefit immensely from earlier reintegration to sports and faster recovery times, not to mention the economic benefit for both the player and their corresponding club.

The overall conclusion of this chapter is that the use of standard treatments has been directed toward restoring the anatomy and functional recovery. With the use of PRGF, it has been demonstrated that the natural evolution of orthopedic surgery and traumatology can move toward biological enhancement of standardized treatments, and therefore it can be said that the coming years will show that the field of regenerative medicine and biology will play a major role in orthopedic surgery, traumatology, and sports medicine (Figs. 27.1, 27.2, 27.3, 27.4, and 27.5).

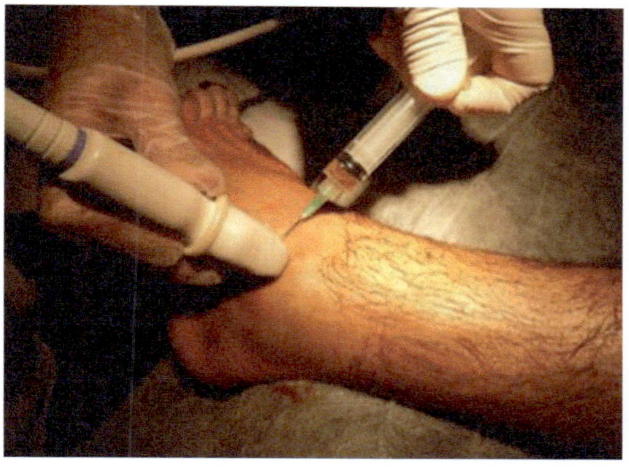

Fig. 27.1 Application of PRGF-Endoret guided by ultrasound in a patient with injury to the distal tibiofibular syndesmosis

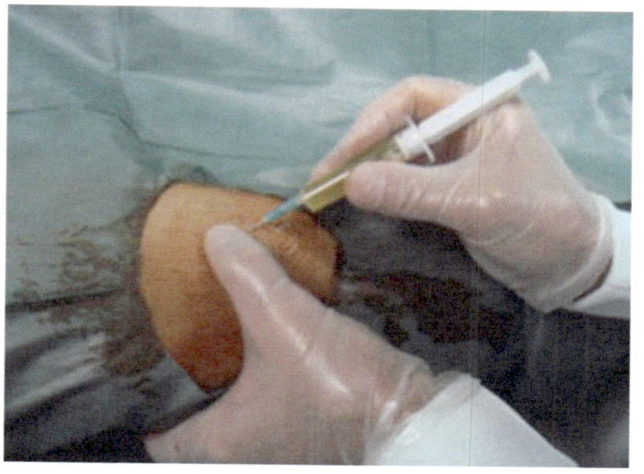

Fig. 27.2 Application of PRGF-Endoret throughout the injured medial collateral ligament

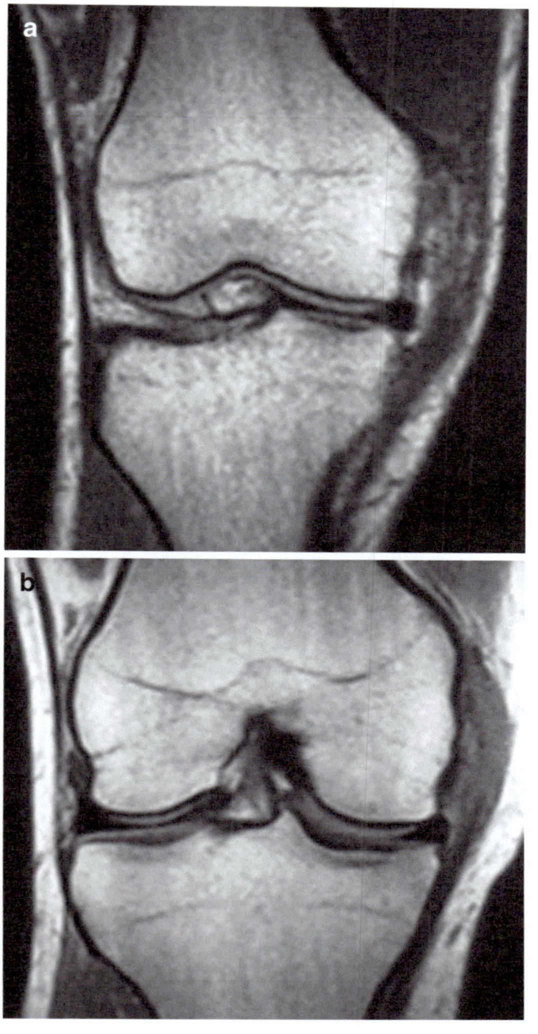

Fig. 27.3 MRI medial collateral ligament. Image of pre- and postinjection PRGF-Endoret in MCL illustrating healing postinjection. (**a**) Pr-injection, (**b**) postinjection

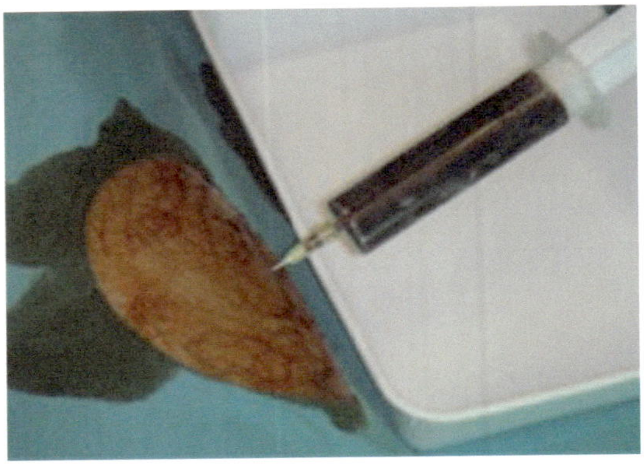

Fig. 27.4 Muscle injury. Evacuation of hematoma secondary to muscle injury and application of the protocol recommended in Table 27.2

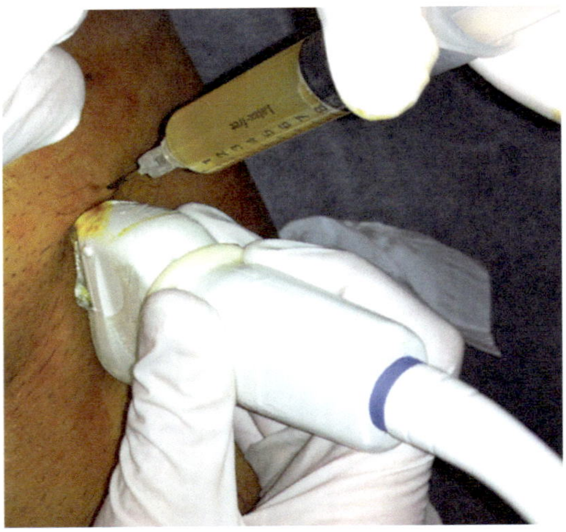

Fig. 27.5 Hip. Application of PRGF-Endoret in the intracapsular hip space guided by ultrasound

References

1. Aim A, Liljedahl SO, Stromberg B (1979) Clinical and experimental experience in the reconstruction of the anterior cruciate ligament. Orthop Clin North Am 7:181–189
2. Allen D, Beaulé PE, Ramadan O, Doucette S (2009) Prevalence of associated deformities and hip pain in patients with cam-type femoroacetabular impingement. J Bone Joint Surg Br 91(5):589–594
3. Anderson K, Seneviratne AM, Izawa K, Atkinson BL, Potter HG, Rodeo SA (2001) Augmentation of tendon healing in an intraarticular bone tunnel with use of a bone growth factor. Am J Sports Med 29(6): 689–698
4. Anitua E (1999) Plasma rich in growth factors: preliminary results of use in the preparation of sites for implants. Int J Oral Maxillofac Implants 14:529–535
5. Anitua E, Andia I, Ardanza B, Nurden P, Nurden AT (2004) Autologous platelets as a source of proteins for healing and tissue regeneration. Thromb Haemost 91:4–15
6. Anitua E, Sanchez M, Nurden AT, Zalduendo M, de la Fuente M, Azofra J, Andia I (2007) Reciprocal actions of platelet-secreted TGF-beta1 on the production of VEGF and HGF by human tendon cells. Plast Reconstr Surg 119(3):950–959
7. Anitua E, Sanchez M, Nurden AT, Zalduendo M, de la Fuente M, Orive G, Azofra J, Andia I (2006) Autologous fibrin matrices: a potential source of biological mediators that modulate tendon cell activities. J Biomed Mater Res A 77(2):285–293
8. Arnoczky SP, Tarvin GB (1982) Anterior cruciate ligament replacement using patellar tendon: an evaluation of graft revascularization in the dog. J Bone Joint Surg Am 64:217–224
9. Aspenberg P, Virchenko O (2004) Platelet concentrate injection improves Achilles tendon repair in rats. Acta Orthop Scand 75(1):93–99
10. Audenaert EA, Peeters I, Vigneron L, Baelde N, Pattyn C (2012) Hip morphological characteristics and range of internal rotation in femoroacetabular impingement. Am J Sports Med 40:1329–1336
11. Backus JD, Viens NA, Nunley JA (2012) Arthroscopic treatment of osteochondral lesions of the talus: microfracture and drilling versus debridement. J Surg Orthop Adv 21(4):218–222
12. Badekas T, Takvorian M, Souras N (2013) Treatment principles for osteochondral lesions in foot and ankle. Int Orthop 37(9):1697–1706
13. Barnes CJ, Ferkel RD (2003) Arthroscopic debridement and drilling of osteochondral lesions of the talus. Foot Ankle Clin 8(2):243–257
14. Battaglia M, Guaraldi F, Vannini F, Buscio T, Buda R, Galletti S, Giannini S (2011) Platelet-rich plasma (PRP) intra-articular ultrasound-guided injections as a possible treatment for hip osteoarthritis: a pilot study. Clin Exp Rheumatol 29(4):754
15. Beaufils P, Gaudot F, Drain O, Boisrenoult P, Pujol N (2011) Mini-invasive technique for bone patellar tendon bone harvesting: its superiority in reducing anterior knee pain following ACL reconstruction. Curr Rev Musculoskelet Med 4(2):45–51
16. Beck M, Kalhor M, Leunig M, Ganz R (2005) Hip morphology influences the pattern of damage to the acetabular cartilage: femoroacetabular impingement as a cause of early osteoarthritis of the hip. J Bone Joint Surg Br 87:1012–1018
17. Bedi A, Dolan M, Leunig M, Kelly BT (2011) Static and dynamic mechanical causes of hip pain. Arthroscopy 27(2):235–251
18. Bennett NT, Schultz GS (1993) Growth factors and wound healing: biochemical properties of growth factors and their receptors. Am J Surg 165(6): 728–737

19. Bennett NT, Schultz GS (1993) Growth factors and wound healing: part II. Role in normal and chronic wound healing. Am J Surg 166(1):74–81
20. Birmingham PM, Kelly BT, Jacobs R, McGrady L, Wang M (2012) The effect of dynamic femoroacetabular impingement on pubic symphysis motion: a cadaveric study. Am J Sports Med 40:1113–1118
21. Burns J, Rosenbach B (1989) Osteochondrosis dissecans of the talus. Results of a follow-up study. Z Orthop Ihre Grenzgeb 127(5):549–555
22. Braun HJ, Wasterlain AS, Dragoo JL (2013) The use of PRP in ligament and meniscal healing. Sports Med Arthrosc 21(4):206–212
23. Cervellin M, de Girolamo L, Bait C, Denti M, Volpi P (2012) Autologous platelet-rich plasma gel to reduce donor-site morbidity after patellar tendon graft harvesting for anterior cruciate ligament reconstruction: a randomized, controlled clinical study. Knee Surg Sports Traumatol Arthrosc 20(1):114–120
24. Cimino F, Volk BS, Setter D (2010) Anterior cruciate ligament injury: diagnosis, management and prevention. Am Fam Physician 82(8):917–922
25. Clanton TO, Coude KJ (1998) Hamstring strains in athletes: diagnosis and treatment. J Am Acad Orthop Surg 6:237–248
26. Copland ST, Tipton JS, Fields KB (2009) Evidence-based treatment of hamstring tears. Curr Sports Med Rep 8:308–314
27. Creaney L, Hamilton B (2008) Growth factor delivery methods in the management of sports injuries: the state of play. Br J Sports Med 42:314–320
28. Cugat R (2009) Platelet growth factors: experience in soft tissue injuries and in joint trauma. ISAKOS, Osaka, 5–9 Apr 2009
29. De Almeida AM, Demange MK, Sobrado MF, Rodrigues MB, Pedrinelli A, Hernandez AJ (2012) Patellar tendon healing with platelet-rich plasma: a prospective randomized controlled trial. Am J Sports Med 40(6):1282–1288
30. Drezner JA (2003) Practical management hamstring muscle injuries. Clin J Sport Med 13:48–52
31. de Mos M, van der Windt AE, Jahr H, van Schie HT, Weinans H, Verhaar JA, van Osch GJ (2008) Can platelet-rich plasma enhance tendon repair? A cell culture study. Am J Sports Med 36(6):1171–1178
32. Dvorak J, Junge A (2006) F-MARC: manual de medicina del fútbol. Federación Internacional de Fútbol Asociación (FIFA), Zurich
33. Edwards SG, Calandruccio JH (2003) Autologous blood injection for refractory lateral epicondylitis. J Hand Surg [Am] 28(2):272–278
34. Ekstrand J, Hägglund M, Walden M (2011) Epidemiology of muscle injuries in professional football (soccer). Am J Sports Med 39:1226–1232
35. Engebretsen L, Steffen K, Alsousou J, Anitua E, Bachl N, Devilee R, Everts P, Hamilton B, Huard J, Jenoure P, Kelberine F, Kon E, Maffulli N, Matheson G, Mei-Dan O, Menetrey J, Philippon M, Randelli P, Schamasch P, Schwellnus M, Vernec A, Verrall G (2010) IOC consensus paper on the use of platelet-rich plasma in sports medicine. Br J Sports Med 44:1072–1081
36. Falconiero RP, DiStefano VJ, Cook TM (1998) Revascularization and ligamentization of autogenous anterior cruciate ligament grafts in humans. Arthroscopy 14:197–205
37. Fernandez-Sarmiento JA, Dominguez JM, Granados MM et al (2013) Histological study of the influence of plasma rich in growth factors (ORGF) on the healing of divided Achilles tendons in sheep. J Bone Joint Surg Am 95(3):246–255
38. Filardo G, Kon E, Della Villa S, Vincentelli F, Fornasari PM, Marcacci M (2010) Use of platelet rich plasma for the treatment of refractory jumper's knee. Int Orthop 34(6):909–915
39. Fong DT, Hong Y, Chan LK, Yung PS, Chan KM (2007) A systematic review on ankle injury and ankle sprain in sports. Sports Med 37(1):73–94
40. Foster TE, Puskas BL, Mandelbaum BR et al (2009) Platelet-rich plasma. From basic science to clinical applications. Am J Sports Med 37:2259–2272
41. Ganz R, Parvizi J, Beck M, Leunig M, Notzli H, Siebenrock KA (2003) Femoroacetabular impingement: a cause for osteoarthritis of the hip. Clin Orthop Relat Res 417:112–120
42. Garret WE (2000) Principles & practice of orthopaedic sports medicine. Lippincott Williams & Wilkins, Philadelphia, p 888
43. Gaweda K, Tarczynska M, Krzyzanowski W (2010) Treatment of Achilles tendinopathy with platelet-rich plasma. Int J Sports Med 31(8):577–583
44. Gerhardt MB, Romero AA, Silvers HJ, Harris DJ, Watanabe D, Mandelbaum BR (2012) The prevalence of radiographic hip abnormalities in elite soccer players. Am J Sports Med 40(3):584–588
45. Giannini S, Buda R, Battaglia M, Cavallo M, Ruffilli A, Ramponi L, Pagliazzi G, Vannini F (2013) One-step repair in talar osteochondral lesions: 4-year clinical results and t2-mapping capability in outcome prediction. Am J Sports Med 41(3):511–518
46. Giordano B (2010) The effect of platelet enriched plasma on early clinical outcomes in patients with femoroacetabular impingement following arthroscopic labral repair and femoral neck osteplasty. ISHA 2010, Cancun
47. Giza E, Sullivan M, Ocel D, Lundeen G, Mitchell ME, Veris L, Walton J (2010) Matrix-induced autologous chondrocyte implantation of talus articular defects. Foot Ankle Int 31(9):747–753
48. Gobbi A, Francisco RA, Lubowitz JH, Allegra F, Canata G (2006) Osteochondral lesions of the talus: randomized controlled trial comparing chondroplasty, microfracture, and osteochondral autograft transplantation. Arthroscopy 22(10):1085–1092
49. Golightly YM, Marshall SW, Callahan LF, Guskiewicz K (2009) Early-onset arthritis in retired National Football League players. J Phys Act Health 6(5):638–643
50. Gosens T, Peerbooms JC, van Laar W, den Oudsten BL (2011) Ongoing positive effect of platelet-rich plasma

versus corticosteroid injection in lateral epicondylitis: a double-blind randomized controlled trial with 2-year follow-up. Am J Sports Med 39(6):1200–1208
51. Griffin LY, Agel J, Albohm MJ et al (2000) Noncontact anterior cruciate ligament injuries: risk factors and prevention strategies. J Am Acad Orthop Surg 8(3):141–150
52. Hack K, Di Primio G, Rakhra K, Beaulé PE (2010) Prevalence of cam-type femoroacetabular impingement morphology in asymptomatic volunteers. J Bone Joint Surg Am 92(14):2436–2444
53. Hangody L (2003) The mosaicplasty technique for osteochondral lesions of the talus. Foot Ankle Clin 8(2):259–273
54. Hankemeier S, Müller EJ, Kamisnski A, Muhr G (2003) 10-year results of bone marrow stimulating therapy in the treatment of osteochondritis dissecans of the talus. Unfallchirurg 106(6):461–466
55. Hembree WC, Wittstein JR, Vinson EN, Queen RM, Larose CR, Singh K, Easley ME (2012) Magnetic resonance imaging features of osteochondral lesions of the talus. Foot Ankle Int 33(7):591–597
56. Hildebrand KA, Woo SL, Smith DW, Allen CR, Deie M, Taylor BJ, Schmidt CC (1998) The effects of platelet-derived growth factor-BB on healing of the rabbit medial collateral ligament. An in vivo study. Am J Sports Med 26(4):549–554
57. Howell SM, Clark JA, Blasier RD (1991) Serial magnetic resonance imaging of hamstring anterior cruciate ligament autografts during the first year of implantation. Am J Sports Med 19:42–47
58. Insall JN, Scott WN (2007) Surgery of the knee, 3rd edn. Philadelphia, Elsevier pp 600–650
59. Jarvinen TAH, Jarvinen TLN, K€a€ari€ainen M, A€arimaa V, Vaittinen S, Kalimo H, Jarvinen M (2007) Muscle injuries: optimising recovery. Best Pract Res Clin Rheumatol 21:317–331
60. Junge A, Dvorak J (2004) Soccer injuries: a review on incidence and prevention. Sports Med 34(13):929–938
61. Kajikawa Y, Morihara T, Sakamoto H, Matsuda K, Oshima Y, Yoshida A, Nagae M, Arai Y, Kawata M, Kubo T (2008) Platelet-rich plasma enhances the initial mobilization of circulation-derived cells for tendon healing. J Cell Physiol 215(3):837–845
62. Kang AC, Gooding AJ, Coates MH, Goh TD, Armour P, Rietveld J (2010) Computed tomography assessment of hip joints in asymptomatic individuals in relation to femoroacetabular impingement. Am J Sports Med 38(6):1160–1165
63. Kennedy JC, Willis RB (1976) The effects of local steroid injections on tendons: a biomechanical and microscopic correlative study. Am J Sports Med 4:11–21
64. Kleinman M, Gross A (1983) Achilles tendon rupture following steroid injection. Report of three cases. J Bone Joint Surg Am 65:1345–1347
65. Kon E, Filardo G, Di Martino A, Marcacci M (2011) Platelet-rich plasma (PRP) to treat sports injuries: evidence to support its use. Knee Surg Sports Traumatol Arthrosc 19(4):516–527
66. Kondo E, Yasuda K, Yamanaka M et al (2005) Effects of administration of exogenous growth factors on biomechanical properties of the elongation-type anterior cruciate ligament injury with partial laceration. Am J Sports Med 33:188–196
67. Kovacevic D, Rodeo SA (2008) Biological augmentation of rotator cuff tendon repair. Clin Orthop 466:622–633
68. Laborie LB, Lehmann TG, Engesaeter IO, Eastwood DM, Engesaeter LB, Rosendahl K (2011) Prevalence of radiographic findings thought to be associated with femoroacetabular impingement in a population-based cohort of 2081 healthy young adults. Radiology 260(2):494–502
69. Larson CM, Giveans MR, Taylor M (2011) Does arthroscopic FAI correction improve function with radiographic arthritis? Clin Orthop Relat Res 469(6):1667–1676
70. Lopez-Vidriero E, Goulding KA, Simon DA, Sanchez M, Johnson DH (2010) The use of platelet-rich plasma in arthroscopy and sports medicine: optimizing the healing environment. Arthroscopy 26(2):269–278
71. Loredo R, Sanders TG (2001) Imaging of osteochondral injuries. Clin Sports Med 20(2):249–278
72. Lyras DN, Kazakos K, Verettas D et al (2009) The effect of platelet-rich plasma gel in the early phase of patellar tendon healing. Arch Orthop Trauma Surg 129(11):1577–1582
73. Lyras DN, Kazakos K, Verettas D, Chronopoulos E, Folaranmi S, Agrogiannis G (2010) Effect of combined administration of transforming growth factor-b1 and insulin-like growth factor I on the mechanical properties of a patellar tendon defect model in rabbits. Acta Orthop Belg 76(3):380–386
74. Magnussen RA, Carey JL, Spindler KP (2011) Does autograft choice determine intermediate-term outcome of ACL reconstruction? Knee Surg Sports Traumatol Arthrosc 19(3):462–472
75. Mair SD, Seaber AV, Glisson RR et al (1996) The role of fatigue in susceptibility to acute muscle strain injury. Am J Sports Med 24:137–143
76. Mardones R (2011) Effects of Platelet-Rich Plasma (PRP) on the management of early postoperative pain and inflammation following hip arthroscopy in patients with femoroacetabular impingement: a prospective, double blinded, randomized, placebo controlled, clinical trial. ISHA 2011, Paris
77. Matava M (1996) Patellar tendon ruptures. J Am Acad Orthop Surg 4:287–296
78. Mei-Dan O, Lopez V, Carmont MR, McConkey MO, Steinbacher G, Alvarez PD, Cugat RB (2013) Adductor tenotomy as a treatment for groin pain in professional soccer players. Orthopedics 36(9):e1189–e1197
79. Mintz DN, Tashjian GS, Connell DA, Deland JT, O'Malley M, Potter HG (2003) Osteochondral lesions of the talus: a new magnetic resonance grading system with arthroscopic correlation. Arthroscopy 19(4):353–359

80. Mishra A, Pavelko T (2006) Treatment of chronic elbow tendinosis with buffered platelet-rich plasma. Am J Sports Med 34(11):1774–1778
81. Molsa J, Airaksinen O, Nasman O, Torstilla I (1997) Ice hockey injuries in Finland: a prospective epidemiologic study. Am J Sports Med 25:495–499
82. Murawski CD, Kennedy JG (2013) Operative treatment of osteochondral lesions of the talus. J Bone Joint Surg Am 95(11):1045–1054
83. Nakasa T, Adachi N, Shibuya H, Okuhara A, Ochi M (2013) Evaluation of joint position sense measured by inversion angle replication error in patients with an osteochondral lesion of the talus. J Foot Ankle Surg 52(3):331–334
84. Navid DO, Myerson MS (2002) Approach alternatives for treatment of osteochondral lesions of the talus. Foot Ankle Clin 7(3):635–649
85. Niemeyer P, Salzmann G, Schmal H, Mayr H, Südkamp NP (2012) Autologous chondrocyte implantation for the treatment of chondral and osteochondral defects of the talus: a meta-analysis of available evidence. Knee Surg Sports Traumatol Arthrosc 20(9):1696–1703
86. Nin JR, Gasque GM, Azcárate AV et al (2009) Has platelet-rich plasma any role in anterior cruciate ligament allograft healing? Arthroscopy 25(11): 1206–1213
87. Noyes FR, Butler DL, Grood ES (1984) Biomechanical analysis of human ligament grafts used in knee-ligament repairs and reconstructions. J Bone Joint Surg Am 66(3):344–352
88. Nurden AT (2011) Platelets, inflammation and tissue regeneration. Thromb Haemost 105(Suppl 1):S13–S33
89. Orr JD, Dutton JR, Fowler JT (2012) Anatomic location and morphology of symptomatic, operatively treated osteochondral lesions of the talus. Foot Ankle Int 33(12):1051–1057
90. Orrego M, Larrain C, Rosales J et al (2008) Effects of platelet concentrate and bone plug on the healing of hamstring tendons in bone tunnel. Arthroscopy 24:1373–1380
91. Paul J, Sagstetter M, Lämmle L, Spang J, El-Azab H, Imhoff AB, Hinterwimmer S (2012) Sports activity after osteochondral transplantation of the talus. Am J Sports Med 40(4):870–874
92. Peerbooms JC, Sluimer J, Bruijn DJ, Gosens T (2010) Positive effect of an autologous platelet concentrate in lateral epicondylitis in a double-blind randomized controlled trial: platelet rich plasma versus corticosteroid injection with a 1-year follow-up. Am J Sports Med 38(2):255–262
93. Peetrons P (2002) Ultrasound of muscles. Eur Radiol 12(1):35–43
94. Peterson L, Renstrom P (1986) Sports injuries: their prevention and treatment. Year Book Medical Publishers, Chicago
95. Philippon M, Schenker M, Briggs K, Kuppersmith D (2007) Femoroacetabular impingement in 45 professional athletes: associated pathologies and return to sport following arthroscopic decompression. Knee Surg Sports Traumatol Arthrosc 15(7):908–914
96. Pollard TC, Villar RN, Norton MR, Fern ED, Williams MR, Simpson DJ, Murray DW, Carr AJ (2010) Femoroacetabular impingement and classification of the cam deformity: the reference interval in normal hips. Acta Orthop 81(1):134–141
97. Radice F, Yánez R, Gutiérrez V et al (2010) Comparison of magnetic resonance imaging findings in anterior cruciate ligament grafts with and without autologous platelet-derived growth factors. Arthroscopy 26(1):50–57
98. Raikin SM, Elias I, Zoga AC, Morrison WB, Besser MP, Schweitzer ME (2007) Osteochondral lesions of the talus: localization and morphologic data from 424 patients using a novel anatomical grid scheme. Foot Ankle Int 28(2):154–161
99. Randelli PS, Arrigoni P, Cabitza P et al (2008) Autologous platelet rich plasma for arthroscopic rotator cuff repair: a pilot study. Disabil Rehabil 30(20–22):1584–1589
100. Reed GL, Fitzgerald ML, Polgár J (2000) Molecular mechanisms of platelet exocytosis: insights into the "secrete" life of thrombocytes. Blood 96(10):3334–3342
101. Rougraff BT, Shelbourne KD (1999) Early histologic appearance of human patellar tendon autografts used for anterior cruciate ligament reconstruction. Knee Surg Sports Traumatol Arthrosc 7:9–14
102. Sánchez M, Anitua E, Andia I (2005) Application of autologous growth factors on skeletal muscle healing. Presented at 2nd world congress on regenerative medicine, Liepzig, 18–20 May 2005
103. Sánchez M, Anitua E, Azofra J, Andía I, Padilla S, Mujika I (2007) Comparison of surgically repaired Achilles tendon tears using platelet-rich fibrin matrices. Am J Sports Med 35(2):245–251
104. Sánchez M, Anitua E, Azofra J, Prado R, Muruzabal F, Andia I (2010) Ligamentization of tendon grafts treated with an endogenous preparation rich in growth factors: gross morphology and histology. Arthroscopy 26(4):470–480
105. Sánchez M, Guadilla J, Fiz N, Andia I (2012) Ultrasound-guided platelet-rich plasma injections for the treatment of osteoarthritis of the hip. Rheumatology (Oxford) 51(1):144–150
106. Schimmer RC, Dick W, Hintermann B (2001) The role of ankle arthroscopy in the treatment strategies of osteochondritis dissecans lesions of the talus. Foot Ankle Int 22(11):895–900
107. Schnabel LV, Mohammed HO, Miller BJ, McDermott WG, Jacobson MS, Santangelo KS, Fortier LA (2007) Platelet rich plasma (PRP) enhances anabolic gene expression patterns in flexor digitorum superficialis tendons. J Orthop Res 25(2):230–240
108. Scranton PE Jr, Frey CC, Feder KS (2006) Outcome of osteochondral autograft transplantation for type-V cystic osteochondral lesions of the talus. J Bone Joint Surg Br 88(5):614–619
109. Seijas R, Alvarez P, Ares O, Steinbacher G, Cuscó X, Cugat R (2010) Osteocartilaginous lesions of the

talus in soccer players. Arch Orthop Trauma Surg 130:329–333

110. Seijas R, Ares O, Catala J, Alvarez-Diaz P, Cusco X, Cugat R (2013) Magnetic resonance imaging evaluation of patellar tendon graft remodelling after anterior cruciate ligament reconstruction with or without platelet-rich plasma. J Orthop Surg (Hong Kong) 21(1):10–14
111. Seijas R, Ares O, Cuscó X, Alvarez P, Steinbacher G, Cugat R (2014) Partial anterior cruciate ligament tears treated with intraligamentary plasma rich in growth factors. World J Orthop 5(3):373–378
112. Seijas R, Rius M, Ares O, García-Balletbó M, Serra I, Cugat R (2015) Healing of donor site in bone-tendon-bone ACL reconstruction accelerated with plasma rich in growth factors: a randomized clinical trial. Knee Surg Sports Traumatol Arthrosc 23(4):991–997
113. Seil R, Rupp S, Pape D, Dienst M, Kohn D (2001) Approach to open treatment of osteochondral lesions of the talus. Orthopade 30(1):47–52
114. Seo SS, Park JY, Kim HJ, Yoon JW, Park SH, Kim KH (2012) Percutaneous osteoplasty for the treatment of a painful osteochondral lesion of the talus: a case report and literature review. Pain Physician 15(5):E743–E748
115. Skendzel JG, Philippon MJ, Briggs KK, Goljan P (2014) The effect of joint space on midterm outcomes after arthroscopic hip surgery for femoroacetabular impingement. Am J Sports Med 42(5): 1127–1133
116. Silvis ML, Mosher TJ, Smetana BS, Chinchilli VM, Flemming DJ, Walker EA, Black KP (2011) High prevalence of pelvis and hip magnetic resonance imaging findings in asymptomatic collegiate and professional hockey players. Am J Sports Med 39(4):715–721
117. Stellos K, Kopf S, Paul A, Marquardt JU, Gawaz M, Huard J, Langer HF (2010) Platelets in regeneration. Semin Thromb Hemost 36(2):175–184
118. Stone DK (1998) Receptors: structure and function. Am J Med 105(3):244–250
119. Stroud CC, Marks RM (2000) Imaging of osteochondral lesions of the talus. Foot Ankle Clin 5(1):119–133
120. Struijs PA, Tol JL, Bossuyt PM, Schuman L, van Dijk CN (2001) Treatment strategies in osteochondral lesions of the talus. Review of the literature. Orthopade 30(1):28–36
121. Takao M, Uchio Y, Kakimaru H, Kumahashi N, Ochi M (2004) Arthroscopic drilling with debridement of remaining cartilage for osteochondral lesions of the talar dome in unstable ankles. Am J Sports Med 32(2):332–336
122. Taylor DW, Petrera M, Hendry M, Theodoropoulos JS (2011) A systematic review of the use of platelet-rich plasma in sports medicine as a new treatment for tendon and ligament injuries. Clin J Sport Med 21(4):344–352
123. Thermann H, Becher C (2004) Microfracture technique for treatment of osteochondral and degenerative chondral lesions of the talus 2-year results of a prospective study. Unfallchirurg 107(1):27–32
124. Tol JL, Strijs PA, Bossuyt PM, Verhagen RA, van Dijk CN (2000) Treatment strategies in osteochondral defects of the talar dome: a systematic review. Foot Ankle Int 21(2):119–126
125. Tsitskaris K, Sharif K, Meacock LM, Bansal M, Ayis S, Li PLS, Elias DA (2012) The prevalence of cam-type femoroacetabular morphology in young adults and its effect on functional hip scores. Hip Int 22(1):68–74
126. van Dijk CN, Reilingh ML, Zengerink M, van Bergen CJ (2010) The natural history of osteochondral lesions in the ankle. Instr Course Lect 59:375–386
127. Vaquerizo V, Plasencia MÁ, Arribas I, Seijas R, Padilla S, Orive G, Anitua E (2013) Comparison of intra-articular injections of plasma rich in growth factors (PRGF-Endoret) versus Durolane hyaluronic acid in the treatment of patients with symptomatic osteoarthritis: a randomized controlled trial. Arthroscopy 29(10):1635–1643
128. Vega JA, García-Suárez O, Martínez Almagro A (2000) Cartílago articular y factores de crecimiento (primera parte). Mapfre Medicina 11:212–225
129. Verhagen RA, Struijs PA, Bossuyt PM, van Dijk CN (2003) Systematic review of treatment strategies for osteochondral defects of the talar dome. Foot Ankle Clin 8(2):233–242, viii–ix
130. Wang-Saegusa A, Cugat R, Ares O, Seijas R, Cuscó X, Garcia-Balletbó M (2011) Infiltration of plasma rich in growth factors for osteoarthritis of the knee short-term effects on function and quality of life. Arch Orthop Trauma Surg 131(3):311–317
131. Weibrich G, Kleis WK (2002) Curasan PRP kit vs PCCS PRP system: collection efficiency and platelets counts of two different methods for the preparation of platelet rich plasma. Clin Oral Implants 13:437–443
132. Weiler A, Förster C, Hunt P et al (2004) The influence of locally applied platelet-derived growth factor–BB on free tendon graft remodeling after anterior cruciate ligament reconstruction. Am J Sports Med 32:881–891
133. Wong P, Hong Y (2005) Soccer injury in the lower extremities. Br J Sports Med 39(8):473–482
134. Woods C, Hawkins RD, Maltby S, Hulse M, Thomas A, Hodson A (2004) The football association medical research programme. An audit of injuries in professional football-analysis of hamstring injuries. Br J Sports Med 38(1):36–41
135. Wright-Carpenter T, Klein P, Schaferhoff P, Appell HJ, Mir LM, Wehling P (2004) Treatment of muscle injuries by local administration of autologous conditioned serum: a pilot study on sportsmen with muscle strains. Int J Sports Med 25:588–593
136. Xie X, Wu H, Zhao S, Xie G, Huangfu X, Zhao J (2013) The effect of platelet-rich plasma on patterns of gene expression in a dog model of anterior cruciate ligament reconstruction. J Surg Res 180(1):80–88

137. Yasuda K, Tomita F, Yamazaki S, Minami A, Tohyama H (2004) The effect of growth factors on biomechanical properties of the bone-patellar tendon-bone graft after anterior cruciate ligament reconstruction: a canine model study. Am J Sports Med 32(4):870–880
138. Zengerink M, Szerb I, Hangody L, Dopirak RM, Ferkel RD, van Dijk CN (2006) Current concepts: treatment of osteochondral ankle defects. Foot Ankle Clin 11(2):331–359, vi

Knee Arthritis in Ex-Footballers

28

Stefano Zaffagnini, Tommaso Roberti di Sarsina, F. Raggi, A. Grassi, T. Bonanzinga, G. Marcheggiani Muccioli, and M. Marcacci

28.1 Etiology

Elite soccer players are at a considerable risk of obtaining joint knee and ankle injuries and in addition to this high injury rate, they are exposed to a sport that is both high intensity and extensive.

Being exposed to high-intensity and prolonged sports activity, footballers are particularly vulnerable to osteoarthritis as a long-term effect of such vigorous physical stress, resulting in irreversible pathological changes in affected joints.

Osteoarthritis is the most common joint disease. The main symptoms are joint pain, stiffness, dysfunction, instability, deformity, swelling, and crepitus. Those symptoms can be presented early in an athlete career and lead to sport dismissal.

The etiology of osteoarthritis is multifactorial and not fully understood. Age is the major independent risk factor of osteoarthritis; however, aging and osteoarthritis are interrelated, not interdependent. Cartilage senescence is related to other factors, both intrinsic (e.g., alignment, overloading) and extrinsic (e.g., genetics) to the joint [1]. In the young patient, the pathogenesis of knee osteoarthritis is predominantly related to an unfavorable biomechanical environment at the joint, which results in mechanical demand that exceeds the ability of a joint to repair and maintain itself, predisposing the articular cartilage to premature degeneration [2].

Systemic risk factors are thought to make the joint vulnerable to local factors and are thereby associated with the development of OA. They include age, gender, hormonal status, and genetics. Local risk factors cause abnormal biomechanical loading on joints and include occupational activities (squatting, kneeling, lifting), joint injury, and high-level sports participation.

28.2 Injury Mechanism

28.2.1 Malalignment

Various studies tried to analyze the relationship between soccer and lower limb alignment, given a higher prevalence of bowlegs among soccer players [3].

Varus alignment has been shown to increase the risk of OA, especially in the medial condyle, and also accelerate disease progression in knees with existing OA. Due to varus alignment, the knee experiences higher loads through a larger adduction moment during gait that increases loading through the medial condyle and reduces loads passing through the lateral condyle, thus causing or exacerbating the problems of OA on the medial condyle.

S. Zaffagnini (✉) • T. Roberti di Sarsina • F. Raggi
A. Grassi • T. Bonanzinga • G. Marcheggiani Muccioli
M. Marcacci
Clinica Ortopedica e Traumatologica II,
Laboratorio di Biomeccanica ed Innovazione
Tecnologica, Istituto Ortopedico Rizzoli,
Via pupilli, 40100 Bologna, Italy
e-mail: stefano.zaffagnini@biomec.ior.it;
tommaso.robertidisarsina@hotmail.com

P. Volpi (ed.), *Football Traumatology: New Trends*, DOI 10.1007/978-3-319-18245-2_28

Varus or valgus malalignment of the lower extremity results in an abnormal load distribution across the medial and lateral tibiofemoral compartment. For example, a 4–6 % increase in varus alignment increases loading in the medial compartment by up to 20 % [4].

Articular cartilage and subchondral bone are subjected to an increased stress, suggesting axial malalignment plays an important role in the development of early OA.

However, studies examining the relationship between malalignment and early knee osteoarthritis have produced conflicting results.

A possible relationship between the incidence of early osteoarthritic changes and axial malalignment is only supported by limited evidence so far.

In contrast, the correlation between the progression of early osteoarthritic changes and axial malalignment has been well established. Both conventional radiological and MRI [5] studies found that axial malalignment is a potent risk factor for progression of early osteoarthritic changes in patients with axial malalignment. Articular cartilage loss and subchondral bone changes may lead to an increased malalignment. Cicuttini et al. [6] reported that the degree of varus knee angle was associated with a reduction in the volume of both femoral and tibial articular cartilage in the medial tibiofemoral compartment of the knee over a 1.9-year follow-up period. Similar results were seen in the lateral tibiofemoral compartment.

The rationale for high tibial osteotomy (HTO) is slowing or preventing early osteoarthritic changes by restoring a more favorable biomechanical situation, thereby reducing local compartmental overload, via correction of malalignment.

Everything suggests that malalignment is related to increased occurrence and faster progression of osteoarthritic changes, and high tibial osteotomy shows promising results even though there is not evidence of such changes prevention. Such practice must be studied deeper to increase our knowledge and to justify this practice.

28.2.2 Loss of Meniscal Tissue

Any substantial loss of meniscal tissue from injury or iatrogenic meniscectomy permanently alters knee joint biomechanics and biology [7]. Subtotal or total meniscectomy increases the risk of secondary osteoarthritic changes by a factor 14 when compared to matched controls [8], eventually resulting in radiographic changes in 30–70 % of patients [9]. The role of concomitant cartilage damage related to the trauma that resulted in meniscal injury in the first place or of iatrogenic damage related to the meniscectomy procedures has not been determined, but is likely to play a role as well. The younger the patients, the worse the outcomes, especially in those with associated articular comorbidities such as chondral damage, ligamentous instability, and malalignment [10].

28.2.3 Meniscectomy

Initially described as vestigial, nonfunctional tissue, the menisci have since been found to play a vital role in load transmission in the knee. They transmit 50 % and 70 % of the medial and lateral compartment load, respectively, with the knee in extension. This increases to almost 85 % when the knee is flexed to 90° [11]. The menisci also serve as an important secondary restraint to anteroposterior joint translation in unstable knees, that is, knees with deficient anterior cruciate ligament. Biomechanical studies have demonstrated significant alteration in load transmission with meniscal deficiency or mismatch [10].

Biomechanical and animal models of meniscal repair demonstrated near-normal load transmission [12], providing a rationale for meniscal repair when possible. The same study, however, pointed out the challenges posed by radial tears, which even after successful healing demonstrated decreased contact area.

Clinical data reflect the biomechanical changes observed experimentally. Radiographic changes in the knee joint after meniscectomy were noticed as early as 1939; however, Fairbank was the first to describe in 1948 a consistent pattern of ridge formation, femoral flattening, and joint space narrowing in 107 patients that had undergone open, most likely complete meniscectomy [13]. Jackson in 1968 reviewed 577 meniscectomized knees, demonstrating increasing numbers of patients with degenerative changes and osteoarthritic symptoms with longer follow-up, reaching 67 % and 33 %, respectively, at 30 years follow-up [14]. These findings were confirmed subsequently by multiple authors, supporting Fairbank's theory that meniscectomy predisposes the knee to osteoarthritis, especially when concomitant injuries or abnormalities are present, such as instability or malalignment. Relatively few experimental studies on this subject have been performed in vivo besides Voloshin et al. [15] who were able to demonstrate a 20 % reduction in the shock absorption capacity of the knee after meniscectomy.

28.2.4 Meniscal Transplantation

The changes in biomechanical and biological environment of the knee joint following loss of meniscal tissue, either traumatic or following meniscectomy, and the deleterious consequences of those changes on the articular cartilage are well known.

This leads to meniscal transplantation rationale, to restore the optimal biomechanical environment that has demonstrated an improved contact area and peak stresses, and a reduction in tibial translation and thus in ACL strains, the menisci being a secondary stabilizer of the knee.

Of course sizing, positioning, and fixation technique for meniscal transplants appear to have important impact on biomechanical results.

In literature, it is reported that even though degenerative changes were not avoided, they were reduced in comparison to meniscectomized controls.

Overall, patients needing a meniscal transplant without malalignment or following high tibial osteotomy had far better results.

28.2.5 Cartilage Defects

Cartilage lesions should be evaluated carefully in order to assess their depth: they are divided into partial-thickness and full-thickness defects, plus osteochondral lesions.

Partial-thickness lesions are usually less symptomatic (symptoms are usually related to bone and periarticular tissue changes) and there is little evidence regarding their progression onto osteoarthritis, while full-thickness chondral or osteochondral lesions are believed to predispose to premature osteoarthritis [16–18].

This kind of lesions are of common finding in asymptomatic patients (up to 20 % during arthroscopy and up to 40 % as MRI findings) and it's not clear which lesion and under which circumstances progress to osteoarthritis.

Various animal models have helped us to understand the biology of cartilage repair; however, due to the anatomical and biomechanical differences, they cannot give evidence on the natural history of cartilage defects in humans.

An unanswered issue still remains: do our cartilage repair strategies stop or slow down osteoarthritis process?

At present, only the classical autologous chondrocyte implantation (ACI) technique has a prospective follow-up of over 10 years.

What we know is that the repair tissue does not have the mechanical properties of native hyaline cartilage, leaving the rim of the defect exposed to increased stress. Clinical data with sufficient long-term follow-up regarding different treatment options are not yet available. However, what seems to be the aim of treatment still remains the restoration of the biomechanical environment to near normal.

28.2.6 Joint Instability or Laxity

We can define instability as a shift from the primary load-bearing areas to a different location, resulting in overloading of part of the articular cartilage, with a change in both static and dynamic loading with increased stress through the articular cartilage.

The ACL is the most commonly injured knee ligament and it is a primary constraint to anteroposterior joint translation, and isolated lesions are uncommon. Frequently other ligamentous structures or the menisci are affected, leading to further compromission of joint stability.

However, there is a lack of evidence that anterior cruciate ligament reconstruction or meniscus repair prevents the development of osteoarthritis in the long term. There is evidence of radiographic osteoarthritic changes in 50–80 % of injured knees even after adequate ACL reconstruction [19].

This can be due to a persistent excessive tibial rotation during demanding activity. This is the case of athletes whose return to high functional demanding sport is allowed by ACL reconstruction.

In conclusion, joint instability or laxity seems to play an important role in the development of early osteoarthritis even though more studies are needed to better understand and justify our everyday handling of ligamentous injuries.

28.3 Diagnosis

The classification criteria, used typically as inclusion criteria in clinical trials worldwide, are mostly the combination of clinical and radiographic findings. They include one of the following three findings, age above 50, stiffness less than 30 min, and crepitus, together with structural changes, i.e., osteophytes and joint space narrowing (Kellgren II on standardized radiographs). These classification criteria display a 91 % sensitivity and 86 % specificity. Recently, in an attempt to harmonize studies addressing the underlying genetic basis of OA, Kerkhof HJ et al. [20] published recommendations on standardization of OA phenotypes, suggesting that at least one definite osteophyte with possible joints space narrowing is needed to establish the diagnosis of radiological knee OA. Additional issues around the OA knee phenotype have been reported in other publications, highlighting the pitfalls in defining symptomatic and radiological OA [21].

Defining classification criteria of symptomatic early knee OA is certainly challenging, but is obviously based on the fact that the patient cannot be classified as established OA. To make it clinically relevant, and to help classifying patients for clinical trials, would still imply the combination of symptoms, signs, and structural changes. However, strict radiographic criteria as defined by Kellgren will not suffice to capture an early OA population. Therefore, a more comprehensive classification allowing other methods of structural assessment such as arthroscopy and MRI is proposed.

As suggested above, and in view of the existing classification criteria for OA, the following criteria are proposed. A patient can be classified as having early OA of the knee based on clinical and imaging findings and should fulfill the following three criteria:

1. Pain in the knee
2. Standard radiographs Kellgren–Lawrence grade 0 or I or II (osteophytes only)
3. At least one of the two following structural criteria:
   - Arthroscopic findings of cartilage lesions
   - MRI findings demonstrating articular cartilage
   - Degeneration and/or meniscal degeneration and/or subchondral BMLs

28.4 Treatment Strategy

There are two approaches to early osteoarthritis, conservative and surgical.

Conservative approach is usually the first choice in early knee degenerative processes, with no clear lesions or associated abnormalities requiring surgical procedures.

If we exclude the oral medication (NSAIDs, COX inhibitors) and exercise, of which we will not cover here, conservative treatment trend nowadays involves injective treatments.

Corticosteroid intra-articular therapy was firstly described in 1951 by Hollander [22], and the first clinical trial was performed by Miller et al. [23]. Since then short-term benefits of i.a. corticosteroids are well established and universally accepted; however, long-term benefits have not been confirmed and repeated use is controversial, since they might facilitate tissue atrophy, joint destruction, or cartilage degeneration.

Viscosupplementation, which involves the use of i.a. injections of hyaluronic acid (HA), adds this glycosaminoglycan to the joint, providing lubrication and shock adsorbency, and acts as a backbone for the proteoglycans of the extracellular matrix.

HAs on the market differ in molecular weight, method of preparation, dose instructions, biologic characteristics, and possible clinical outcome. Clinical trials do not confirm that differences in molecular weight have any impact on clinical efficacy, and it has not been shown that higher molecular weight is related to higher efficacy [24].

Another injective procedure based on the use of autologous blood derivatives have been developed since the mid-1990s in order to obtain an injectable material enriched with endogenous interleukins or growth factors that can lead to cartilage repair or at least reduced cartilage degeneration.

Platelet-rich plasma (PRP) is gaining more and more attention due to the pools of growth factors stored in platelet α-granules that take part in cartilage regulation.

Blood is harvested and centrifuged to separate and concentrate platelets, which are injected into the joint. Kon et al.[25] published a pilot study on 100 patients, with evidence of safety, pain reduction, and improved function. The evaluation performed at 2 years follow-up [26] showed an overall worsening and showed a median duration of the beneficial effect of 9 months. It is interesting that better results were found in patients with no clear signs of osteoarthritis, suggesting indication for early osteoarthritis.

However, no well-designed high-level studies have been found in literature to support its efficacy, and one of the main reasons can be found in the heterogeneous products used.

Conservative management with physical therapy should be prescribed for at least 3–6 months before thinking about surgery, and it must comprehend activity modification and weight normalization.

Injective therapy must be considered especially for those patients eligible for joint replacement within few years.

Preoperative counseling is fundamental in order to find the best patient-fitting solution and to set reasonable expectation.

Surgical intervention is considered after failure of conservative management and lack of other alternatives. Moreover, patients with systemic inflammatory disease and who are heavy smokers and obese are not good candidates for cartilage repair.

28.5 Surgical Treatment

As stated before varus or valgus malalignment of the lower extremity results in an abnormal load distribution across the medial and lateral tibiofemoral compartment, thus leading to unicompartmental OA. It is caused by local overload exceeding the resilience of the osteochondral unit, resulting in accelerated tissue degeneration.

Osteotomy is a very old surgical technique that remains an important procedure for salvage surgery in patients with unicompartmental OA, cartilage defects, and ACL or meniscal lesions. Surgical treatment of such lesions without malalignment correction leads often to poor results.

Indications for osteotomy are malalignment associated with unicompartmental OA, cartilage or meniscal lesions, and ligament instability.

Generalized OA affecting multiple compartments is considered a contraindication, and such patients should be considered for arthroplasty.

This procedure does not require permanent activity restriction thus being suitable for young active patients, even though it's not indicated during an elite football career as it has long rehabilitation and it is often performed bilaterally and could compromise a sportsman career.

However, it is indicated early after football dismissal in order to prevent rapid OA progression, leading the ex-footballer to an early joint replacement.

Closing-wedge high tibial osteotomy in association with ACL reconstruction and/or meniscal allograft transplantation has shown good results in varus angulated knees (combine ACL reconstruction and closing-wedge HTO for varus angulated ACL-deficient knees).

Postoperatively, patients are instructed to wear a long leg brace for the first 4 weeks after surgery.

Rehabilitation protocol, starting from the day after surgery, comprehends quadriceps muscle isometric exercises, straight leg raises, patellar mobilization, and electric muscle stimulation.

After 2 weeks, passive range of motion exercises (0°–90°) with motorized hardware. Complete range of motion should be achieved at week 6. Patients are allowed to toe-touch weight-bearing for the first 4 weeks to prevent excessive forces on the osteotomy site and, then, progressive weight-bearing. Swimming pool exercise and stationary bike should start from week 5, running 4 months after surgery, and a return to sport activity after 8 months [27].

To address focal chondral defects, osteochondral autograft transfer represents a good single-stage technique that involves harvesting and implantation of autologous osteochondral plugs.

From a small incision plugs are harvested from lesser weight-bearing regions such as the medial and lateral margins of the trochlea, the intercondylar notch, or the sulcus terminalis of the lateral femoral condyle [28].

Patients shouldn't be over 50 and present with a full-thickness focal chondral defect that should be smaller than 4 cm^2. This procedure should not be performed in case of advanced OA, inflammatory disease, uncorrectable ligamentous instability, or malalignment.

Rehabilitation, starting from day 1 after surgery, should engage in passive motion without ROM limitations, except in case of patellofemoral lesions.

Toe-touch weight-bearing for the first 6 weeks and then progressive.

If muscle mass is restored and ROM is complete, full athletic activity is permitted 4 months after surgery, and a return to sport at the preoperative level should be achieved after 6–8 months.

However, donor site morbidity has been reported, and up to 50 % of patients after surgery reported pain in the donor site.

Marcacci et al. [29] focused on the correlation between lesion size and outcomes suggesting to apply only a limited number of plugs. However, in literature good results have been reached in lesions up to 4 cm^2. Also, clinical trials showed that this technique is superior to microfracture and as good or better than autologous chondrocyte implantation (ACI) in small to medium lesions [30, 31].

In patients with bigger lesions, results are expected to be inferior than for focal lesion; however, they have few alternative treatment options. Autologous chondrocyte implantation (ACI) is one of those.

This technique developed almost 20 years ago addresses large chondral defects. This technique utilizes nowadays biodegradable scaffold, mostly collagen or hyaluronan based, as cell carriers, facilitating implantation and maintaining chondrocyte-differentiated phenotype, which is mostly done arthroscopically.

This surgical technique is indicated for young active patients with large chondral lesions, after a careful evaluation of comorbidities such as malalignment and meniscal or ligamentous insufficiency that should be addressed concurrently or before ACI.

The implant is very delicate and vulnerable for at least the first 6 weeks, so weight-bearing restriction and limited motion are suggested.

A CPM machine is used for 6 weeks in association with isometric exercise for the quadriceps. Strengthening and proprioceptive exercises are added after 6 weeks, when the use of a stationary bike and elliptical trainer is also allowed. Return to running and contact sports is delayed until at least 12–18 months to allow graft maturation.

Cavallo et al. [32] showed that hyaluronan is able to recreate an ideal environment for the cells. Their results suggest that the scaffold might favor the activation of anabolic factors, which induce chondrocyte differentiation and reduce the expression and production of catabolic molecules, thus negating the differences between cells derived from normal and degenerated cartilage. Histological and biochemical analysis showed that OA does not inhibit the regeneration process, confirming an important role for bioengineering.

Filardo et al. [33] analyzed a group of patients with degenerative cartilage lesions treated with arthroscopic second-generation hyaluronan scaffold ACI. All the scores evaluated showed a statistically significant improvement at medium-term follow-up. However, the number of failures was quite high: 18,5 % at 6 years follow-up.

Aging and joint overuse in footballers may lead to degenerative or traumatic meniscal lesions. Treatment may include meniscal resection, meniscal suture, or meniscal replacement using scaffolds or allografts.

Meniscal scaffolds are indicated in case of history of meniscal injury with loss of >25 % of meniscal tissue, both traumatic and iatrogenic, in the absence of minimal chondral damage. They require some residual meniscal tissue for attachment, thus being contraindicated in meniscectomized patients without anterior/posterior horn attachments and a circumferential rim.

Meniscal allograft transplantation is indicated in a young patient with a history of meniscectomy and pain in the meniscus-deficient compartment, in ACL-deficient patients with previous medial meniscectomy who can benefit from this second stabilizer, and in young athletic patients to avoid early joint degeneration, prior to symptom onset.

In patients with advanced chondral degeneration or evidence of significant osteophyte formation or femoral condyle flattening, this procedure is contraindicated. Other contraindications are obesity, instability, synovial defects, inflammatory disease, and previous joint infection.

Rehabilitation guidelines for meniscal scaffolds include limited weight-bearing and motion for the first 6–8 weeks and a return to sport after 6 months.

In case of meniscal allograft transplantation, weight-bearing is not permitted for 3 weeks followed by 3 weeks of partial weight-bearing and progression to full weight-bearing between week 6 and week 10.

ROM is limited to 30° during the first 2 weeks and increased by 30° every 2 weeks. Proprioceptive training is started after week 3. Swimming is allowed after week 6 and biking after week 12. Running shouldn't be introduced before week 2.

Meniscal scaffold has the general risks associated with meniscal repair, and allografts have specific risks related to the transplant itself, that is, disease transmission from the donor and injury to the patellar tendon due to the anterior approach.

Zaffagnini et al. [34] reported a 10-year follow-up in 33 male patients after either Menaflex (ReGen Biologics, USA) or partial medial meniscectomy (PMM) alone based on patient choice. The Menaflex group showed significantly lower pain and higher objective IKDC, Tegner index, and SF-36 scores; the Lysholm score did not show any significant difference. Radiographic evaluation showed significantly less medial joint space narrowing in Menaflex patients, and MRI scores remained constant between 5 and 10 years after surgery.

Verdonk et al. reported on 52 patients after Actifit (Orteq, UK) implantation. At 3 months postimplantation, MRI showed evidence of tissue ingrowth in the peripheral half of the scaffold in 86 % of patients. At 12 months MRI showed stable or improved cartilage scores compared to baseline, and statistically significant improvements were reported for IKDC functionality, Lysholm, VAS knee pain, and KOOS subscale at 6, 12, and 24 months after surgery.

There is clinical evidence to support meniscus allograft transplantation in meniscectomized painful knees. Significant pain reduction and functional improvement have been reported in a high percentage of patients and appear to be long-lasting, preventing further cartilage degeneration [35, 36]. There seems to be a strong rationale for adding meniscal transplantation to cartilage repair procedures motivated by the well-known deleterious effects of meniscal loss and positive outcomes.

Marcacci M. and Zaffagnini et al. published the results after 36 months follow-up after arthroscopic meniscus allograft transplantation in male professional soccer players. What they showed is that at 36 months from surgery 92 % of the players were able to return to play soccer and 75 % were able to return to their preinjury level of activity (Tegner score of 10) after arthroscopic meniscus allograft transplantation without bone plugs. It was to our knowledge the first study to report outcomes of arthroscopic MAT in male professional soccer players, suggesting its feasibility even in high demanding athletes but with some limitations: the small sample size and the broad range of concomitant knee injuries, due to such complex patient knee comorbidities.

28.6 Conclusion

High functional demand and limited treatment options make early OA a challenging pathology to deal with. Conservative measures as physical therapy and injections are only palliatives that can provide short-term pain relief.

Cartilage repair represent a promising treatment option for such patients. We are seeing a rapid development of new promising technologies whose aim is to provide easier application techniques, less demanding rehabilitation, and better outcomes. Normalizing knee biomechanics with concurrent procedures such as meniscal transplantation and osteotomy still remains a crucial procedure to provide an adequate environment for these new technologies, and such procedures should be performed early after football career dismissal, in order to prevent the progression of early OA.

Literature shows that the prevalence of knee OA in former elite soccer players is high compared to the general population and to other occupations. To identify players at risk for OA, a health surveillance program could be implemented in elite soccer, and preventive measures for injuries should be made. Additionally, whether the risk of developing OA varies among different subgroups of elite soccer players, for example, among different positions or age groups, remains to be explored. In this way, adequate prevention can focus on these high-risk subgroups. Furthermore, it should be determined what the consequences of knee OA in former elite soccer players are. It could be determined if retired players diagnosed with OA encounter any limitations in their activities and daily function and if OA affected the quality and length of their professional careers [37].

Joint replacement, indicated in older population, is controversial in younger patients, who are less satisfied and experience a higher failure rate, because of a higher functional demand and thus a higher consumption and revision rate.

28.6.1 Practical Implications

- As the prevalence of knee and/or ankle OA in former elite soccer players is high, health surveillance program should be implemented in elite soccer, and preventive measures for injuries should be made to identify players at risk for OA.
- Whether the risk of developing OA varies among different subgroups of elite soccer players, for example, among different positions or age groups, should be explored in order to develop and implement adequate prevention programs.
- With regard to the high prevalence of knee and/or ankle OA in former elite soccer players, it should be determined if retired players diagnosed with OA encounter any limitations in their activities and daily function and if OA affected the quality and length of their professional careers.

References

1. Loeser RF (2010) Age-related changes in the musculoskeletal system and the development of osteoarthritis. Clin Geriatr Med 26:371–386
2. Buckwalter JA, Martin JA, Brown TD (2006) Perspectives on chondrocyte mechanobiology and osteoarthritis. Biorheology 43:603–660
3. Yaniv M, Becker T, Goldwirt M, Khamis S, Steinberg DM, Weintroub S (2006) Prevalence of bowlegs among child and adolescent soccer players. Clin J Sport Med 16(5):392–396
4. Tetsworth K, Paley D (1994) Malalignment and degenerative arthropathy. Orthop Clin North Am 25:367–377
5. Brouwer GM, van Tol AW, Bergink AP, Belo JN, Bernsen RM, Reijman M, Pols HA, Bierma-Zeinstra SM (2007) Association between valgus and varus alignment and the development and progression of radiographic osteoarthritis of the knee. Arthritis Rheum 56:1204–1211
6. Cicuttini F, Wluka A, Hankin J, Wang Y (2004) Longitudinal study of the relationship between knee angle and tibiofemoral cartilage volume in subjects with knee osteoarthritis. Rheumatology (Oxford) 43:321–324
7. Heijink A, Gomoll AH, Madry H, Drobnič M, Filardo G, Espregueira-Mendes J, Van Dijk CN (2012) Biomechanical considerations in the pathogenesis of osteoarthritis of the knee. Knee Surg Sports Traumatol Arthrosc 20(3):423–435
8. Roos EM, Ostenberg A, Roos H, Ekdahl C, Lohmander LS (2001) Long-term outcome of meniscectomy: symptoms, function, and performance tests in patients with or without radiographic osteoarthritis compared to matched controls. Osteoarthritis Cartilage 9:316–324
9. Alford JW, Lewis P, Kang RW, Cole BJ (2005) Rapid progression of chondral disease in the lateral compartment of the knee following meniscectomy. Arthroscopy 21:1505–1509
10. van Dijk CN, Tol JL, Struijs PAA (1997) Complications, rehabilitation and results of arthroscopic meniscectomy and meniscal repair: a review of the literature. J Sports Traumatol Relat Res 19:43–50

11. Ahmed AM, Burke DL (1983) In vitro measurement of static pressure distribution in synovial joints – part I: tibial surface of the knee. J Biomech Eng 105:216–225
12. Baratz ME, Fu FH, Mengato R (1986) Meniscal tears: the effect of meniscectomy and of repair on intraarticular contact areas and stress in the human knee. A preliminary report. Am J Sports Med 14:270–275
13. Fairbank TJ (1948) Knee joint changes after meniscectomy. J Bone Joint Surg Br 30B:664–670
14. Jackson JP (1968) Degenerative changes in the knee after meniscectomy. Br Med J 2:525–527
15. Voloshin AS, Wosk J (1983) Shock absorption of meniscectomized and painful knees: a comparative in vivo study. J Biomed Eng 5:157–161
16. Buckwalter JA (2002) Articular cartilage injuries. Clin Orthop Relat Res 402:21–37
17. Ding C, Cicuttini F, Scott F, Boon C, Jones G (2005) Association of prevalent and incident knee cartilage defects with loss of tibial and patellar cartilage: a longitudinal study. Arthritis Rheum 52:3918–3927
18. Heir S, Nerhus TK, Rotterud JH, Loken S, Ekeland A, Engebretsen L, Aroen A (2010) Focal cartilage defects in the knee impair quality of life as much as severe osteoarthritis: a comparison of knee injury and osteoarthritis outcome score in 4 patient categories scheduled for knee surgery. Am J Sports Med 38:231–237
19. Lohmander LS, Ostenberg A, Englund M, Roos H (2004) High prevalence of knee osteoarthritis, pain, and functional limitations in female soccer players twelve years after anterior cruciate ligament injury. Arthritis Rheum 50:3145–3152
20. Kerkhof HJ, Meulenbelt I, Akune T, Arden NK, Aromaa A, Bierma-Zeinstra SM et al (2011) Recommendations for standardization and phenotype definitions in genetic studies of osteoarthritis: the TREAT-OA consortium. Osteoarthritis Cartilage 3:254–264
21. Felson DT, Niu J, Guermazi A, Sack B, Aliabadi P (2011) Defining radiographic incidence and progression of knee osteoarthritis: problems with the Kellgren and Lawrence scale. Ann Rheum Dis 70:1884–1886
22. Hollander JL (1951) The local effects of compound F (hydro cortisone) injected into joints. Bull Rheum Dis 2:3–4
23. Miller JH, White J, Norton TH (1958) The value of intraarticular injections in osteoarthritis of the knee. J Bone Joint Surg Br 40-B:636–643
24. Kon E, Filardo G, Drobnic M, Madry H, Jelic M, van Dijk N, Della Villa S (2012) Non-surgical management of early knee osteoarthritis. Knee Surg Sports Traumatol Arthrosc 20(3):436–449
25. Kon E, Buda R, Filardo G, Di Martino A, Timoncini A, Cenacchi A, Fornasari PM, Giannini S, Marcacci M (2010) Platelet-rich plasma: intra-articular knee injections produced favorable results on degenerative cartilage lesions. Knee Surg Sports Traumatol Arthrosc 18:472–479
26. Filardo G, Kon E, Buda R, Timoncini A, Di Martino A, Cenacchi A, Fornasari PM, Giannini S, Marcacci M (2011) Platelet-rich plasma intra-articular knee injections for the treatment of degenerative cartilage lesions and osteoarthritis. Knee Surg Sports Traumatol Arthrosc 19:528–535
27. Gomoll AH, Filardo G, Almqvist FK, Bugbee WD, Jelic M, Monllau JC, Puddu G, Rodkey WG, Verdonk P, Verdonk R, Zaffagnini S, Marcacci M (2012) Surgical treatment for early osteoarthritis. Part II: allografts and concurrent procedures. Knee Surg Sports Traumatol Arthrosc 20(3):468–486
28. Gomoll AH, Filardo G, de Girolamo L, Espregueira-Mendes J, Marcacci M, Rodkey WG, Steadman JR, Zaffagnini S (2012) Kon E surgical treatment for early osteoarthritis. Part I: cartilage repair procedures. Knee Surg Sports Traumatol Arthrosc 20(3):450–466
29. Marcacci M, Kon E, Delcogliano M, Filardo G, Busacca M, Zaffagnini S (2007) Arthroscopic autologous osteochondral grafting for cartilage defects of the knee: prospective study results at a minimum 7-year follow-up. Am J Sports Med 35:2014–2021
30. Dozin B, Malpeli M, Cancedda R, Bruzzi P, Calcagno S, Molfetta L, Priano F, Kon E, Marcacci M (2005) Comparative evaluation of autologous chondrocyte implantation and mosaicplasty: a multicentered randomized clinical trial. Clin J Sport Med 15:220–226
31. Hangody L, Dobos J, Baló E, Pánics G, Hangody LR, Berkes I (2010) Clinical experiences with autologous osteochondral mosaicplasty in an athletic population: a 17-year prospective multicenter study. Am J Sports Med 38:1125–1133
32. Cavallo C, Desando G, Facchini A, Grigolo B (2010) Chondrocytes from patients with osteoarthritis express typical extra- cellular matrix molecules once grown onto a three-dimensional hyaluronan-based scaffold. J Biomed Mater Res A 93:86–95
33. Filardo G, Kon E, Di Martino A, Patella S, Altadonna G, Balboni F, Visani A, Bragonzoni L, Marcacci M (2011) Second- generation arthroscopic autologous chondrocyte implantation for the treatment of degenerative cartilage lesions. A prospective 6-year follow-up study. Knee Surg Sports Traumatol Arthrosc. doi:10.1007/s00167-011-1732-5
34. Zaffagnini S, Marcheggiani Muccioli GM, Lopomo N, Bruni D, Giordano G, Ravazzolo G, Molinari M, Marcacci M (2011) Prospective long-term outcomes of the medial collagen meniscus implant versus partial medial meniscectomy: a minimum 10-year follow-up study. Am J Sports Med 39:977–985
35. Zaffagnini S, Marcheggiani Muccioli GM, Grassi A, Bonanzinga T, Filardo G, Canales Passalacqua A, Marcacci M (2011) Arthroscopic lateral collagen meniscus implant in a professional soccer player. Knee Surg Sports Traumatol Arthrosc 19:1740–1743
36. Marcacci M, Marcheggiani Muccioli GM, Grassi A, Ricci M, Tsapralis K, Nanni G, Bonanzinga T, Zaffagnini S (2014) Arthroscopic meniscus allograft transplantation in male professional soccer players: a 36-months follow-up study. Am J Sports Med 42:382
37. Kuijt MT, Inklaar H, Gouttebarge V, Frings-Dresen MH (2012) Knee and ankle osteoarthritis in former elite soccer players: a systematic review of the recent literature. J Sci Med Sport 15(6):480–487. doi:10.1016/j.jsams.2012.02.008, Epub 8 May 2012

29 Groin Pain

Nicola Maffulli, Alessio Giai Via, and Francesco Oliva

29.1 Introduction

Groin pain is well known among both athletes and physicians. Groin injuries account for about 6 % of all athletes' injuries, and the incidence increases up to 13 % in specific sport such as soccer [13]. The incidence ranges from 12 % to 16 % of all injuries per season in a recent prospective study of hip and groin injuries in professional soccer players, with a mean absence from competitions of 15 days [61]. This is probably due to typical soccer movements like jumps, dribbling and rapid twisting which cause high stress to the pubic symphysis and muscular imbalance. Kicking and running on uneven surfaces, male gender and preseasonal training are considered risk factors for developing groin pain [26].

N. Maffulli, MD, MS, PhD, FRCS (Orth) (✉)
Department of Musculoskeletal Disorders, School of Medicine and Surgery, University of Salerno, Salerno, Italy

Barts and the London School of Medicine and Dentistry, Centre for Sports and Exercise Medicine, Mile End Hospital, Queen Mary University of London, 275 Bancroft Road, London E1 4DG, UK
e-mail: n.maffulli@qmul.ac.uk

A. Giai Via, MD • F. Oliva, MD, PhD
Department of Orthopaedic and Traumatology, University of Rome "Tor Vergata", School of Medicine, Viale Oxford 81, 00133 Rome, Italy
e-mail: alessiogiaivia@hotmail.it; olivafrancesco@hotmail.com

Diagnosis and management are major challenges for physicians because the aetiopathogenesis is not clear yet. Diagnosis is difficult because of the anatomical complexity of the groin area, the biomechanics of the pubic symphysis region and the large number of potential sources of groin pain (Table 29.1). A recent review reported that 30–90 % of patients are affected by different coexisting groin pathologies [56]. This condition justifies the term 'groin pain syndrome' (GPS). The nomenclature is also confusing. Many athletes with a diagnosis of 'sport hernia' or 'athletic pubalgia' have a spectrum of related pathologic conditions resulting from musculotendinous injuries and subsequent instability of the pubic symphysis without any finding of inguinal hernia at physical examination. For this reason, the term 'groin pain disruption' introduced by Gilmore is becoming more popular [19].

Management of groin pain is difficult, and patients usually undergo prolonged rest and many different treatments. The management of groin pain is multidisciplinary and consists of rehabilitation, physical therapies or surgery for patients who do not respond to conservative treatments [55].

29.2 Groin Anatomy

Knowledge of groin anatomy is of great importance in understanding the causes of groin pain. The groin region consists of ligaments, tendons, muscles and fascia which all insert to the pubic

P. Volpi (ed.), *Football Traumatology: New Trends*, DOI 10.1007/978-3-319-18245-2_29

Table 29.1 Differential diagnosis of groin pain

Intra-articular pathologies	Extra-articular pathologies	Non-musculoskeletal disorders
Femoroacetabular impingement (FAI) syndrome	Insertional adductor and rectus abdominis tendinopathy	***Intra-abdominal pathologies***
Acetabular labral tears	Groin pain disruption	Appendicitis
Chondral lesions	Osteitis pubis	Diverticulitis/diverticulosis
Femoral neck stress fractures	Greater trochanter pain syndrome	Lymphadenitis
Osteoarthrosis	Lumbar radiculopathy	Inflammatory bowel disease
Transitory synovitis	Pubic ramus stress fracture	Inguinal hernia
Osteonecrosis of the femoral head	Apophyseal avulsion fractures	
Osteochondritis dissecans	Sacroiliac joint disorders	***Genitourinary***
Legg-Calvè-Perthes disease	Nerve entrapment	Adnexal torsion
Epiphysiolysis of the femoral head	Snapping hip syndrome	Nephrolithiasis
Septic arthritis		Orchitis
Oncologic process		Ovarian cysts
		Pelvic inflammatory disease
		Urinary tract infections
		Endometriosis
		Prostatitis
		Testicular cancer

bone and symphysis. The inguinal region consists of the inferior part of large flat muscular sheets (obliquus externus, internus and transversus abdominis), the rectus abdominis, the pyramidalis, the inguinal canal, the symphysis pubis and the femoral triangle. Central to the groin area is the inguinal ligament. The inguinal ligament is an important connective tissue structure which supports soft tissues in the groin as well as the external abdominal oblique muscle. It arises from the inferior aponeurosis of the external abdominal oblique and runs obliquely across the pelvis. On its superior and lateral end, it connects to the anterior iliac spine of the ilium and extends to the pubic tubercle of the pubis bone on its inferior and medial end. The inguinal ligament supports the muscles that run inferior to its fibres, including the iliopsoas and pectineus muscles of the hip. It also supports the nerves and blood vessels of the leg as they pass through the groin, including the femoral artery, femoral vein and femoral nerve. The support provided by the inguinal ligament is important to maintain the flexibility of the hip region while allowing vital blood and nerve supply to the leg. A small opening in the muscles and connective tissues of the abdomen, the superficial inguinal ring, is located just superior to the inguinal ligament. This opening is part of the inguinal canal and permits the spermatic cord in males and the round ligament of the uterus in females to exit the abdominopelvic cavity and pass through the external tissues of the pelvis. The pubic symphysis is an amphiarthrodial joint with limited mobility (it can be moved roughly 2 mm with 3° of rotation) but with good capacity of load absorption, thanks to the presence of hyaline and fibrous cartilage and connective tissue on its surface. The abdominal and paravertebral muscles act synergistically to stabilize the symphysis pubis during movements, particularly during static or dynamic single-leg stance [4]. The adductor muscles act as antagonists and exert opposing traction and rotation on the pubic symphysis. The femoral triangle is located in the upper inner thigh, and several structures pass through it: the femoral nerve, the femoral vessels and the sartorius, the iliopsoas, the pectineus and the adductor longus muscles. The adductor muscles also comprise the adductor brevis, the adductor magnus and the gracilis. Many peripheral nerves cross or innervate the anatomic structures of the inguinal region. These include the ilioinguinal nerve (T8–L1); the obturator nerve (L2–L4); the medial and intermediate cutaneous nerve of the thigh (L2–L3), with sensory function; and the femoral nerve (L2–L4) [4].

29.3 Insertional Adductors and Rectus Abdominis Tendinopathy

Insertional tendinopathy of the adductors and rectus abdominis is a frequent cause of groin pain in athletes. It involves the adductor muscles and/or the rectoabdominal muscles [57]. The incidence of insertional adductors tendinopathy is about 2.5–3 % in athletes and is more frequent in soccer, basketball, hockey and rugby players and long-distance runners [44]. More than 70 % of patients are males. Even if insertional adductor tendinopathy can develop independently, in most of the cases, it occurs in association with osteitis pubis. Hiti et al. suggested that groin pain and pubic osteitis are the most common causes of chronic groin pain in athletes [21].

The aetiopathogenesis is multifactorial. It is related to functional overuse and repeated microtraumas caused by torsion and traction of abdominal and adductor tendon insertions. The overloading of the pubic symphysis and insertional tendons could be induced by the strength imbalance between the hypertonic adductor muscle and hypotonic large flat muscular sheets of the abdomen [42]. Other authors suggest that this condition could also be induced by the hypertonia of the quadriceps femoris muscle [57]. Some intrinsic and extrinsic factors may predispose athletes to develop insertional adductor tendinopathy. The muscular imbalance is the main intrinsic factor, while reduced flexibility of the posterior chain muscles and/or iliopsoas-lumbar hyperlordosis; sacroiliac, sacrolumbar and hip arthropathy; and marked asymmetry and/or dissymmetry of lower limbs are other risk factors. Incorrect athletic training, unsuitable footwear and unfavourable conditions of the playground are considered as extrinsic factors [57].

29.3.1 Clinical Examination and Diagnosis

The main symptom is groin or lower abdominal pain, with radiation to the medial aspect of the thigh, abdomen and, in some cases, perianal area. The symptoms are unilateral at the beginning and occur after sport but this condition is progressive in nature, limiting or stopping the sporting activities. In advanced stages, the pathology could progress bilaterally and could affect social life and everyday activities such as climbing stairs and getting up from a bed or a chair. Sometimes sneezing, coughing, defecating and sexual activity can reproduce the symptoms [48].

Diagnosis is based on clinical examination and supported by imaging. Painful points such as tendon insertions of adductor, rectoabdominal and iliopsoas muscles, the pubic symphysis and iliac spines are evaluated. Pain can also be reproduced with adduction or contraction of the abdominal, the iliopsoas, the rectus femoris and the adductor muscles against resistance and with passive stretching of the adductors and iliopsoas muscle. The mobility of the hips on all planes should be assessed. Specific tests show the shortening of the anterior chain (test of Thomas), the posterior chain (hamstring muscles) and sacroiliac joint (test of Patrick and test of Gaenslen). Finally, a peripheral neurological examination should be conducted.

Plain radiographs, ultrasound scan and MRI are useful to confirm the diagnosis. Plain radiographs are useful to exclude different causes of groin pain, including femoroacetabular impingement (FAI), hip osteoarthritis or fractures. Flamingo stress views are used to assess pelvic stability, which is measured as the amount of vertical displacement observed at the symphysis [18]. Flamingo stress views are obtained with the patient bearing weight alternately on each leg. If a displacement greater than 2 mm at the symphysis pubis is observed, a macro-instability of the symphysis pubis can be diagnosed. Other indirect signs of pelvic instability can be observed at plain radiography, such as spurs of the cortical bone, subchondral cysts and associated widening of the sacroiliac joint (Fig. 29.1). Ultrasound evaluation allows to assess musculotendinous structures, soft tissues and insertional area of tendons and ligaments. MRI usually shows bone marrow oedema, insertional tendinopathy of the adductors and rectus abdominis [45] and

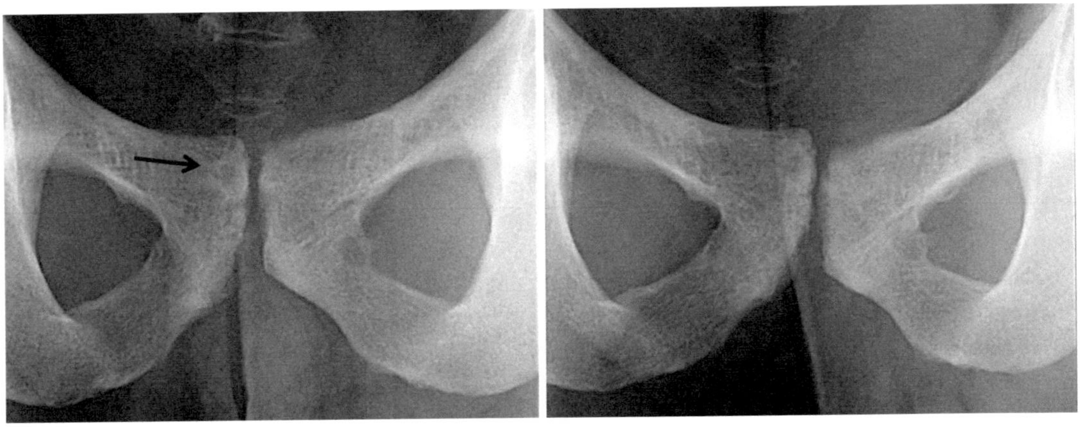

Fig. 29.1 Flamingo stress views show pelvic instability with displacement at the symphysis pubis greater than 2 mm. Note the subchondral cyst (*black arrow*) which is an indirect sign of degenerative changes

symphysis capsular disruption; central disc protrusion may also be present, in particular in soccer players [7].

29.3.2 Treatment

The management is multidisciplinary. Treatment includes rest and focused rehabilitation. Rehabilitation phases can be divided in acute, subacute and return to sport [57]. The first goal during acute phase is pain reduction. For this purpose, pharmacological, instrumental, physical and manual therapies are recommended. Laser therapy and extracorporeal shock wave therapy are useful to relieve pain. Rehabilitation measures consist of postural balance techniques through global and site-specific stretching, the use of mechanical and proprioceptive orthotic insoles and global postural re-education [60]. In the early stages, physical therapy involves isometric strengthening of the abdominal muscles and adductor muscles in the gym or in a therapeutic swimming pool. In the subacute phase, muscle strengthening is increased by the introduction of concentric and eccentric exercises and by cardiovascular reconditioning. Core stability exercises are useful in this phase [39]. Finally, running is gradually introduced, at first on a treadmill. The return-to-sport phase of rehabilitation consists of aerobic running with increasing speed.

If conservative measures have failed for at least 3 months, surgical intervention may be necessary [57]. Adductor longus tenotomy is commonly performed in order to reduce the stress of the hypertonic adductor muscle on the pubic symphysis and to reduce the muscular imbalance of the adductor-abdomino. Many authors reported good results and high rate of return to sport after adductor longus tenotomy. In a large series of professional soccer players, Mei-Dan et al. reported good or excellent results in 80 % of patients with a mean return to sport in 11 weeks (range, 4–36 weeks) [37]. Robertson et al. reported improvements in 91 % of patients (99/109) in particular in patients with the worst preoperative symptoms [49]. More recently good results have been reported with bilateral mini-invasive adductor tenotomy for athletes suffering from unilateral adductor longus tendinopathy refractory to nonoperative management [35]. At the time of the latest follow-up, 76 % of patients returned to their pre-injury level of sport or higher levels, with a median time to return to sport of 18 weeks. However, 3 of 29 patients ceased to participate in sport. Concern following adductor tenotomy is the potential for loss of hip adductor strength, although this does not seem to influence participation in high-level sport [1, 37].

29.4 Femoroacetabular Impingement Syndrome

Femoroacetabular impingement (FAI) syndrome is a common cause of pain and discomfort in young active non-dysplastic patients [16].

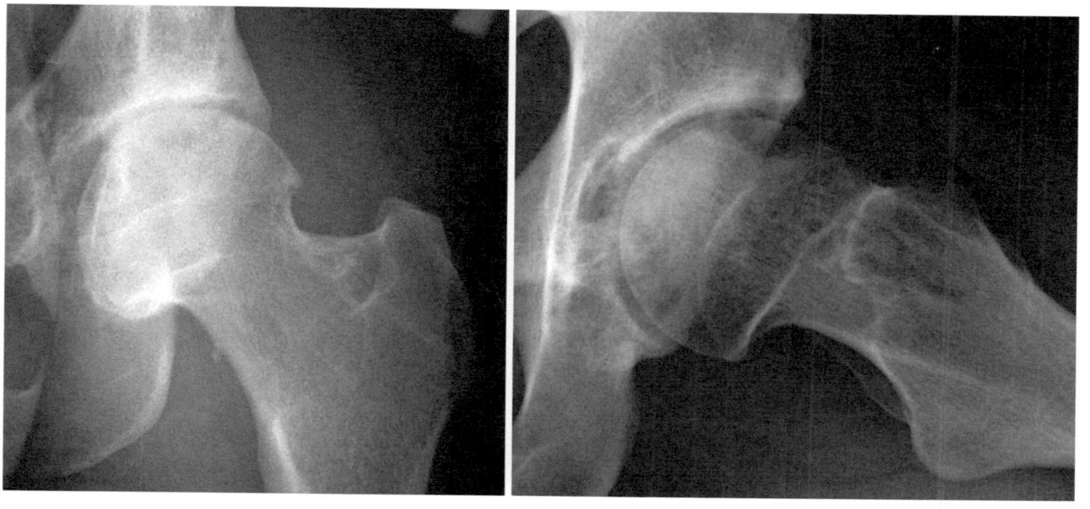

Fig. 29.2 FAI of a 31-year-old soccer player. Large chondral lesions are evident at plain radiographs

Two types of impingement have been described, namely, cam impingement and pincer impingement. Cam impingement is caused by an abnormal morphology of the femoral head with increasing radius into the acetabulum during forceful motion, especially flexion. Pincer impingement is the result of an altered anatomy of the acetabulum, as coxa profunda or abnormal retroversion or anteversion of the acetabular rim, which cause pathological contact between the acetabular rim and the femoral head-neck junction [16]. Dynamic pincer impingement can occur in normal hips if the required range of movement is large or translated, as in dancers, gymnasts and hockey players [5]. Cam-type impingement is more common in young and athletic males, while the pincer-type impingement is more common in middle-aged females [16]. However, a minority of patients present pure FAI (14 %): most patients have a combination of both forms (86 %), the so-called mixed pincer and cam impingement.

FAI alters the biomechanics of the hip resulting in painful and limited range of motion, mostly in flexion and internal rotation. In cam impingement, the nonspherical portion of the femoral head adducting against the acetabular rim leads to deep chondral lesions and extensive labral tears. In pincer-type impingement, the first structure to fail is the acetabular labrum, leading to ossification of the rim and additional deepening of the acetabulum and worsening of the coverage. In pincer impingement, chondral lesions are smaller than in cam type and often limited to a small rim area [16]. However, FAI is not symptomatic in all cases. FAI in healthy young adults may be asymptomatic up to 35 % of cases [30].

29.4.1 Diagnosis

Groin pain and limited hip motion are the clinical key symptoms and signs of FAI. A decreased ROM, in particular of internal rotation, is the most common sign in case of FAI. People with asymptomatic FAI also demonstrate reduced ROM compared with people with no evidence of FAI [11]. Many specific clinical tests have been developed to support clinical diagnosis of FAI. A recent systematic review showed that hip-specific tests have high sensitivity but poor specificity and that only the FADIR test (flexion, adduction and internal rotation test) and the flexion-internal rotation test are valuable screening tests for FAI and acetabular labral tears [47].

Standard anteroposterior pelvic and lateral cross-table radiographs supported the first clinical suspicion of FAI disease (Fig. 29.2). MRI arthrography with gadolinium is important for assessing the status and extent of labral and cartilage lesions (Fig. 29.3) [22].

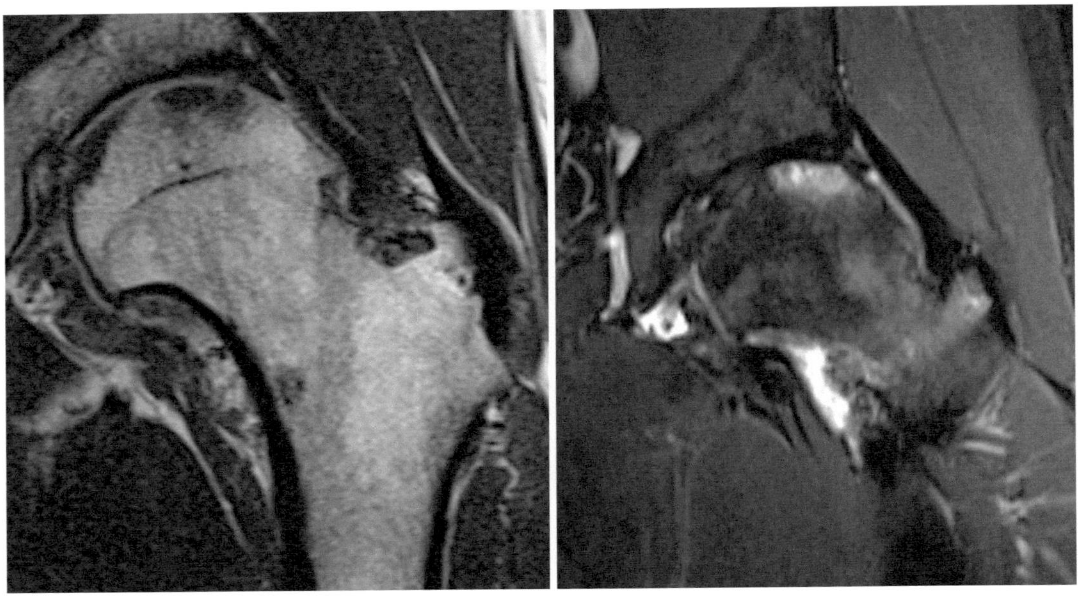

Fig. 29.3 T1- and T2-weighted MRI with gadolinium of the same patient showing "Large osteochondral lesions and labral tear

29.4.2 Treatment

The management of FAI is still controversial. The appropriate timing for surgery is also debated, even though recent studies showed that delayed surgery may lead to progression of the disease to the point where joint preservation is no longer indicated [34]. Some authors suggest that patients should undergo surgery within 6 months of symptom onset [3].

Surgery is indicted to relieve symptoms, to treat concomitant degenerative joint disease and to encourage return to sport. According to present data, arthroscopy, open surgery and arthroscopic followed by mini-open surgery are comparable for functional results, biomechanics and return to sport [46]. Hip dislocation and open osteochondroplasty were considered the gold standard treatment, with good to excellent results in 70–80 % of patents [16, 34, 41]. These authors suggest that complex bony abnormalities including extra-articular impingement, major deformities and global pincer FAI are better treated by open techniques, which also allow femoral osteotomies or acetabular reorientations when they seem appropriate. Heterotopic ossification is the most frequent complication after open surgery [46].

Recent studies reported good results after less invasive arthroscopic treatment in terms of time to recovery and allowing 93 % of patients to return to their pre-injury sport [46]. In a study on more than 600 patients, the quality of life scores improved in 76.6 % of cases after hip arthroscopy at 3 years follow-up [36]. However, arthroscopy is more technically demanding. A need for a revision hip arthroscopy has been reported for persistent symptoms, further debridement, lysis of adhesions and advanced osteoarthritis. A recent study showed that, in patients who undergo revision hip arthroscopy for persistence of groin pain, findings of FAI are still evident at imaging and revision surgery [20].

Finally, it is difficult to state whether surgery modifies the evolution of osteoarthritis in young patients and contributes to prevent the development of osteoarthritis. Open dislocation and debridement show a higher rate of conversion to total hip arthroplasty, particularly in patients with pre-existing severe osteoarthritis and cartilage lesions [46]. Concomitant cartilage lesions and degenerative changes result in lower clinical and functional scores, short-term pain relief, no evidence of long-term satisfactory outcomes and higher rate of conversion to total hip arthroplasty [46].

Table 29.2 Stages of osteitis pubis according to Rodriguez et al.

	Side of pain	Side of pain	Characteristics of pain
Stage 1	Unilateral symptoms	Inguinal, with radiation to adductors. Usually involve the dominant leg	Mechanical, settles after rest, returns after training
Stage 2	Bilateral symptoms	Inguinal pain involving the adductor muscles	Increases after training
Stage 3	Bilateral symptoms	Groin, adductor region, suprapubic, abdominal muscles	During training, kicking, sprinting, turning. Cannot achieve training goals, forced to withdraw
Stage 4	Generalized symptoms	Generalized, pelvic girdle and radiation to lumbar region	Walking, getting up, straining at stool, simple activities of daily living. Pain with defecation and sneezing

29.5 Osteitis Pubis

Osteitis pubis is a painful degenerative condition of the pubic symphysis, surrounding soft tissues and tendons. It was first described by Beer in 1924 [53], and it is currently considered as one of the most debilitating syndromes to affect athletes [50]. The incidence in the general athletic population has been reported as 0.5–7 %. It mostly affects basketball players, distance runners and athletes participating in kicking sport, such as soccer or football, where the incidence is up to 13 % in patients with groin pain [9]. It affects more often males, while it has been reported in females in about 5 % of cases [58].

Even though the pathogenesis is still debated, currently the new concepts of 'sport-related chronic groin injury' and 'groin disruption injury' describe a condition of chronic groin pain associated with pubic instability [58]. Muscle imbalance between the abdominal and hip adductor muscles is considered the most important pathogenetic factor in the development of this condition [14]. The abdominal muscles act synergistically with the posterior paravertebral muscles to stabilize the symphysis, allowing single-leg stance while maintaining balance and contributing to the power and precision of the kicking leg. The adductors are antagonists to the abdominal muscles. Imbalances between abdominal and adductor muscle groups disrupt the equilibrium of forces around the symphysis pubis, predisposing the athlete to a subacute periostitis caused by chronic microtrauma.

29.5.1 Clinical Presentation and Diagnosis

Athletes with osteitis pubis commonly present with anterior and medial groin pain and, in some cases, may have pain centred directly over the pubic symphysis. Pain may also be felt in the adductor region, lower abdominal muscles, perineal region, inguinal region or scrotum. The pain is usually aggravated with running, cutting, hip adduction and flexion against resistance and loading of the rectus abdominis [6].

The diagnosis is clinical, based on clinical history, physical examination and functional assessment. Physical examination findings include tenderness to palpation of the pubic symphysis and pain with resisted strength testing of the adductor and lower abdominal muscle groups.

Imaging studies include plain radiography, MRI and CT scan, and they are advocated to exclude concomitant pathologies. MRI can show bone marrow oedema, and MRI findings were graded according to subchondral bone oedema, fluid in the pubic symphysis and periarticular oedema [29]. Osteitis pubis has been classified according to the severity of symptoms by Rodriguez et al. (Table 29.2) [50].

29.5.2 Treatment

Management is conservative first, while surgery is indicated in unresponsive patients. Many studies proposed different treatment options depending on the severity of symptoms. However, a recent systematic review showed that no level 1 studies are reported in literature. Current treatment of osteitis pubis is based on level 4 evidence studies, making it difficult to compare the efficacy of different treatment protocols [9].

A progressive rehabilitation programme produces good results [24]. Patients are moved through the protocol stages after they are able to perform exercises without pain and have achieved adequate levels of movement and core stability grading. The first stage is to focus on pain control and improve lumbo-pelvic stability. Gentle prolonged stretching, except for the adductors and ischiopubic muscles, is started. Cycling on an exercise bike is introduced as cardiovascular training. In the second stage, Swiss balls and other aids are indicated to perform resistance and strength contraction exercises of the pelvic floor, transversus abdominis and multifidus muscles. Gluteal strengthening is started. In the third and final stage, eccentric work on the sliding board is started. Running time is gradually increased, and changes of pace and direction are introduced. To reproduce the sport requirements, athletes start training on the field performing exercises mimicking their sport. Kicking is allowed only at the end of this stage. Eccentric abdominal wall strengthening exercises are started. Good results have been reported with this progressive rehabilitation programme, and most of the athletes diagnosed with stages III and IV returned to sport within 3 months (10–13 weeks).

Surgery is indicated in 5–10 % of cases which do not respond to conservative treatment [62]. Different surgical techniques have been described, such as curettage of the pubic symphysis, polypropylene mesh placement into the preperitoneal retropubic space and pubic symphysis stabilization. Satisfying results have been reported in a systematic review with these techniques (72 % of return to sport for curettage of the pubic symphysis, 92 % for polypropylene mesh placement into the preperitoneal retropubic space and 100 % for pubic symphysis stabilization) [9]. However, it is difficult to state which is the best treatment strategy for osteitis pubis because of lack of level 1 randomized controlled trials. Osteitis pubis has a negative impact on the career of an athlete, who may be obliged to stop their sporting activities. Prevention programmes based on specific sport-related demands should be tailored to the needs of each individual athlete. A correct diagnosis and an early treatment are fundamental for the management because patients diagnosed earlier experience fewer symptoms and faster return to play [64].

29.6 Sportsman Hernia/Athletic Pubalgia

Sportsman hernia is a syndrome characterized by chronic groin pain in athletes that is associated with a small direct inguinal hernia [32]. The term athletic pubalgia is currently used to describe the disruption and/or separation of the more medial common aponeurosis from the pubis, usually with insertional tendinopathy of the adductors and rectus abdominis muscles. In advanced phases, it can be associated with osteitis pubis and FAI. Currently, there is little consensus concerning this condition about aetiopathogenesis and even the nomenclature. While many authors distinguish between the terms ‘sport hernia’ and ‘athletic pubalgia’, others consider them different aspects of the same pathology considering the close relationship between structures implicated in the development of this condition [12, 31]. Different terms have also been used to describe this condition, including sport hernia, athletic pubalgia, Gilmore’s groin [19], footballers’ groin injury complex, pubic inguinal pain syndrome (PIPS) and syndrome of muscle imbalance of the groin [40]. As recent studies showed that this pathology rarely arises as a single condition but multiple coexisting pathologies are often present, such as posterior inguinal canal wall deficiency and intra- and extra-articular pathologies, the term ‘groin pain disruption’ (GPD) has become more popular [17].

GPD is more frequent in males, but an increasing number of female patients are being diagnosed [38]. The aetiology is debatable. Currently, many authors believe that the underlying aetiology is muscular imbalance and pelvic instability [31, 40, 38], although isolated traumatic tears of the conjoint tendon are occasionally diagnosed.

29.6.1 Clinical Presentation and Diagnosis

Athletes typically complain of gradually increasing activity-related lower abdominal and proximal adductor-related pain. The pain is typically located over the lower lateral edge of the rectus abdominis muscle and may radiate towards the testis, suprapubic region or adductor longus origin. The onset is usually insidious, but in some cases it can involve an initial sudden 'tearing' sensation. GPD pain is often aggravated by sudden acceleration, twisting and turning, cutting and kicking, sit-ups, coughing or sneezing [2].

Diagnosis is dependent upon concordance between the patient history, physical examination and imaging investigation. Palpation for a positive inguinal cough impulse is usually either negative or equivocal. Valsalva manoeuvres such as coughing and sneezing can occasionally reproduce symptoms. Fifty percent of the hernias became more apparent with Valsalva manoeuvre, and imaging obtained during Valsalva manoeuvre aids in the detection and characterization of suspected abdominal wall hernias [23].

29.6.2 Management

The first approach to GPD is traditionally nonsurgical. However, there are issues unique to the athlete regarding timing, sport seasons and level of athlete. Physical therapy is focused on core stabilization, postural retraining and normalization of the dynamic relationship of the hip and pelvic muscles [31]. After a period of rest, a gradual pain-free progression to sport may be possible. However, there are very little data about the effectiveness of nonsurgical treatment. Physical therapy and laparoscopic surgical repair have been compared in a recent RCT [43]. The authors found that only 50 % returned to sport in the nonsurgical group at 1-year follow-up. Surgery is indicated after 3–6 months of failed conservative treatments and when the athlete is limited in season and unable to participate. A number of different surgical techniques have been described, including repair of the external oblique, transversus abdominis and transversalis fascia, repairs with mesh reinforcement, laparoscopic repairs, mini-open repairs and broad pelvic floor repairs with or without adductor releases and neurectomies [31]. Surgical repair of the sportsman hernia is associated with good functional outcomes, and 80–100 % return-to-sport rates have been reported [28, 43]. After surgery, a 3-month programme of post-operative physiotherapy is indicated to maintain pelvic stability and restore function.

29.7 Greater Trochanter Pain Syndrome

Lateral hip pain is a debilitating condition characterized by pain located at or around the greater trochanter. This is the site of confluence of three bursae, the hip abductor-lateral thigh muscles and the iliotibial band (ITB). Described for years as trochanteric bursitis, advanced imaging and surgical findings evidenced disorders involving partial tear or avulsion of the anterior aspect of the gluteus medius and minimus tendons, external snapping hip and insertional tendinopathies with no real bursal involvement [10]. For these reasons, the term 'greater trochanteric pain syndrome' (GTPS) is now used to better define this clinical condition [54]. GTPS is more frequent in women (F-M=4:1) aged 40–60 years and affects from 10 % to 25 % of the general population and up to 35 % in patients who have leg length discrepancies and low back pain [63]. Abnormal force vectors acting across the hip, leading to abnormal hip biomechanics, are predisposing factors and also age, gender, ipsilateral ITB pain, knee osteoarthritis, obesity, low back pain and specific sporting activities. The higher prevalence in women could be related to the configuration of their pelvis. Though common in sedentary patients, runners are also particularly predisposed [2].

29.7.1 Clinical Presentation and Diagnosis

Diagnosis of GTPS is clinical. Patients usually report pain anterior or posterior to the greater trochanter from several months. Local tenderness over the greater trochanteric area can be noted at palpation and positive single-leg stance and resisted external rotation tests [33]. Plain radiography excludes concomitant hip or knee joint disease and can detect insertional calcific deposits at the greater trochanter. Ultrasound scans can be indicated to assess abductor tendon thickening, tendinopathy and partial- or full-thickness tears [27]. When there is suspicion of involvement of the gluteus muscle tendons, MRI is effective to recognize partial- and full-thickness tears, tendon calcification and muscle fatty atrophy.

29.7.2 Management

Conservative measures including relative rest, anti-inflammatory medication, ice, stretching and strengthening, physical therapy, shock wave therapy, ultrasound and local corticosteroid injection are commonly used [10]. However, often symptoms linger and recurrence occurs, and symptomatic athletes need to modify training for prolonged periods. Corticosteroid injections have been used for many years, but recurrence of symptoms and incomplete relief have been commonly recorded [10]. An RCT evaluated three treatment procedures, home training, corticosteroid injection and shock wave therapy [51]. Corticosteroid injections were found to be effective in the short term, with declining effectiveness over a few months. Repetitive low-energy radial SWT without local anaesthesia did not result in early pain relief, but provides a beneficial effect over several months, with a success rate of 68 % at 4 months and 74 % at 15 months. Home training exercises included progressive exercise including piriformis stretch, iliotibial band stretch standing, straight leg raise, wall squat with ball and gluteal strengthening. Their effects were evident after 4 months, with a 41 % success rate, increasing to 80 % at 15 months. Home training exercises were more effective in the longer term. In a case control study, Furia et al. found that 76.5 % of patients who participated in regular sporting activities and were treated with SWT were able to return to sport at their pre-injury levels, compared to the 66.7 % in the control group [15]. At the final follow-up, the number of patients with excellent and good results was significantly higher after SWT.

Several surgical procedures have been described for patients' refractory to conservative treatments. Brooker reported on five patients treated with fenestration or T-shaped incision of the iliotibial band [8]. At 1 year, patients were satisfied and had near-normal function, with a Harris Hip Score of 88 compared with a baseline score of 46. Slawski and Howard performed a simple longitudinal incision of the iliotibial band (ITB) and bursectomy [52]. All the patients were satisfied. Kagan firstly described rotator cuff tears of the hip [25]. He reported good outcomes after open repair and suture reattachment of the gluteus medius at a median follow-up of 45 months. Recently, Voss et al. also reported successful short-term outcomes on 10 patients who underwent endoscopic repair of gluteus medius tears [59]. However, despite the good results reported after open and arthroscopic procedures, all the studies are small and retrospective case series reporting success rates difficult to compare.

29.8 Summary

Evaluation and treatment of groin pain in athletes is challenging. It is important to remember that 'groin pain' means 'pain in the groin area' and is not a diagnosis. The groin anatomy is complex, and pain is often caused by the association of different conditions. Frequently, groin pain is a component of a more extensive pattern of 'groin pain disruption' which involves several concurrent pathologies. These may include not only intra-articular and extra-articular pathologies around the hip but also lumbar spine diseases, nerve entrapments and intra-abdominal and genitourinary pathologies. Muscular imbalance and pelvic instability seem to be the common denominator for many conditions causing athlete's groin pain. Correct diagnosis is mandatory for appropriate management. As the differential diagnosis for chronic groin pain is wide, thorough clinical examination is paramount. Symptoms may overlap, and no high-specificity tests are available.

Many different treatment protocols and strategies have been proposed to manage groin pain. Conservative management is indicated to stabilize the pelvis and pubic symphysis. Core stability exercises and muscle stretching and strengthening exercises of the abdominal, adductor, flexor and extensor hip muscles are effective for this purpose. Better results have been reported after surgical treatment for FAI and sportsman hernia. Surgery is also indicted for patients who do not respond to conservative management. However, given the complexity of the pathology, proper treatment should be multidisciplinary.

References

1. Akermark C, Johansson C (1992) Tenotomy of the adductor longus tendon in the treatment of chronic groin pain in athletes. Am J Sports Med 20(6): 640–643
2. Anderson K, Strickland SM, Warren R (2001) Hip and groin injuries in athletes. Am J Sports Med 29: 521–533
3. Aprato A, Jayasekera N, Villar R (2012) Timing in hip arthroscopy: does surgical timing change clinical results? Int Orthop 36:2231–2234
4. Bhosale PR, Patnana M, Viswanathan C, Szklaruk J (2008) The inguinal canal: anatomy and imaging features of common and uncommon masses. Radiographics 28:819–835
5. Bizzini M, Notzli HP, Maffiuletti NA (2007) Femoroacetabular impingement in professional ice hockey players: a case series of 5 athletes after open surgical decompression of the hip. Am J Sports Med 35:1955–1959
6. Beatty T (2012) Osteitis pubis in athletes. Curr Sports Med Rep 11:96–98
7. Branci S, Thorborg K, Bech BH, Boesen M, Nielsen MB, Hölmich P (2014) MRI findings in soccer players with long-standing adductor-related groin pain and asymptomatic controls. Br J Sports Med 49:681–691
8. Brooker AF Jr (1979) The surgical approach to refractory trochanteric bursitis. Johns Hopkins Med J 145:98–100
9. Choi H, McCartney M, Best TM (2011) Treatment of osteitis pubis and osteomyelitis of the pubic symphysis in athletes: a systematic review. Br J Sports Med 45:57–64
10. Del Buono A, Papalia R, Khanduja V, Denaro V, Maffulli N (2012) Management of the greater trochanteric pain syndrome: a systematic review. Br Med Bull 102:115–131
11. Diamond LE, Dobson FL, Bennell KL, Wrigley TV, Hodges PW, Hinman RS (2015) Physical impairments and activity limitations in people with femoroacetabular impingement: a systematic review. Br J Sports Med 49:230–242
12. Economopoulos KJ, Milewski MD, Hanks JB, Hart JM, Diduch DR (2013) Sports hernia treatment: modified bassini versus minimal repair. Sports Health 5:463–469
13. Ekstrand J, Ringborg S (2001) Surgery versus conservative treatment in soccer players with chronic groin pain: a prospective randomised study in soccer players. Eur J Sports Traumatol 23:141–145
14. Fricker PA, Taunton JE, Ammann W (1991) Osteitis pubis in athletes. Infection, inflammation or injury? Sports Med 12:266–279
15. Furia JP, Rompe JD, Maffulli N (2009) Low-energy extracorporeal shock wave therapy as a treatment for greater trochanteric pain syndrome. Am J Sports Med 37:1806–1813
16. Ganz R, Parvizi J, Beck M, Leunig M, Notzli H, Siebenrock KA (2003) Femoroacetabular impingement: a cause for osteoarthritis of the hip. Clin Orthop Relat Res 417:112–120
17. Garvey JF, Hazard H (2014) Sports hernia or groin disruption injury? Chronic athletic groin pain: a retrospective study of 100 patients with long-term follow-up. Hernia 18:815–823
18. Garvey JF, Read JW, Turner A (2010) Sportsman hernia: what can we do? Hernia 14:17–25
19. Gilmore J (1998) Groin pain in the soccer athlete: fact, fiction, and treatment. Clin Sports 17:787–793
20. Haviv B, Singh PJ, Takla A, O'Donnell J (2010) Arthroscopic femoral osteochondroplasty for cam lesions with isolated acetabular chondral damage. J Bone Joint Surg Br 92:629–633
21. Hiti CJ, Stevens KJ, Jamati MK, Garza D, Matheson GO (2011) Athletic osteitis pubis. Sport Med 41: 361–376
22. Ito K, Minka MA II, Leunig M, Werlen S, Ganz R (2001) Femoroacetabular impingement and the cam-effect. A MRI-based quantitative anatomical study of the femoral head-neck offset. J Bone Joint Surg Br 83:171–176
23. Jaffe TA, O'Connell MJ, Harris JP, Paulson EK, Delong DM (2005) MDCT of abdominal wall hernias: is there a role for valsalva's maneuver? AJR Am J Roentgenol 184:847–851
24. Jardí J, Rodas G, Pedret C et al (2014) Osteitis pubis: can early return to elite competition be contemplated? Transl Med UniSa 10:52–58, 8
25. Kagan A 2nd (1999) Rotator cuff tears of the hip. Clin Orthop Relat Res 368:135–140
26. Karlsson MK, Dahan R, Magnusson H, Nyquist F, Rosengren BE (2014) Groin pain and soccer players: male versus female occurrence. J Sports Med Phys Fitness 54:487–493
27. Kong A, Van der Vliet A, Zadow S (2007) MRI and US of gluteal tendinopathy in greater trochanteric pain syndrome. Eur Radiol 17:1772–1783
28. Kopelman D, Kaplan U, Hatoum OA et al (2014) The management of sportsman's groin hernia in professional and amateur soccer players: a revised concept. Hernia. [Epub ahead of print]

29. Kunduracioglu B, Yilmaz C, Yorubulut M, Kudas S (2007) Magnetic resonance findings of osteitis pubis. J Magn Reson Imaging 25:535–539
30. Laborie LB, Lehmann TG, Engesæter I et al (2011) Prevalence of radiographic findings thought to be associated with femoroacetabular impingement in a population-based cohort of 2081 healthy young adults. Radiology 260:494–502
31. Larson CM (2014) Sports hernia/athletic pubalgia: evaluation and management. Sports Health 6:139–144
32. LeBlanc KE, LeBlanc KA (2003) Groin pain in athletes. Hernia 7:68–71
33. Lequesne M, Djian P, Vuillemin V, Mathieu P (2008) Prospective study of refractory greater trochanter pain syndrome. MRI findings of gluteal tendon tears seen at surgery. Clinical and MRI results of tendon repair. Joint Bone Spine 75:458–464
34. Leunig M, Beaulé PE, Ganz R (2009) The concept of femoroacetabular impingement: current status and future perspectives. Clin Orthop Relat Res 467:616–622
35. Maffulli N, Loppini M, Longo UG, Denaro V (2012) Bilateral mini-invasive adductor tenotomy for the management of chronic unilateral adductor longus tendinopathy in athletes. Am J Sports Med 40:1880–1886
36. Malviya A, Stafford GH, Villar RN (2012) Impact of arthroscopy of the hip for femoroacetabular impingement on quality of life at a mean follow-up of 3.2 years. J Bone Joint Surg Br 94:466–470
37. Mei-Dan O, Lopez V, Carmont MR, McConkey MO, Steinbacher G, Alvarez PD, Cugat RB (2013) Adductor tenotomy as a treatment for groin pain in professional soccer players. Orthopedics 36:1189–1197
38. Meyers WC, McKechnie A, Philippon MJ, Horner MA, Zoga AC, Devon ON (2008) Experience with "sports hernia" spanning two decades. Ann Surg 248: 656–665
39. Marshall PW, Murphy BA (2005) Core stability exercises on and off a swiss ball. Arch Phys Rehabil 86: 242–249
40. Morales-Conde S, Socas M, Barranco A (2010) Sportsmen hernia: what do we know? Hernia 14: 5–15
41. Naal FD, Miozzari HH, Wyss TF, Notzli HP (2011) Surgical hip dislocation for the treatment of femoroacetabular impingement in high-level athletes. Am J Sports Med 39:544–550
42. Orchard J, Read JW, Verrall GM, Slavotinek JP (2000) Pathophysiology of chronic groin pain in the athlete. Int J Sports Med 1:1–16
43. Paajanen H, Brinck T, Hermunen H, Airo I (2011) Laparoscopic surgery for chronic groin pain in athletes is more effective than nonoperative treatment: a randomized clinical trial with magnetic resonance imaging of 60 patients with sportsman's hernia (athletic pubalgia). Surgery 150:99–107
44. Paajanen H, Ristolainen L, Turunen H, Kujala UM (2011) Prevalence and etiological factors of sport-related groin injuries in top-level soccer compared to non-contact sports. Arch Orthop Trauma Surg 131: 261–266
45. Palisch A, Zoga AC, Meyers WC (2013) Imaging of athletic pubalgia and core muscle injuries: clinical and therapeutic correlations. Clin Sports Med 32:427–447
46. Papalia R, Del Buono A, Franceschi F, Marinozzi A, Maffulli N, Denaro V (2012) Femoroacetabular impingement syndrome management: arthroscopy or open surgery? Int Orthop (SICOT) 36:903–914
47. Reiman MP, Goode AP, Cook CE, Hölmich P, Thorborg K (2014) Diagnostic accuracy of clinical tests for the diagnosis of hip femoroacetabular impingement/labral tear: a systematic review with meta-analysis. Br J Sports Med. 2014 Dec 16. pii: bjsports-2014-094302. doi:10.1136/bjsports-2014-094302. [Epub ahead of print]
48. Robertson BA, Barker PJ, Fahrer M, Schache AG (2009) The anatomy of the pubic region revisited: implications for the pathogenesis and clinical management of chronic groin pain in athletes. Sports Med 39:225–234
49. Robertson IJ, Curran C, McCaffrey N, Shields CJ, McEntee GP (2011) Adductor tenotomy in the management of groin pain in athletes. Int J Sports Med 32:45–48
50. Rodriguez C, Miguel A, Lima H, Heinrichs K (2001) Osteitis pubis syndrome in the professional soccer athlete: a case report. J Athl Train 36(4):437–440
51. Rompe JD, Segal NA, Cacchio A, Furia JP, Morral A, Maffulli N (2009) Home training, local corticosteroid injection, or radial shock wave therapy for greater trochanter pain syndrome. Am J Sports Med 37: 1981–1990
52. Slawski DP, Howard RF (1997) Surgical management of refractory trochanteric bursitis. Am J Sports Med 25:86–89
53. Schnute WJ (1961) Osteitis pubis. Clin Orthop 20:187–192
54. Segal NA, Felson DT, Torner JC et al (2007) Greater trochanteric pain syndrome: epidemiology and associated factors. Arch Phys Med Rehabil 88: 988–992
55. Serner A, van Eijck CH, Beumer BR, Hölmich P, Weir A, de Vos RJ (2015) Study quality on groin injury management remains low: a systematic review on treatment of groin pain in athletes. Br J Sports Med. 2015 Jan 29. pii: bjsports-2014-094256. doi:10.1136/bjsports-2014-094256. [Epub ahead of print]
56. Suarez JC, Ely EE, Mutnal AB et al (2013) Comprehensive approach to the evaluation of groin pain. J Am Acad Orthop Surg 21:558–570
57. Valent A, Frizziero A, Bressan S, Zanella E, Giannotti E, Masiero S (2012) Insertional tendinopathy of the adductors and rectus abdominis in athletes: a review. Muscles Ligaments Tendons J 10(2):142–148
58. Verrall GM, Slavotinek JP, Fon GT, Barnes PG (2007) Outcome of conservative management of athletic chronic groin injury diagnosed as pubic bone stress injury. Am J Sports Med 35:467–474
59. Voos JE, Shindle MK, Pruett A, Asnis PD, Kelly BT (2009) Endoscopic repair of gluteus medius tendon tears of the hip. Am J Sports Med 37:743–747

60. Weir A, Jansen J, van Keulen J, Mens J, Backx F, Stam H (2010) Short and mid-term results of a comprehensive treatment program for longstanding adductor-related groin pain in athletes: a case series. Phys Ther Sport 11:99–103
61. Werner J, Hägglund M, Waldén M, Ekstrand J (2009) UEFA injury study: a prospective study of hip and groin injuries in professional football over seven consecutive seasons. Br J Sports Med 43: 1036–1040
62. Williams PR, Thomas DP, Downes EM (2000) Osteitis pubis and instability of the pubic symphysis. When nonoperative measures fail. Am J Sports Med 28:350–355
63. Williams BS, Cohen SP (2009) Greater trochanteric pain syndrome: a review of anatomy, diagnosis and treatment. Anesth Analg 108:1662–1670
64. Wollin M, Lovell G (2006) Osteitis pubis in four young football players: a case series demonstrating successful rehabilitation. Phys Ther Sport 7:153–160

Femoroacetabular Impingement (FAI) in Football Traumatology

30

Raul Zini and Manlio Panascì

30.1 FAI

FAI is a pathologic condition due to an abnormal contact between the articular rim of the acetabulum and the proximal femoral portion, at the junction between the neck and the head.

R. Ganz has described the peculiarities of this pathologic condition in the 1990s and in 2008 he underlined that, in order to prevent hip arthritis, a correct therapeutic treatment of FAI has the same importance as a correct treatment of hip dysplasia [1].

The results in a recent study showed that athletes facing impact sports are at an increased risk of physeal abnormalities of the anterosuperior head-neck junction that result in a CAM deformity at skeletal maturity [2].

The CAM-type impingement is sustained by an abnormal conformation of the head-neck junction at the proximal femoral epiphysis, with a loss of the femoral head sphericity and a mechanical limit to the normal range of motion. The loss of sphericity of the femoral head is determined by a bony prominence at the head-neck junction; this bony prominence is usually called "bump," and it causes a precocious contact between the femur and the acetabular edge (and, of course, the acetabular labrum) in the movement of flexion and internal rotation [3, 4].

R. Zini • M. Panascì (✉)
Maria Cecilia Hospital, GVM Care and Research, Cotignola (RA) 48010, Italy
e-mail: raulzini@gmail.com; manliopa@gmail.com

An excess of acetabular surface covering the femoral epiphysis causes PINCER impingement. The excessive acetabular coverage can be localized, in the case of acetabular retroversion, or global and generalized, in the case of "coxa profunda" or "protrusio acetabuli" [5]. Although this abnormal conformation grants a major area of superficial contact between the femoral head and the acetabular cavity, it is easy to understand that it leads to a precocious contact between the acetabular edge and the femoral neck [6].

30.1.1 Clinical Presentation

As previously mentioned, CAM impingement is characterized by a loss of the femoral head sphericity. The continuous pressure that the bump has on the labrum gradually causes an unstable cartilage flap delamination and an enlarging area of exposed subchondral bone at the peripheral board of the acetabulum.

CAM impingement is more frequent in young and active men, with clinical appearance usually before 30 years of age [7].

The very first symptom is pain, usually located at the groin and laterally, in the trochanteric area (C-sign: the patient indicates the painful area using the first two fingers of his hand, thus forming a "C" that embraces the area across the great trochanter, from anterior to posterior). Pain becomes much more continuous and intense as time goes by and is higher in case of long sitting

P. Volpi (ed.), *Football Traumatology: New Trends*, DOI 10.1007/978-3-319-18245-2_30

position and in the movement of flexion and internal rotation of the hip (the latter consisting in the "anterior impingement test"). At the objective examination, internal rotation is often very poor or completely absent, just as the combined movement of flexion, abduction and external rotation (FABER test). At the beginning of the symptoms caused by CAM impingement, very often the acetabular cartilage damage, which is peculiar of this pathologic condition, is already present, as it is sensibly precocious although clinical symptoms may be very occasional [8]. On the contrary, in the case of PINCER impingement, the compression of the acetabular labrum activates the proprioceptive fibers belonging to the labrum itself, so pain precociously appears and patients affected by PINCER impingement usually consult an orthopedic surgeon before a cartilage damage has occurred. Obviously, in the case of PINCER impingement, the acetabular labrum is the very first component to be involved in the contact between the femoral neck and the prominent acetabular edge, and this contusive trauma leads to labrum tear and degeneration. Moreover, PINCER impingement causes a recoil damage in the posteroinferior portion of the acetabulum, because the contact between the prominent acetabular edge and the femoral neck acts as a fulcrum that shifts the femoral head frontward, till hitting the inferior portion of the cavity: this pathologic mechanism leads to the creation of the so-called contrecoup lesion. PINCER impingement is more frequent in active women, and symptoms are developed later compare to Cam FAI, at about 40 years of age. Differently from CAM impingement, the articular movement which mostly evocates pain is extension and external rotation of the hip, thus creating the "posterior impingement test" [1, 6]. Pain can be either localized at the groin, trochanteric area, or, typically in the case of PINCER-type FAI, gluteal area, specifically because of the contrecoup lesion previously mentioned above.

30.1.2 Instrumental Exams

Because FAI is due to an abnormal contact between the articular surfaces, a complete and accurate radiological evaluation is essential [9]. It is mandatory to obtain a correct AP X-ray evaluation: 120 cm between the origin of the X-rays and the patient, whose inferior limbs have to be internally rotated for 15°, in order to compensate the physiological femoral neck anteversion. An axial projection is necessary, for a better evaluation of the anterior edge of the head-neck junction. Various radiological techniques have been described to obtain a correct axial view of the hip. One of the most efficient and easily obtainable axial projection is the "modified Dunn view," which is an AP projection to the hip in slight abduction (20°) and flexion (45°); another common technique for the axial view is an AP projection in "frog leg position" of the patient's lower limbs [10]. In the normal hip, the anterior edge of the acetabulum remains in a medial position in comparison to the posterior edge. On the contrary, in case of acetabular retroversion or excessive coverage by the acetabular walls toward the femoral head (i.e., in the anatomic condition that leads to a PINCER impingement) in AP projections, the anterior edge of the acetabulum stands in a more external position than the posterior edge. Sometimes, a figure of "8" appears, designed by the lines of the two acetabular edges, the anterior and the posterior ones, crossing each other: such a radiographic finding is called the "crossover sign" and is pathognomonic of an acetabular retroversion [11]. In case of CAM impingement, the presence of the "bump" at the head-neck junction appears as a prominence that, in axial X-ray projections, make the femoral epiphysis similar to a pistol grip. In axial projections, the bump is detected trough the head-neck offset [12] or the alpha-angle measurement. The higher the alpha angle appears, the bigger the bump determining the CAM impingement. In normal hips, the alpha angle is always <50°, while in the case of CAM impingement, the presence of the bump alters the profile of the neck-head junction, increasing the value of alpha angles to always >50°, sometimes up to nearly 90°[13].

MRI gives a great help for the articular anatomopathology evaluation in case of FAI. Contrasting solution (gadolinium) is directly injected inside the joint (arthro-MRI), in order to evaluate the condition of the acetabular labrum; arthro-MRI proved to be very sensible and precise in detecting the status of the labrum and the gravity of its lesions, from the very precocious alterations of its structure till the complete detachment from the bony edge of the acetabulum [14–16].

3D CT static reconstructions offer beautiful and intuitive images of the anatomic structures, but they can offer no more information than a well-performed X-ray exam and an arthro-MRI.

On the opposite, new devices with 3D CT dynamic reconstruction could actually change the way we have been treating patients, by identifying areas and degree of hip impingement between the pelvis and femur, automating measurements and providing adjustable ROM simulations that allow the development of a presurgical resection plan, based on a patient's morphology[17].

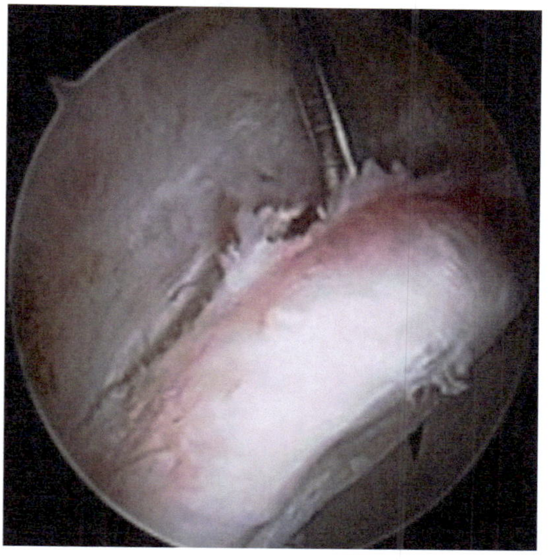

Fig. 30.1 The torn labrum is completely detached

30.2 Isolated Acetabular Labrum Tear

Isolated labral tears have become an increasingly prevalent injury among soccer players. They occur when the labrum becomes pinched and eventually torn. Impingement may predispose to a labrum damage, but it is likely that most labral tears occur due to some underlying factors, of which FAI is but one popular example [18]. Hyperextension combined with femoral external rotation is the injury pattern most commonly associated with the presentation of acetabular labral tears. Repetitive twisting motions and movements to end-range hyperflexion, hyperextension, and abduction are at greater risk. A recurring contact occurs between the anterior femoral head-neck junction and the anterior aspect of the acetabular rim and/or labrum during extreme hip flexion and internal rotation movements that are most prevalent in soccer.

30.2.1 Surgical Technique

Supine position is preferred in our routine. Traction is given with a dedicated system to obtain sufficient space and to perform arthroscopy without risk for the intra-articular structures. We routinely use a 20 cm post pad in order to minimize risk of pudendal neuropraxia. Time of traction should always be no more than 2 h [19].

Standard anterolateral and mid-anterior portals are usually sufficient to perform the entire surgical procedure. We always start with a central compartment evaluation and we routinely perform interportal capsulotomy, which allows a safer and easier instrument movement around the hip joint. Every structure is assessed to look for any pathologic sign and treatment of every possible cause of pain is achieved. Diagnostic central compartment arthroscopy is performed with a 70° arthroscope to identify any labral or acetabular chondral lesions as well as the impingement. In case of a labrum tear, we usually reattach it with resorbable suture anchors (Figs. 30.1 and 30.2); a debridement is a second choice only in case of degenerative lesions. Labral repair with a simple looped stitch, labral base stitch, or a vertical mattress technique is chosen depending on labrum dimensions. It represents an evolution for orthopedic sport medicine, and although reports of labral debridement have been promising, restoring the normal chondrolabral junction with suture-anchor repair techniques can potentially provide a more viable option for healing potential of the labrum [20–22].

Chondral pathologies are treated with shaving, micro-fractures, or biomimetic scaffold

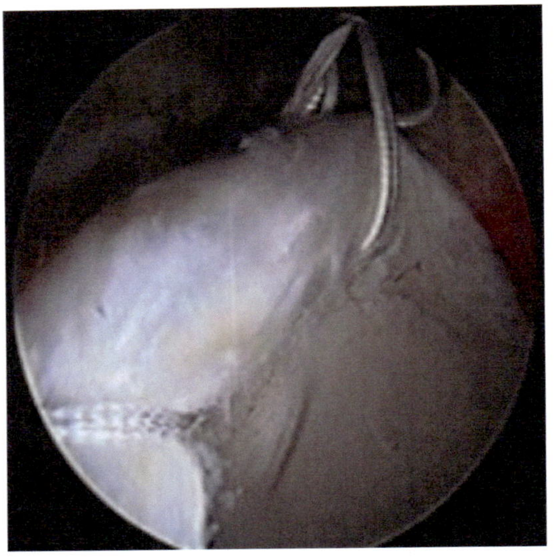

Fig. 30.2 Labrum refixation using multiple reabsorbable anchors

Table 30.1 Surgical technique scheme: complexity arises together with the gesture required

Simple	Diagnostic
	Removal loose body
	Labral debridement
	Ligamentum Teres debridement
Intermediate	CAM decompression
	Iliotibial band release
	Iliopsoas release
Complex	Acetabular rim trimming + labral repair + CAM decompression
	Microfracture
Very complex	Acetabular rim trimming + labral repair + CAM decompression + capsular plication

positioning depending on the age of the patient and the size of the defect.

PINCER-type impingement decompression is achieved under fluoroscopic control. After detaching the labrum from the bone with a beaver blade, trimming of the rim with a 5.5-mm round-tip burr is performed; if a subspine impingement is present, arthroscopic decompression is achieved. In patients who had showed relief from psoas injections, trans-capsular evaluation of the iliopsoas tendon is executed just before removing traction. A correlation between the psoas tendon and the status of the anterior labrum at approximately the 3 o'clock position is performed. In case of fraying or an erythematous, contusion-type lesion of the labrum, we perform fractional release of the tendinous portion of the iliopsoas musculotendinous unit with a radiofrequency probe. A fractional lengthening of the psoas is also performed in case of impingement with the medial portion of the acetabular rim.

CAM-type impingement treatment is possible without traction and a 45° hip flexion. It is sometimes indicated to make a longitudinal capsulotomy to better reach the head-neck junction. Scope is inserted from the anterolateral portal, while the instruments (shaver, burr) are inserted from the mid-anterior portal, but switching is common and very useful for a better three-dimensional assessment. Lateral-based lesions are challenging due to the intimate location of the retinacular vessels; thus proper attention should be given to the vascular anatomy. Osteochondroplasty should include all pathologically appearing cartilage but shall not go higher or more proximally to the epiphyseal scar, which can be confirmed fluoroscopically. It is also fundamental to perform a dynamic evaluation to ensure an adequate decompression, and this should be the last gesture before arthroscopy can be considered completed (See Table under section 30.2.2).

30.2.2 Technical Notes

Consider preoperative planning to evaluate the amount of acetabular trimming and femoroplasty (3D CT dynamic reconstruction)
Careful portal placement when entering the joint (labrum penetration, femoral head scuffing)
If rim trimming is not appreciated on intraoperative fluoroscopic imaging, direct arthroscopic visualization, dynamic testing, and preoperative X-rays should guide further resection
Divergent suture-anchor placement orientation is recommended to prevent screw penetration of the acetabulum
"T" capsulotomy is useful in case of a wide femoral bump
Address lateral retinacular vessels before starting femoral decompression
Fluoroscopy and dynamic evaluation are mandatory to confirm the amount of bone resection

30.2.2.2 Rehabilitation

After hip arthroscopy, athletes wish to return to a fully active lifestyle and to practice their preferred sport as soon as possible. Currently, the best evidence for postoperative rehabilitation is based upon few scientific productions; thus communication with the specialist is vital to the treating physical therapist in order to give an individualized and evaluation-based program [23, 24].

Before starting rehabilitation it is fundamental to know the exact procedure and operative findings, to plan a truly customized rehabilitation program both for simple and complex procedures (Table 30.1)

Rehabilitation can be divided into four phases. The timeline for each phase is based on clinical findings. If clinical presentation meets the established criteria, the athlete may move to the next phase. Progression in terms of type and intensity of the workout should be function based, not time based (Table 30.2).

It would be helpful to see the player preoperatively to prepare the affected joint and explain process and timescales involved. It should also be mandatory to give written rehabilitation indications at discharge.

Time recovery for a full activity is usually four months, but it may last longer depending on operative findings or prolonged rehabilitation.

It is fundamental not to force recovery [25]. Possible risks of a premature return to sport activity are:

- Persistent pain
- Prolonged rehabilitation time
- Low performance
- Re-injury(new labral tear, articular cartilage lesion)
- New injuries

Table 30.2 Rehabilitation schedule

Phase I	Start mobilization and isometric exercises, avoid swelling
Phase II	Continue recovery of range of motion and isometric exercises
Phase III	Recovery of full strength
Phase IV	Recovery of balance and neuromuscular control
Phase V	Functional recovery and return to sport

30.2.3 Outcome and Return to Play

Several published articles have been written on an athletic patient population after hip arthroscopy.

Results of this studies show that athletes with FAI can return to high-level competitive sport following this procedure.

Philippon has published a cohort study of 28 professional players who underwent hip arthroscopy for FAI. The return to sport was 3.8 months (range 1–5 months) with MHHS of 95 at follow-up. Patients with symptoms lasting less than 1 year returned to sport at 3 months, but patients who delayed surgery over 1 year returned to sport at 4.1 months [26].

Brunner et al. in 2009 reported values return to full sporting activity in 68.8 % of cases [27].

Byrd in 2009 reported its results with a mean follow-up of 27 months. In 90 % of professional athletes and 85 % of college, there was a return to full sports activity [28].

Another study by Nho et al. estimated the return to sport in patients undergoing hip arthroscopy up to 83 % [29].

A recent systematic review showed a high rate of return to pre-injury activity level in athletes treated for FAI. Results achieved a 92 % rate of return to activity, observed in athletic populations across a variety of sports, with 88 % of athletes returning to pre-injury activity levels of participation [30].

Arthroscopic management among athletes is very favorable but often performed when an important damage has occurred. Substantial secondary damage is frequently present that cannot be completely reversed. In fact, FAI is very often not recognized, leading to a delay for a precise diagnosis. Early recognition and treatment have been demonstrated to have a tremendous impact on outcome; Phillipon has showed that patients with symptoms lasting less than 1 year returned to sport at 3 months, but patients who delayed surgery over 1 year returned to sport at 4.1 months. Because early treatment is the only change for full recovery, athletes that decide to delay treatment should be aware of the risk [31].

Rehabilitation after hip arthroscopy is long and has its own peculiarity; thus it is fundamental to follow the patient during the entire post-op protocol. Data suggest that professional athletes may show quicker return to sports than recreational athletes but the hip scores and rate of return seem to be analogous. Villar recently published his result showing a quicker recovery in pros, with no statistical difference when comparing the overall return both in recreational and professional athletes [32].

30.3 Rectus Femoris Tendon Calcification

Calcification of the proximal rectus femoris tendon has been described following avulsion (with or without bony fragment) or tendon rupture (partial or complete) of the rectus femoris origin in young people, especially in kicking athletes and in football players [33].

Ouellette et al. found a 0.5 % incidence of rectus femoris origin injuries on a retrospective revision of 3,160 pelvis and hip magnetic resonance images, and it has been shown that after the acute phase, an injury of rectus femoris origin could lead to HC, resulting in pain and loss of function [34–36].

A similar condition has been described after an avulsion of the anterior inferior iliac spine (AIIS). The healing process could lead to an extra bony mass extending inferiorly and resulting in a prominent AIIS that eventually will impinge on the femoral neck when the hip is flexed over 90°. This has been referred to as iliac spine impingement, AIIS impingement, or subspine impingement [37]. A recent paper described a new pathological entity, the hip anterosuperior labral tear with avulsion of rectus femoris (HALTAR). This entity combines the labral tear with an injury of the rectus femoris, similarly to what happens in superior labral anterior-posterior (SLAP) lesions of the shoulder. Since the insertion of the rectus femoris tendon is close to the acetabular labrum, a sudden and powerful eccentric contraction of the rectus femoris muscle or a sudden knee flexion may cause an avulsion injury of the rectus femoris as well as a concomitant labral tear [38] (Fig. 30.3)

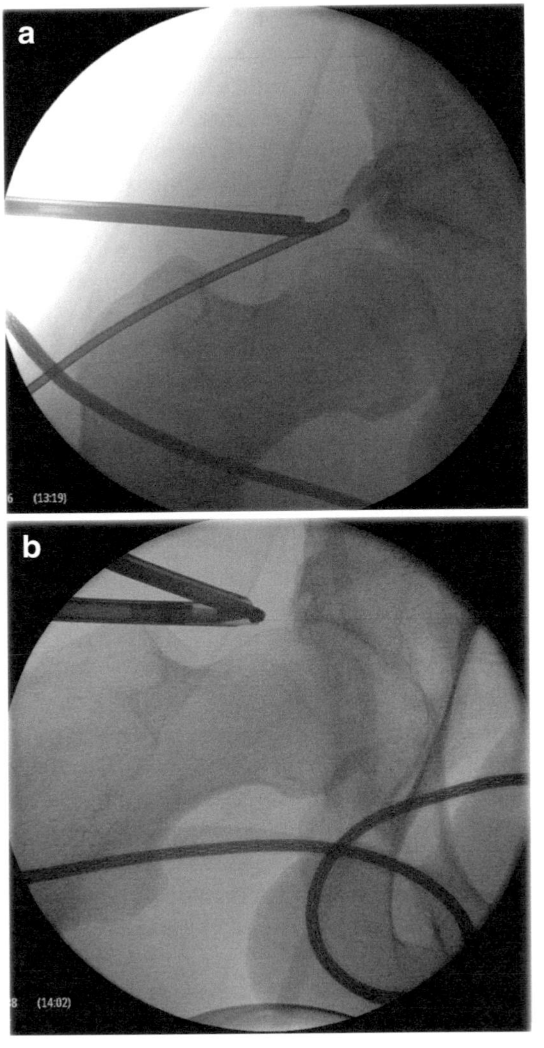

Fig. 30.3 (**a**) Fluoroscopy during the endoscopic decompression at the AIIS: the ossification is no more present (**b**)

Calcification of the rectus femoris tendon has been traditionally addressed by local injection of anesthetic and corticosteroids or by open excision of the lesion through an anterior approach (Smith-Petersen). The same approach is used for subspine impingement. In recent years, hip arthroscopy has been proposed, with satisfactory outcomes, as a less invasive surgical alternative for both conditions [39].

30.3.1 Surgical Technique

In case of a rectus femoris tendon calcification, the central compartment is addressed first. Concomitant lesions (labral tear, chondral lesion, impingement) are evaluated and eventually treated. After central compartment examination and treatment is completed, the traction is removed and attention is focused to the calcification of the rectus femoris. A shaver is used to clear all soft tissues from the overhanging acetabulum and to better delimit the plane between the acetabular rim and the calcification. Using an extra-long, 5.5-mm full-radius shaver and a radiofrequency device, complete exposure of the calcification is achieved (Fig. 30.3). When possible, care is taken in detaching the minimum amount of fibers of the direct head of the rectus femoris from its insertion site. Using the image intensifier as a guide, the calcification is removed using a 5.5-mm bur. During the entire procedure, both dynamic direct visualization and fluoroscopic evaluation of the amount of resection are performed.

30.3.2 Rehabilitation

Weight bearing is permitted as tolerated, but extension of the hip is forbidden for 3 weeks to avoid excessive elongation of the rectus femoris tendon. To avoid recurrence, a course of celecoxib is ordered (200 mg/d for 4 weeks).

References

1. Ganz R, Leunig M, Leunig-Ganz K, Harris WH (2008) The etiology of osteoarthritis of the hip: an integrated mechanical concept. Clin Orthop Relat Res 466:264–272
2. Nepple JJ et al (2015) What is the association between sports participation and the development of proximal femoral cam deformity? A systematic review and meta-analysis. Am J Sports Med
3. Johnston TL, Scheker BS, Phillippon MJ et al (2008) Relationship between offset angle alpha and hip chondral injury in femoroacetabular impingement. Arthroscopy 24(6):669–675
4. Gosvig KK, Jacobsen S, Sonne-Holm S, Gebuhr P (2008) The prevalence of cam-type deformity of the hip joint: a survey of 4151 subjects of the Copenhagen Osteoar- thritis study. Acta Radiol 49:436–441
5. Steppacher SD, Tannast M, Werlen S, Siebenrock KA (2008) Femoral morphology differs between deficient and excessive acetabular coverage. Clin Orthop Relat Res 466:782–790
6. Tanzer M, Noiseux N (2004) Osseus abnormalities and early osteoarthritis: the role of hip impingement. Clin Orthop Relat Res 428:170–177
7. Hack K, Di Primio G, Rakhra K, Beaule PE (2010) Prevalence of cam-type femoroacetabular impingement morphology in asymptomatic volun- teers. J Bone Joint Surg Am 92(14):2436–2444
8. Lorentzon R, Wedren J, Pietila T (1998) Incidence, nature and cause of ice hockey injuries: a three-year prospective study of a Swedish elite ice hockey team. Am J Sports Med 16:392–396
9. Dudda M, Albers C, Mamisch TC, Werlen S, Beck M (2009) Do normal radiographs exclude asphericity of femoral head-neck junction? Clin Orthop Relat Res 467(3):651–659
10. Tannast M, Siebenrock KA, Anderson SE (2007) Femoroacetabular impingement: radiographic diagnosis—what the radiologist should know. AJR Am J Roentgenol 188(6):1540–1552
11. Meyer DC, Beck M, Ellis T, Ganz R, Leunig M (2006) Comparison of six radiographic projections to assess femoral head/neck asphericity. Clin Orthop Relat Res 445:181–185
12. Nötzli HP, Wyss TF, Stoecklin CH, Schmid MR, Treiber K, Hodler J (2002) The contour of the femoral head-neck junction as a predictor for the risk of anterior impingement. J Bone Joint Surg Br 84:556–560
13. Siebenrock KA, Wahab KH, Werlen S, Kalhor M, Leunig M, Ganz R (2004) Abnormal extension of the femoral head epiphysis as a cause of cam impingement. Clin Orthop Relat Res 418:54–60
14. Werlen S, Leunig M, Ganz R (2005) Magnetic resonance arthrogra- phy of the hip in femoroacetabular impingement: technique and findings. Oper Tech Orthop 15:191–203
15. Czerny C, Hofmann S, Neuhold A et al (1996) Lesions of the acetabular labrum: accuracy of MR imaging and MR arthrog- raphy in detection and staging. Radiology 200:225–230
16. Ito K, Minka MA, Leunig M et al (2001) Femoroacetabular impinge- ment and the cam effect. A MRI-based quantitative anatomical study of the femoral head-neck offset. J Bone Joint Surg Br 83:171–176
17. Khan O, Witt J (2014) Evaluation of the magnitude and location of cam deformity using three dimensional CT analysis. Bone Joint J 96-B(9):1167–1171. doi:10.1302/0301-620X.96B9.33555
18. Byrd JW (2014) Primary repair of the acetabular labrum: outcomes with 2 years' follow-up J. W. T. Arthroscopy 30(5):588–592

19. Clarke MT, Villar RN (2003) Hip arthroscopy: complications in 1054cases. Clin Orthop Relat Res 406:84–88
20. Philippon MJ, Arnoczky SP, Torrie A (2007) Arthroscopic repair of the acetabular labrum: a histologic assessment of healing in anovine model. Arthroscopy 23:376–380
21. Kelly BT, Shapiro GS, Digiovanni CW, Buly RL, Potter HG, Hannafin JA (2008) Vascularity of the hip labrum: a cadaveric investigation. Arthroscopy 21:3–11
22. Bedi A, Chen N, Robertson W, Kelly BT (2008) The management of labral tears and femoroacetabular impingement of the hip in young, active patient. Arthroscopy 24:1135–1145
23. Cheatham SW, Kolber MJ (2012) Rehabilitation after hip arthroscopy and labral repair in a high school football athlets. Int J Sports Phys Ther 7(2):173–184
24. Bennell KL, O'Donnell JM, Takla A, Spiers LN, Hunter DJ, Staples M, Hinman RS (2014) Efficacy of a physiotherapy rehabilitation program for individuals undergoing arthroscopic management of femoroacetabular impingement – the FAIR trial: a randomised controlled trial protocol. BMC Musculoskelet Disord 26(15): 1471-2474-15-58
25. Emery CA, Meeuwisse WH (2001) Risk factors for groin injuries in hockey. Med Sci Sports Exerc 33(9): 1423–1433
26. Philippon MJ, Wiess DR, Kuppersmith DA, Briggs KK, Hay CJ (2010) Arthroscopic labral repair and treatment of femoroacetabular impingement in professional hockey players. Am J Sports Med 38(1): 99–104
27. Brunner A, Horisberger M, Herzog RF (2009) Sports and recreation activity of patients with femoroacetabular impingement before and after arthroscopic osteoplasty. Am J Sports Med 37(5):917–922
28. Byrd JW, Jones KS (2009) Arthroscopic femoroplasty in the management of cam-type femoroacetabular impingement. Clin Orthop Relat Res 467(3):739–746
29. Nho SJ et al (2011) Outcomes after the arthroscopic treatment of femoroacetabular impingement in a mixed group of high-level athletes. Am J Sports Med 39(Suppl):14S–19S
30. Alradwan H, Philippon MJ, Farrokhyar F et al (2012) Return to preinjury levels after surgical management of femoroacetabular impingement in athletes. Arthroscopy 28(10):1567–1576
31. Philippon M et al (2007) Femoroacetabular impingement in 45 professional athletes: associated pathologies and return to sport following arthroscopic decompression. Knee Surg Sports Traumatol Arthrosc 15(7):908–914
32. Malviya A, Paliobeis CP, Villar RN (2013) Do professional athletes perform better than recreational athletes after arthroscopy for femoroacetabular impingement? Clin Orthop Relat Res 471(8): 2477–2483
33. Gamradt SC, Brophy RH, Barnes R, Warren RF, Thomas Byrd JW, Kelly BT (2009) Nonoperative treatment for proximal avulsion of the rectus femoris in professional American football. Am J Sports Med 37:1370–1374
34. Ouellette H, Thomas BJ, Nelson E, Torriani M (2006) MR imaging of rectus femoris origin injuries. Skeletal Radiol 35:665–672
35. Kim YS, Lee HM, Kim JP (2013) Acute calcific tendinitis of the rectus femoris associated with intraosseous involvement: a case report with serial CT and MRI findings. Eur J Orthop Surg Traumatol 23(suppl 2):S233–S239
36. Sarkar JS, Haddad FS, Crean SV, Brooks P (1996) Acute calcific tendinitis of the rectus femoris. J Bone Joint Surg Br 78:814–816
37. Larson CM, Kelly BT, Stone RM (2011) Making a case for anterior inferior iliac spine/subspine hip impingement: three representative case reports and proposed concept. Arthroscopy 27:1732–1737
38. Hosalkar HS, Pennock AT, Zaps D, Schmitz MR, Bomar JD, Bittersohl B (2012) The hip anterosuperior labral tear with avulsion of rectus femoris (HALTAR) lesion: does the SLAP equivalent in the hip exist? Hip Int 22:391–396
39. Zini R, Panascì M (2014) Rectus femoris tendon calcification: arthroscopic excision in 6 top amateur athletes. Orthop J Sports Med 2(12):15–24

Achilles Tendon Lesions in Soccer Players

31

Jón Karlsson, Nicklas Olsson, and Katarina Nilsson Helander

31.1 Introduction

The Achilles tendon is the thickest and strongest tendon in the human body and needs to resist forces of up to 9 kN (approximately 12 times the weight of the body) during running [1]. For optimal function, the tendon must be capable of resisting high tensile forces with limited elongation and at the same time storing elastic energy when activated. Despite its strength, it is susceptible to both overuse injury and acute injury, such as a complete rupture.

Functional deficits are commonly described after an Achilles tendon rupture [2–5], and several studies have shown that only approximately 50 % of the patients return to previous activity level and sports [2, 6, 7]. Accordingly, an Achilles tendon rupture might be career-ending for the professional athlete [8].

A large number of medical reports have been published in the field of Achilles tendon rupture, but there is still a lack of consensus in terms of the best treatment.

J. Karlsson (✉) • N. Olsson, MD, PhD
K.N. Helander, MD, PhD
Department of Orthopaedics,
Sahlgrenska University Hospital,
Sahlgrenska Academy, Gothenburg University,
413 85 Gothenburg, Sweden
e-mail: Jon.karlsson@telia.com;
Nicklas.olsson@gu.se; Ina.nilsson@telia.com

31.2 Epidemiology

The annual incidence of Achilles tendon ruptures in the population is increasing with a peak incidence of 37 per 100,000 persons [9–11]. A bimodal age distribution has been reported with the highest incidence in the 30–39-year age group [9, 12]. A study by Houshian et al. [9] showed that 73 % of the injuries were sports-related and the peak of sports-related injuries occurred in the 30–49-year age group. There is a second non-sports-related peak in incidence occurring at a mean age of 53 years [10]. Epidemiological studies generally show much a higher incidence of Achilles tendon ruptures in men, and the ratio between men and women is between 3:1 and 18:1, in general approximately 10:1 [9, 13].

A recently published study of the UEFA Champions League injury showed that Achilles tendon disorders (tendinopathies and ruptures) accounted for 2.5 % of all injuries and 3.8 % of layoff times in male professional football players [14]. In this cohort of 203 football players, only 4 % were classified as partial or total ruptures.

31.3 Etiology

The etiology of Achilles tendon ruptures is regarded as multifactorial, and many factors have been proposed, but the pathology still remains unclear.

P. Volpi (ed.), *Football Traumatology: New Trends*, DOI 10.1007/978-3-319-18245-2_31

Degenerative changes have been found in ruptured Achilles tendons [15–17]. Aging reduces the collagen fiber diameter [18], and this change, combined with a high activity level, may partly explain the sports-related peak of increased incidence in the middle-aged group. Overuse (microtrauma) and imbalance between muscle power and tendon elasticity might lead to permanent tendon weakening and incomplete tendon regeneration [19]. In especially young patients, healthy tendon may rupture under violent muscular strain (macrotrauma) in the presence of certain anatomical and functional conditions [20].

The midsection has less vascularization than the proximal and distal tendon ends and is consequently the most common rupture site [21, 22]. There is limited evidence that oral corticosteroids and local steroid injections are risk factors for Achilles tendon ruptures [23, 24]. The use of fluoroquinolones is also associated with Achilles tendinopathy and tendon ruptures [25], and the administration of fluoroquinolones should be carefully considered, especially in patients undergoing corticosteroid treatment [26]. Achilles tendon rupture can also be associated with systemic diseases such as gout, lupus erythematosus, and rheumatoid arthritis.

31.4 Injury Mechanism

The Achilles tendon fibers are at rest in a curly configuration but become fully stretched at a strain of 1–3 %. At this stage, the tendon is able to return to its initial length when the force is released. When the tendon is stressed and elongated more than approximately 4 %, some fibers start to break. Further stress on the tendon will cause the failure of the rest of the fibers in an unpredictable manner, and this will result in a complete tendon rupture [27]. There is a variation between studies of tendon strain at failure of 4–16 % [27, 28]; however, 8 % [29] is often used as the strain level at which macroscopic failure occurs.

The most common injury mechanisms for Achilles tendon ruptures have been classified into three main categories, all with a very distinct patient history [30]. In the first mechanism, the patient pushes off with the weight-bearing forefoot while the knee is extended. The rupture occurs in an elongated tendon when the force is greater than the ultimate tensile strength. This mechanism is described by the majority of patients and is seen in sprint starts, jumping, and racket sports. The second mechanism is a sudden, unexpected dorsiflexion of the ankle, which occurs when the patient slips into a hole or falls down stairs. The third mechanism is a violent dorsiflexion of a plantar-flexed foot, which may occur after a fall from height.

31.5 Clinical and Diagnostic Examination

Patients who sustain an Achilles tendon rupture have a typical history of a sudden pain in the Achilles tendon without any previous symptoms. Less than 10 % of the patients have complained of previous symptom from the Achilles tendon. Many patients report that they feel as they had been struck by something/someone from behind, often accompanied by an audible snap. In the typical case, the diagnosis is clear. The diagnosis is clinical, and there is a palpable gap at the site of the rupture in the mid-substance, 2–6 cm proximal to the calcaneal insertion site. The ability to plantar flex the ankle is absent or very weak. In the literature, numerous of different clinical diagnostic tests are described [31].

Sensitivity and specificity have been evaluated for these various clinical tests [31]. The calf squeeze test and Matles test had the highest sensitivity (0.96 and 0.88, respectively) and specificity (0.93 and 0.85, respectively), and these tests are also noninvasive, simple, and inexpensive [31].

The calf squeeze test is also known as Thompson's or Simmonds' test [32]. The patient lies in a prone position, and the examiner squeezes the affected calf muscle from side-to-side, and, if the tendon is intact, the foot will plantar flex, but, if the tendon is ruptured, there will be minimal or no reaction in the foot, and the test is said to be positive (Fig. 31.1). In the Matles

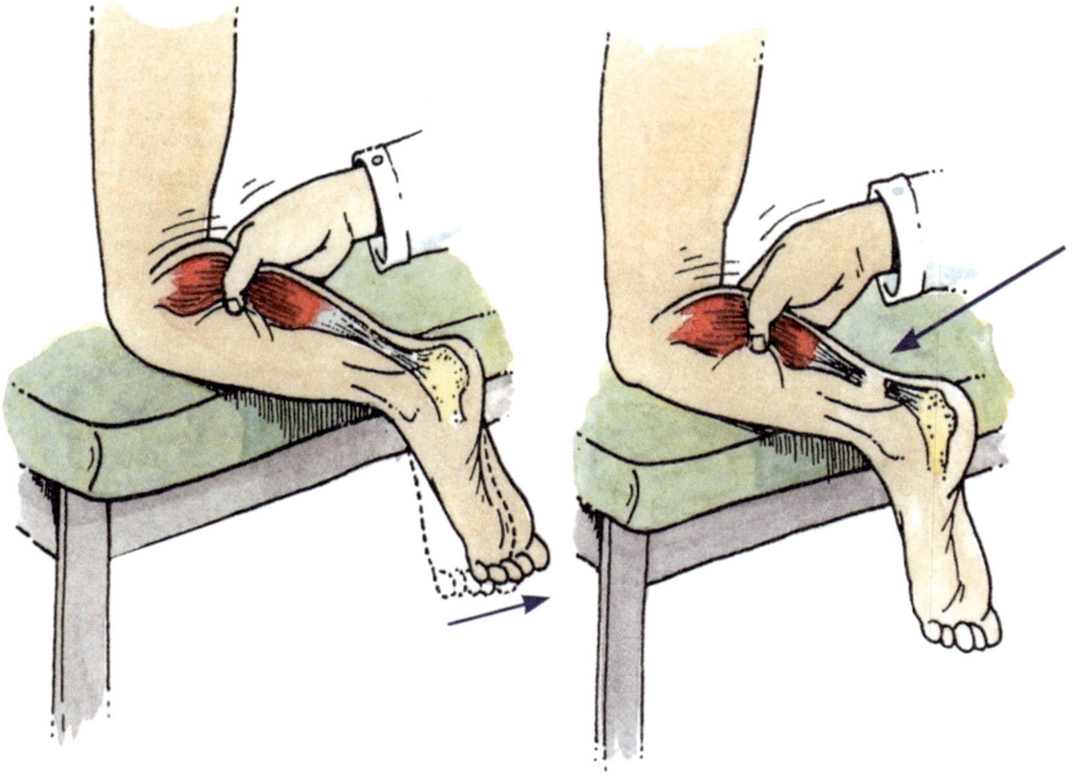

Fig. 31.1 Calf-squeeze (Simmonds' or Thompson's) test

test, also in the prone position, the patient actively flexes both knees, and a change in foot position is observed. The test is positive if the foot on the injured side moves into neutral or dorsiflexion (Fig. 31.2).

Partial ruptures are very uncommon, at least after typical acute trauma. However, these are frequently seen in patients with previous tendinopathy and no distinct trauma.

Ultrasound (US) and/or magnetic resonance imaging (MRI) are not recommended for routine use to establish the diagnosis in acute ruptures [33]. Nevertheless, additional investigations can be useful in certain cases, especially in planning the surgical procedure in chronic cases.

Chronic ruptures refer to ruptures with a delay in treatment (either patient's delay or doctor's delay) and diagnosis of more than 4 weeks. Patients with a chronic rupture commonly complain of pain in contrast to patients with an acute injury [34].

31.6 Tendon Healing

At the moment of injury, the body initiates a process of healing. Tendon healing is a highly complex process with interaction between blood- and tissue-derived cells, matrix molecules, and inflammatory mediators. The aim of the healing and repair process is to achieve hemostasis, tissue integrity, and load-bearing capacity. After an acute tendon injury (complete rupture), three phases of healing occur [17, 35].

Inflammation is the *first* phase and lasts for up to 1 week after injury. During this phase, a cascade of pro-inflammatory mediators leads to angiogenesis and recruitment of inflammatory cells to the injury site. The inflammatory cells degenerate the blood clot and debris in the injured tissue.

The *second* phase also known as the proliferative phase is characterized by profuse synthetic activity and lasts 6–8 weeks. During this phase,

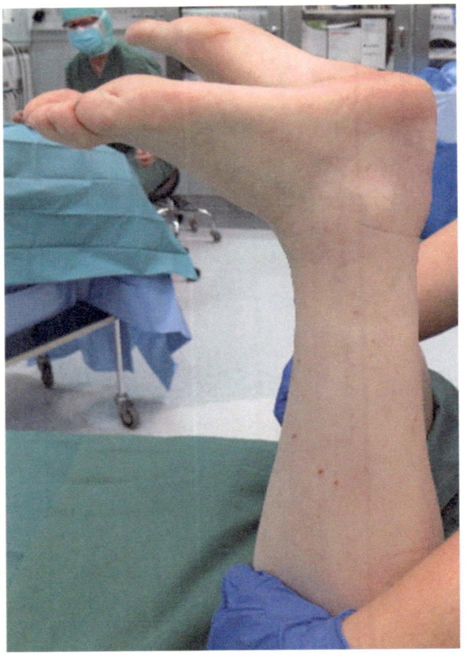

Fig. 31.2 Matles test

a temporary stability is achieved by the fibroblasts producing mostly collagen III.

The *third* and last phase is called the remodeling phase and lasts for more than a year. During this phase, the tensile strength, elasticity, and internal structure of the tendon are improved and matured. At the end of this phase, a mature scar tissue is formed even though there are signs of incomplete recovery of the tendon.

31.7 Treatment Strategy

It is necessary to distinguish between ruptures at the insertion site, proximal ruptures, and the most frequent ruptures in the midportion of the tendon, 2–6 cm from the calcaneal insertion. The uncommon ruptures at the insertion site are almost always treated with surgery, and the proximal ruptures are generally treated nonsurgically.

The optimal treatment for Achilles tendon rupture is still a subject of debate and can be broadly classified as either surgical (open or mini-invasive/percutaneous) and nonsurgical (cast or functional brace). Even closed approach using the arthroscope to visualize the tendon ends is reported today. Several high-quality, randomized, controlled studies have been published, and they all concluded that surgical treatment involves an approximately 2–4 times lower risk of rerupture but disadvantages related to increased risks of complications, such as scar problems, sural nerve dysfunction, and infection are reported [5, 7, 36–40]. These studies are not subgrouped into high level sports or football, mainly due to the small sample size. Therefore, the data should be interpreted with caution even though the functional outcome data are inconclusive, and no treatment can therefore be strongly recommended over the other. Young active athletes are in the majority of cases treated with surgery [41].

When surgical treatment has been selected, the important issue is to make a choice of the technique and approach. Classically, an end-to-end repair is performed (Fig. 31.3). Open primary repair can probably be performed up to approximately 3 weeks after the injury. End-to-end sutures are generally not acceptable to treat chronic ruptures and reruptures where reconstruction with reinforcement is recommended [42].

In an open surgical approach, the patient should always be placed in a prone position, with the feet over a pillow or outside the operating table in order to avoid excessive plantar flexion, as over-tightening of the repair will be risk of shortening of the tendon and loss of motion. On the other hand, lengthening of the tendon (as this will most probably cause reduced plantar flexion strength) should be avoided at any cost. The procedure can be carried out in local, regional, or general anesthesia. Bloodless field is not needed. When considering the position of the foot, in order to avoid shortening or lengthening of the tendon, it is wise to compare the position to the other foot (the resting angle) in neutral position and dorsiflexion [43]. It is important to judge the tension of the repair and the balance between the dorsiflexors and the plantarflexors. A posteromedial skin incision is preferred in order to minimize any risk of injury to the branches of the sural nerve. The ends of the tendon are debrided and thereafter carefully approached with different suture selections and suture techniques generally due to the surgeon's

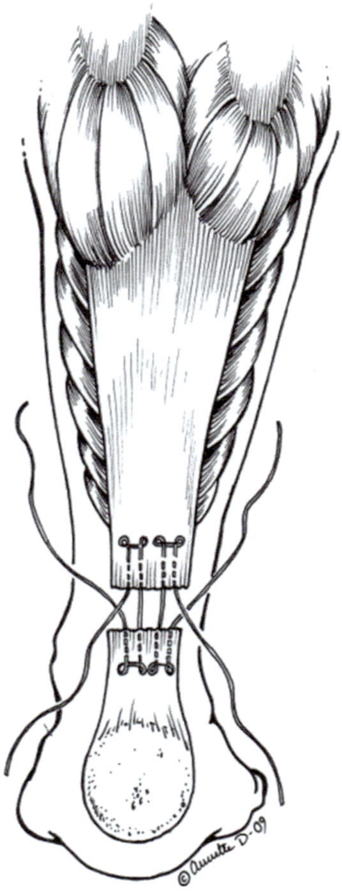

Fig. 31.3 Modified Kessler suture

preference. A recent study has shown a very low risk of rerupture (as low as 0 %) using a strong suture technique [39] (Fig. 31.4).

Postoperatively, the leg is immobilized either using a short leg plaster cast or brace or a combination. Provided the suture strength is judged as satisfactory, range of motion exercises are generally started after approximately 10–14 days. Weight-bearing should be started as early as possible.

Several techniques have been described to treat chronic and reruptures. Turn-down flaps are commonly used. Another option is augmentation with a free flap from the gastrocnemius aponeurosis, with generally good results. Advantage of this technique is to avoid a large tissue mass at the surgical area [34] (Fig. 31.5).

31.8 Rehabilitation and Return to Play

The issue of immobilization is of major concern. The trend is without doubt toward a shorter immobilization period. Early range of motion training, using movable brace, and early weight-bearing have been advocated recently as well. In fact, it has been shown that early, well-protected range of motion training and at least moderately aggressive rehabilitation will result in better outcomes after surgical treatment.

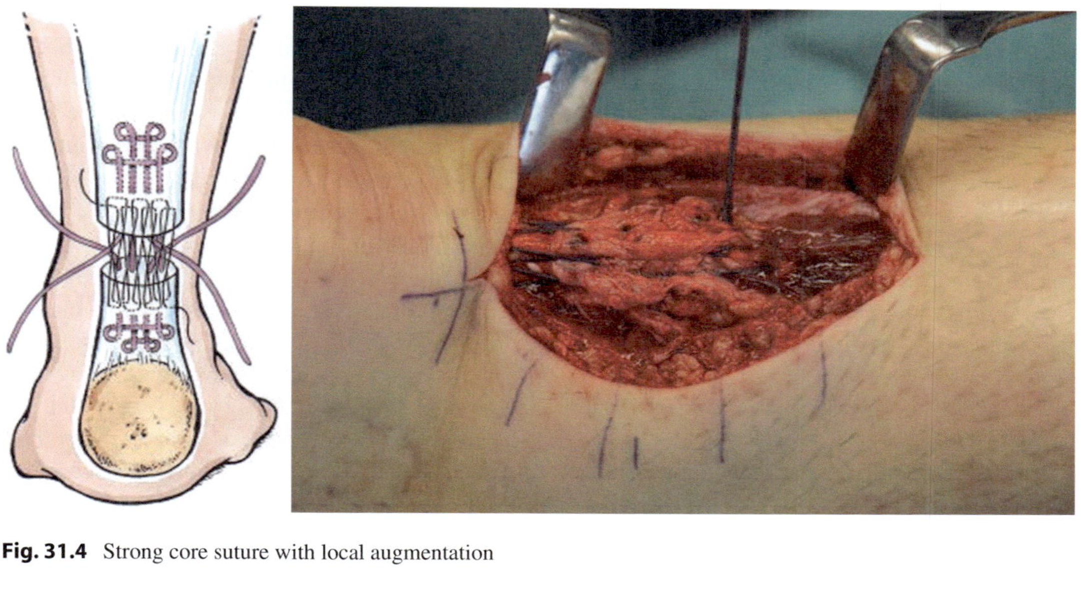

Fig. 31.4 Strong core suture with local augmentation

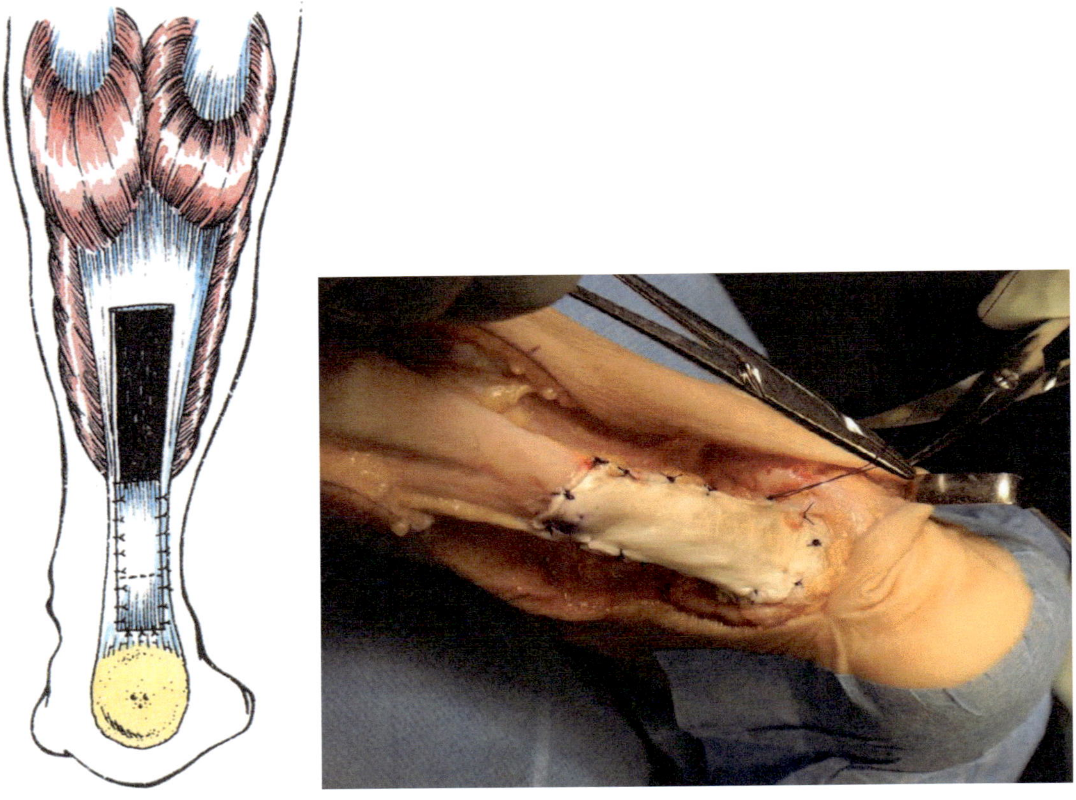

Fig. 31.5 Augmentation with a free gastrocnemius aponeurosis flap after an end-to-end suture

In general, the tendency is that the immobilization has been shortened and the motion of the ankle started earlier [44–46].

Most studies and clinical guidelines recommend return to running and non-contact sports between weeks 16 and 20 [41, 46]. In general, most of the guidelines are time-based and do not include any specific criteria with regard to return of strength or lower leg function. Costa et al. [45] reported a median time of 12.5–18 weeks (depending of treatment) to return to normal walking. The Achilles Tendon Study Group has on the other hand a functional perspective rather than a time perspective, and this is probably of major importance when rehabilitation is advanced. In the given guidelines for sport resumption in their book "*Achilles Tendon Rupture – current concepts*" [47], the recovery is divided into four levels of increasing activity: walking, running, return to non-contact sport, and return to contact sport. Each phase must be fully accomplished prior to entering the next one. The first level ends when the patient is able to walk normally again. To achieve that, the difference in strength is said to be less than 25 % compared to the uninjured side in repeated single-heel raises, and also, toe walking should be possible. The proposed time for this level is 12 weeks but 8 weeks for operative treatment with a functional brace, even though another study [48] has shown that only half of the patients were able to achieve a single-heel raise 12 weeks after a surgically treated rupture.

Complete Achilles tendon rupture leads to long layoff from football playing, with a median absence period of 169 days for professional football players [14]. The same thing has been reported in professional rugby players (mean 186 days) [49]. In professional American Football League (AFL), 32 % of the players did not return to the NFL, and of the players who did return, they returned to play an average of 11 months after the injury [8].

References

1. Komi PV, Fukashiro S, Järvinen M (1992) Biomechanical loading of Achilles tendon during normal locomotion. Clin Sports Med 11(3):521–531
2. Keating JF, Will EM (2011) Operative versus non-operative treatment of acute rupture of tendo Achillis: a prospective randomised evaluation of functional outcome. J Bone Joint Surg Br 93(8):1071–1078. doi:10.1302/0301-620X.93B8.25998
3. Moller M, Lind K, Movin T, Karlsson J (2002) Calf muscle function after Achilles tendon rupture. A prospective, randomised study comparing surgical and non-surgical treatment. Scand J Med Sci Sports 12(1):9–16
4. Olsson N, Nilsson-Helander K, Karlsson J, Eriksson BI, Thomee R, Faxen E, Silbernagel KG (2011) Major functional deficits persist 2 years after acute Achilles tendon rupture. Knee Surg Sports Traumatol Arthrosc 19(8):1385–1393. doi:10.1007/s00167-011-1511-3
5. Willits K, Amendola A, Bryant D, Mohtadi NG, Giffin JR, Fowler P, Kean CO, Kirkley A (2010) Operative versus nonoperative treatment of acute Achilles tendon ruptures: a multicenter randomized trial using accelerated functional rehabilitation. J Bone Joint Surg Am 92(17):2767–2775
6. Metz R, Verleisdonk EJ, van der Heijden GJ, Clevers GJ, Hammacher ER, Verhofstad MH, van der Werken C (2008) Acute Achilles tendon rupture: minimally invasive surgery versus nonoperative treatment with immediate full weightbearing–a randomized controlled trial. Am J Sports Med 36(9):1688–1694
7. Moller M, Movin T, Granhed H, Lind K, Faxen E, Karlsson J (2001) Acute rupture of tendon Achillis. A prospective randomised study of comparison between surgical and non-surgical treatment. J Bone Joint Surg Br 83(6):843–848
8. Parekh SG, Wray WH 3rd, Brimmo O, Sennett BJ, Wapner KL (2009) Epidemiology and outcomes of Achilles tendon ruptures in the National Football League. Foot Ankle Spec 2(6):283–286. doi:10.1177/1938640009351138
9. Houshian S, Tscherning T, Riegels-Nielsen P (1998) The epidemiology of Achilles tendon rupture in a Danish county. Injury 29(9):651–654
10. Leppilahti J, Puranen J, Orava S (1996) Incidence of Achilles tendon rupture. Acta Orthop Scand 67(3): 277–279
11. Nyyssonen T, Luthje P, Kroger H (2008) The increasing incidence and difference in sex distribution of Achilles tendon rupture in Finland in 1987–1999. Scand J Surg 97(3):272–275
12. Maffulli N, Waterston SW, Squair J, Reaper J, Douglas AS (1999) Changing incidence of Achilles tendon rupture in Scotland: a 15-year study. Clin J Sport Med 9(3):157–160
13. Cretnik A, Frank A (2004) Incidence and outcome of rupture of the Achilles tendon. Wien Klin Wochenschr 116(Suppl 2):33–38
14. Gajhede-Knudsen M, Ekstrand J, Magnusson H, Maffulli N (2013) Recurrence of Achilles tendon injuries in elite male football players is more common after early return to play: an 11-year follow-up of the UEFA Champions League injury study. Br J Sports Med 47(12):763–768. doi:10.1136/bjsports-2013-092271
15. Maffulli N, Longo UG, Maffulli GD, Rabitti C, Khanna A, Denaro V (2010) Marked pathological changes proximal and distal to the site of rupture in acute Achilles tendon ruptures. Knee Surg Sports Traumatol Arthrosc. doi:10.1007/s00167-010-1193-2
16. Arner O, Lindholm A, Orell SR (1959) Histologic changes in subcutaneous rupture of the Achilles tendon; a study of 74 cases. Acta Chir Scand 116(5–6):484–490
17. Jozsa L, Kannus P (1997) Histopathological findings in spontaneous tendon ruptures. Scand J Med Sci Sports 7(2):113–118
18. Sargon MF, Ozlu K, Oken F (2005) Age-related changes in human tendo calcaneus collagen fibrils. Saudi Med J 26(3):425–428
19. Jozsa LG, Kannus P (1997) Human tendons: anatomy, physiology, and pathology. Human Kinetics, Champaign/Leeds
20. Maffulli N, Almekinders L (2007) The Achilles tendon. Springer, New York/London
21. Chen TM, Rozen WM, Pan WR, Ashton MW, Richardson MD, Taylor GI (2009) The arterial anatomy of the Achilles tendon: anatomical study and clinical implications. Clin Anat 22(3):377–385. doi:10.1002/ca.20758
22. Theobald P, Benjamin M, Nokes L, Pugh N (2005) Review of the vascularisation of the human Achilles tendon. Injury 36(11):1267–1272. doi:10.1016/j.injury.2005.02.012
23. Mahler F, Fritschy D (1992) Partial and complete ruptures of the Achilles tendon and local corticosteroid injections. Br J Sports Med 26(1):7–14
24. Newnham DM, Douglas JG, Legge JS, Friend JA (1991) Achilles tendon rupture: an underrated complication of corticosteroid treatment. Thorax 46(11): 853–854
25. Seeger JD, West WA, Fife D, Noel GJ, Johnson LN, Walker AM (2006) Achilles tendon rupture and its association with fluoroquinolone antibiotics and other potential risk factors in a managed care population. Pharmacoepidemiol Drug Saf 15(11):784–792. doi:10.1002/pds.1214
26. Melhus A (2005) Fluoroquinolones and tendon disorders. Expert Opin Drug Saf 4(2):299–309
27. Maganaris CN, Narici MV, Maffulli N (2008) Biomechanics of the Achilles tendon. Disabil Rehabil 30(20–22):1542–1547.doi:10.1080/09638280701785494
28. Wren TA, Yerby SA, Beaupre GS, Carter DR (2001) Mechanical properties of the human Achilles tendon. Clin Biomech (Bristol, Avon) 16(3):245–251
29. Wang JH (2006) Mechanobiology of tendon. J Biomech 39(9):1563–1582. doi:10.1016/j.jbiomech.2005.05.011
30. Arner O, Lindholm A (1959) Subcutaneous rupture of the Achilles tendon; a study of 92 cases. Acta Chir Scand Suppl 116(Supp 239):1–51
31. Maffulli N (1998) The clinical diagnosis of subcutaneous tear of the Achilles tendon. A prospective study in 174 patients. Am J Sports Med 26(2):266–270
32. Thompson TC, Doherty JH (1962) Spontaneous rupture of tendon of Achilles: a new clinical diagnostic test. J Trauma 2:126–129

33. Chiodo CP, Glazebrook M, Bluman EM, Cohen BE, Femino JE, Giza E, Watters WC 3rd, Goldberg MJ, Keith M, Haralson RH 3rd, Turkelson CM, Wies JL, Raymond L, Anderson S, Boyer K, Sluka P (2010) Diagnosis and treatment of acute Achilles tendon rupture. J Am Acad Orthop Surg 18(8):503–510
34. Nilsson-Helander KN-K (2008) A new surgical method to treat chronic ruptures and reruptures of the Achilles tendon. Knee Surg Sports Traumatol Arthrosc 16(6):614
35. Enwemeka CS (1989) Inflammation, cellularity, and fibrillogenesis in regenerating tendon: implications for tendon rehabilitation. Phys Ther 69(10):816–825
36. Jiang N, Wang B, Chen A, Dong F, Yu B (2012) Operative versus nonoperative treatment for acute Achilles tendon rupture: a meta-analysis based on current evidence. Int Orthop 36(4):765–773. doi:10.1007/s00264-011-1431-3
37. Khan RJ, Carey Smith RL (2010) Surgical interventions for treating acute Achilles tendon ruptures. Cochrane Database Syst Rev(Online) 9, CD003674. doi:10.1002/14651858.CD003674.pub4
38. Nilsson-Helander K, Silbernagel KG, Thomee R, Faxen E, Olsson N, Eriksson BI, Karlsson J (2010) Acute Achilles tendon rupture: a randomized, controlled study comparing surgical and nonsurgical treatments using validated outcome measures. Am J Sports Med 38(11):2186–2193. doi:10.1177/0363546510376052, 0363546510376052 [pii]
39. Olsson N, Silbernagel KG, Eriksson BI, Sansone M, Brorsson A, Nilsson-Helander K, Karlsson J (2013) Stable surgical repair with accelerated rehabilitation versus nonsurgical treatment for acute Achilles tendon ruptures: a randomized controlled study. Am J Sports Med 41(12):2867–2876. doi:10.1177/0363546513503282
40. Soroceanu A, Sidhwa F, Aarabi S, Kaufman A, Glazebrook M (2012) Surgical versus nonsurgical treatment of acute Achilles tendon rupture: a meta-analysis of randomized trials. J Bone Joint Surg Am 94(23):2136–2143. doi:10.2106/JBJS.K.00917
41. Maffulli N, Longo UG, Maffulli GD, Khanna A, Denaro V (2011) Achilles tendon ruptures in elite athletes. Foot Ankle Int 32(1):9–15. doi:10.3113/FAI.2011.0009, 50047363 [pii]
42. Gerdes MH, Brown TD, Bell AL, Baker JA, Levson M, Layer S (1992) A flap augmentation technique for Achilles tendon repair. Postoperative strength and functional outcome. Clin Orthop Relat Res 280:241–246
43. Carmont MR, Silbernagel KG, Mathy A, Mulji Y, Karlsson J, Maffulli N (2013) Reliability of Achilles tendon resting angle and calf circumference measurement techniques. Foot Ankle Surg 19(4):245–249. doi:10.1016/j.fas.2013.06.007
44. Kerkhoffs GM, Struijs PA, Raaymakers EL, Marti RK (2002) Functional treatment after surgical repair of acute Achilles tendon rupture: wrap vs walking cast. Arch Orthop Trauma Surg 122(2):102–105. doi:10.1007/s004020100312
45. Costa ML, MacMillan K, Halliday D, Chester R, Shepstone L, Robinson AH, Donell ST (2006) Randomised controlled trials of immediate weight-bearing mobilisation for rupture of the tendo Achillis. J Bone Joint Surg Br 88(1):69–77. doi:10.1302/0301-620X.88B1.16549, 88-B/1/69 [pii]
46. Suchak AA, Bostick GP, Beaupre LA, Durand DC, Jomha NM (2008) The influence of early weight-bearing compared with non-weight-bearing after surgical repair of the Achilles tendon. J Bone Joint Surg Am 90(9):1876–1883
47. Maayke N. van Sterkenburg BGD, van Dijk CN (2008) Guidelines for sport resumption. In: van Dijk CN, Nicola Maffuli JK, Thermann H (ed) Achilles tendon rupture, current concepts. DJO Publications, pp 108–117
48. Olsson N, Karlsson J, Eriksson BI, Brorsson A, Lundberg M, Silbernagel KG (2012) Ability to perform a single heel-rise is significantly related to patient-reported outcome after Achilles tendon rupture. Scand J Med Sci Sports. doi:10.1111/j.1600-0838.2012.01497.x
49. Sankey RA, Brooks JH, Kemp SP, Haddad FS (2008) The epidemiology of ankle injuries in professional rugby union players. Am J Sports Med 36(12):2415–2424. doi:10.1177/0363546508322889

32 Ankle Ligament Lesions

C. Niek van Dijk and Gwendolyn Vuurberg

32.1 Etiology

32.1.1 Lateral Ankle Ligaments

Ankle ligament lesions are reported as the most common injuries in football, especially lateral ligament sprains [1, 2]. They count for about 14 % of all sport-related injuries [3]. Ligament injuries are usually sustained in sports involving running, cutting, jumping, diving, landing, and contact with others [4], which explains the high incidence and recurrence rate among footballers [1–3]. In football, player to player contact has shown to be responsible for 59 % of the injuries, and noncontact injuries counted for 39 %. In goalkeepers 79 % occurred during noncontact situations [2]. The two most common causes of lateral ligament lesions were the impact of an opponent on the medial side of the leg just before or at foot strike, causing a laterally directed force after which the player lands with the ankle in an inverted position, and secondly forced plantar flexion when the player hits the foot of an opponent when attempting to shoot the ball [3]. The most common mechanisms of sustaining an ankle sprain during contact situations are defined as tackling (36 %) and being tackled (18 %). Most common during noncontact situations were landing (36 %), twisting/turning (21 %), and diving (10 %) [2].

C.N. van Dijk • G. Vuurberg (✉)
Department of Orthopaedic Surgery, Amsterdam Medical Centre, Amsterdam, The Netherlands
e-mail: g.vuurberg@amc.nl

32.1.2 Tibiofibular Syndesmosis

Isolated total ruptures of the syndesmosis are relatively rare, but are reported in football as well as American football, dancing, and skiing. More common are ruptures of the syndesmosis with concomitant injuries like deltoid ligament lesions, fractures, and soft-tissue injuries [2]. Ruptures of the syndesmotic ligaments are always present in patients with Weber C ankle fractures, a fracture following pronation-exorotation. This movement mechanism can also injure the tibiofibular ligaments [1].

32.2 Injury Mechanism

32.2.1 Lateral Ankle Ligaments

The fibula extends further to the lateral malleolus, compared to the tibia to the medial malleolus, blocking eversion. Allowing a larger range of inversion than eversion, makes inversion sprains more common than eversion sprains. Most common is a supination sprain, a movement combination of inversion, internal rotation of the foot, and plantar flexion with the

P. Volpi (ed.), *Football Traumatology: New Trends*, DOI 10.1007/978-3-319-18245-2_32

subtalar joint adducting and inverting [5, 6]. This usually happens when the athlete's center of gravity is shifted over the lateral border of the weight-bearing leg, causing the ankle to roll inward at high velocity [4]. Something that might happen when the foot is incorrect positioned at landing, causing a medially deviated vertical projected ground reaction force, causing an explosive supination moment in the subtalar joint [7].

The anterior talofibular ligament (ATFL) is often injured during plantarflexion and possesses the lowest ultimate load [5], whereas the calcaneofibular ligament (CFL) is often injured during dorsiflexion [6]. Among 80 % are ligamentous sprains caused by explosive inversion or supination [8] and mostly occur during systematic loading and unloading. They rarely occur while the ankle is fully loaded, due to articular restraints [3].

32.2.2 Tibiofibular Syndesmosis

Syndesmotic sprains are also known as high ankle sprains. They are more prevalent in high-energy contact sports or in sports that involve wearing a stiff boot or skate, such as ice hockey or skiing [4]. Compared to lateral ligament injury, they are rare as they have the highest load to failure. Several mechanisms causing syndesmotic injury have been described including pronation-abduction, pronation-eversion, supination-eversion, external rotation, supination-abduction, and dorsiflexion, but most often the mechanism consists of hyperdorsiflexion and external rotation of the ankle [9]. This mechanism leads to disruption of the syndesmotic ligaments and possibly a rupture of the deltoid ligament [4]. In the field a rupture of the syndesmotic ligaments is most commonly experienced when a footballer rapidly twists internally with the foot planted in external rotation with lateral impact on the leg, or when a blow to the lateral aspect of the heel forces the foot and ankle into external rotation while the athlete lies on the ground [10].

32.3 Clinical and Diagnostic Examination

Ankle ligament injuries are often classified as grade I (mild), grade II (moderate/micro lesions), and grade III (severe/full lesion) [11]. Both clinical and diagnostic examination can contribute to classifying ankle injuries. First of all serious injuries should be treated [6]. Harmon [12] presented a systematic approach that consists of five steps to avoid missing potentially serious injuries: (1) palpation of bony structures, (2) palpation of ligamentous structures, (3) assessment of range of motion (ROM) of the ankle, (4) testing of ankle muscles, and (5) specific testing. To exclude ankle fractures the Ottawa Ankle and Foot Rules can be used to determine if radiography is indicated [6]. Urgent evaluation is recommended for patients with a high level of pain, rapid onset of swelling, coldness or numbness in the injured foot, inability to bear weight, or complicating conditions (e.g., diabetes). Excessive swelling and pain can limit adequate examination up to 48 h after injury [1]. The specificity and sensitivity of delayed physical examination for the presence or absence of a lesion of an ankle ligament were found to be 84 % and 96 %, respectively [13, 14], whereas clinical examination within 48 h had a sensitivity of 71 % and a specificity of 33 % [15]. This is why, after the ankle is examined and a fracture is excluded, reexamination 3–5 days after injury is important in distinguishing partial tears from full ligament ruptures [13, 14]. It is important to distinguish a simple distortion from an acute ankle ligament rupture as adequate treatment is associated with a better prognosis.

32.3.1 Acute Lateral Ligament Injury

In the acute setting most athletes recall having "rolled over" the outside of the ankle [6]. Clinically the most important features of physical examination are swelling, hematoma, and pain on palpation [4].

In the acute setting the anterior drawer test and palpation cannot be correctly performed due to pain. After a few days pain is more localized and reexamination is possible and more reliable [13]. Pain on palpation over the ATFL in combination with hematoma gives a high raise of suspicion to a lateral ankle ligament rupture with an 80 % predictive value. The third component of the physical examination is the anterior drawer test (see Fig. 32.1). Having all three of these symptoms, pain on palpation on the ATFL, hematoma discoloration, and a positive anterior drawer test, means a lateral ligament rupture in 96 % of the patients. The reliability of this delayed physical examination is similar to arthrography in identifying lateral ligament rupture [1].

In 40 % of patients with an isolated lateral ankle ligament rupture, there is also pain on palpation over the syndesmotic ligaments without a syndesmotic ligament rupture! 65 % of patients with supination trauma resulting in a lateral ligament rupture also have pain on palpation on the medial side of the joint due to compression [22].

Additional diagnostics to demonstrate laxity in the ankle joint are by means of stress radiographs [16]. Stress radiographs, however, are difficult to perform for acute ankle sprains due to pain, edema, and muscle spasms. If a stress film is needed for an accurate preoperative diagnosis, this should be done under local anesthesia [17]. MRI and ultrasound are used to diagnose concomitant injury (bone, chondral, or tendon), provide a superior soft-tissue resolution diagnosing ligament lesions, and are routine investigations in professional athletes [18]. MRI might be able to show injury to individual components of the ligaments and has a sensitivity and specificity of, respectively, 95 % and 90 %. Ultrasound has been demonstrated to be an accurate investigation that leads to little discomfort in patients, but requires technical expertise, and data may be difficult to interpret on retrospective review by other physicians. The sensitivity and specificity of ultrasound investigation for a ligament rupture are 92 % and 64 %, respectively. A computed tomography (CT) scan is a useful modality if injury to the articular surface, avulsion fractures, or abnormal osseous anatomy is suspected [15].

32.3.2 Chronic Lateral Ankle Instability

Progressing to chronicity might be caused by inadequate treatment or diagnosis, but might also occur despite an adequate rehabilitation program. The main complaint patients will present in chronic ankle instability is "giving way." Other possible symptoms are persistent discomfort, swelling, pain or tenderness, or anterolateral impingement [19]. As the anterior talofibular ligament is the most important stabilizer of the ankle joint, it is the first ligament to rupture during an inversion trauma and is the weak link in chronic lateral ankle instability. This makes the anterior drawer test the most important test to detect acute and chronic ankle instability, together with the talar tilt test which is less reliable [20]. These tests are performed with the patient sitting and the feet hanging free. Radiographs are often used to decide whether surgery is indicated to treat chronic ankle instability. Radiographs can also be used as assessment of therapy. CT, MRI, and ultrasonography are not used in chronic ligament injury as they are unable to demonstrate ligament laxity [21].

32.3.3 Acute Syndesmotic Ligament Injury

In the acute setting it is difficult to distinguish between lateral and syndesmotic ligament injury as 40 % of patients with lateral ligament injury also present with pain on palpation over the anterior distal tibiofibular ligament without a rupture of these syndesmotic ligaments to be present [22]! Tenderness should be tested taking membrana interossea into account, and pain reaching higher means a greater extent of the lesion. Additional tests are the fibular translation test, the cotton test, the external rotation test, the tibia and fibula squeeze test, the crossed leg test, and the stabilization test [4, 6].

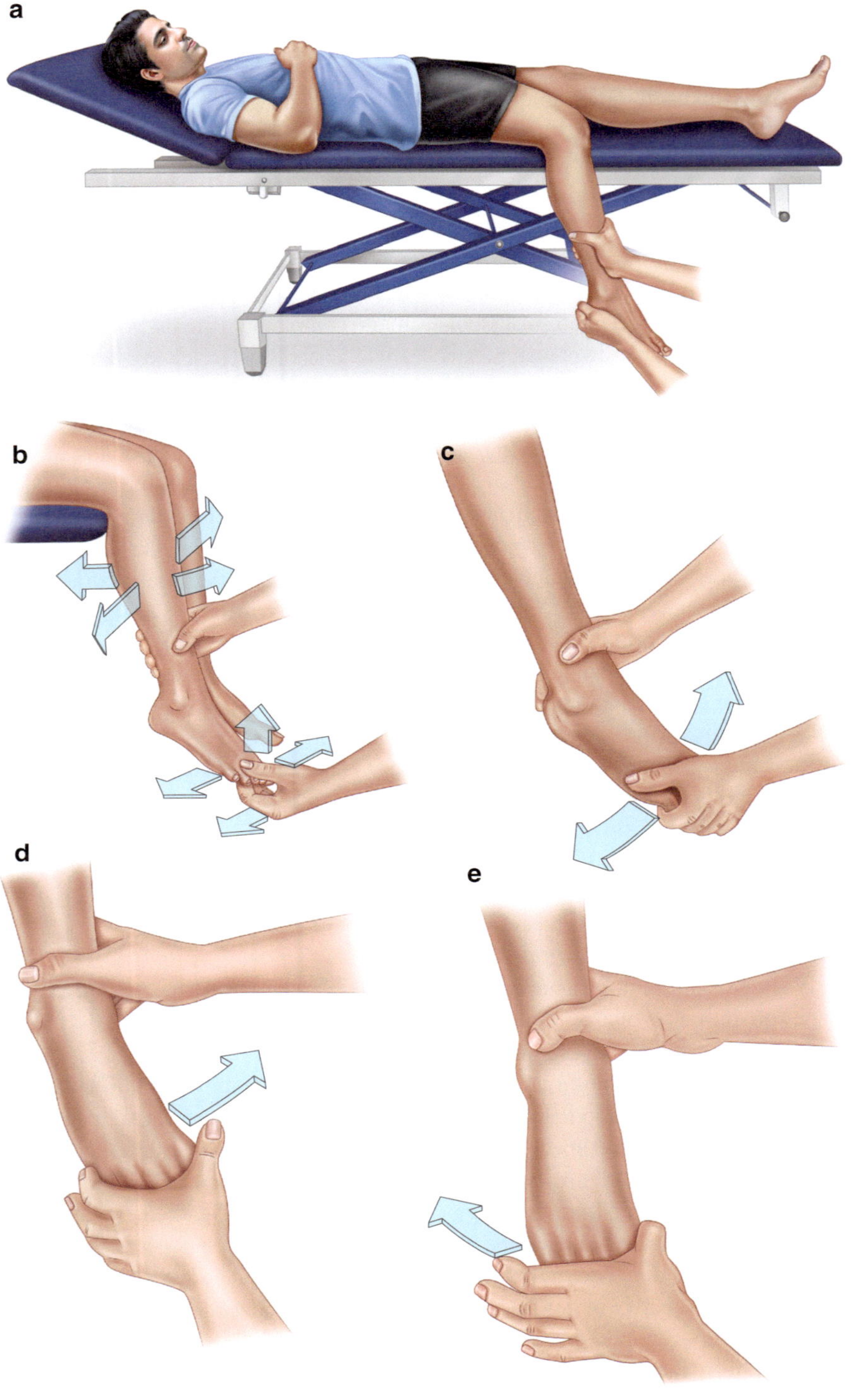

Fig. 32.1 Correct positioning of patient for performing anterior drawer test. (**a**) The patient is in the supine position. The upper leg supported by the table, the knee joint is flexed. The ankle joint is held in 10°–15° of plantar flexion. (**b**) When the patient is very apprehensive, relaxation is stimulated by grasping patients free hanging forefoot/toes loosening the ankle and foot by gentle manipulation in all directions. This includes exo- and endorotation of the hip and flexion and extension of the knee. (**c**) Gentle flexion and extension of the toes and ankle joint. (**d**) Gentle inversion and eversion (**e**) to check if the patient has relaxed all muscles that can control the anterior drawer

Radiographic imaging must include an AP view and a mortise view of the syndesmosis to rule out the tibiofibular clear space, medial clear space overlap, tibial width, and fibular width. MRI should be the second imaging tool to be used [23], as it has a sensitivity and specificity of, respectively, 95 % and 90 % for syndesmotic ligament injuries [10, 24].

Isolated syndesmotic injury can be classified as stable or unstable. The stable ankle sprain (grade I) is characterized by a lesion of the anterior inferior tibiofibular ligament (AITFL) with or without the interosseous ligament (IOL) with an intact deltoid ligament. If physical examination is inconclusive, additional diagnostics are needed to evaluate the stability of the ankle syndesmosis (grade IIa being stable, IIb being unstable). The proven unstable ankle sprain (grade III) should be classified in latent or frank diastasis. The latent diastasis is characterized by a rupture of the AITFL with or without IOL and a rupture of the deltoid ligament. It can be detected on MRI imaging and/or arthroscopic assessment. The frank diastasis is characterized by a rupture of all the syndesmotic including the deltoid ligaments, and it is visible on standard radiographs [24].

32.3.4 Subacute and Chronic Syndesmotic Injury

Even though syndesmotic injury heals slowly, residual disability with recurrent instability episodes is rare. Patients typically have a sensation of giving way and have difficulty to walk on uneven grounds and "pushing" off when running. On clinical examination, stiffness, limited dorsiflexion, and sometimes swelling on the anterolateral aspect, just proximal to the ankle joint, can be observed [10]. In case of suspicion of chronic syndesmotic injury, a positive squeeze test, positive fibular translation test, and testing for local recognizable palpation pain should be done. In experienced hands these tests are highly specific for chronic syndesmotic injury [25].

32.4 Treatment Strategy

Therapy for acute ankle sprains firstly focuses on controlling pain and swelling and complete recovery without residual symptoms on the long term [8]. PRICE (Protection, Rest, Ice, Compression, and Elevation) is a well-established protocol for the treatment [26]. As evidence on relative effectiveness of RICE therapy is insufficient, treatment decisions should be made on an individual basis [27, 28]. There is, however, some evidence that applying ice and using nonsteroidal anti-inflammatory drugs (NSAIDs) improves healing and speeds recovering [26].

32.4.1 Acute Lateral Ligament Injury

Treatment of lateral ankle ligament injury consists of immobilization, functional rehabilitation, or surgery (as described in Sect. 34.4.2) [8, 29]. Treatment options differ according to the grade of injury. Grade I and II sprains usually respond to rest and immobilization, early use of RICE, maintenance of ROM, weight bearing, neuromuscular training, and usage of ankle support, while grade III sprains require tape or brace treatment and, possibly, surgery [8, 30]. Early motion and mobility are recommended especially in athletes, but ligamentous strength does not return until months after an ankle sprain [31].

Functional rehabilitation is preferred over immobilization and is most effective in isolated ligament injuries [32–34]. Functional treatment consists of exercise, mobilization, and using semirigid supports up to 6 weeks [27]. A short period of plaster immobilization or similar rigid support could facilitate a rapid decrease of pain and swelling in selected cases [11].

In the general population and in athletes, good results have been achieved by both conservative treatment and reconstructive surgery [35–37]. Pijnenburg et al. [35] showed that operative treatment leads to better results than functional treatment and functional treatment leads to better results than cast immobilization for 6 weeks [38].

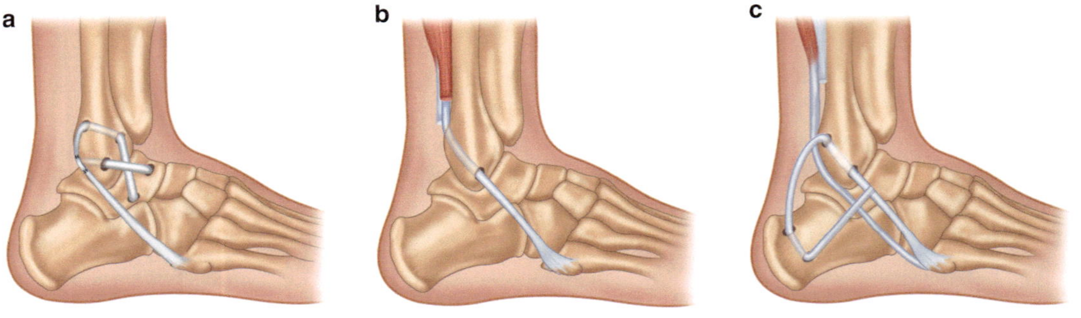

Fig. 32.2 Tenodesis procedures: Watson-Jones procedure (**a**), Evans procedure (**b**), Chrisman-Snook procedure (**c**)

In the general population, functional treatment is preferred over surgical therapy [14]. However, in professional footballers surgery is preferred as it gives a better chance of regaining joint stability. It is the only treatment with direct anatomic repair of ruptured ligaments without lengthening, loss of strength, or delaying return to participation in sports [39, 40].

32.4.2 Chronic Lateral Ankle Instability

The initial treatment of chronic ankle instability consists of neuromuscular training, restoring active stability by training which might provide good results in a short time. If ankle instability remains despite appropriate rehabilitation, this is an indication for surgery. In surgery there is a choice between anatomic and nonanatomic reconstruction. Anatomic reconstruction of the ankle ligaments usually results in good stability, diminishes symptoms, and in most cases leads to a normal functional capacity [16, 41]. Tenodesis on the other hand is a nonanatomic reconstruction and is not recommended as it can lead to functional and mechanical instability, restricted ROM, a higher number of reoperations, chronic pain, degenerative changes, and impaired athletic performance [42–44]. Increasing interest in arthroscopy might not only improve diagnosing lesions but may also replace the open approaches that are currently performed [39]. The question remains if current surgical strategies are the best practice for ligament and functional recovery and if anatomic reconstruction is fully anatomic (Figs. 32.2 and 32.3).

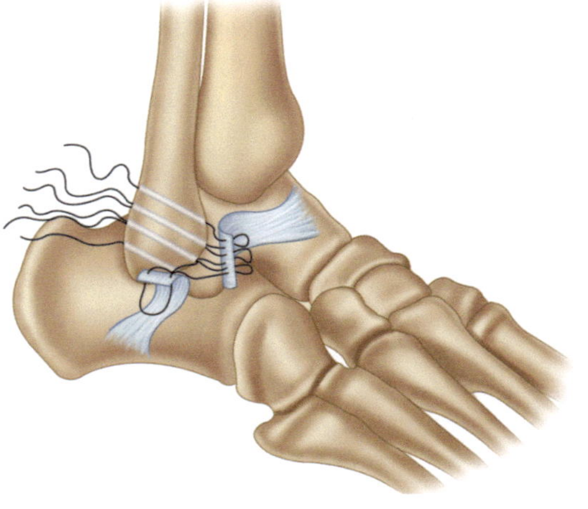

Fig. 32.3 Anatomic reconstruction of the lateral ankle ligaments using the Duquennoy technique [45]

32.4.3 Acute Syndesmotic Ligament Injury

For isolated syndesmotic sprains additional treatment strategies have to be taken into account. The treatment should include 3 weeks non-weight bearing, a below the knee cast, rest, and ice. Return to normal activities should be done as tolerated by pain and disability. After 3 weeks of non-weight bearing, proprioceptive exercises are recommended [22]. A walking boot is prescribed for 4–6 weeks, so the interosseous tibiofibular ligament can heal [3].

Surgery is indicated when there is instability based on a disruption of normal tibiofibular relationships on radiographs or if the deltoid ligament is ruptured (grade IIb and all grade III lesions) [10]. For the professional footballer with a grade II syndesmotic injury and clinical suspicion of dynamic instability, examination under anesthesia and arthroscopy with assessment of the syndesmosis is recommended. Grade III injuries are uncommon in professional football players and are often associated with other injuries around the ankle. In case of dynamic diastasis of 2 mm or more, fixation is needed. The use of a suture button repair in a syndesmosis injury is preferred as it leads to similar functional outcome, but implant removal is less frequently needed compared to the use of a syndesmotic screw [22].

32.4.4 Subacute and Chronic Syndesmotic Injury

Subacute syndesmotic injuries mean syndesmotic lesions that are detected > 6 weeks after trauma. These lesions usually do not respond to conservative treatment and require surgical treatment. Surgical intervention may include arthroscopic debridement, screw fixation, and anatomic reconstruction of the syndesmotic ligaments. Chronic syndesmotic ruptures are ruptures > 6 month old. These best can be treated by means of a synostosis [46].

32.5 Rehabilitation and Return to Play

32.5.1 Lateral Ligament Injury

The functional rehabilitation protocol for acute ligament injury consists of three phases. Firstly the PRICE protocol [6] is initiated within 24 h of injury to minimize pain and swelling up till 1 week after injury [3]. When needed, crutches can be used for a few days and weight bearing should be modulated [47]. The second phase consists of restoring ROM and strength, early weight bearing after 4–7 days, normalizing gait, functions in daily living, and neuromuscular training exercises [6]. This usually begins within 1 week of injury, and usage of brace, tape, or elastic bandage is advised possibly up till 6 weeks post-injury [14]. The final phase consists of endurance training, sport-specific drills, and training to improve balance [1]. The goal is to prepare the footballer for return to full sports participation. More advanced neuromuscular training, agility drills, and sport-specific tasks are the central components of this phase [10].

Rehabilitation for chronic lateral ankle ligament injury tries to restore the stability using neuromuscular training. In case this last recourse fails, surgery is indicated. The rehabilitation program after ankle surgery is similar to functional rehabilitation for acute ligament injury apart from the first phase. After surgery treatment consists of wearing a lower-leg cast for 1 or 2 weeks followed by 2–4 weeks in a walking boot. Partial to full weight bearing commences when pain complaints have subsided after approximately 2 weeks post-surgery. Active-assisted physiotherapy focuses on ROM and proprioception exercises. Progression to the next phase is guided by players' complaints. Full weight bearing, strength training, and proprioception are emphasized, and thereafter sport-specific functional exercises are started [48].

32.5.2 Syndesmotic Ligament Injury

In case of conservative management of isolated syndesmotic ligament injury (grade I and grade IIa), a patient will have to rest, apply ice, and wear a non-weight-bearing cast for 3 weeks. This way inflammation and swelling can improve. After 3 weeks the patient should be able to return to normal activities as tolerated by pain and disability. In case of surgery the patient can resume partial weight bearing 6 weeks after surgery. Rehabilitation after surgery is similar to that used in nonsurgical management, but might progress more slowly [10, 49, 50]. A sign of a healing syndesmosis is the ability to repeatedly single-leg hop. Return to sporting activity is permitted when the athlete is able to single-leg hop without significant pain. The time to pain-free full recovery is variable, but a syndesmotic sprain may require a treatment period almost twice as long as a grade III lateral ankle sprain [4].

32.5.3 Sport-Specific Rehabilitation

Best is to use a protocol specified for the football player, a rehabilitation program with a variety of exercises in which propriocepsis, strength, coordination, and function of the extremity are maintained. This as a disturbance of propriocepsis may cause functional instability [27]. ROM must be regained before functional rehabilitation is initiated. As the patient achieves full weight bearing without pain, proprioceptive training is initiated for the recovery of balance and postural control. When the distance walked by the patient is no longer limited by pain, the next step is a regimen of 50 % walking and 50 % jogging. Using the same criteria, jogging eventually progresses to running, backward running, and pattern running [10]. Circles and figures of 8 are commonly employed patterns. The final phase of the rehabilitation process is documentation that the athlete can perform sport-specific exercises pain-free at a level consistent with pre-injury status [51]. Before being allowed to return to full competition, the athlete should be put through a functional test that simulates all requirements of his or her sport [52]. Proprioceptive and strength training should be continued even after players have returned to the field, as an increased error in accuracy of ankle position was still present compared with the healthy ankle 12 weeks after the injury [53].

32.5.4 Return to the Field

Functional rehabilitation is effective for all grades of ankle sprain; however, the time required to return to full athletic function will increase as the severity of injury increases. For competitive athletes with a lateral ankle sprain, complete immobilization, even for short periods, may greatly extend rehabilitation time required for full return to activity [52]. Comparing functional rehabilitation with surgery followed by functional rehabilitation, the time to return to sport with external ankle support ranged from 3 to 12 weeks c.q. 3–8 weeks. Return to the full athletic activity with no external ankle support ranged from 8 to 48 weeks for functional treatment alone and 8–15 weeks for surgery followed by functional treatment [54].

In syndesmosis injury in football players, injury severity on physical examination and player position can help predict the time to return to unrestricted athletic activity [55]. The best predictor for time to return to sport is the external rotation test, and in association with other test results, it predicted an extended time taken to return to competitive sports. Two or three positive tests were significantly more likely to take 7 or more days to walk 10 m without pain than subjects with none or one positive test result [56].

References

1. Ivins D (2006) Acute ankle sprain: an update. Am Fam Physician 74(10):1714–1720
2. Woods C et al (2003) The football association medical research programme: an audit of injuries in professional football: an analysis of ankle sprains. Br J Sports Med 37(3):233–238
3. Fong DT et al (2009) Understanding acute ankle ligamentous sprain injury in sports. Sports Med Arthrosc Rehabil Ther Technol 1:14
4. Dubin JC et al (2011) Lateral and syndesmotic ankle sprain injuries: a narrative literature review. J Chiropr Med 10(3):204–219
5. Hertel J (2002) Functional anatomy, pathomechanics, and pathophysiology of lateral ankle instability. J Athl Train 37(4):364–375
6. Lynch SA, Renstrom PA (1999) Treatment of acute lateral ankle ligament rupture in the athlete. Conservative versus surgical treatment. Sports Med 27(1):61–71
7. Fuller EA (1999) Center of pressure and its theoretical relationship to foot pathology. J Am Podiatr Med Assoc 89(6):278–291
8. Verhagen RA, de Keizer G, van Dijk CN (1995) Long-term follow-up of inversion trauma of the ankle. Arch Orthop Trauma Surg 114(2):92–96

9. Mulligan EP (2011) Evaluation and management of ankle syndesmosis injuries. Phys Ther Sport 12(2): 57–69
10. Williams GN, Allen EJ (2010) Rehabilitation of syndesmotic (high) ankle sprains. Sports Health 2(6): 460–470
11. Konradsen L, Holmer P, Sondergaard L (1991) Early mobilizing treatment for grade III ankle ligament injuries. Foot Ankle 12(2):69–73
12. Harmon KG (2004) The ankle examination. Prim Care 31(4):1025–1037, x
13. van Dijk CN et al (1996) Physical examination is sufficient for the diagnosis of sprained ankles. J Bone Joint Surg Br 78(6):958–962
14. van Dijk CN (2002) Management of the sprained ankle. Br J Sports Med 36(2):83–84
15. van Dijk CN et al (1996) Diagnosis of ligament rupture of the ankle joint. Physical examination, arthrography, stress radiography and sonography compared in 160 patients after inversion trauma. Acta Orthop Scand 67(6):566–570
16. Ruedi T, Huggler A (1981) [Fresh ligament injuries of the ankle joint]. Helv Chir Acta 47(6):763–772
17. Zinman C et al (1979) Acute rupture of the lateral ligaments of the ankle joint, diagnosis and surgical treatment. Am Surg 45(7):465–470
18. O'Neill PJ, Van Aman SE, Guyton GP (2010) Is MRI adequate to detect lesions in patients with ankle instability? Clin Orthop Relat Res 468(4):1115–1119
19. Gerstner Garces JB (2012) Chronic ankle instability. Foot Ankle Clin 17(3):389–398
20. Kerkhoffs GM et al (2002) An instrumented, dynamic test for anterior laxity of the ankle joint complex. J Biomech 35(12):1665–1670
21. Tourne Y et al (2010) Chronic ankle instability. Which tests to assess the lesions? Which therapeutic options? Orthop Traumatol Surg Res 96(4):433–446
22. McCollum GA et al (2013) Syndesmosis and deltoid ligament injuries in the athlete. Knee Surg Sports Traumatol Arthrosc 21(6):1328–1337
23. Howard DR et al (2012) Magnetic resonance imaging as a predictor of return to play following syndesmosis (high) ankle sprains in professional football players. Sports Health 4(6):535–543
24. Brown KW et al (2004) MRI findings associated with distal tibiofibular syndesmosis injury. AJR Am J Roentgenol 182(1):131–136
25. Sman AD, Hiller CE, Refshauge KM (2013) Diagnostic accuracy of clinical tests for diagnosis of ankle syndesmosis injury: a systematic review. Br J Sports Med 47(10):620–628
26. Inklaar H, van Beek PA (2011) Guideline for diagnosis and treatment of acute inversion trauma of the ankle in athletes. Ned Tijdschr Geneeskd 155(33): A3324
27. Kerkhoffs GM et al (2012) Diagnosis, treatment and prevention of ankle sprains: an evidence-based clinical guideline. Br J Sports Med 46(12):854–860
28. van den Bekerom MP et al (2012) What is the evidence for rest, ice, compression, and elevation therapy in the treatment of ankle sprains in adults? J Athl Train 47(4):435–443
29. Petersen W et al (2013) Treatment of acute ankle ligament injuries: a systematic review. Arch Orthop Trauma Surg 133(8):1129–1141
30. Wexler RK (1998) The injured ankle. Am Fam Physician 57(3):474–480
31. Wolfe MW et al (2001) Management of ankle sprains. Am Fam Physician 63(1):93–104
32. Kerkhoffs GM et al (2002) Different functional treatment strategies for acute lateral ankle ligament injuries in adults. Cochrane Database Syst Rev 3:CD002938
33. Kerkhoffs GM et al (2001) Immobilisation for acute ankle sprain. A systematic review. Arch Orthop Trauma Surg 121(8):462–471
34. Jones MH, Amendola AS (2007) Acute treatment of inversion ankle sprains: immobilization versus functional treatment. Clin Orthop Relat Res 455:169–172
35. Pijnenburg AC et al (2003) Operative and functional treatment of rupture of the lateral ligament of the ankle. A randomised, prospective trial. J Bone Joint Surg Br 85(4):525–530
36. Kaikkonen A, Kannus P, Jarvinen M (1996) Surgery versus functional treatment in ankle ligament tears. A prospective study. Clin Orthop Relat Res 326: 194–202
37. Wening JV, Raabe S, Jungbluth KH (1991) [Comparative study between conservative and surgical therapy of fibular ligament ruptures of the upper ankle joint]. Zentralbl Chir 116(18):1047–1060
38. Pijnenburg AC et al (2000) Treatment of ruptures of the lateral ankle ligaments: a meta-analysis. J Bone Joint Surg Am 82(6):761–773
39. Schmitz R, Jager E (1992) Benefits and risks of surgical therapy of acute lateral fibular ligament rupture of the upper ankle joint. Results of a retrospective study. Aktuelle Traumatol 22(6):276–280
40. Kerkhoffs GM, Van Dijk CN (2013) Acute lateral ankle ligament ruptures in the athlete: the role of surgery. Foot Ankle Clin 18(2):215–218
41. Lassus J et al (2001) Anatomical reconstruction of ruptured lateral ligaments of upper ankle joint. Ann Chir Gynaecol 90(3):213–217
42. Maffulli N, Ferran NA (2008) Management of acute and chronic ankle instability. J Am Acad Orthop Surg 16(10):608–615
43. Krips R et al (2002) Anatomical reconstruction and Evans tenodesis of the lateral ligaments of the ankle. Clinical and radiological findings after follow-up for 15 to 30 years. J Bone Joint Surg Br 84(2): 232–236
44. Krips R et al (2001) Long-term outcome of anatomical reconstruction versus tenodesis for the treatment of chronic anterolateral instability of the ankle joint: a multicenter study. Foot Ankle Int 22(5):415–421
45. Muijs SP, Dijkstra PD, Bos CF (2008) Clinical outcome after anatomical reconstruction of the lateral ankle ligaments using the Duquennoy technique in chronic lateral instability of the ankle: a long-term follow-up study. J Bone Joint Surg Br 90(1):50–56

46. van den Bekerom MP, Raven EE (2009) Arthrex tightrope distal tibiofibular syndesmotic stabilization. Foot Ankle Int 30(6):577–578, author reply 578
47. Hubbard TJ, Wikstrom EA (2010) Ankle sprain: pathophysiology, predisposing factors, and management strategies. Open Access. J Sports Med 1:115–122
48. de Vries JS et al (2011) Interventions for treating chronic ankle instability. Cochrane Database Syst Rev 8:CD004124
49. Parlamas G et al (2013) Treatment of chronic syndesmotic injury: a systematic review and meta-analysis. Knee Surg Sports Traumatol Arthrosc 21(8):1931–1939
50. Taylor DC et al (2007) Aggressive surgical treatment and early return to sports in athletes with grade III syndesmosis sprains. Am J Sports Med 35(11):1833–1838
51. Mattacola CG, Dwyer MK (2002) Rehabilitation of the ankle after acute sprain or chronic instability. J Athl Train 37(4):413–429
52. Safran MR et al (1999) Lateral ankle sprains: a comprehensive review part 2: treatment and rehabilitation with an emphasis on the athlete. Med Sci Sports Exerc 31(7 Suppl):S438–S447
53. Konradsen L, Olesen S, Hansen HM (1998) Ankle sensorimotor control and eversion strength after acute ankle inversion injuries. Am J Sports Med 26(1): 72–77
54. Takao M et al (2012) Functional treatment after surgical repair for acute lateral ligament disruption of the ankle in athletes. Am J Sports Med 40(2):447–451
55. Miller BS et al (2012) Time to return to play after high ankle sprains in collegiate football players: a prediction model. Sports Health 4(6):504–509
56. Alonso A, Khoury L, Adams R (1998) Clinical tests for ankle syndesmosis injury: reliability and prediction of return to function. J Orthop Sports Phys Ther 27(4):276–284

Ankle Osteochondral Lesions

33

Sandro Giannini, Roberto Buda, Laura Ramponi,
Francesco Castagnini, Silvio Caravelli,
Giuseppe Gianluca Costa, and Francesca Vannini

33.1 Definition

Osteochondral lesion (OCL) of the ankle joint is an injury involving the chondral layer and, secondarily, the subchondral bone. It is usually localized on the talar dome, less frequently on the tibial plafond [1, 2].

33.1.1 Etiology

Ankle OCLs are usually traumatic in origin, mostly subsequent to ankle sprains or repetitive microtraumas [1]. Chondral lesions are present in 50 % of the acute ankle sprains and may be traced in 23 % of the lateral chronic instability of the ankle, causing persisting pain even after ligament reconstruction [3, 4]. Regarding the location, lateral lesions recognize a traumatic etiology in 93–98 % of the cases, whereas medial defects reported an ankle injury in only 60–71 % [1]. In a recent work by Orr, OCLs were centro-lateral (49 %) or centro-medial (33 %): specifically, the centro-lateral lesions were sent to surgery more frequently than the medial ones, which, nevertheless, tended to be larger [5]. The nontraumatic etiology encounters for a small amount of cases, which have been addressed to various hypothesis as, for example, embolic, hereditary, endocrine, idiopathic, or vascular etiology but still scarcely investigated [6, 7]. Due to the overwhelming percentage of traumatic etiology, football has definitely one of the highest occurrence rates of osteochondral lesion due to the high frequency of ankle sprains. It is generally accepted that the weight-bearing ankle while landing is be more susceptible to injury because of a relative inability to respond to rotational forces [8]. Finally, osteochondral lesions are more likely to occur if there is a preexisting abnormality in the ankle or remainder of the lower limb kinetic chain (muscles, knee, and hip joints).

S. Giannini (✉) • R. Buda
Orthopaedics and Traumatology,
University of Bologna, Bologna, Italy

I Clinic, Rizzoli Orthopaedic Institute, Bologna, Italy
e-mail: giannini@ior.it; roberto.buda@ior.it

L. Ramponi, MD • F. Castagnini, MD
S. Caravelli, MD • G.G. Costa, MD • F. Vannini, MD
I Clinic, Rizzoli Orthopaedic Institute, Bologna, Italy
e-mail: gpagliazzi@libero.it;
francescocastagnini@hotmail.it;
silvio.caravelli@ior.it;
giuseppegianluca.costa@ior.it;
france_vannini@yahoo.it

33.1.2 Injury Mechanism and Natural History

While playing football, the ankle is exposed to stresses during sprinting, sudden changes of direction ("cutting-in"), tackling, and kicking mechanism. During normal gait, the joint reaction forces generated are equivalent to 5 times body weight, but they can increase to 13 times

P. Volpi (ed.), *Football Traumatology: New Trends*, DOI 10.1007/978-3-319-18245-2_33

body weight on jogging with further increases on sprinting, cutting-in, or stumbling [9, 10].

Traumas causing lateral OCLs are ankle inversion or inversion-dorsiflection [1, 11]. As described by Berndt-Hardy, the forced inversion causes the talar dome to impact on fibular surface, damaging the articular surface through a shearing force. In this case, the lesion looks superficial and oval [1, 11].

Medial OCL is less correlated to traumas; nevertheless, a combined torsional impaction and axial loading (plantar flexion, anterior displacement, and internal rotation of the talus on tibia during inversion) is the advocated preponderant etiology. It usually appears deeper than the lateral one and is described as cup shaped [11]. The most affected areas are the centro-medial and centro-lateral, with the last localization seriously injured by the rotational forces. So, the centro-lateral lesions are more prone to a surgical treatment, despite the lower surface involved [5].

Among the causes of injury specifically correlated to football are inferior playing surfaces and inappropriate footwear. Incorrect footwear which cannot provide sufficient frictional force will eventually lead to slipping. On the other hand, too much frictional force will produce large torque when twisting and turning, which may also lead to injury [12].

The kicking mechanism in soccer can vary, but the most common actions of controlled passing and dead ball striking are performed with the inside (medial) aspect of the foot [9, 13]. On ball strike, the ankle is forced into plantar flexion that often exceeds the normal range of passive plantar flexion [13]. These features have several influences on potential mechanisms for acute and chronic osteochondral injury. It is proposed that repeated traumatic forces (average 1020 N) to the anterior tibiotalar joint can cause chronic osteochondral and capsular injury resulting in an anterior impingement, which was originally termed "footballer's ankle" [13, 14].

Tackling is the most common injury mechanism [15], resulting in chronic sequelae that include mechanical instability, osteochondral lesions, and impingement (anterolateral and anterior) [16]. The forces generated during tackling can frequently extend medially and obliquely, resulting in a higher incidence of direct medial structure, compared with other sports [8]. Medial forces causing aversion and leading to medial ligamentous, capsular, and osteochondral injuries can also be generated on striking the ball or cutting-in [13, 17]. When the planted foot is tackled with an external rotation force, the rest of the limb and body continues to move forward, resulting in dorsiflexion and a subsequent distraction force to the syndesmosis. This combination of forces can also produce talar chondral injury (usually posterolateral). This mechanism of injury can also occur with impact at the knee that results in forced internal rotation of the femur and relative external rotation of the tibia and distal syndesmosis. This mechanism commonly results in acute morbidity from the syndesmosis injury, with potential chronic symptoms related to chondral injury.

33.2 Clinical and Diagnostic Examination

Swelling, pain, and symptoms related to lateral ligament lesions may be present. Locking, or catching, is associated with displaced fragments. Pain and limited range of motion (ROM) usually persist over 4–6 weeks after the acute event [1, 11, 18].

Chronic OCL's most frequent symptom is a mild, continuous pain, mostly associated with physical activity [1, 11, 18]. Asymptomatic cases are not uncommon. Walking on uneven ground may increase the symptoms. Swelling, stiffness, weakness, and reduced ROM may be present, mostly in degenerated OCL. Patients may complain for the inability to load on the joint and, in case of loose bodies, for catching, locking, or clicking [1, 11, 18].

Palpation often evokes tenderness on posterior-medial or anterior-lateral areas of the talus [1, 11, 18]. The range of motion may be limited in half of the cases. Limpness, or antalgic gait, is relatively common. Anterior drawer and talar tilt test should be performed as sprains usually underlie OCL. Other tendon, vascular, and neurological pathologies should be ruled out.

The OCL may be limited to the chondral tissue, or it may involve the subchondral bone, or, after intense traumas, it may even isolate a loose body [1]. From a histological perspective, after the impact, the chondral layer is found to be softened, with a significant chondrocyte apoptosis and matrix degeneration. The hyaline cartilage is progressively replaced by fibrocartilage during the healing process. The subchondral bone is strongly reshaped by an increased osteoclastic activity, with an ultimate bone stock loss [19]. The presence of bone bruise is a significant prognostic factor of chondral damage, causing cartilage irregularities, chondrocytes apoptosis, and matrix degeneration [20]. Classically, OCL may evolve to osteoarthritis and, when symptomatic and large defects are found, should be addressed to surgery in order to avoid progression [6, 7, 11]. The work by Guettler highlighted that not only OCL provides a local osteochondral disruption but alters the biomechanics of the surrounding cartilage as well, predisposing to arthritis [21].

Routine X-ray is the first-line diagnostic tool, also in order to rule out a fracture in acute cases [22]. Nevertheless, apart from large lesions, OCL can easily be undiagnosed [23].

CT is valuable for the detection of subchondral bone injuries (Fig. 33.1): it may clearly detect the size, shape, and extent of the localization [24].

MRI is the gold standard for OCL diagnosis (Fig. 33.2), providing information about bone bruise, cartilage status, and soft tissues [24]. The sensitivity of MRI is high when correlated to arthroscopic findings (81–83 % or even higher) [25]. The most frequent features compatible with OCL are decreased signal intensity on T1-weighted images and increased intensity on T2-weighted images. In case of incomplete separation of the fragment, T2-weighted images may be confusing due to a high signal, with lower percentage of correlation with arthroscopic findings (55,6 %). In this case, the cartilage break discriminates [25].

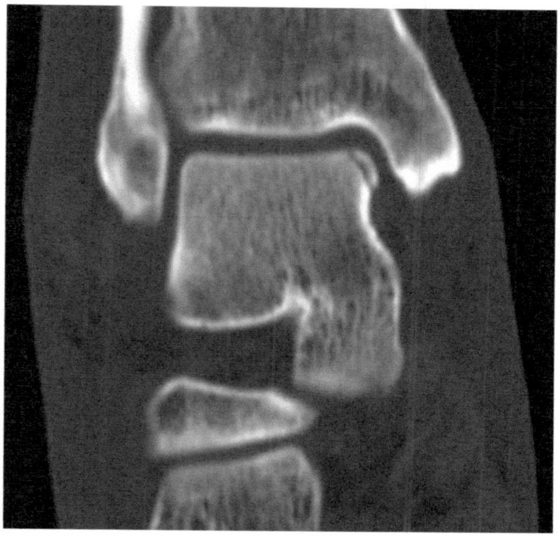

Fig. 33.1 Coronal view of a CT scan performed for OCL preoperative evaluation. CT scan is very useful to improve subchondral bone visualization

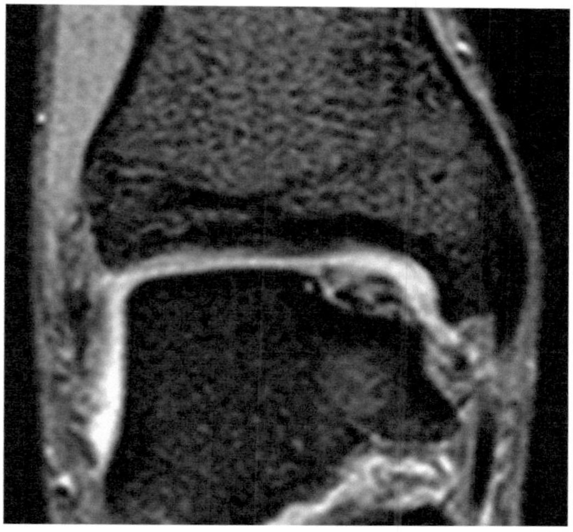

Fig. 33.2 Coronal view of MRI scan performed for chronic medial OCL. MRI is the best diagnostic tool, as it can visualize the cartilage and the subchondral bone, as well as other soft tissues as ligaments

33.3 Treatment Strategy

No widely shared guidelines exist for OCL treatment [23, 26, 27]. A valid classification, focused on arthroscopic/MRI findings and corresponding treatments, considering the area and the depth of the lesions as well, was made by Giannini (Table 33.1) [28].

33.3.1 Acute Lesions

Conservative treatment is not successful in acute lesions, requiring arthroscopic procedures.

Table 33.1 OCL classification according to Giannini divides the lesions into acute and chronic ones. The area and the depth of the OCL are taken into account. For every kind of lesion, the most suitable treatment is suggested

	Surface	Extension	Treatment
Acute			
Type I	Damaged	< 1 cm^2	Debridement
Type II	Damaged	> 1 cm^2	Fixation
Chronic			
Type 0	Intact	Any	Retrograde drilling
Type I	Damaged	< 1.5 cm^2	Microfractures
Type II	Damaged	> 1.5 cm^2	Cartilage replacement
Type IIA	Damaged	> 1.5 cm^2 >5mm	CR+bone graft
Type III	Damaged	Anatomy disruption	Massive graft

Debridement and fragment excision are advised in case of acute lesions with fragment's dimensions inferior to 1 cm [28, 29]. Fragment fixation is performed in case of larger OCL using bioresorbable screws: good long-term results are achieved thanks to an effective vascular restoration [30]. Excision for larger fragment can dramatically raise osteoarthritis rates at long-term follow-up [29]. Recently, osteochondral autografts have been adopted, with good results even in acute lesions [30].

33.3.2 Chronic Lesions

33.3.2.1 Conservative Treatment

The aim of conservative treatment is unloading the osteochondral layer, preventing the necrosis and resolving the bone edema. To date, it should be reserved to small lesions with no fragment isolation in almost-asymptomatic patients [23, 26, 31]. In these cases, 45 % of the patients may benefit from a conservative approach. A possible beneficial approach in athletes may consist in rest, with sport activity restriction and even a limited period of non-weight bearing, lasting only a few weeks, according to the gravity of the lesion. In a work by Mei-Dan, hyaluronate and platelet-rich plasma (PRP) were injected intra-articularly in OCL, improving the clinical outcomes, with long-lasting results for PRP (at least 6 months) [32]. Intra-articular injections may be functional in athletes to delay the surgical treatment even in symptomatic lesions with no fragment isolation.

33.3.2.2 Retrograde Drilling

Retrograde drilling is mostly effective in lesions 0 according to Giannini's classification, with modest subchondral bone involvement and chondral layer continuity and viability [28]. The rationale consists in a stimulation of the repair depending on subchondral bone marrow cells [27, 28, 33]. The approach is made through sinus tarsi, drilling the subchondral bone without damaging the articular surfaces. An autologous calcaneal bone graft is then performed. Retrograde drilling may avoid the necrotic effect of the anterograde approach, preserving the chondral tissue [27]. Good results were reached in case of viable cartilage; nevertheless, it has been applied even in revision surgery [27].

33.3.2.3 Microfractures

Widely diffused, microfractures are effective in OCL inferior to 1,5 cm^2 [6, 7, 28, 34]. The technique can be easily performed arthroscopically, penetrating the subchondral bone every 3–4 mm, using an awl [34]. Thanks to bone marrow stimulation, this procedure allows a good and rapid restoration of the osteochondral layer, but it generates fibrocartilage, with lower biomechanical properties and durability [23, 33]. Good clinical outcomes were reported by many authors, but medial lesions and larger and deep OCL tended to worsen over the time [34, 35].

33.3.2.4 Mosaicplasty

Osteochondral plugs, obtained from non-weight-bearing areas of the knee and, possibly, ankle, are implanted to restore the proper osteochondral layer [31, 33, 36]. This procedure often requires a malleolar osteotomy to improve the exposure. In the report by Hangody [31], the best OCL to treat is defined as approximately 10-mm large, positioned on the medial or lateral dome (not the central part of the talus), in a non-arthritic ankle. Clinical and bioptic results were promising,

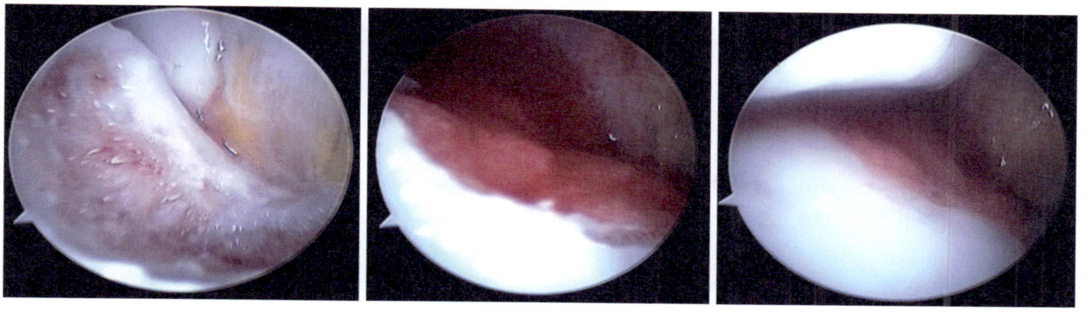

Fig. 33.3 Intraoperative arthroscopic images during BMDCT. This procedure can be performed using an arthroscopic one-step technique. First, the lesion is debrided, reaching a healthy subchondral bone. Then the biomaterial, a collagen membrane loaded with autologous mesenchymal stem cells, is implanted. Then a layer of PRF is sprayed on the biomaterial, to improve the stability of the implant and the cell differentiation and growth

achieving remarkable outcomes even in athletes (63 % of the patients came back to sport activity at the same level, only 9 % gave up sport), with a slight deterioration over time, at around 10 years from the surgical procedure [36]. Nevertheless, mosaicplasty faces some drawbacks. First, it is a technically demanding technique, which includes a donor site morbidity. Between osteochondral plugs, fibrocartilage is frequently found; moreover, not all lesions are successfully treated due to challenging locations [31, 33, 36].

33.3.2.5 Autologous Chondrocytes Implantation

Autologous chondrocytes implantation (ACI) has been intensively applied for OCL of the ankle, with successful clinical outcomes (90 %) [27]. Although no clear superiority has been established, ACI is considered the gold standard in regenerative procedures [27, 28]. The first-generation procedure was technically demanding, requiring an open-field approach, a malleolar osteotomy, and a periosteal flap suture [37, 38]. The second-generation procedure was performed arthroscopically, thanks to the development of specific instrumentation and scaffold [38]. Arthroscopic technique is performed with a two-step approach, with a first arthroscopy to debride the lesion and harvest the autologous chondrocytes doomed to expansion. A source of viable chondrocytes is the osteochondral fragment, the area around the OCL, or even a non-weight-bearing area of the knee [38, 39]. After the first arthroscopy, the chondrocytes are expanded in culture and seeded on a hyaluronate membrane. After 3 weeks, the second step takes place, and the biomaterial is arthroscopically implanted onto the lesion. The hyaline regeneration was confirmed by histological and radiological outcomes [38, 39].

33.3.2.6 Bone Marrow-Derived Cell Transplantation

Bone marrow-derived cell transplantation (BMDCT) is a regenerative technique for bony and chondral layer, based on mesenchymal stem cells [28, 33, 40]. This technique may be performed one step, in a same surgical session, or with more steps, with cell culture and enrichment: good results were achieved also in degenerated joints [28, 33, 40]. In the one-step technique, the cells are harvested from the iliac crest using a bone marrow needle (Fig. 33.3). During the concentration, a standard arthroscopy of the ankle is performed, and the joint and the defect are debrided. The cell concentrate is loaded on a collagen (or hyaluronate) membrane, then implanted in the joint using a specific instrumentation [40]. Then, a layer of platelet-rich fibrin (PRF) is sprayed on the biomaterial, to improve growth and differentiation and stability of the implant. Clinical results at medium-term follow-up are encouraging, with excellent outcomes even in athletes. Hyaline cartilage regeneration has been appreciated in bioptic samples and MRI qualitative scans. [28, 40].

33.3.2.7 Allograft

Ankle allograft is a biological reconstruction, which should be reserved to highly degenerated joints: it can be partial or total [28, 33]. Ankle may be approached laterally or anteriorly, with a fixation of both the articular surfaces using articular pins. The clinical and radiological outcomes are encouraging, and there is evidence of hyaline cartilage presence and colonization of host cells [28, 33]. Nevertheless, the indications of this procedure are selective and encompass young, active people with destroyed anatomy of the ankle [28].

33.4 Rehabilitation and Return to Play

Very few evidences about rehabilitation and return to play exist in literature and many confounding factors may vary the outcomes [41]. Youth, small lesions, and lower BMI have been advocated as positive prognostic factors in a precocious sport comeback [41]. Nowadays, the two key points in cartilage rehabilitation are continuous passive motion, which may provide a good chondral nutrition, and careful weight bearing, which may avoid the deleterious effects of overloading. Positive results may be achieved thanks to pulse electromagnetic fields, biphosphonates, or injective therapy with hyaluronate or platelet-rich plasma [32, 41]. A personalized program should always be recommended in athletes.

33.4.1 Fragment Fixation

A posterior splint or cast is advised in the first 2 weeks; then passive continuous motion is recommended, and a partial weight bearing, possibly with ankle in brace, is allowed not before 4 weeks [30].

33.4.2 Drilling

Active movements are encouraged since the day after surgery, while weight bearing is proscribed for 6 weeks [27].

33.4.3 Microfractures

Rehabilitation after microfractures requires non-weight bearing in ankle brace for 3 weeks. A progressive weight bearing is then allowed, promoting exercises for proprioception and range of motion. Return to sport was advised not before 12 weeks [34]. In a work by Lee, early or delayed weight bearing (after 1 week or 6 weeks) after microfractures for OCL did not influence the final outcome [42].

33.4.4 Mosaicplasty

Continuous passive motion is allowed the day after surgery, but the ankle is kept non-weight bearing for 3 weeks (6 weeks in case of osteotomy), which are necessary for graft incorporation [31, 36]. A progressive, partial weight bearing is allowed. After 6 weeks, complete weight bearing is allowed, and athletic activities can be started after 6 months after surgery [31, 36].

33.4.5 ACI and BMDCT

Regenerative techniques require a specific timetable for rehabilitation, due to biological properties of the implanted cells [43]. For a large division and initial incorporation, chondrocytes requires 6 weeks. Between 3 and 6 months, a primitive extracellular matrix is produced [28, 33, 43]. After 6 months, a progressive integration of the biomaterial with the subchondral bone occurs. Remodeling and maturation continues for 2–3 years [43]. The rehabilitation protocol for regenerative techniques should take into account this process, resulting in a mix of continuous passive motion, progressive weight bearing, and muscular strengthening. Personalized schemes should be encouraged but they have to share a precise program. The day after surgery, continuous passive motion is advised, and a Walker ankle brace is applied [43]. The period of non-weight bearing lasts about 6 weeks, and then a period of partial, progressive weight bearing of 2 weeks follows. After 4 months from surgery, low-impact sport activities (swimming, cycling, etc.) can be safely performed. A progressive return to running and high-impact sport activities is not allowed before 10 months.

Conclusions

Athletes required effective treatments for OCL, with a rapid sport comeback. This aim is quite difficult to be achieved, as a good restoration of qualitative and durable hyaline cartilage can be achieved only through regenerative techniques. These procedures, due to biological reasons, need longer time to heal. Although clear guidelines for OCL in athletes do not exist, conservative treatment should be proposed only in very small, not painful OCL. Debridement in small acute OCL and fixation in larger defects are two effective procedures. Microfractures could be advised in symptomatic, small chronic OCL (1,5–2 cm^2). Larger chronic lesions may pose a serious challenge: microfractures, although widely used due to the possibility of an early return to play, may not achieve satisfying results nor long lasting and may spoil the athlete career especially in young and promising players. Up to now instead regenerative techniques, ACI in particular, permit a tissue regeneration closer to hyaline with superior mechanical quality and more stable results over time; still athletes should be clearly warned of the longer times needed for rehabilitation after such procedures [44]. Nevertheless, BMDC transplantation showed the capability to regenerate a tissue extremely similar to hyaline both at bioptic harvest and qualitative MRI [39, 40] and, in a population of more than 100 athletes (data in press), permitted an early return to play (6 months) with good and satisfactory results mid term. This may be the future solution for the football player capable to combine a regeneration of quality and an early return to play.

References

1. van Dijk CN, Reilingh ML, Zengerink M et al (2010) Osteochondral defects in the ankle: why painful? Knee Surg Sports Traumatol Arthrosc 18(5):570–580. doi:10.1007/s00167-010-1064-x
2. Schachter AK, Chen AL, Reddy PD, Tejwani NC (2005) Osteochondral lesions of the talus. J Am Acad Orthop Surg 13(3):152–158
3. Saxena A, Eakin C (2007) Articular talar injuries in athletes: results of microfracture and autogenous bone graft. Am J Sports Med 35(10):1680–1687
4. Choi WJ, Park KK, Kim BS, Lee JW (2009) Osteochondral lesion of the talus: is there a critical defect size for poor outcome? Am J Sports Med 37(10):1974–1980. doi:10.1177/0363546509335765
5. Orr JD, Dutton JR, Fowler JT (2012) Anatomic location and morphology of symptomatic, operatively treated osteochondral lesions of the talus. Foot Ankle Int 33(12):1051–1057. doi:10.3113/FAI.2012.1051
6. Murawski CD, Kennedy JG (2013) Operative treatment of osteochondral lesions of the talus. J Bone Joint Surg Am 95(11):1045–1054. doi:10.2106/JBJS.L.00773
7. Talusan PG, Milewski MD, Toy JO et al (2014) Osteochondritis dissecans of the talus: diagnosis and treatment in athletes. Clin Sports Med 33(2):267–284. doi:10.1016/j.csm.2014.01.003
8. Giza E, Fuller C, Junge A, Dvorak J (2003) Mechanisms of foot and ankle injuries in soccer. Am J Sports Med 31:550–554
9. Lees A, Nolan L (1998) The biomechanics of soccer: a review. J Sports Sci 16:211–234
10. Self BP, Paine D (2001) Ankle biomechanics during four landing techniques. Med Sci Sports Exerc 33:1338–1344
11. Canale ST, Belding RH (1980) Osteochondral lesions of the talus. J Bone Joint Surg Am 62(1):97–102
12. Wong P, Hong Y (2005) Soccer injury in the lower extremities. Br J Sports Med 39:473–482
13. Tol JL, Slim E, van Soest AJ, van Dijk CN (2002) The relationship of the kicking action in soccer and anterior ankle impingement syndrome. A biomechanical analysis. Am J Sports Med 30:45–50
14. Robinson P, White LM (2002) Soft-tissue and osseous impingement syndromes of the ankle: role of imaging in diagnosis and management. Radiographics 22:1457–1469, discussion 1470–1471
15. Hawkins RD, Hulse MA, Wilkinson C et al (2001) The association football medical research programme: an audit of injuries in professional football. Br J Sports Med 35:43–47
16. Hintermann B, Boss A, Schafer D (2002) Arthroscopic findings in patients with chronic ankle instability. Am J Sports Med 30:402–409
17. Chomiak J, Junge A, Peterson L, Dvorak J (2000) Severe injuries in football players. Influencing factors. Am J Sports Med 28(5 suppl):S58–S68
18. van Dijk CN, Reilingh ML, Zengerink M et al (2010) The natural history of osteochondral lesions in the ankle. Instr Course Lect 59:375–386
19. Koch S, Kampen WU, Laprell H (1997) Cartilage and bone morphology in osteochondritis dissecans. Knee Surg Sports Traumatol Arthrosc 5(1):42–45
20. Johnson DL, Urban WP Jr, Caborn DN et al (1998) Articular cartilage changes seen with magnetic

resonance imaging-detected bone bruises associated with acute anterior cruciate ligament rupture. Am J Sports Med 26(3):409–414
21. Guettler JH, Demetropoulos CK, Yang KH et al (2004) Osteochondral defects in the human knee: influence of defect size on cartilage rim stress and load redistribution to surrounding cartilage. Am J Sports Med 32(6):1451–1458
22. Dheer S, Khan M, Zoga AC et al (2012) Limitations of radiographs in evaluating non-displaced osteochondral lesions of the talus. Skeletal Radiol 4:415–421
23. Navid DO, Myerson MS (2002) Approach alternatives for treatment of osteochondral lesions of the talus. Foot Ankle Clin 7(3):635–649
24. Ferkel RD, Flannigan BD, Elkins BS (1991) Magnetic resonance imaging of the foot and ankle: correlation of normal anatomy with pathologic conditions. Foot Ankle 11:289–305
25. Bae S, Lee HK, Lee K et al (2012) Comparison of arthroscopic and magnetic resonance imaging findings in osteochondral lesions of the talus. Foot Ankle Int 33(12):1058–1062. doi:10.3113/FAI.2012.1058
26. Verhagen RA, Struijs PA, Bossuyt PM et al (2003) Systematic review of treatment strategies for osteochondral defects of the talar dome. Foot Ankle Clin 8(2):233–242, viii-ix
27. Taranow WS, Bisignani GA, Towers JD et al (1999) Retrograde drilling of osteochondral lesions of the medial talar dome. Foot Ankle Int 20:474–480
28. Giannini S, Buda R, Faldini C et al (2005) Surgical treatment of osteochondral lesions of the talus in young active patients. J Bone Joint Surg Am 87(Suppl 2):28–41
29. Badekas T, Takvorian M, Souras N (2013) Treatment principles for osteochondral lesions in foot and ankle. Int Orthop 37(9):1697–1706. doi:10.1007/s00264-013-2076-1
30. Liu W, Liu F, Zhao W et al (2011) Osteochondral autograft transplantation for acute osteochondral fractures associated with an ankle fracture. Foot Ankle Int 32(4):437–442. doi:10.3113/FAI.2011.0437
31. Hangody L (2003) The mosaicplasty technique for osteochondral lesions of the talus. Foot Ankle Clin 8(2):259–273
32. Mei-Dan O, Carmont MR, Laver L et al (2012) Platelet-rich plasma or hyaluronate in the management of osteochondral lesions of the talus. Am J Sports Med 40(3):534–541. doi:10.1177/0363546511431238
33. Giannini S, Vannini F (2004) Operative treatment of osteochondral lesions of the talar dome: current concepts review. Foot Ankle Int 25(3):168–175
34. Ventura A, Terzaghi C, Legnani C et al (2013) Treatment of post-traumatic osteochondral lesions of the talus: a four-step approach. Knee Surg Sports Traumatol Arthrosc 21(6):1245–1250. doi:10.1007/s00167-012-2028-0
35. Yoshimura I, Kanazawa K, Takeyama A et al (2013) Arthroscopic bone marrow stimulation techniques for osteochondral lesions of the talus: prognostic factors for small lesions. Am J Sports Med 41(3):528–534. doi:10.1177/0363546512472979
36. Hangody L, Dobos J, Baló E et al (2010) Clinical experiences with autologous osteochondral mosaicplasty in an athletic population: a 17-year prospective multicenter study. Am J Sports Med 38(6):1125–1133. doi:10.1177/0363546509360405
37. Niemeyer P, Salzmann G, Schmal H et al (2012) Autologous chondrocyte implantation for the treatment of chondral and osteochondral defects of the talus: a meta-analysis of available evidence. Knee Surg Sports Traumatol Arthrosc 20(9):1696–1703. doi:10.1007/s00167-011-1729-0
38. Giannini S, Buda R, Ruffilli A et al (2014) Arthroscopic autologous chondrocyte implantation in the ankle joint. Knee Surg Sports Traumatol Arthrosc 22(6):1311–1319. doi:10.1007/s00167-013-2640-7
39. Battaglia M, Vannini F, Buda R et al (2011) Arthroscopic autologous chondrocyte implantation in osteochondral lesions of the talus: mid-term T2-mapping MRI evaluation. Knee Surg Sports Traumatol Arthrosc 19(8):1376–1384. doi:10.1007/s00167-011-1509-x
40. Giannini S, Buda R, Battaglia M et al (2013) One-step repair in talar osteochondral lesions: 4-year clinical results and t2-mapping capability in outcome prediction. Am J Sports Med 41(3):511–518. doi:10.1177/0363546512467622
41. van Eekeren IC, Reilingh ML, van Dijk CN (2012) Rehabilitation and return-to-sports activity after debridement and bone marrow stimulation of osteochondral talar defects. Sports Med 42(10):857–870. doi:10.2165/11635420-000000000-00000
42. Lee DH, Lee KB, Jung ST (2012) Comparison of early versus delayed weightbearing outcomes after microfracture for small to midsized osteochondral lesions of the talus. Am J Sports Med 40(9):2023–2028. doi:10.1177/0363546512455316
43. Nho SJ, Pensak MJ, Seigerman DA et al (2010) Rehabilitation after autologous chondrocyte implantation in athletes. Clin Sports Med 29(2):267–282. doi:10.1016/j.csm.2009.12.004, viii
44. Giannini S, Buda R, Cavallo M, Ruffilli A, Cenacchi A, Cavallo C, Vannini F (2010) Cartilage repair evolution in post-traumatic osteochondral lesions of the talus: from open field autologous chondrocyte to bone-marrow-derived cells transplantation. Injury 41(11):1196–1203. doi:10.1016/j.injury.2010.09.028, Epub 2010 Oct 8

Ankle Osteoarthritis in Ex-Professional Footballers

34

Vincent Gouttebarge and Gino M.M.J. Kerkhoffs

Osteoarthritis (OA) is the most important reason for pain of the musculoskeletal system and the leading cause of disability in Europe and the United States [7, 8, 14]. OA is a "degenerative joint disease" resulting from the interaction of several factors such as joint integrity, genetics, local inflammation, mechanical forces, and cellular and biochemical processes [7, 8, 14]. Being a normal consequence of aging, OA is caused by overuse of the joint's cartilage and results in irreversible pathologic changes in affected joints [7, 8, 14]. Distinction is made between primary and secondary OA [7, 8, 14]. Primary OA is seen as an idiopathic phenomenon related to the aging process including previously healthy joints and having no apparent cause or initiating factor. Secondary OA is easier to understand and refers to a joint disease resulting from clear predisposing and initiating factors such as obesity, prior traumatic event that causes cartilage damage, and excessive repetitive injury. In contrast to primary OA, secondary OA can occur in relatively young individuals, especially in ex-professional footballers.

V. Gouttebarge (✉)
Department of Orthopaedic Surgery, Academic Medical Center (AMC), Meibergdreef 9, Amsterdam 1105 AZ, The Netherlands

World Players' Union (FIFPro), Hoofddorp, The Netherlands
e-mail: v.gouttebarge@fifpro.org

G.M.M.J. Kerkhoffs
Department of Orthopaedic Surgery, Academic Medical Center (AMC), Meibergdreef 9, Amsterdam 1105 AZ, The Netherlands

34.1 Ankle OA Occurrence in Ex-Professional Footballers

Ankle OA in ex-professional footballers involves a progressive degeneration of articular cartilage characterized by the formation of impinging bone spurs, loose bodies, and joint space narrowing [7, 8, 14]. Because degenerative changes in the joint are not consistently associated with clinical OA, determining the prevalence of ankle OA remains difficult. While epidemiological researches related to hip and knee OA have been largely performed among various study populations among which former elite athletes, studies related to ankle OA are scarce, especially among ex-professional footballers [9].

Nearly 20 years ago, 6 % of ex-professional footballers were found to have been admitted to hospital for OA of the weight-bearing joints of the lower limbs (hip, knee, ankle, foot) [20]. When it comes specifically to ankle joint, recent epidemiological evidence about the occurrence of ankle OA among ex-professional footballers remains scarce as acknowledged recently in a systematic literature review [19]. Only two empirical studies were retrieved from the recent scientific literature in which the prevalence of ankle OA was presented. Among 185 retired

P. Volpi (ed.), *Football Traumatology: New Trends*, DOI 10.1007/978-3-319-18245-2_34

English professional footballers who had played professional football on average for nearly 14 years, the prevalence of ankle OA (diagnosed by clinician) was found to be 5.7 % in the right ankle and 6.3 % in the left ankle [19]. In this study, the mean age at diagnosis was 29.5 years for the right ankle and 31.6 years for the left ankle. A second study explored 284 ex-professional footballers from the United Kingdom who had played professional football on average for nearly 13.5 years. Forty-nine percent of these ex-professional footballers indicated that they had been diagnosed (by clinician) at an average age of 40 years with OA on at least one anatomical site, 29 % in two or more joints, and 15 % in three or more joints [19]. Especially, the ankle joints accounted for 17 % of all 314 OA diagnoses among these 284 ex-professional footballers, whereof 11 % in the right ankle and 6 % in the left ankle [19]. A latest published study by Armenis et al. [3] explored the prevalence of ankle/foot OA in a group of 105 retired Greek professional footballers (older than 40 years) who had played professional football for 8–10 years. Clinical signs of OA were found in 4.1 % of these ex-professional footballers, while radiographic OA was found in nearly 9 %.

Whether the occurrence of ankle OA in ex-professional footballers is alarming can be put into perspective when compared to former athletes from other sport disciplines and to the general population (Table 34.1). However, epidemiological evidence about the occurrence of ankle OA among former elite athletes from other sport disciplines is scarce as acknowledged recently in a systematic literature review [9]. Among 40 former elite high jumpers, prevalence of OA was found to be 2.5 % in the right ankle as well as in the left ankle [9]. An older study from Kujala et al. [20] acknowledged that the prevalence of ankle OA ranged from 0 % to 1.8 % in former elite athletes that were involved during their career in different sport disciplines (long-distance running, cross-country skiing, ice hockey, boxing, and weight lifting). Worldwide, approximately 1–4 % of the adult general population has OA of the ankle. Then, despite the limited information available from the scientific literature, it is clear that the prevalence of ankle OA in ex-professional footballers is higher than in former athletes from other sport disciplines and the general population.

Table 34.1 Prevalence of ankle osteoarthritis: overview among ex-professional footballers, former elite athletes from other sport disciplines, and the general population

Sports	Prevalence (%)
Football	9–17
Athletics	0.2
Basketball	0
Boxing	0.4
Cross-country skiing	0
High Jump	2.5
Ice hockey	1.8
Long-distance running	0
Volleyball	0
Weight lifting	0.9
General population	1–4

34.2 Etiology

Age, gender, obesity, lifestyle, joint injury, and abnormal biochemical load on joints during occupational (squatting, kneeling, lifting) and sport activities have been acknowledged as risk factors for developing OA [14, 24]. Within professional football, it remains unknown whether the cumulative exposure to intense and prolonged physical demands (running, sprinting, jumping and landing, dribbling and passing, duel forms with opponents) during both training and competition contributes solely on the long-term to the high prevalence of ankle OA among retired professional footballers. Despite the lack of empirical studies involving large sample sizes and suitable controls matched for football exposure, ankle OA in ex-professional footballers seems principally attributed to the occurrence and recurrence of ankle injury during a football career.

As in many sport disciplines, the ankle joint is after the hamstring, the most common injury localization in (professional) football. Ankle ligament (medial and lateral bands) and cartilage injuries are common during training and competition, accounting approximately for 20–30 % of all injuries [2, 6, 10]. While mild acute ankle sprains do not impair recovery and return to sport on short notice, recurrent or severe ankle injuries might have more drastic consequences during a football career in terms of related surgery, rehabilitation, and long-term disability. In addition, causing persistent symptoms for months or even years that might even lead to early retirement, i.e., end of professional career, these recurrent or severe ankle injuries, in combination with their surgical treatment, are seen as risk factors for ankle OA in ex-professional footballers.

Recent empirical studies in which the association between previous injury and ankle OA was investigated among retired professional football players (both in study and control groups) are lacking. However, older studies or studies performed among elite athletes from other sports disciplines indicate that the occurrence of ankle injuries is a relevant determinant for ankle OA. Larsen et al. [21] examined the incidence of ankle OA in injured and uninjured elite football players, with a mean time from injury of 25 years. OA was present in 33 % of the injured ankles, whereas the incidence of OA in uninjured players was 18 % in the ankle. On a series of more than 300 ankle fractures treated with open reduction and internal fixation, Lindsjö [22] found that the prevalence of post-traumatic OA was 14 %, which was directly correlated with the fracture pattern. Reviewing retrospectively data from 30 patients (mean age 59 years, 33 ankles) with ankle OA, Valderrabano et al. [36] found that 55 % had a history of sports injuries (33 % from soccer) and 85 % had a lateral ankle ligament injury. Even more, the same author [37] found in a study of 406 ankles with end-stage OA that the underlying etiology in this group was post-traumatic ankle OA in 78 % of cases. Within these post-traumatic OA cases, 62 % were attributable to fracture events (malleolar fractures and tibial plafond fractures) and 16 % to ligamentous injuries. Some studies indicate that severity of the initial injury and initial cartilage damage may play a role in the development of ankle OA.

In summary, the high prevalence of ankle OA among ex-professional footballers is predominantly of post-traumatic origin, being associated with the occurrence and recurrence of ankle injury and related surgery during a football career. Even if empirical evidence is lacking, the cumulative exposure to intense and prolonged physical demands (running, sprinting, jumping and landing, dribbling and passing, duel forms with opponents) during both training and competition might also contribute on the long-term to the high prevalence of ankle OA among ex-professional footballers.

34.3 Diagnostic: Clinical and Radiographic Examination

34.3.1 Clinical Examination

In order to determine the presence of ankle OA, a good anamnesis and careful physical examination are essential. During the anamnesis, the physician strives to retrieve important information related to ankle symptoms, exploring several aspects such as:

- Duration of the symptoms
- Joint stiffness in the morning
- Past (recurrent) trauma, sprain, surgery
- Contribution of sport activities to the symptoms
- Contribution of occupational activities to the symptoms
- Contribution of daily living activities to the symptoms
- Family history
- Any general symptoms (fatigue, weight loss, fever, etc.) affecting the whole body

During the physical examination, the physician evaluates several aspects of the ankle(s) such as:

- Presence of swelling, warmth, abnormal skin, and soft tissues
- Presence of tender areas, synovitis, effusion, bony knobs, and loose bodies
- Ankles pattern (if only one affected)

- Ankle instability (anterior draw and talar tilt test)
- Ankle impingement (Molloy impingement test)
- Remaining movement in the subtalar and midtarsal joints
- Range of motion
- Signs of muscle weakness or atrophy
- Signs of unequal leg lengths
- Alignment of the tibia to the hind foot, the midfoot, and the forefoot
- Other joints and limb alignment
- Gait

34.3.2 Radiographic Examination

While the presence of OA is often suggested by anamnesis and physical examination, ankle OA diagnosis is usually confirmed by routine radiographic evaluation. In addition, radiological diagnostic assesses OA severity and serves as an initial evaluation to monitor the worsening of the disease.

A routine radiographic evaluation of the ankle consisting of a weight-bearing AP view, a mortise view, and a lateral view is made in order to identify radiologic signs of OA, including asymmetrical narrowing of the joint space (indicating loss of cartilage), development of osteophytes, and subchondral sclerosis (Fig. 34.1). On a true AP view, the talus overlaps a portion of the lateral malleolus, obscuring the lateral aspect of the ankle joint. The mortise view is obtained with the foot in 15–20° endorotation, making visualization of both the lateral and medial joint spaces possible. An additional hind foot alignment radiograph can be considered in situations where the ankle has coronal plane tilting and the heel is in varus or valgus position.

The Kellgren and Lawrence (K&L) criteria have been widely used to grade OA and were chosen as reference by the World Health Organizations to characterize OA in the hip and knee joints [15]. By now, the K&L criteria have been also validated for the ankle joints [13], consisting in the assessment of three radiological ankle features (osteophyte formation, joint space narrowing, and bone end sclerosis). According to the K&L criteria, ankle OA can be classified as follows:

- Grade 0: Normal joint
- Grade 1: Unlikely or doubtful narrowing of joint space and possible osteophytes
- Grade 2: Definite osteophytes and possible narrowing of joint space
- Grade 3: Multiple moderately sized osteophytes, definite narrowing of joint space, some sclerotic areas, and possible deformation of bone contour
- Grade 4: Large osteophytes, marked narrowing of joint space, severe sclerosis, and defined deformation of bone contour

It is worth noticing that the radiological diagnosis of ankle OA has some limitations. First, the evaluation of the thickness of ankle articular cartilage is difficult, second, the correlation between radiological findings and symptoms is poor, and third, the lack of radiological sign does not rule out the presence of OA. Consequently, attempting to diagnose ankle OA exclusively by radiographic evaluation is limited and should be therefore combined with anamnesis and physical examination, exploring thoroughly the functional consequences of the joint disease.

34.4 Functional Consequences of Ankle OA in Ex-Professional Footballers

Being primarily associated with previous traumatic injuries, ankle OA is a frequent health concern among ex-professional footballers, condition that might even appear in the early years after the end of a football career. The adverse impacts of ankle OA on the quality of life and functioning (work and daily living) of ex-professional footballers cannot be neglected, even if empirical evidence about the long-term consequences of this health condition is limited.

In a recent systematic review [11], only two original studies exploring the consequences of ankle OA in ex-professional footballers were

Fig. 34.1 Radiographs of a healthy ankle joint and an ankle joint affected by OA

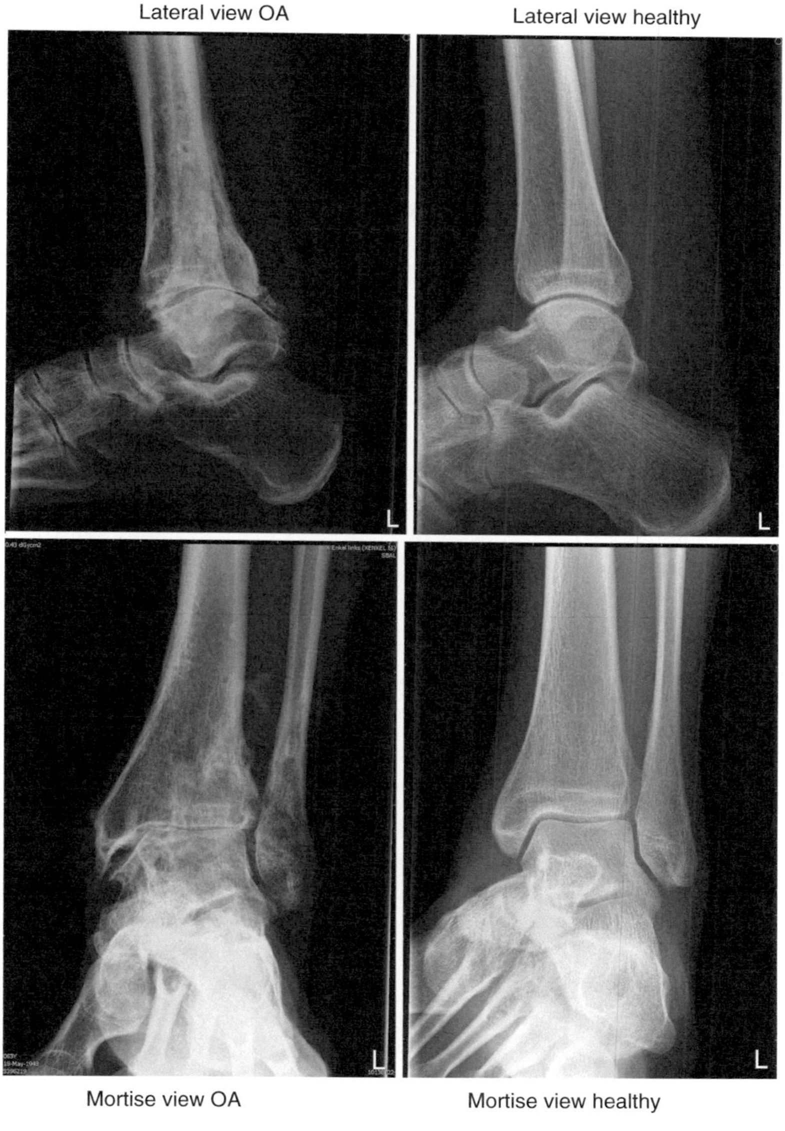

identified. A cross-sectional survey was conducted in the United Kingdom (UK) among 284 retired professional footballers who had played professional football on average for nearly 14 years. One hundred and thirty eight of these ex-professional footballers suffered from OA in a lower limb joint (hip, knee, ankle, and/or foot), from which 33 from OA in the right ankle and 20 from OA in the left ankle. From the retired professional footballers suffering from OA (not solely of the ankle), nearly 90 % reported to have moderate or severe joint pain and discomfort, while around 65 % indicated to experience moderate or severe problems with mobility and performing usual activities (work, study, house, etc.). In addition, 37 % of them reported moderate or severe problems with anxiety/depression because of their medical condition. Based on this study, the authors conducted 2 years later a qualitative study by interviewing 12 ex-professional footballers who were suffering from hip, knee, and/or ankle OA. With regard to pain, some retired players reported that their conditions were chronically very painful and that the pain was significantly affecting their lives. With regard to restricted mobility and movement, some ex-professional footballers reported that the lack of mobility was a major issue in their lives, moving being hardly possible, especially bending, kneeling, and long standing. With regard to employment, some ex-professional footballers reported that no employer wanted to employ them with their conditions and that they abandoned their jobs for this reason.

In summary, despite the limited evidence in the scientific literature, ex-professional footballers with ankle OA seem to suffer from joint pain and discomfort during several activities, reporting that their health condition affects both their daily lives and their work functioning. These findings are not surprising given that OA is the most important cause of pain of the musculoskeletal system and leading cause of disability worldwide.

34.5 Treatment and Management Strategies

The treatment and management of ankle OA involves a multidisciplinary approach striving to relieve symptoms and improve joint function [17, 18, 26, 30, 31, 33]. Therefore, it might rely on strategies related to conservative treatment, surgical treatment, and self-management. With regard to safety, invasiveness, and costs, conservative treatment should be preferred, and surgical treatment should be reserved to the patients who do not improve with conservative treatment and who have seriously affected quality of life.

34.5.1 Conservative Strategies

Aiming to relieve and control the pain associated with ankle OA and improve the function of the joint, conservative treatment relies on the following strategies [17, 23, 25, 27, 30, 31]:

- Medications, especially the short-term use (because of side effects) of nonsteroidal anti-inflammatory drugs (NSAIDs) to relieve and control ankle pain
- Dietary supplements, especially glucosamine and chondroitin as safe and effective option for the management of ankle OA symptoms
- Judiciously timed intra-articular injection of corticosteroids into the ankle joint to decrease inflammation and pain for the enjoyment of a particularly important life event
- Modified footwear (rocker-bottom sole, solid ankle cushion heel, polypropylene ankle-foot orthosis, lace-up ankle support, ankle brace)
- Physical therapy to preserve range of motion
- Specific exercises to increase muscle and neuromuscular, i.e., proprioceptive, functions in order to enhance ankle functions and stability
- Healthy lifestyle, especially related to weight control through general physical, i.e., fitness programs

It has been shown that the application of the aforementioned single approaches in isolation has negligible effects and should be consequently combined in order to reach an optimal effect [4, 16].

34.5.2 Surgical Treatment

The decision for surgical treatment of ankle OA requires a grounded evaluation of the patient's functional needs and problems. As surgical techniques continuously change and evidence for effectiveness accumulates, the indications for surgery treatment of ankle OA have been evolving in time. For ankle OA, surgery is seen as a treatment option when conservative and nonsurgical strategies have failed to control the patient's symptoms in such a way that the patient's quality of life and daily living or work activities are seriously affected. Surgical options (see previous chapters for details of technique procedures) for ankle OA include joint-preserving surgery, arthrodesis, and (total) ankle replacement [18, 26, 29, 32, 34, 35].

Joint-preserving surgery, including arthroscopic débridement and articular distraction, aims to delay more invasive and extensive surgery. Being commonly achieved through arthroscopy, ankle débridement is performed in case of impinging osteophytes, loose bodies, and chondral defects. For severe end-stage of OA, articular distraction based on an external articulated fixation frame and a distraction force applied across the ankle has been recently advocated for patients being candidate for arthrodesis in order to decrease joint pain and improve movements.

Ankle arthrodesis has been seen for several decades as the gold standard treatment of end-stage ankle OA. Ankle arthrodesis can be done with numerous techniques and approaches. Several methods of stabilization can be used such as external fixation, internal fixation with screws, plates, and onlay or dowel bone grafts, and cast fixation alone. Despite several limitations such as a disturbed gait pattern and reduced functionality after ankle fusion, most patients are satisfied with ankle arthrodesis. However, it remains unclear to which extent ankle arthrodesis contributes to progressive degeneration of adjacent joints.

34.5.3 Self-Management Strategy

For chronic health conditions such as rheumatic diseases (including OA), self-management strategies have been identified as effective in order to engage and promote a healthful and active behavior of patients in managing their disease [5, 28]. For ankle OA, analogously to other joints, self-management interventions covering aspects such as self-awareness (information provision and patient education) and cognitive and behavioral therapy might be helpful to manage the disease, prevent its worsening, and improve both social and self-care capabilities [4]. However, self-management interventions being specifically developed for ex-professional footballers are lacking, which appear to be peculiar.

Professional footballers are workers in the eyes of the law and should be seen as any other employees from any occupational sectors. Consequently, as stated by the World Health Organization (WHO) and the International Labour Organization (ILO), professional football clubs and responsible (inter)national bodies should be aware that they are responsible for "the protection, promotion, surveillance and maintenance of the highest degree of physical, mental and social well-being of players during their career but also long after their retirement years." Being applicable to any workers and thus to professional footballers, such a statement puts the physical, mental, and social well-being of any player in a life span perspective, which is in line with the view and needs toward improvement in medical care and support previously expressed by the most important stakeholders in this occupational category, namely, the professional footballers [1, 12]. The specific development of self-management interventions for ex-professional footballers seems relevant, especially with regard to ankle OA because it may impair their sustainable health and functioning in their post-sport life.

References

1. Akturk A, Inklaar H, Gouttebarge V et al (2014) Medical examination in Dutch professional football (soccer): a qualitative study. Int Sports Med J 15(4): 343–351
2. Aoki H, O'Hata N, Kohno T et al (2012) A 15-year prospective epidemiological account of acute traumatic injuries during official professional soccer league matches in Japan. Am J Sports Med 40: 1006–1014
3. Armenis E, Pefanis N, Tsiganos G et al (2011) Osteoarthritis of the ankle and foot complex in former Greek soccer players. Foot Ankle Spec 4:338–343
4. Bennell K, Hunter DJ, Vicenzino B (2012) Long-term effects of sport: preventing and managing OA in athletes. Nat Rev Rheumatol 8:747–752
5. Coleman S, Briffa NK, Carroll G et al (2012) A randomised controlled trial of a self-management education program for osteoarthritis of the knee delivered by health care professionals. Arthritis Res Ther 14:R21
6. Eirale C, Faroop A, Smiley FA et al (2012) Epidemiology of football injuries in Asia: a prospective study in Qatar. J Sci Med Sport 16:113–117
7. Felson DT (2004) An update on the pathogenesis and epidemiology of osteoarthritis. Radiol Clin North Am 42:1–9
8. Garstang SV, Stitik TP (2006) Osteoarthritis: epidemiology, risk factors, and pathophysiology. Am J Phys Med Rehabil 85:S2–S11
9. Gouttebarge V, Inklaar H, Backx F et al (2014) Prevalence of osteoarthritis in former elite athletes: a systematic overview of the recent literature. Rheumatol Int 35:405–418
10. Gouttebarge V, Hughes Schwab BA, Vivian A et al (2015) Injuries, match missed and effect of Minimum

Medical Standards in the A-LEAGUE professional football: a 5-year prospective study. Asian J Sports Med 6(2). In press
11. Gouttebarge V, Inklaar H, Frings-Dresen MHW (2014) Risk and consequences of osteoarthritis after a professional football career: a systematic review of the recent literature. J Sports Med Phys Fitness 54:494–504
12. Gouttebarge V, Aoki H (2014) Life span perspective of professional footballers' health. Asian J Sports Med 5:e23813
13. Holzer N, Salvo D, Marijnissen AK et al (2012) How to assess ankle osteoarthritis: comparison of the Kellgren and Lawrence scale with functional outcome and digital image analysis. J Bone Surg Br 94-B:Supp XXXVII
14. Hunter DJ, McDougall JJ, Keefe FJ (2008) The symptoms of OA and the genesis of pain. Rheum Dis Clin North Am 34:623–643
15. Kellgren JH, Lawrence JS (1957) Radiological assessment of osteo-arthrosis. Ann Rheum Dis 16:494–502
16. Kirkendall DT, Garrett WE (2012) Management of the retired athlete with osteoarthritis of the knee. Cartilage 3:69S–76S
17. Koh J, Dietz J (2005) Osteoarthritis in other joints (hip, elbow, foot, ankle, toes, wrist) after sports injuries. Clin Sports Med 24:57–70
18. Koopman WJ, Moreland LW (eds) (2004) Arthritis and allied conditions: a textbook of rheumatology. Lippincott Williams & Wilkins, Philadelphia
19. Kuijt M-TK, Inklaar H, Gouttebarge V et al (2012) Knee and ankle osteoarthritis in former elite soccer players: a systematic review. J Sci Med Sports 15:480–487
20. Kujala UM, Kaprio J, Sarna S (1994) Osteoarthritis of weight bearing joints of lower limbs in former elite male athletes. BMJ 308:231–234
21. Larsen E, Jensen PK, Jensen PR (1999) Long-term outcome of knee and ankle injuries in elite football. Scand J Med Sci Sports 9:285–289
22. Lindsjö U (1985) Operative treatment of ankle fracture-dislocations. A follow-up study of 306/321 consecutive cases. Clin Orthop Relat Res 199:28–38
23. McAlindon TE, LaValley MP, Gulin JP et al (2000) Glucosamine and chondroitin for treatment of osteoarthritis: a systematic quality assessment and meta-analysis. JAMA 283:1469–1475
24. McWilliams DF, Leeb BF, Muthuri SG, Doherti M, Zhang W (2011) Occupational risk factors for osteoarthritis: a meta-analysis. Osteoarthr Cartil 19:829–839
25. Migliore A, Giovannangeli F, Bizzi E et al (2011) Viscosupplementation in the management of ankle osteoarthritis: a review. Arch Orthop Trauma Surg 131:139–147
26. Moskowitz RW, Altman RD, Hochberg MC et al (eds) (2007) Osteoarthritis. Wolters Kluwer/Lippincott Williams & Wilkins, Philadelphia
27. Nakasone Y, Watabe K, Watanabe K et al (2011) Effect of a glucosamine-based combination supplement containing chondroitin sulfate and antioxidant micronutrients in subjects with symptomatic knee osteoarthritis: a pilot study. Exp Ther Med 2:893–899
28. Nolte S, Osborne RH (2012) A systematic review of outcomes of chronic disease self-management interventions. Qual Life Res 22:1817
29. Pagenstert G, Leumann A, Hintermann B et al (2008) Sports and recreation activity of varus and valgus ankle osteoarthritis before and after realignment surgery. Foot Ankle Int 29:985–993
30. Rao S, Ellis SJ, Deland JT et al (2010) Nonmedical therapy in the management of ankle osteoarthritis. Cur Opinion Rheumatology 22:223–228
31. Roos EM, Juhl CB (2012) Osteoarthritis 2012 year in review: rehabilitation and outcomes. Osteoarthritis Cartilage 20:1477–1483
32. Saltzman CL, Hillis SL, Stolley MP et al (2012) Motion versus fixed distraction of the joint in the treatment of ankle osteoarthritis. J Bone Joint Surg Am 94:961–970
33. Semanik PA, Chang RW, Dunlop DD (2012) Aerobic activity in prevention and symptom control of osteoarthritis. PM R 4:S37–S44
34. Sinusas K (2012) Osteoarthritis: diagnosis and treatment. Am Fam Phys 85:49–56
35. Thomas RH, Daniels TR (2003) Ankle arthritis. J Bone Joint Surg 85:923–936
36. Valderrabano V, Hintermann B, Horisberger M et al (2006) Ligamentous posttraumatic ankle osteoarthritis. Am J Sports Med 34:612–620
37. Valderrabano V, HorisbergerM RI et al (2009) Etiology of ankle osteoarthritis. Clin Orthop Relat Res 467:1800–1806

35 Foot Problems in Football

Pieter PRN d'Hooghe

35.1 Introduction

A higher proportion of foot injuries in football occur as a result of foul play and involved direct contact with the injured foot. The majority of foot injuries are caused by tackles from the side involving lateral or medial forces on the foot that create a corresponding inversion or eversion of this foot. The weight-bearing status of the injured foot is a significant risk factor. Although the severity of injury to the weight-bearing footballer's foot is generally higher than that observed for the non-weight-bearing foot, referees are no more likely to rule that these tackles represent foul play [1–3].

The footballer's foot has already some troubles when considering the ground on which the game is performed: grass. The foot has to undergo atmospheric constraints and adapt to smooth, hard, dry, (un)stable or synthetic terrain [4–7]. The specific entities of the football shoe also need to be modified in this regard. Although the classic foot lesions that are encountered in football are mainly linked with trauma, shoes (untapped at the tibiotarsal level), the ambient environment and the relative hygiene of some players can be as important determinants for problems also [8].

P. PRN. d'Hooghe, MD, MSc
Department of Orthopaedic Surgery,
Aspetar Orthopaedic and Sports Medicine Hospital,
Aspire Zone, Sportscity Street, 29222, Doha, Qatar
e-mail: pieter.dhooghe@aspetar.com

35.2 The Football Shoe

The kick and the ballistic conduct of the ball require a great freedom of the tibiocrural joint and a great stability in the subtalar and midfoot joints.

Thus, the modern shoe is low necked and the hind foot stabilisers stop at the crop of the malleolar edges. The shoe will 'expose' further the ligaments in contrast with higher models from the past that protected ligaments and tendons more but also significantly restricted the foot/ankle mobility.

This explains the facilitation of abnormal movements (hammer/anvil) causing degenerative ankle lesions, painful kicking wounds and contusions of the periosteum that require significant healing time. The leather used in the modern football shoe is light, smooth and soft and aims to create a natural 'skin feeling'. The disadvantage is that it facilitates direct shocks of the inlay soles onto the foot and microtrauma on the (dorsal) foot area.

Also, the Chopart joint area and its surrounding ligaments of the foot are well known to suffer from this repetitive kicking in football [6].

The tip end of the shoe has become smooth, the kick and its effects have improved, the players 'feel' the ball more natural than before with more beautiful goals scored, but the foot has to pay the prize: subungual hematomas, overuse syndromes, early joint degeneration, avulsions, stress fractures, big toe hallux rigidus etc.

P. Volpi (ed.), *Football Traumatology: New Trends*, DOI 10.1007/978-3-319-18245-2_35

35.3 The Inlay Soles

Football is one of the most popular sports and one in which the feet are most exposed to injury. Statistics show that between 2 and 9.4 players per 1,000 h of exposure suffer injury to their feet. Of these injuries, we most commonly find sprains, fractures and torn ligaments as well as various blows and bruises. The type of foot is considered to be an intrinsic factor when taking injury into consideration, while at the same time the football shoe is considered an extrinsic factor.

The inlay sole or foot orthosis (FO) has been used for many years as a tool for health professionals in the treatment and prevention of injury to the feet and lower limbs among football players. The principal objectives are improvement in sports performance, optimization of biomechanics and reduction of pain.

The evolution of the materials used in FO – and at the same time the making of the moulds and the techniques employed in their manufacturing – has evolved at a rapid pace over the last few years. It's not so long ago that metal inlays were beaten into shape with a hammer. Compare that to the carbon fibre ones (or the composites formed under high temperatures) we have nowadays, and you will know what an evolution football inlay soles have gone through over the last decennia.

The advances in technology and the materials used in the fabrication have enabled more and better results, thanks to the wide range of options now available. Furthermore, weight and size are now no longer a problem for the adaptation of the football shoe.

The importance of the foot in the mechanics of the lower extremities is an undeniable reality, and custom-made FOs are possibly the best option for the treatment and prevention of injuries, through the optimization of the biomechanics of the Football player

The manufacturing of Foot Orthoses (FOs) has been susceptive to major changes in the last decennium with the emergence of 3D scanners and software designs. They offer a variety of options to improve the design of corrective or accommodative orthotic insoles. Particularly the latest generation of customised FOs is widely recognised and is used in elite football. Digitalization facilitates further the FO design and manufacturing processes. It also offers a reliable, precise and comfortable FO to the player, compared to the thermo-formed moulded techniques. Nowadays, FO materials are used with special mechanical properties that offer the player flexible, lightweight and comfortable FOs. The challenge remains to reduce the FO thickness even more in the future, occupying minimal space in the football shoe (enabling the player to maintain a natural feeling) without compromising the FO's therapeutic goals [9].

35.4 The Studs

The height and the positioning of the studs change according to the terrain and play an important role in injury prevention of the foot. A continuous referee control of the cylindrical studs is mandatory since aggressive cone-shaped or point-shaped studs can cause potential injury during gameplay.

Bad stud positioning can create disastrous torsion forces to the balance of the foot and subsequently cause injury to the lower limb and its ligaments.

We all know the mechanism of a locked foot onto the ground with a combined knee rotation, resulting in severe ligament and meniscal damage to the knee.

Studs that are too high and too few have shown to be most harmful for the footballer's foot. The positioning of the studs is considered in relation with the major zone of support to the foot, and the positioning of the studs can compensate in the absence of rigid shoe inlays.

When we study a modern footballer's shoe, tailored with six studs, they serve in pairs: two anterior, two middle and two posterior ones.

The anteromedial stud is situated below the interphalangeal joint of the big toe and the anterolateral in the pulp of the third toe without overhang. Together they serve to snatch the foot with the ground in order to optimise the initiation of a spurt.

The two middle studs toggle the roll of the foot and its course over the ground. They also play a role as brakes in a sudden stop during a moderate run. The middle medial stud is positioned slightly behind the sesamoids and the mediolateral under the fifth metatarsal head.

The two posterior studs serve as standoffs and further as stabilisers when landing and sudden brutal deceleration.

Off course, a prefabricated shoe cannot accommodate to the individual foot deformations: hallux valgus, metatarsus varus or accessorius, etc. Eventually, contact bursitis problems of the feet can occur.

Hammertoes or too long toes can create horns and hyperkeratosis. Too high and too widely positioned posterior studs will favour heel problems on hard surfaces. Still it's advised to slightly elevate the posterior studs compared to the anterior and middle pairs in order to relieve the Achilles tendon.

Furthermore, rigid hind foot shoe support can trigger annoying retrocalcaneal bursitis. Painful plantar callus formation can be set off under the big toe by a too externally located stud or also frequently due to wear over the shoe at the area of the base of the middle medial stud.

The first conclusion is evidently that every elite football player needs a tailored shoe with the possibility of half sizes. The second conclusion is that we need to mitigate the inconveniences that present with the use of new shoes.

Deformations due to frequent usage can be prevented by humid brushing and regular lubrication of the shoe. Rational maintenance guidelines can alter these deformations with simple measures. Finally, the interior of the shoe is controlled over the major support points, especially the base area of the studs (mousse lamellae).

The author found it always interesting to talk with veteran players about their tips and tricks. Although science has helped us hugely the last decade in order to optimise the footballer's shoe, some tricks remain helpful over time:

- Quintus varus: Strapping
- Skin horns: Circular soft washers
- Partridge eye prevention: 'Cigarette paper' between the toes
- Hallux valgus: Interphalangeal orthosis
- Skin crease and compression prevention: Careful foot positioning during strapping
- According to some experts, a double pair of dry and slightly tight football socks (one in cotton, one in wool) can improve the sliding problems in the shoe significantly.

35.5 The Footballer's Foot and Static Problems

Hollow feet frequently create certain conflicts in the footballer's shoe and relate to the occurrence of painful lower limbs, the so-called shin splints.

They even disturb the chain balances of the mechanical lower limb axis from the knee over the pelvis towards the spine.

The nature of the footballer's shoe condemns all voluminous orthosis. Therefore, the inlays need to be light, flexible and precise. To individualise the necessary adaptations to the inlays, we use collars, bowls, 'pelottes', pronators, supinators and (un)winged retro-capital bars [10].

35.6 Dermatological and Cutaneous Lesions

Precocious disinfecting strategies can prevent chronic foot problems in football through simple protocols.

In order to avoid lymphangitis, adenitis and cellulitis problems, it's important that young football players get acquainted with the habit to show all hematomas, wounds and blisters over the foot to the club's physiotherapist or medical doctor immediately after every match or training (Figs. 35.1 and 35.2).

Frequently encountered football-related foot problems that require specific medical (dermatological) care are:

- Bulbs and blisters
- Ingrown toenail
- Subungual hematoma
- Plantar warts
- Hyperhidrosis

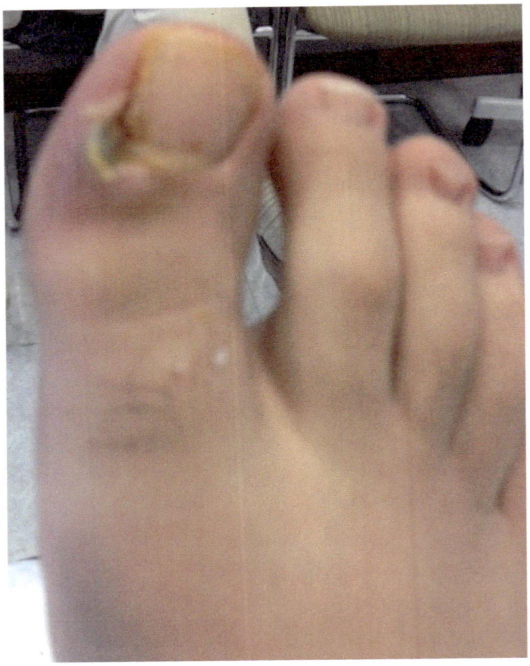

Fig. 35.1 Image of a chronic ingrown toenail in a football player with progressive infectious evolution

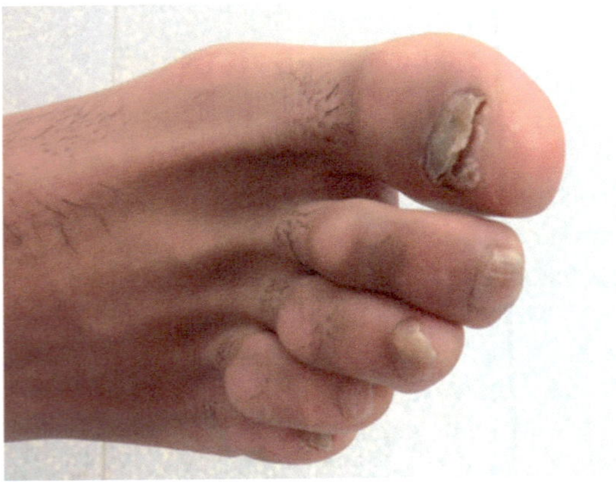

Fig. 35.2 Image of football-related chronic toe onychomycosis

35.7 Common Traumatic Foot Injuries in Football

35.7.1 Turf Toe (First Ray Metatarsophalangeal Sprain)

- Aetiology: Injuries to the first metatarsophalangeal joint are commonly encountered in football players who participate on hard surfaces while wearing flexible shoes. Recent data suggest that turf toe injuries occur more commonly in football players with an associated decreased MTP motion and an increased hallucal peak pressure.
- Injury mechanism: Forced hyperextension of the first metatarsophalangeal joint tears the plantar portion of the capsuloligamentous complex at its origin from the metatarsal head and neck (Fig. 35.3).
- Clinical and diagnostic examination: A turf toe is a debilitating football injury because the hallux is pivotal to a football player's ability to accelerate and cut. Immediately after trauma, the initial swelling and pain can be minor, but it then worsens over the next 24 h. In addition to the soft tissue injury, there can be a combined presentation of metatarsal head

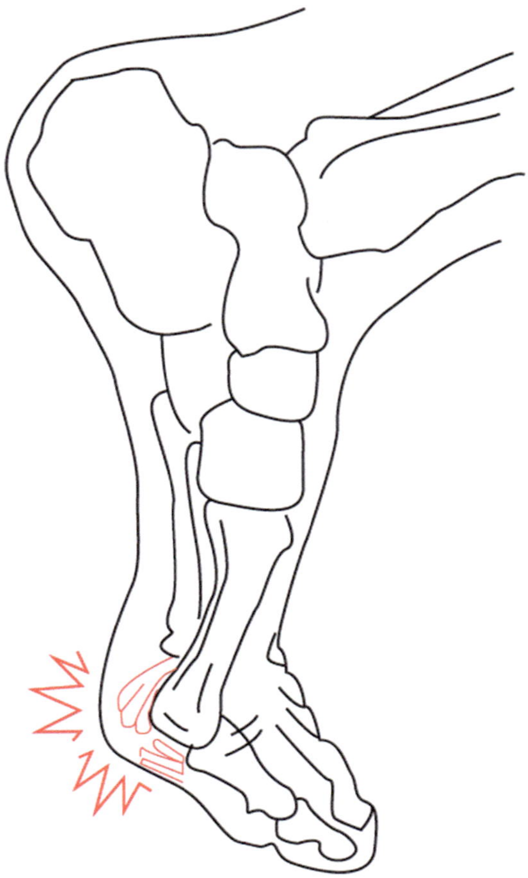

Fig. 35.3 Digital image of a turf toe injury mechanism

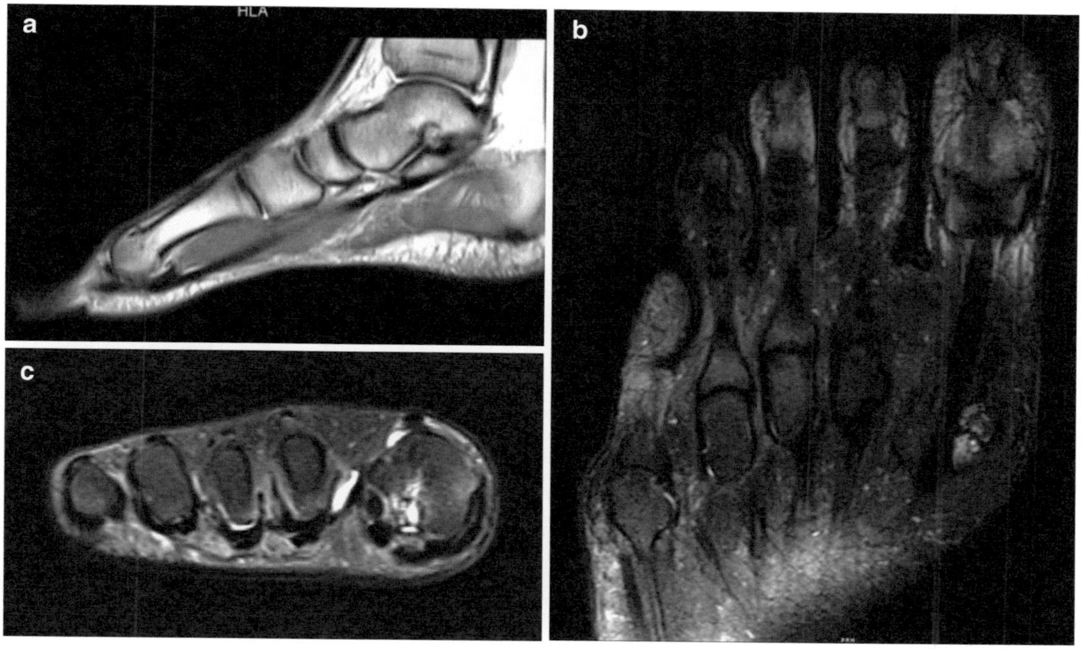

Fig. 35.4 (a) Sagittal T1 MRI image of a retractile plantar plate hallux injury. (b) Axial T2 MRI image of a medial sesamoid fracture. (c) Coronal T2 MRI image of a sesamoid bursitis

impaction, fractured or unstable bipartite sesamoid (Fig. 35.4a–c).

– Treatment strategy: Most turf toes can be treated nonoperatively. A tailored football shoe and an individualised inlay sole – which limits the hyperextension of the first metatarsophalangeal joint – can give adequate support to the soft tissue injury. Nevertheless, it's advised to tape the toe for football training and gameplay. Severe injuries can require temporary restriction from football and can require the need of protected weight-bearing with crutches for several days. Only in case of irreducible dislocation or full rupture of the plantar plate (with sesamoid retraction), a surgical intervention can be indicated. These injuries warrant appropriate acute and long-term management to prevent long-term dysfunction [11–17].

35.7.2 Metatarsal Fractures/Tarsometatarsal Dislocations

– Injury mechanism: A direct blow or twisting injury with severe foot pain, immediate impossible weight-bearing and the need to be removed from play is classic presentations of a metatarsal fracture during fieldside assessment.
– Clinical and diagnostic examination: The foot can rapidly swell up to twice its normal size; there's a localised or global tenderness over the injured areas (in case of additional midfoot/Lisfranc/forefoot injury). A classic X-ray can usually reveal the specific diagnosis.
– Treatment strategy: A classic stable metatarsal shaft fracture can be treated with a partial weight-bearing boot or a stiff-soled shoe and crutches. In case of a Jones fracture, it's advised to consult your orthopaedic surgeon since transverse fractures of the shaft of the fifth metatarsal need individualised treatment, especially in elite football players (Fig. 35.5a–d). The treatment should be based upon the player's needs, and early internal fixation is shown to be frequently indicated in this regard, since it provides stability for reliable healing, allows accelerated rehabilitation and thus decreases the time lost from football (Fig. 35.5e).

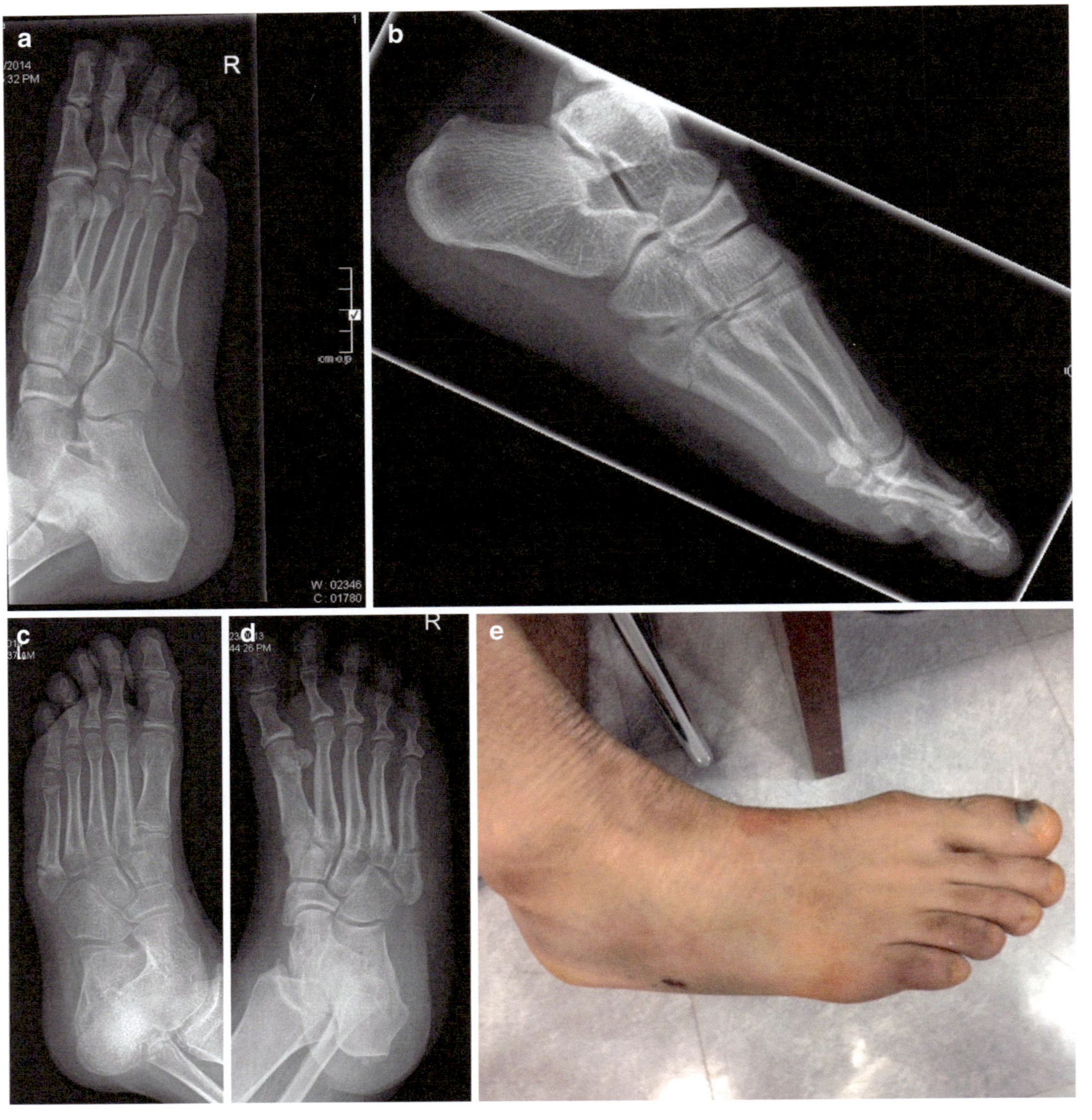

Fig. 35.5 (**a**) Oblique X-ray image of a proximal MT5 fracture.(**b**) Lateral X-ray image of a proximal MT5 fracture. (**c**) Oblique X-ray image of another proximal MT5 fracture presentation. (**d**) Oblique X-ray image of another proximal MT5 fracture type presentation. (**e**) Postoperative image of the minimal invasive character of a surgical percutaneous MT5 fracture fixation

Tuberosity fractures of the fifth metatarsal are treated with a boot until the player is asymptomatic, and supportive taping/cuboid pad can be used to relieve the pressure from the fracture site.

Intra-articular fractures (with a displacement of 2 mm or more), unstable spiral fracture, Lisfranc fracture/dislocation and presentation of two or more metatarsal fractures in the foot are usually treated with open reduction and internal surgical fixation.

– Rehabilitation and return to play: Rehabilitation can start upon sufficient fracture healing. Progressive weight-bearing activities can be initiated within pain limits. Particularly important exercises are plantar fascia stretching and the strengthening of the intrinsic foot musculature. Full participation towards football is usually allowed when the fracture healing is complete and the strength and flexibility have returned to approximately 90–95 % of the opposite, uninjured foot [17–19].

35.7.3 Midfoot Sprains (Lisfranc Injuries)

– Aetiology: The Lisfranc joint is a complex skeletal and capsuloligamentous structure that provides significant stability while maintaining the transverse arch of the foot. Football players suffer a much higher rate of midfoot sprains, compared to the general population. They are the second most commonly documented foot injury in football after injury to the metatarsophalangeal joint and occur in 4 % of football players per year.
– Injury mechanism: In contrast with the high-velocity roadside Lisfranc injuries, football-related midfoot sprains occur by means of an indirect low-velocity force. Most football players describe an axial longitudinal force sustained while the foot was plantarflexed and slightly rotated.
– Diagnostic examination: Weight-bearing radiographs and bone scintigrams are commonly used to diagnose midfoot sprains in football players. In case of doubt about the stability aspects of the sprain, clinical examination together with contralateral foot X-ray comparisons can be found very helpful.
– Treatment strategy: The management of stable undisplaced midfoot sprains in football players is not controversial. They respond successfully to nonoperative management. However, the appropriate management of midfoot sprains with diastasis is controversial. Although these sprains represent a true Lisfranc injury, its management can differ from the classic surgical anatomical reduction that is the standard treatment for high-velocity Lisfranc injuries. Restoration and maintenance of the anatomic alignment of the Lisfranc joint is the key to appropriate treatment of midfoot sprains (Fig. 35.6).

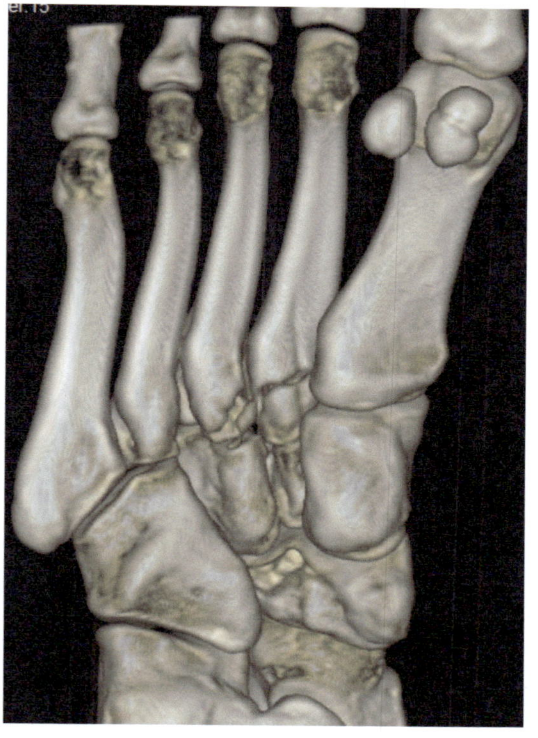

Fig. 35.6 3D CT image of a plantar base metatarsal 2 and 3 fracture that was initially misdiagnosed as midfoot sprain on X-ray

– Rehabilitation and return to play: Midfoot sprains in football are associated with an acute disability that can require prolonged restriction from competition (up to 3 months) although most lesions recover quickly (4–6 weeks) and long-term residual problems are minor [2].

35.8 Common Nontraumatic Foot Injuries in Football

35.8.1 Stress Fractures

– Aetiology: Repetitive cyclical loading after sudden increase in intensity, frequency and duration of training usually cause stress fractures over the foot (Fig. 35.7).
– Clinical and diagnostic examination: The football player presents with swelling, pain and localised tenderness over the foot. AP, lateral and oblique X-rays do not always exclude

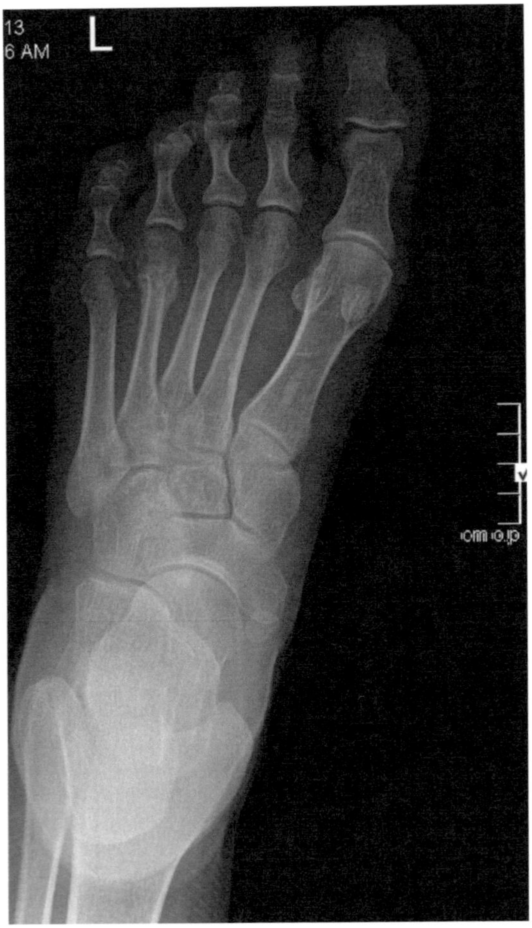

Fig. 35.7 Anteroposterior X-ray image of the healing process after a distal metatarsal four stress fracture

a stress fracture, and an MRI or bone scan can be indicated to acquire a definitive diagnosis (Fig. 35.8).

– Treatment strategy: Stress fractures in the foot of football players are notoriously known for difficult and slow healing, especially in the areas of the talar neck, the tarsal navicular and Jones fifth metatarsal. Boot immobilisation, electromagnetic pulse stimulation and non-weight-bearing are started, but surgical fixation (with or without bone grafting and drilling) can be indicated in case of delayed union or displaced fractures.
– Rehabilitation and return to play: Weeks/months of restricted weight-bearing are usually needed during the rehabilitation phase.

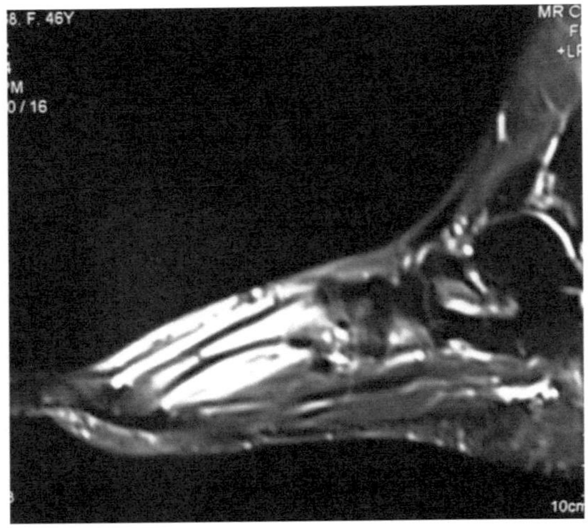

Fig. 35.8 Sagittal T2 MRI image of a midshaft metatarsal stress fracture

Pool exercises can be started early with further gradual progressive rehabilitation protocols within pain limits to be followed. A football player with an asymptomatic but incomplete fracture is allowed to regain training after 6 weeks using appropriate protective orthoses (steel shank and arch support) for at least 6 months more. It can take up to 6–9 months though in case of required surgical intervention before the player is allowed to play full throttle again [9, 17, 20–28].

35.8.2 Hallux Rigidus

– Aetiology and injury mechanism: Hallux rigidus is a disabilitating degenerative disease of the first metatarsophalangeal joint. In football, the disease arises from the repetitive dorsiflexion/jamming of the foot's first row. Together with trauma, systemic arthropathies, hyperpronation, elevated metatarsal, poor footwear and unusually long first metatarsal can also initiate the degenerative changes.
– Clinical and diagnostic examination: The football player complains of pain, swelling and decreased motion over the great toe. The diagnosis is made by X-ray showing joint space narrowing, osteophytes and metatarsal

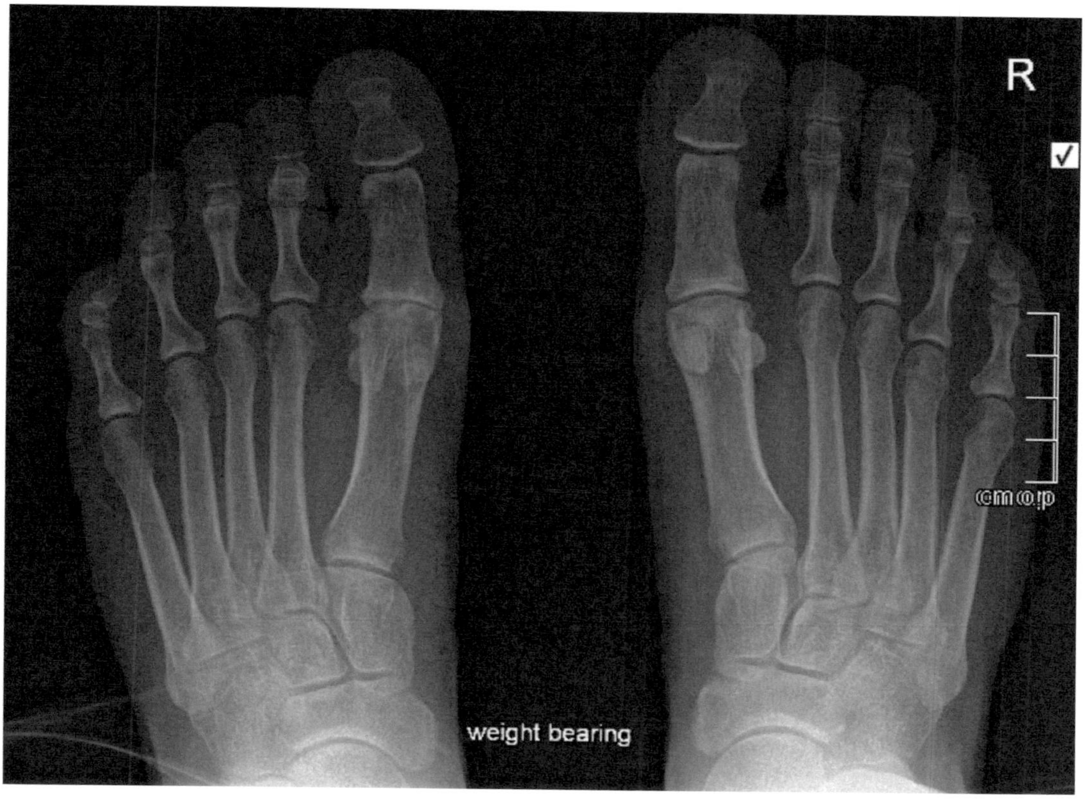

Fig. 35.9 Anteroposterior X-ray image of a football player with a left foot hallux rigidus

head flattening (Fig. 35.9). Ankylosis of the joint may also occur but is usually present at a later stage of the disease.

– Treatment strategy: Adjustments to the football shoe/inlays and podiatric modifications (to limit the motion of the first metatarsophalangeal joint) are the initial preferred type of treatment in football players with hallux rigidus. As an adjuvant to the biomechanical corrections of the footballer's foot made, an oral NSAID or intermediate-acting steroid intra-articular injection can help to relieve the synovial joint inflammation. In case of failed conservative treatment, most players are treated surgically with a cheilectomy that removes the dorsal joint impingement of the bone and soft tissue. Other surgical options available are dorsiflexion osteotomy of the proximal phalanx, decompression osteotomy and arthrodesis.
– Rehabilitation and return to play: Conservative treatment aims at restoring the motion of the joint and strength of the intrinsic foot muscles. After cheilectomy, the football player is allowed to weight-bear as tolerated in a protective rigid postoperative shoe. After about 10 weeks postoperatively, running can be initiated, but caution needs to be taken that the shoes can accommodate any occurring postoperative swelling. This swelling may persist for 6–9 months after surgery [17, 29]. Further in-depth information on football-related stress fractures will be covered in Chap. 36.

35.8.3 Plantar Fasciitis

– Aetiology: Plantar fasciitis is the most common cause of heel pain in adult football. It refers to a chronic inflammation at the origin of the plantar medial calcaneal tuberosity on the anteromedial portion of the heel. Analogous to the adult form, in children, it's referred to as calcaneal apophysitis (Sever's disorder). In chronic cases, there can occur combined entrapments of the first branch of the lateral plantar nerve, contributing to the pain.

- Clinical and diagnostic examination: The affected football player usually reports pain that worsens after resting and also reports morning pain and stiffness. Typically the pain increases during rest and decreases during activity. A combined stress fracture can clinically present through swelling over the lateral side of the heel. The symptoms arise from the plantar fascia's microscopic tears and inflammation, not from the bony spurs that occur over the calcaneal edge. Frequently in plantar fasciitis with local tenderness over the heel, a tight Achilles tendon is encountered. Although malalignment is not commonly associated with plantar fasciitis, hind foot valgus with pronation increases the peak stresses over the medial plantar fascia.
- Treatment strategy: A nonoperative treatment protocol is commonly used for plantar fasciitis, even in a chronic setting (up to 8 months). Podiatric soft heel pads, custom orthosis (with a medial heel wedge and a first metatarsal lift to relieve the stress on the medial fascia and correct the pronation deformity) and arch taping, NSAIDS and eccentric Achilles tendon stretching exercises (4 min, four times a day) help in decreasing symptoms during football. Long-acting steroid injections (maximum 3 per year) may benefit the in-season football player with plantar fasciitis but should be used judiciously since an overuse can lead to atrophy of the fat pad and make the heel pain worse [30]. Operative treatment is used for chronic cases >9 months that have failed conservative treatment with a return to sport between 3 and 4 months after a gradual increase of impact activities during rehabilitation. Due to the huge amount of different surgical techniques for chronic plantar fasciitis and due to the unsatisfactory results in elite football, the author only recommends a surgical approach in limited and individualised plantar fasciitis cases. After the recovery treatment, it's advised to continue a preventative and rigorous stretching programme throughout the football player's subsequent career [17].

35.9 Sesamoid Dysfunction

- Aetiology: Football players with cavus feet and associated plantarflexed first metatarsal head are most prone to this entity. Dorsiflexion of the first metatarsophalangeal joint causes the pain, and combined sesamoid stress fractures are usually caused by training error itself.
- Injury mechanism: Usually repetitive microtrauma lies at the origin of sesamoid dysfunction. The cause of pain symptoms can come from a fracture, sesamoiditis (inflammation and swelling over the peritendinous structures around the sesamoids) (Fig. 35.4b), plantar keratosis, medial digital nerve compression, osteochondritis or bursitis (Fig. 35.4c).
- Clinical and diagnostic examination: The player presents with localised tenderness and pain plantar to the first metatarsal head. Sometimes it's difficult to clinically differ sesamoiditis from inflammation over the adjacent flexor halluces longus (FHL) tendon. If active plantar flexion of the interphalangeal joint against resistance exacerbates the pain, the FHL tendon is probably involved. A sesamoid view X-ray and bone scan are good tools in the diagnostic setup (Fig. 35.10). It can sometimes be challenging to differentiate a bipartite sesamoid from a fractured sesamoid on X-ray. A fracture will normally appear as a straight radiolucent line, while a congenital bipartite sesamoid will have more irregular lines.
- Treatment strategy: It will depend on the cause of the sesamoid dysfunction but is most commonly through nonoperative measures. Custom orthosis, NSAID, shoe modification and padding are used in the treatment of sesamoiditis, especially in the case of bursitis where the main intention is to relieve the

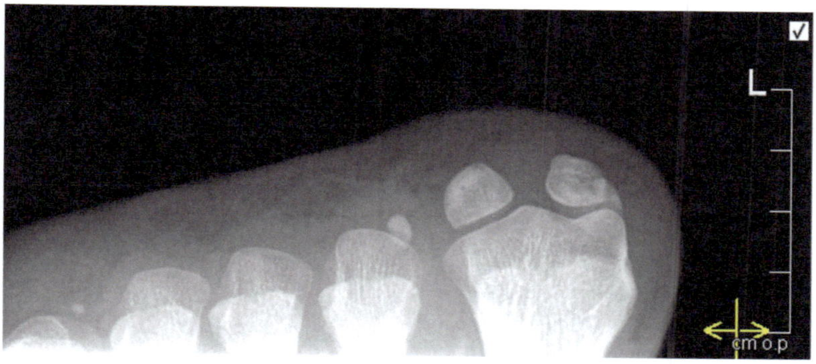

Fig. 35.10 X-ray image of a sesamoid view

pressure under the first metatarsal head. Cortisone injections should be used judiciously in chronic cases, and only rarely, an excision of a sesamoid bone in the foot of a football player is needed. This excision can induce other problems again like progression of a pre-existing hallux valgus deformity. Total sesamoidectomy in the football player is disadvised because of the significant biomechanical abnormalities that it can induce. Non-displaced sesamoid fractures are generally treated with a below-knee boot or cast for 4–6 weeks followed by a customised orthosis. Surgery is only indicated after failure with conservative therapy for over 6 months. In football players, both bone grafting and sesamoid excision have yielded satisfactory surgical results in chronic nonunion cases [17, 31].

35.10 Rehabilitation of the Injured Footballer's Foot

After every injury (with or without temporary immobilisation), the foot has to regain its flexibility towards a normal gait and its adaptations to unflat surfaces. Manual postural physiotherapy techniques aim at mobilising again the tibiocrural joint, the subtalar joint and the midfoot joint. Every foot injury generates a muscular atrophy and a loss of proprioception. Neuromuscular training, mobilisations, tonifications and gait rehabilitation strategies have been shown very beneficial towards rapid recovery in foot/ankle football problems.

Troubled alignment problems will benefit from specific readaptation protocols. If the traumatic constraints and the degenerative processes can be prevented during the treatment, a perfect recovery towards football with normal flexibility, normal force and adequate proprioception of the foot can be achieved. The football player also has its responsibility in this by respecting the treatment compliance, the adaptations to the shoe (support areas) and the strict pedagogical/pedicure protocols.

References

1. Giza E, Fuller C, Junge A, Dvorak J (2003) Mechanisms of foot and ankle injuries in soccer. Am J Sports Med 31(4):550–554
2. Fuller C, Smith G, Junge A, Dvorak J (2004) The influence of tackle parameters on the propensity for injury in international football. Am J Sports Med 32(1):43S–53S
3. Andersen T, Floerenes T, Arnason A, Bahr R (2004) Video analysis of the mechanisms for ankle injuries in football. Am J Sports Med 32(1):69S–79S
4. Taylor S, Fabrikant P, Khair M, Haleem A, Drakos M (2012) A review of synthetic playing surfaces, the shoe-surface interface, and lower extremity injuries in athletes. Phys Sportsmed 40(4):66–72
5. Williams S, Hume P (2011) A review of football injuries on third and fourth generation artificial turfs compared to natural turf. Sports Med 41(11):903–923
6. Bentley J, Ramanathan A, Arnold G, Wang W, Abboud R (2011) Harmful cleats of football boots: a biomechanical evaluation. Foot Ankle Surg 17(3):140–144
7. Ford K, Manson N, Evans B, Myer G, Gwin R, Heidt R, Hewett T (2006) Comparison of in-shoe foot loading patterns on natural grass and synthetic turf. J Sci Med Sport 9(6):433–440
8. Ekstrand J, Nigg B (1989) Surface-related injuries in soccer. Sports Med 8(1):56–65

9. d'Hooghe P, Kerkhoffs G (2014) The ankle in football. Springer, Heidelberg, pp 253–268, Chap. 21
10. Cain L, Nicholson L, Adams R, Burns J (2007) Foot morphology and foot/ankle injury in indoor football. J Sci Med Sport 10(5):311–319
11. George E, Harris A, Dragoo J, Hunt K (2014) Incidence and risk factors for turf toe injuries in intercollegiate football: data from the national collegiate athletic association injury surveillance system. Foot Ankle Int 35(2):108–115
12. Anandan N, Williams P, Dalavaye S (2013) Turf toe injury. Emerg Med J 30(9):776–777
13. Brophy R, Gamradt S, Ellis S, Barnes R, Rodeo S, Warren R, Hillstrom H (2009) Effect of turf toe on foot contact pressures in professional American football players. Foot Ankle Int 30(5):405–409
14. Childs S (2006) The pathogenesis and biomechanics of turf toe. Orthop Nurs 25(4):276–280
15. Allen R, Flemming D, Sanders T (2004) Turf toe: ligamentous injury of the first metatarsophalangeal joint. Mil Med 169(11):xix–xxiv
16. Watson T, Anderson R, Davis W (2000) Periarticular injuries to the hallux metatarsophalangeal joint in athletes. Foot Ankle Clin 5(3):687–713
17. Michell L, Smith A, Bachl N, Rolf C, Chan K (2001) Team physician manual. Hong Kong, FIMS, Lippincott Williams and Wilkins Asia ltd, pp 406–427, Chap. 17
18. Sikka R, Hunkele T, Sugarman E, Myerson M, Fetzer G, Boyd J (2012) Dorsal dislocation of the great toe in a professional football player: case report. Foot Ankle Int 33(9):798–802
19. Ekstrand J, Van Dijk C (2013) Fifth metatarsal fractures among male professional footballers: a potential career-ending disease. Br J Sports Med 47(12):754–758
20. DeLee JC, Evans J, Julian J (1983) Stress fracture of the fifth metatarsal. Am J Sports Med 11(5):349–353
21. Dimitriou R, Tsiridis E, Giannoudis P (2005) Current concepts of molecular aspects of bone healing. Injury 36(12):1392–1404
22. Ebraheim N, Haman S, Lu J, Padanilam T, Yeasting R (2000) Anatomical and radiological considerations of the fifth metatarsal bone. Foot Ankle Int 21(3):212–215
23. Ekstrand T (2012) Stress fractures in elite male football players. Scand J Med Sci Sports 22:341–346
24. Fazzalari N (2011) Bone fracture and bone fracture repair. Osteoporos Int 22(6):2003–2006
25. Hens J, Martens M (1990) Surgical treatment of Jones fractures. Arch Orthop Trauma Surg 09(5):277–279
26. Kaeding C, Miller T (2013) The comprehensive description of stress fractures: a new classification system. J Bone Joint Surg Am 95(13):1214–1220
27. Kaeding C, Yu J, Wright R, Amendola A, Spindler K (2005) Management and return to play of stress fractures. Clin J Sport Med 15(6):442–447
28. Lee S, Anderson R (2004) Stress fractures of the tarsal navicular. Foot Ankle Clin 9(1):85–104
29. Kubitz E (2003) Athletic injuries of the first metatarsophalangeal joint. Am Podiatr Med Assoc 93(4):325–332
30. Orchard J (2004) Is it safe to use local anaesthetic painkilling injections in professional football? Sports Med 34(4):209–219
31. Kadakia A, Molloy A (2011) Current concepts review: traumatic disorders of the first metatarsophalangeal joint and sesamoid complex. Foot Ankle Int 32(8):834–839

Stress Fractures of the Foot in Footballers

36

Palmanovich Ezequiel, Keltz Eran, Kots Eugene, Marom Niv, Hetsroni Iftach, Nyska Meir, and Mann Gideon

36.1 Etiology

Stress fracture comprises the inability of bone to withstand the repeated stress which athletic activity, military service, or even normal life exerts on a prior strong normal or weakened bone. This failure to repair the microtraumas leads to fatigue microdamage of the bone due to predominance of osteoclastic over the osteoblastic activity.

In 2012, Ekstrand [1] studied the incidence and distribution of stress fractures in elite football players. Stress fracture incidence was observed to be 0.04 injuries/1,000 h of exposure. All fractures affected the lower extremities and 78 % of the fifth metatarsal bone. Less frequent in football players were stress fractures of the navicular, calcaneous, and malleoli. Very rarely, stress fractures were observed in the proximal phalanx of the big toe [2].

Stress fractures in female football players are probably more common than reported in injury surveillance data and are an important cause of time lost from participation [3].

36.2 Risk Factors

In general, risk factors for stress fractures in athletes were reviewed [4] and divided into two categories: *Extrinsic risk factors* are factors in the environment or external to an individual that influence the likelihood of sustaining an injury. These include the training program, equipment, and environmental factors. *Intrinsic risk factors* refer to characteristics within an individual and how their body responds to loading and any damage it generates. These include gender, the endocrine balance, nutritional factors, physical fitness, and neuromusculoskeletal factors.

Specifically for football players, additional risk factors have been proposed: repetitive stress [3], rapid changes of load or changes of surface [3, 5, 6], and negative catabolism due to low energy availability [7, 8].

P. Ezequiel, MD • M. Niv, MD • H. Iftach, MD
N. Meir, MD • M. Gideon, MD (✉)
Unit of Sports Medicine, Department of Orthopaedic Surgery, Meir Medical Centre, Kfar Saba, Tel Aviv University, Tel Aviv, Israel
e-mail: gideon.mann.md@gmail.com

K. Eran, MD
Department of Orthopaedic Surgery, Rambam Medical Centre, Haifa, Israel
e-mail: erankeltz@gmail.com

K. Eugene, MD
Department of Diagnostic Radiology, Meir Medical Centre, Kfar Saba, Tel Aviv University, Tel Aviv, Israel

P. Volpi (ed.), *Football Traumatology: New Trends*, DOI 10.1007/978-3-319-18245-2_36

36.3 Localization of Stress Fractures of the Foot in Football Players

36.3.1 Fifth Metatarsal Bone Stress Fracture

Stewart [9] in 1960 showed a difference in mechanism of injury and in the prognosis for fractures at the junction of the shaft (zone 3), base (Jones fracture) (zone 2), and fractures of the styloid process (zone 1).

The Jones fracture was first described in 1902 by Sir Robert Jones [10]. The fracture occurs at the junction of the diaphysis and the metaphysis of the fifth metatarsal, often involving the articular facet between the fourth and fifth metatarsals but not extending distal to the facet (Figs. 36.1 and 36.2).

The mechanism of an avulsion fracture of the styloid process of the fifth metatarsal has been studied in cadavers. It is suggested that it is caused by the firm attachment of the lateral band of the plantar aponeurosis at the tip of the tuberosity, rather than by the more distal peroneus brevis attachment [11, 12].

Fractures in zones 1 and 2 are not considered as true stress fractures.

The metatarsal stress fracture classically occurs in the shaft. Studies have suggested that stress from the lateral aspect of the fifth metatarsal head occurs in zone 3, where repeated varus forces on the distal end of the bone are believed to be responsible for stress fractures [13, 14]. It may be more prevalent in a supinated foot [15] and has been shown to be associated with metatarsus varus [16], midfoot varus [16], cavovarus deformity of the foot [17, 18], and the fifth metatarsal curvature [18].

Clinical assessment should include a careful search for underlying risk factors, including nutritional and hormonal issues, and should explore training techniques and methods [19–21].

Athletic stress fractures may be missed on initial examination [22]. A high index of suspicion should be maintained [23] and further imaging (computed tomography [CT] or magnetic resonance imaging [MRI]) obtained if necessary to enable early detection [21] Fig. 36.3.

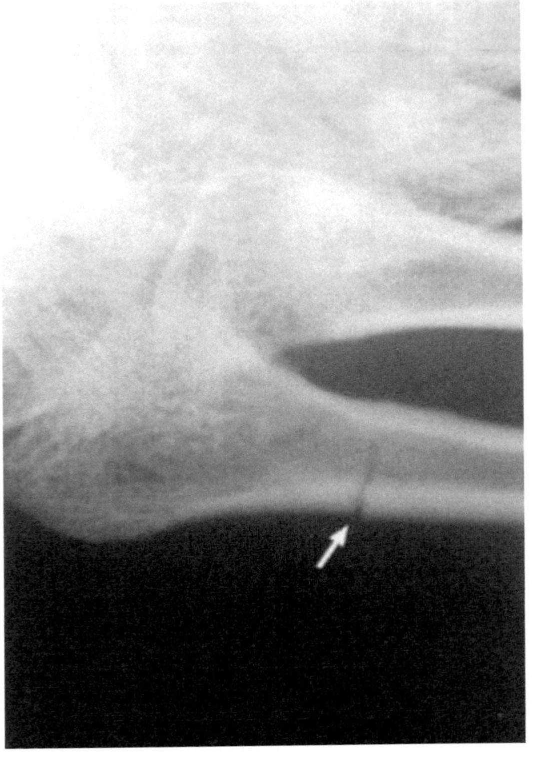

Fig. 36.1 Stress fracture at the diaphysis-metaphysis junction in the fifth metatarsal bone, as seen on common radiography (X-RAY). This is an acute or Torg I fracture

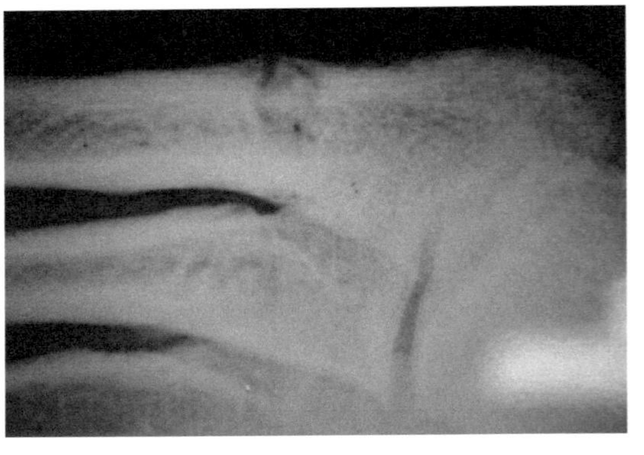

Fig. 36.2 X-ray showing a Torg II scrlerotic stress fracture

In some cases and with ultrasound-dedicated specialist, diagnosis could be shown by ultrasound (Fig. 36.4).

After 2–3 weeks of symptoms also, a simple X-ray can show cortex changes in stress fracture (Fig. 36.5).

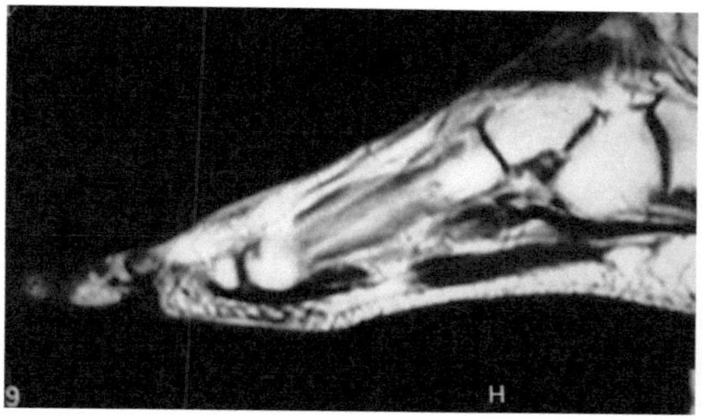

Fig. 36.3 Bone edema and periosteal reaction due to metatarsal stress fracture, as seen on MRI

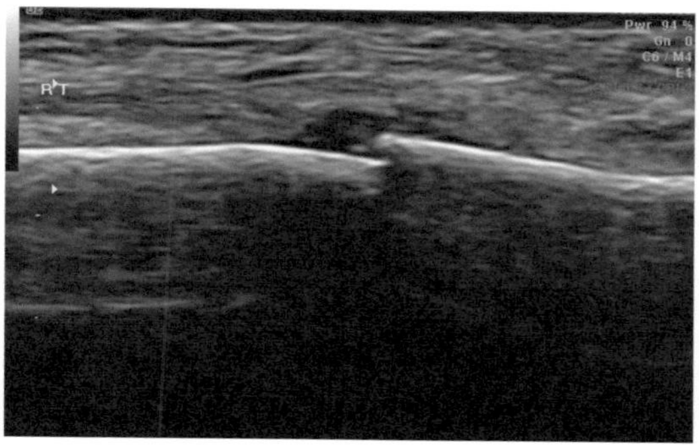

Fig. 36.4 Shown in ultrasound exam a cortex irregularity and periostal edema

Hetsroni et al. [24] evaluated athletes using dynamic plantar foot pressure. They concluded that lateral metatarsal unloading during stance may play a role in the pathogenesis of the injury.

In 1984, Torg and colleagues [25] classified the fractures of the proximal part of the diaphysis into 3 types: acute fracture lacking sclerosis (I), delayed union with fracture line widening and presence of intramedullary sclerosis (II), and nonunion with complete obliteration of the medullary canal with sclerotic bone (III).

36.3.1.1 Acute Fracture Treatment (Torg I) and Delayed Union (Torg II)

Nonoperative Treatment

When applying nonsurgical treatment, concerns have been raised concerning extended healing time, nonunion, and the possibility of refracture.

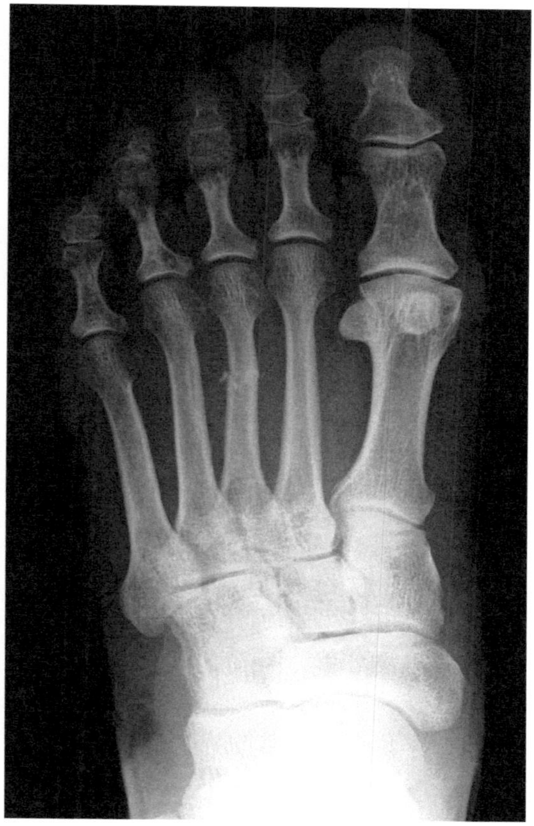

Fig. 36.5 Periostal and cortical reaction at the site of the stress fracture, as seen on X-ray

In the acute Jones fracture and possibly also the subacute (Torg type II), none or very minimally displaced fracture may be treated conservatively with a non-weight-bearing cast for 6–12 weeks [26–31].

Nonoperative treatment has been associated with a higher rate of treatment failure [16, 32, 33], and early fixation in the athlete is widely supported [16, 23, 33–36].

Based on animal models, shock-wave therapy (high-energy acoustic waves) is believed to induce neovascularization, which increases cell proliferation and eventually tissue regeneration. Electromagnetic bone stimulation may also have a possible role in acute fracture healing [37, 38].

As discussed above in a professional athlete, surgical intervention would be considered at an early stage, even when no symptoms are apparent [39]. In the acute stage, when occurring in an athlete, the aim would be to proceed to early surgical intervention which has been shown to be successful in this population [40].

Surgical Treatment

Lee and colleagues [41] retrospectively reviewed 42 patients with acute (Torg I) and subacute (Torg II) fractures treated with modified tension band wiring using two cortical screws. CT evaluation revealed a mean time to union of 75 days (40–150 days), with all patients returning to their previous sporting activity, although there were 4 refractures, 4 delayed unions, and 1 nonunion.

Autologous cancellous bone grafting combined with intramedullary screw fixation has been proposed by Popovic [42]. All cases united and returned to full sports by 12 weeks.

Murawski and Kennedy [43] reported on 26 athletes, 9 of whom were zone 3 injuries, using a fracture-specific percutaneous screw system and bone marrow aspirate concentrate, with a mean overall time to union of 5 weeks (range 5–24 weeks).

There is insufficient evidence to advocate primary bone grafting of acute zone 3 fractures [21].

36.3.1.2 Chronic Fractures (Torg III)

Nonoperative Management

Delayed and nonunion of the fifth metatarsal fractures may not allow return to sport in a reasonable time and thereby may have a profound impact on an athlete's career [21, 44].

Khan et al. [45] retrospectively evaluated fractures distal to the tuberosity, of which 15 were nonunions treated nonoperatively. These investigators showed that although these fractures may eventually unite, this may take up to 20 weeks, thereby supporting the claim for early surgery in athletes.

36.3.1.3 Surgical Treatment

When displacement has occurred [31], delayed union is apparent (Torg III) [27, 28, 30, 31, 46] or the athlete cannot afford the lengthy conservative treatment [27] which may continue up to 5 months [28], surgical treatment should be considered using a large cannulated 4.5 mm intramedullary screw [47] or other method of fixation.

Intramedullary Screw Fixation

Intramedullary screw fixation seems to be the more popular surgical technique in the athletic population Fig. 36.6.

Screw fixation is done as an outpatient procedure, under local or regional anesthesia, guided by fluoroscopy. A cannulated screw is inserted proximal to distal in the intramedullary canal.

Not all agree with the concept of using the thickest intramedullary screw possible. Shah et al. in 2001 found no difference between a 4.5 and a 5.5 mm screw placed intramedullarily in a simulated fracture [48].

The radiological union was 99 % and the mean time to return to sports was 7.5 weeks [47].

Intramedullary screw fixation is the commonest type of fixation for nonunions, although it is not without complications. Porter et al. [47] demonstrated 100 % clinical and radiological union after 4.5 mm cannulated screw fixation in 23 athletes.

Habbu et al. [49] reported a radiological union in all 14 cases in their series, with a mean time to union of 13.3 weeks, and unassisted full pain-free weight-bearing at 10.2 weeks. Complications described included deep infection and sural neuroma.

Nevertheless, there have been a few reported series of failures of intramedullary screw fixation of proximal fifth metatarsal fractures in the form of refracture or screw breakage [50, 51].

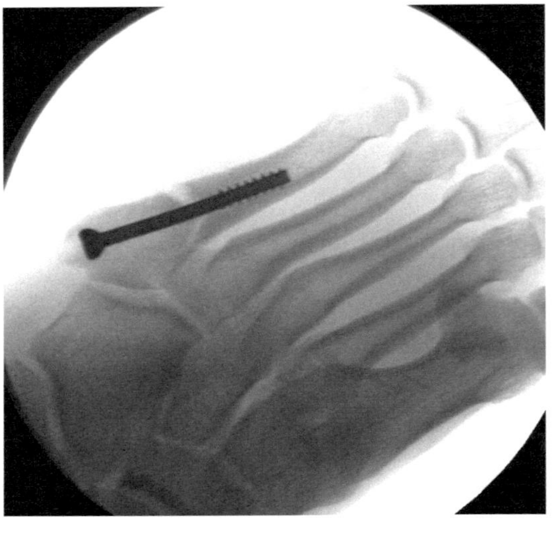

Fig. 36.6 Stress fracture of the fifth metatarsal treated by cortical drilling and intramedullary screw fixation

Tension Band Wiring

Lee et al. presented their results in 42 patients using tension band wiring [18]. Failures occurred in less than 10 % of the cases [41] .

Other Treatment Options

Capacitively coupled electric fields [52, 53], low-intensity pulsed ultrasound [LIPU] [54–56], and shock-wave therapy (SWT) [56, 57] may have a role in treating persistent cases and thus achieving eventual faster consolidation of the fracture or at least alleviation of pain [58].

36.3.2 Navicular Stress Fractures

Navicular stress fracture is a relatively uncommon injury, about 3 % of the foot stress fractures [59]. These have been described in athletes especially in jumping or sprinting, inclusive of figure skating, ball games, and dance [60–62]. These fractures are also seen in long-distance runners using the forefoot in the footstrike [63–68].

The late diagnosis and the tendency for nonunion with or without avascular necrosis [69] have made this fracture unwelcome in sports medicine clinics.

36.3.2.1 Pathophysiology

The navicular bone may be repeatedly "bent" when compressed in the sagittal plane between the talus and the cuneiforms during repeated stress [67, 70]. Some conditions have been suggested as possible contributing factors for navicular stress fractures as reduced dorsiflexion of the ankle [27], short first metatarsal, a long second metatarsal [54], and excessive subtalar pronation [27]. Also avascular area was describe as factor for the stress fractures [27] Fig. 36.7.

36.3.2.2 Clinical Presentation and Diagnosis

Insidious deep pain radiating to the distal forefoot medially and or dorsally, occurring after sprinting, running, or jumping should raise the suspicion of a navicular stress fracture [27, 70–73].

Physical examination will disclose local tenderness of the navicular on the dorsal aspect of the foot [27] and often reduced dorsal flexion and subtalar motion [61, 74].

Imaging includes 3 plane X-rays, which are often of low sensitivity [27, 70], with a positive result for fracture only in 14 % [75].

The technetium bone scan (BS) has shown high sensitivity and low specificity showing a strong reaction of the whole navicular bone [27, 70, 76] Fig. 36.8.

The computerized tomogram (CT) is the most accurate of the imaging methods for the navicular stress fracture. Magnetic resonance (MRI) is not often used in the diagnosis of navicular stress

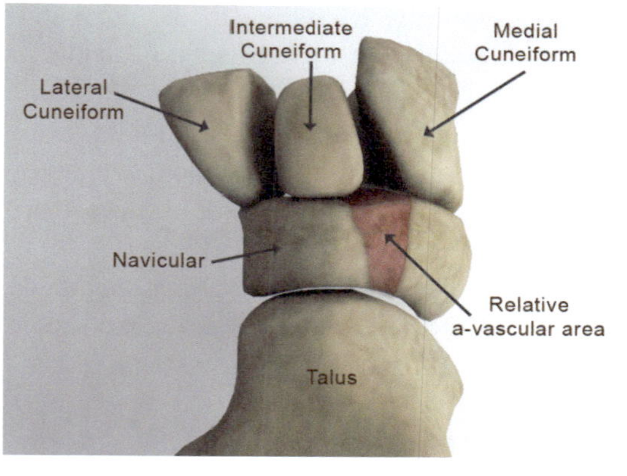

Fig. 36.7 Avascular area described for the navicular bone

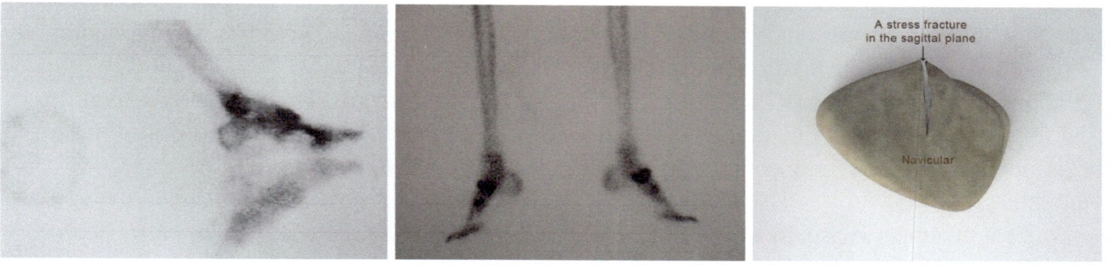

Fig. 36.8 Bone scan showing local reaction over the navicular bone. Schematic view of the stress fracture

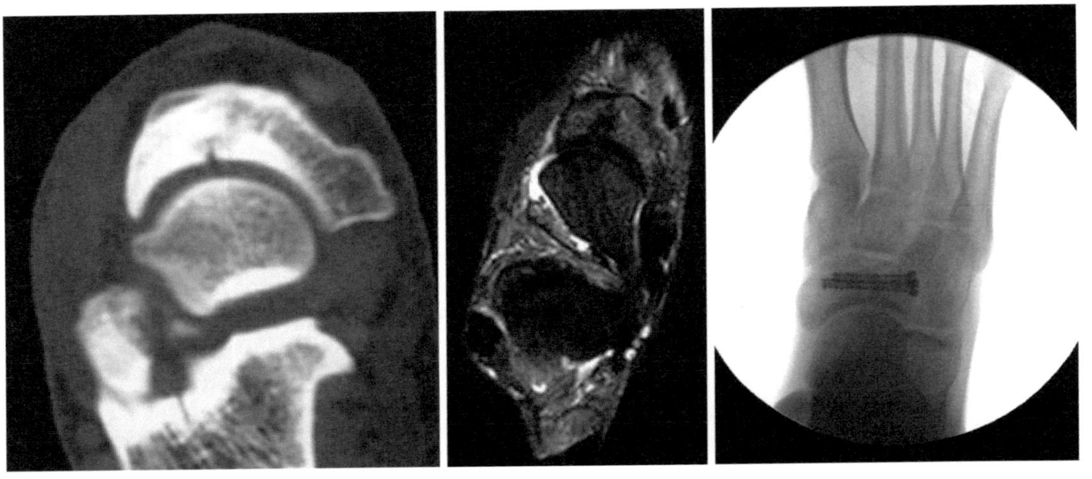

Fig. 36.9 Navicular stress fracture as shown by CT and MRI. Surgical treatment with 2 cannulate screw and bone grafting

fracture though it has been used for serial follow-up of healing [77] Fig. 36.9.

Diagnosis is frequently delayed 4–7 months because of the vague symptoms and frequently normal initial X-rays.

36.3.2.3 Differential Diagnosis

Bipartite navicular according to the computerized tomogram (CT) or accessory navicular is sometimes very difficult to differentiate from a stress fracture. Magnetic resonance (MRI) using T2-weighed images could assist the diagnosis by showing edema in acute trauma or in stress injury [76–78].

Osteochondritis dissecans (OCD), avascular necrosis (AVN), or Kienboeck's disease should be also kept in mind.

36.3.2.4 Treatment

Khan recommended treatment by non-weight bearing with immobilization for 6 weeks, followed by 6 weeks of a rehabilitation program followed up by clinical appearance based on pain on activity and dorsal sensitivity on examination [70]. To follow up union, MRI may be used [77] or CT may be used which might show union beginning at 6 weeks and complete union at 4 months [78].

Surgical treatment is usually not necessary and not recommended [66, 70, 79]. Healing may possibly be assisted by pulsed low-intensity ultrasound [53] or capacitively coupled electric fields [54].

Surgical treatment for painful persistent nonunion remains an option in selected cases [65, 66].

Puddu et al. have suggested the following outline for treatment [62]:

1. *Noncomplicated partial fracture and undisplaced complete fracture*: Non-weight-bearing plaster for 6–8 weeks.
2. *Displaced complete fracture*: Treatment as above or alternatively surgical reduction and fixation followed by non-weight-bearing immobilization in plaster for 6 weeks.
3. *Fracture complicated by delayed union or nonunion*: Curettage and inlaid bone grafting with internal fixation of unstable fragments (without attempting reduction because in general there is already a fibrous union). Any sclerotic fragments found must not be removed but must be fixed. After the operation, a non-weight-bearing cast must be applied for 6–8 weeks. Recovery is monitored by radiographs (sometimes 3–6 months are necessary).
4. *Partial fracture complicated by a small transverse dorsal fracture*: The dorsal fragment may have to be removed.
5. *Complete fracture complicated by a widespread transverse dorsal fracture*: Recovery takes place by immobilization.

Dorsal talar beaks must be removed during surgery.

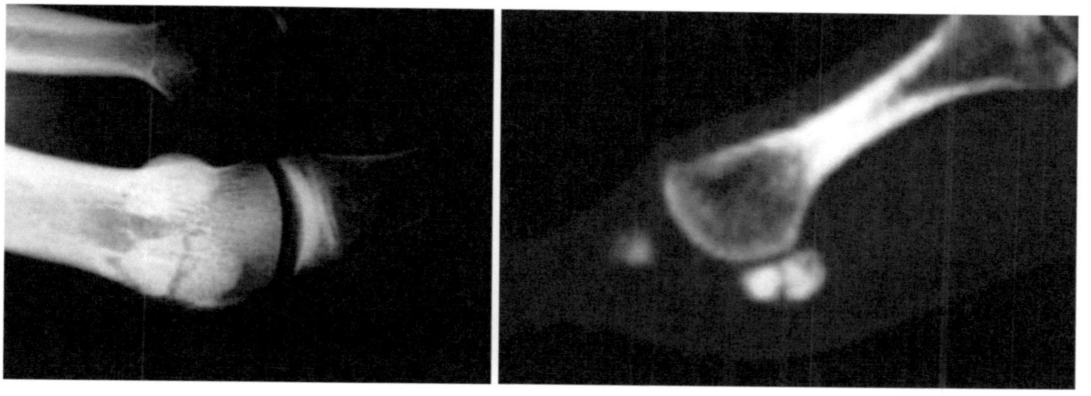

Fig. 36.10 X-ray and CT scan showing a sesamoid stress fracture

Surgical intervention has a relatively high occurrence of failure and complication, and the patient should be informed of possibly less than optimal results, before surgical treatment is initiated.

36.3.3 Sesamoid Stress Fractures

Sesamoid stress fractures occur in a wide variety of sports such as football. Injury of the sesamoid could cause incapacitating pain on athletic activity [80].

36.3.3.1 Pathophysiology

The sesamoid bones are located plantar to the first metatarsal head where they are imbedded within the plantar plate, as part of the tendon of the flexor hallucis brevis. The large forces of weight bearing and traction expose the sesamoids to a variety of pathologies, inclusive of sesamoiditis, chondromalacia, osteochondritis dissecans, avascular necrosis (osteonecrosis), osteoarthritis, osteochondral fractures, and stress fractures [81].

Stress fractures of the sesamoid comprise approximately 5 % of foot stress fractures [59]. The stress fracture involves mostly the medial sesamoid [62, 82, 83].

Sesamoid stress fractures have a strong tendency to nonunion, probably more than any other bone [84].

36.3.3.2 Clinical Presentation

Pain is of insidious onset and unusually long standing. It is poorly localized, occurring during or after activity and relieved by rest [61]. Pain is increased by hyperextension of the great toe and by local pressure.

36.3.3.3 Diagnosis

Diagnosis is confirmed by **X-rays** inclusive of an anterior-posterior projection, a lateral projection, and an axial projection, which would differentiate a fracture from a bipartite sesamoid based on the total length of the fragments. A fractured sesamoid would usually show equal-sized fragments, ragged in texture, while a bipartite sesamoid would have smooth and unequal fragments [61]. 75 % of bipartite sesamoids are bilateral [85, 86].

A *computerized tomogram (CT)* gives an accurate and clear image of the injury [82].

The fracture line would usually be transverse, with osteoporotic edges which would become smoother in time [86]. Both computerized tomograms (CT) [87] and magnetic resonance (MRI) [88] have been suggested for accurate diagnosis. Osteochondritis dissecans or osteonecrosis could occur [89] and radiologically could be difficult to differentiate from a bipartite sesamoid or a fragmented stress fracture (Fig. 36.10).

36.3.3.4 Treatment

Treatment probably should be relatively aggressive, nonsurgical, with orthoses preventing hallux dorsiflexion, and padding along side with relative rest [62] probably for 3–6 weeks. If symptoms are severe, a platform cast for 6 weeks with protection from toe dorsiflexion may be used [59, 61, 90], controlled by repeated X-ray [61]. Others recommend a cast, possibly non-weight bearing, for 6 weeks as the initial treatment [86, 87], with appropriate padding to reduce pressure on the injured bone. To our experience, cast application rarely works and may be harmful, especially in the younger age.

If symptoms persist, bone grafting may be attempted [91], though excision of the fractured sesamoid is probably more often practical [61, 62, 66, 82, 83, 92] a procedure allowing return to full activity after an initial 3 week period of immobilization [66]. Excision could be total or partial [27, 93]. Shaving has been practiced [80]. Excision of both sesamoids is not recommended [80]. Medial partial sesamoidectomy has also been described as an arthroscopic procedure [94].

In summary stress fractures of the sesamoids occur following repeated traction and usually involve the medial sesamoid. Pain is insidious and long standing. Diagnosis is clinical, as pain is caused by both toe dorsiflexion and local pressure. Diagnosis is assisted by X-rays and bone scan and occasional CT or MRI. Radiological differential diagnosis includes bipartite or multipartite sesamoid or osteochondritis. Clinical differential diagnosis includes mainly sesamoid chondromalacia or osteoarthritis, the latter of which could be apparent on x-ray. The sesamoid stress fracture has a strong tendency to nonunion. Treatment should be initiated immediately after diagnosis and includes orthoses or rarely cast for 6 weeks with a platform to prevent toe extension.

If clinical and radiological healing fails to occur, surgical treatment by partial or total excision of the sesamoid should be initiated followed by 3 weeks of immobilization before gradually returning to sports. In selected cases, bone graft to the fracture could be considered.

36.4 Other Different and Relatively Unusual Stress Fractures

36.4.1 The Base of the Fourth Metatarsal Bone

Stress fracture of the base of the fourth metatarsal has been shown to present as a troublesome location of a stress fracture, tending to delayed union and ongoing symptomatology [95–97]. Its similarity to the Jones fracture is rather interesting. Surgical treatment of this injury has been advocated [97] though we never found this necessary Fig. 36.11.

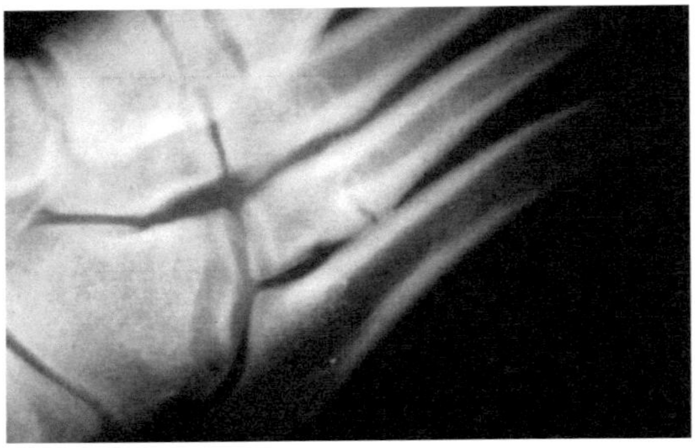

Fig. 36.11 Stress fracture of the base of the 4th metatarsal, as seen on X-ray

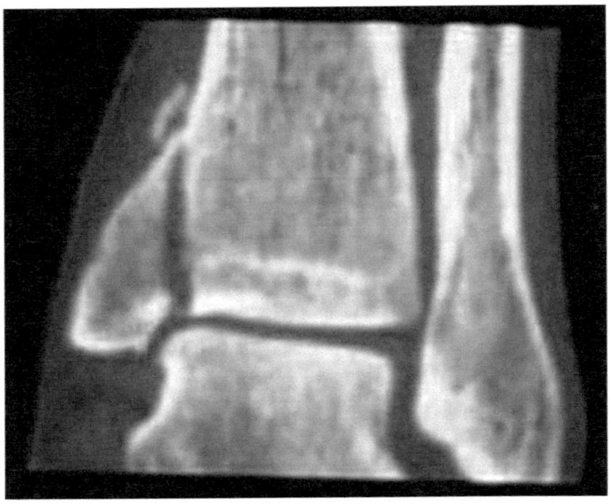

Fig. 36.12 CT scan showing a displaced stress fracture of medial malleolus

36.4.2 Talus Stress Fracture

Stress fractures have also been noted in the talus [98, 99], a rather benign entity well known to physicians working with military personnel. These could also occur as an insufficiency fracture [100].

36.4.3 Tibial Malleolar Stress Fractures

Malleolar stress fractures [101–104] are often seen on bone scans and in the majority of cases will heal uneventfully (Fig. 36.12). Standard radiographs may not reveal the lesion unless displacement has occurred [104] and other imaging as MRI [104] or bone scan should be used. In an occasional case, operative intervention may be required [102]. It should be noted that conservative treatment could lead to displacement [105] and the use of a percutaneous cannulated screw has been described as a surgical option enabling return to training within 24 days [106]. Early surgical intervention is advocated by some authorities in order to prevent displacement and allow early return to full activity [107]. Healing may take 3–4 months [107]. Bilateral occurrence has been described [108].

36.4.4 Calcaneal Stress Fractures

Calcaneal stress fractures are not frequently reported today, though rather common in the past [109].

The incidence of calcaneal stress fractures is highest in military recruits and long-distance runners [110].

A case of bilateral fracture has been reported [111], and a case of stress fracture of the anterior process of the calcaneum has been reported in tarsal coalition [112]. Also described are calcaneal stress fractures during the postoperative period following total knee or total hip arthroplasty [113]. Plain films will often show a sclerotic or radiolucent line after 2–3 weeks of symptoms (Fig. 36.13). MRI probably is the gold standard showing edema and the fracture line (Fig. 36.14).

Diagnosis is difficult and could be confused with plantar fasciitis, Achilles tendinitis, Baxter entrapment, and retrocalcaneal bursitis [110]. Calcaneal stress fractures can be adequately treated with activity modification without casting or surgical intervention.

36.4.5 Base Metatarsal II Stress Fracture

Stress fractures on the base of the second metatarsal are described in ballet dancers [114–117] (Fig. 36.15). It frequently presents with pain over

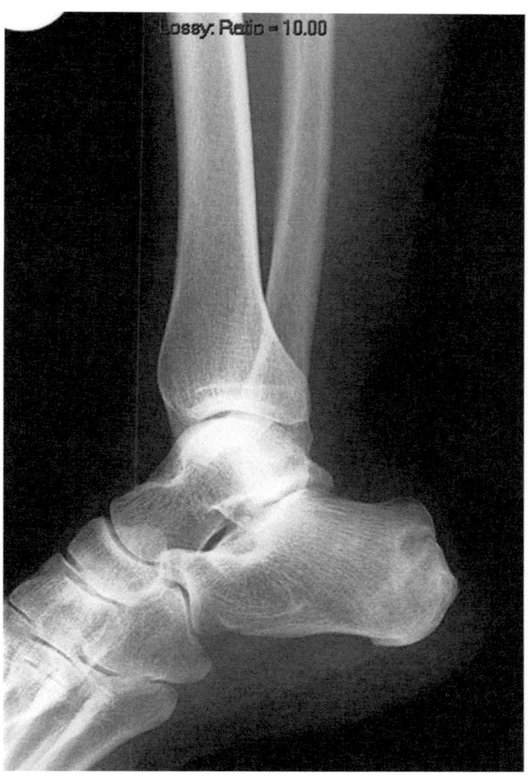

Fig. 36.13 Shows a sclerotic line in the posterior aspect of the calcaneous

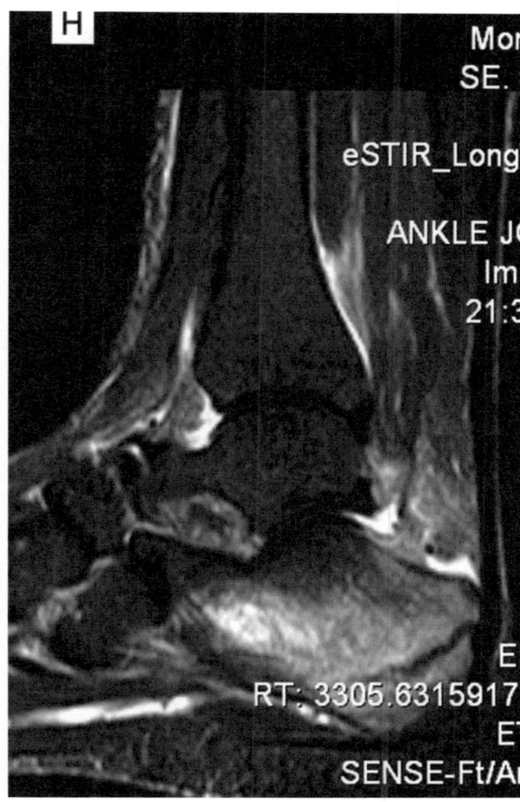

Fig. 36.14 MRI showing the calcaneal edema and the fracture line

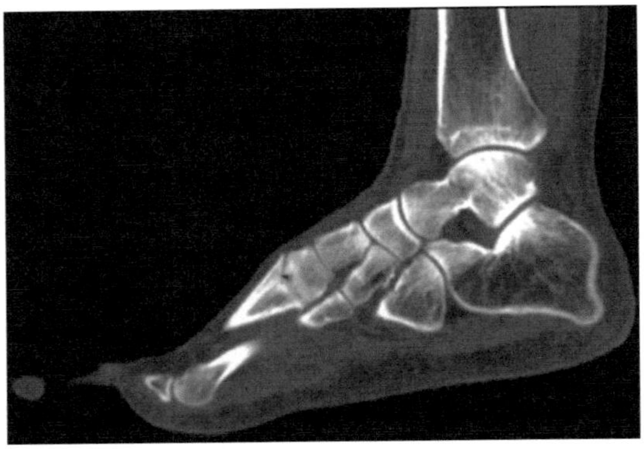

Fig. 36.15 Stress fracture of the base of the second metatarsal with sclerotic and cystic changes as seen in CT scan

the midfoot when jumping or in full-point position. Clinically, it was impossible to differentiate between dancers who had traumatic synovitis of the second tarsometatarsal joint (Lisfranc joint) and stress fracture of the base of the second metatarsal [116]. MRI is the gold standard to differentiate between edema at the metatarsal bone and synovitis. It seems that if the fracture is recognized early and treated appropriately with rest and back gradually to dance, healing should result. Patients returned to performing at an average of 6.2 weeks following diagnosis [114].

36.5 In Summary

Stress fractures in football players are frequent and 78 % occur in the fifth metatarsal. Classically, it occurs in the shaft of the metatarsal and could be classified as in acute, subacute, and chronic. Nonoperative treatment has been associated with a higher rate of treatment failure. Cortical drilling and intramedullar screwing is the most used technique.

Less frequent stress fractures in the football player include navicular and sesamoid stress fracture. Relatively unusual stress fracture of the base of the 2nd, 4th metatarsals, talus, medial maleolar, and calcaneous were described. Guided anamnesis, meticulous physical examination, and correct imaging with a high grade of suspicion would lead to the correct treatment and back to full performance.

References

1. Ekstrand J, Torstveit MK (2012) Stress fractures in elite male football players. Scand J Med Sci Sports 22(3):341–346
2. Shiraishi M, Mizuta H, Kubota K, Sakuma K, Takagi K (1993) Stress fracture of the proximal phalanx of the great toe. Foot Ankle 14(1):28–34
3. Warden SJ, Creaby MW, Bryant AL, Crossley KM (2007) Stress fracture risk factors in female football players and their clinical implications. Br J Sports Med 41(Suppl 1):i38–i43, Epub 2007 Jun 21
4. Warden SJ, Burr DB, Brukner PD (2006) Stress fractures: pathophysiology, epidemiology, and risk factors. Curr Osteoporos Rep 4:103–109
5. Ekstrand J, Gillquist J (1983) The avoidability of soccer injuries. Int J Sports Med 4:124–128
6. Ekstrand J, Gillquist J (1983) Soccer injuries and their mechanisms: a prospective study. Med Sci Sports Exerc 15:267–270
7. Torstveit MK, Sundgot-Borgen J (2005) The female athlete triad: are elite athletes at increased risk? Med Sci Sports Exerc 37:184–193
8. Sundgot-Borgen J, Torstveit MK (2007) The female football player, disordered eating, menstrual function and bone health. Br J Sports Med 41(Suppl 1):i68–i72
9. Stewart IM (1960) Jones fracture: fracture of the base of fifth metatarsal. Clin Orthop 16:190–198
10. Jones R (1902) Fractures for the base of the fifth metatarsal bone by indirect violence. Ann Surg 34:697–700
11. Pritsch M, Heim M, Tauber H et al (1980) An unusual fracture of the base of the fifth metatarsal bone. J Trauma 20(6):530–531
12. Richli WR, Rosenthal DI (1984) Avulsion fracture of the fifth metatarsal: experimental study of the pathomechanics. Am J Roentgenol 143:889–891
13. Kavanaugh JH, Brower TD, Mann RV (1978) The Jones fracture revisited. J Bone Joint Surg Am 60: 776–782
14. Byrd T (1992) Jones fracture: relearning an old injury. South Med J 85:748–750
15. Anderson EG (1990) Fatigue fractures of the foot. Injury 21:275–279
16. Pecina M, Bojanic I, Smoljanovic T et al (2011) Surgical treatment of diaphyseal stress fractures of the fifth metatarsal in competitive athletes: long-term follow-up and computerized pedobarographic analysis. J Am Podiatr Med Assoc 101(6):517–522
17. Bluth B, Eagan M, Otsuka NY (2011) Stress fractures of the lateral rays in the cavovarus foot: indication for surgical intervention. Orthopedics 34(10): e696–e699
18. Lee KT, Kim KC, Park YU, Kim TW, Lee YK (2011) Radiographic evaluation of foot structure following fifth metatarsal stress fracture. Foot Ankle Int 32(8):796–801
19. Goulart M, O'Malley MJ, Hodgkins CW et al (2008) Foot and ankle fractures in dancers. Clin Sports Med 27(2):295–304

20. Monteleone GP Jr (1995) Stress fractures in the athlete. Orthop Clin North Am 26(3):423–432
21. Thevendran G, Deol RS, Calder JD (2013) Fifth metatarsal fractures in the athlete: evidence for management. Foot Ankle Clin 18(2):237–254
22. Gehrmann RM, Rajan S, Patel DV et al (2005) Athletes' ankle injuries: diagnosis and management. Am J Orthop (Belle Mead NJ) 34(11):551–561
23. Brockwell J, Yeung Y, Griffith JF (2009) Stress fractures of the foot and ankle. Sports Med Arthrosc 17(3):149–159
24. Hetsroni I, Nyska M, Ben-Sira D, Mann G, Segal O, Maoz G, Ayalon M (2010) Analysis of foot structure in athletes sustaining proximal fifth metatarsal stress fracture. Foot Ankle Int 31(3):203–211
25. Torg JS, Balduini FC, Zelko RR et al (1984) Fractures of the base of the fifth metatarsal distal to the tuberosity: classification and guidelines for non-surgical and surgical management. J Bone Joint Surg Am 66:209–214
26. Acker JH, Drez D (1986) Non-operative treatment of stress fracture of the proximal shaft for the fifth metatarsal (Jones fracture). Foot Ankle 7(3):152
27. Brukner P, Bennell K, Matheson G (1999) Stress fractures. Blackwell Science, Champaign, pp 178–181
28. Clapper MF, O'Brien TJ, Lyons PM (1995) Fractures of the fifth metatarsal. Analysis of a fracture registry. Clin Orthop Relat Res 315:238–241
29. Lawrence SJ, Botte MJ (1993) Jones fractures and related fractures of the proximal fifth metatarsal. Foot Ankle 14(6):358–365
30. Sammarco GJ (1993) The Jones fracture. Instr Course Lect 42:201–205
31. Strayer SM, Reece SG, Petrizzi MJ (1999) Fractures of the proximal fifth metatarsal. Am Fam Physician 59(9):2516–2522
32. Zogby RG, Baker BE (1987) A review of nonoperative treatment of Jones' fracture. Am J Sports Med 15(4):304–307
33. Polzer H, Polzer S, Mutschler W et al (2012) Acute fractures to the proximal fifth metatarsal bone: development of classification and treatment recommendations based on the current evidence. Injury 43(10):1626–1632
34. DeLee JC, Evans JP, Julian J (1983) Stress fracture of the fifth metatarsal. Am J Sports Med 11(5): 349–353
35. Dameron TB (1975) Fractures and anatomical variations of the proximal portion of the fifth metatarsal. J Bone Joint Surg Am 57:788–792
36. Weinfeld SB, Haddad SL, Myerson MS (1997) Metatarsal stress fractures [review]. Clin Sports Med 16(2):319–338
37. Zelle BA, Gollwitzer H, Zlowodzki M, Bühren V (2010) Extracorporeal shock wave therapy: current evidence. J Orthop Trauma 24(Suppl 1):S66–S70
38. Kesani AK, Gandhi A, Lin SS (2006) Electrical bone stimulation devices in foot and ankle surgery: types of devices, scientific basis, and clinical indications for their use. Foot Ankle Int 27(2):148–156
39. Bergfeld J (2004) FIMS/ISAKOS consensus meeting on Ankle Sprains, Hong Kong, Sept 2004
40. Vertullo CJ, Glisson RR, Nunley JA (2004) Torsional strains in the proximal fifth metatarsal: implications for Jones and stress fracture management. Foot Ankle Int 25(9):650–656
41. Lee KT, Park YU, Young KW et al (2011) Surgical results of 5th metatarsal stress fracture using modified tension band wiring. Knee Surg Sports Traumatol Arthrosc 19(5):853–857
42. Popovic N, Jalali A, Georis P et al (2005) Proximal fifth metatarsal diaphyseal stress fracture in football players. Foot Ankle Surg 11(3):135–141
43. Murawski CD, Kennedy JG (2011) Percutaneous internal fixation of proximal fifth metatarsal fractures (zones II and III) with Charlotte Carolina screw and bone marrow aspirate concentrate: an outcome study in athletes. Am J Sports Med 39(6):1295–1301
44. Ekstrand J, van Dijk CN (2013) Fifth metatarsal fractures among male professional footballers: a potential career-ending disease. Br J Sports Med 47(12):754–758
45. Khan WS, Agarwal M, Warren-Smith C (2005) Management of fractures of the base of the fifth metatarsals distal to the tuberosity. Foot 15:141–145
46. Josefsson PO, Karlsson M, Redlund-Johnell I et al (1994) Jones fracture. Surgical versus non-surgical treatment. Clin Orthop Relat Res 299:252–255
47. Porter DA, Duncan M, Meyer SJ (2005) Fifth metatarsal Jones fracture fixation with a 4.5mm-cannulated stainless steel screw in the competitive and recreational athlete: a clinical and radiographic evaluation. Am J Sports Med 33(5):726–733
48. Shah SN, Knoblich GO, Lindsey DP et al (2001) Intramedullary screw fixation of proximal fifth metatarsal fractures: a biomechanical study. Foot Ankle Int 22(7):581–584
49. Habbu RA, Marsh RS, Anderson JG et al (2011) Closed intramedullary screw fixation for nonunion of fifth metatarsal Jones fracture. Foot Ankle Int 32(6):603–608
50. Wright RW, Fischer DA, Shively RA et al (2000) Refracture of proximal fifth metatarsal (Jones) fracture after intramedullary screw fixation in athletes. Am J Sports Med 28(5):732–736
51. Larson CM, Almekinders LC, Taft TN et al (2000) Intramedullary screw fixation of Jones fractures: analysis of failure. Am J Sports Med 30(1):55–60
52. Beck BR, Matheson GO, Bergman G, Norling T, Fredericson M, Hoffman AR, Marcus R (2008) Do capacitively coupled electric fields accelerate tibial stress fracture healing? A randomized controlled trial. Am J Sports Med 36(3):545–553
53. Benazzo F, Mosconi M, Beccarisi G et al (1995) Use of capacitive coupled electric fields in stress fractures in athletes. Clin Orthop 310:145–149
54. Brand JC, Brindle T, Nyland J et al (1999) Does pulsed low intensity ultrasound allow early return to normal activiites when treating stress fractures? A review of one tarsal navicular and eight tibial stress fractures. Iowa Orthop J 19:26–30

55. de Albornoz PM, Khanna A, Longo UG, Forriol F, Maffuli N (2011) The evidence of low-intensity pulsed ultrasound for in vitro, animal and human fracture healing. Br Med Bull 100:39–57
56. Shindle MK, Endo Y, Warren RF, Lane JM, Helfet DL, Schwartz EN, Ellis SJ (2012) Stress fractures about the tibia, foot, and ankle. J Am Acad Orthop Surg 20(3):167–176
57. Furia JP, Rompe JD, Cacchio A, Maffulli N (2010) Shock wave therapy as a treatment of nonunions, avascular necrosis, and delayed healing of stress fractures. Foot Ankle Clin 25(4):651–662
58. Griffin XL, Smith N, Parsons N, Costa ML (2012) Ultrasound and shockwave therapy for acute fractures in adults. Cochrane Database Syst Rev 2:CD008579. doi:10.1002/14651858.CD008579.pub2
59. Mc Bryde AM (1996) Stress fractures of the foot and ankle. In: De Lee JC, Drez D (eds) Orthopaedic sports medicine. Saunders, Philadelphia, pp 1970–1977
60. Kroening PM, Shelton ML (1963) Stress fractures. Am J Roentgenol 89:1281–1286
61. Linz J, Conti S, Stone D (2001) Foot and ankle injuries. In: Fu F, Stone D (eds) Sports injuries. Lippincott, Williams & Wilkens, Philadelphia, pp 1152–1153
62. Puddu G, Cerulli G, Selvanetti A, De-Paulis F (1998) Stress fractures. In: Harries M, Williams C, Stanish WD, Micheli LJ (eds) Oxford textbook of sports medicine. Oxford University Press, Oxford/New York, p 663
63. Campbell G, Warnekros W (1983) Tarsal stress fracture in a long distance runner. A case report. J Am Podiatry Assoc 73:532–535
64. Davis AW, Alexander IJ (1990) Problematic fractures and dislocations in the foot and ankle of athletes. Clin Sports Med 9:163–181
65. Fitch KD, Blackwell JB, Gilmour WN (1989) Operation for non union of stress fracture of the tarsal navicular. J Bone Joint Surg 71(B):105–110
66. Hulkko A, Orava S, Peltokallio P et al (1985) Stress fracture of the navicular bone. Nine cases in athletes. Acta Orthop Scand 56:503–505
67. Orava S, Karpakka J, Hulkko A et al (1991) Stress avulsion fracture of the tarsal navicular. An uncommon sport related overuse injury. Am J Sport Med 19(4):392–395
68. Towne LC, Blazina ME, Cazen LN (1970) Fatigue fracture of the tarsal navicular. J Bone Joint Surg 52A:376–378
69. Helstad PE, Ringstrom JB, Erdmann BB (1996) Bilateral stress fractures of the tarsal navicular with associated avascular necrosis in a pole vault. J Am Podiatr Med Assoc 86(11):551–554
70. Khan KM, Brukner PD, Kearney C et al (1994) Tarsal navicular stress fractures in athletes. Sports Med 17(1):65–76
71. Alfred R, Belhobek G, Bergfeld JA (1992) Stress fractures of the tarsal navicular. A case report. Am J Sport Med 20(6):766–768
72. Coris EE, Kaeding CC, Marymont JV (2003) Tarsal navicular stress injuries in athletes. Orthopedics 26(7):733–737, quiz 738-9
73. Lee S, Anderson RB (2004) Stress fractures of the tarsal navicular. Foot Ankle Clin 9(1):85–104
74. Torg JS, Pavlov H, Cooley LH et al (1982) Stress fracture of the tarsal navicular. A retrospective review of twenty-one cases. J Bone Joint Surg 64(A):700–712
75. Khan KM, Fuller PJ, Brukner PD et al (1992) Outcome of conservative and surgical management of navicular stress fracture in athletes. Am J Sport Med 20:657–666
76. Sizensky JA, Marks RM (2004) Imaging of the navicular. Foot Ankle Clin 9:181–209
77. Ariyoshi M, Nagata K, Kubo M et al (1998) MRI monitoring of tarsal navicular stress fracture healing – a case report. Kurume Med J 45(2):223–225
78. Kiss ZA, Khan KM, Fuller PJ (1993) Stress fractures of the tarsal navicular bone: CT findings in 55 cases. Am J Roentgenol 160:111–115
79. Mann G (2000) Stress fractures. In Doral MN (ed) Sports injuries. Arthroscopy and joint surgery, current trends and concepts, Ankara, p 307
80. Richardson EG (1999) Hallucal sesamoid pain: causes and surgical treatment. J Am Acad Orthop Surg 7(4):270–278
81. Boike A, Schnirring-Judge M, McMillin S (2011) Sesamoid disorders of the first metatarsophalangeal joint. Clin Podiatr Med Surg 28(2):269–285
82. Biedert R, Hintermann B (2003) Str ess fractures of the medial great toe sesamoids in athletes. Foot Ankle Int 24(2):137–141
83. McBryde AM (1989) Stress fractures in runners. In: D'Amrosia R, Drez D (eds) Prevention and treatment of running injuries, 2nd edn. Slack, Thoroughfare
84. Orava S, Hulkko A (1988) Delayed unions and nonunions of stress fractures in athletes. Am J Sports Med 16:378–382
85. Golding C (1960) Museum pages V: the sesamoids of the hallux. J Bone Joint Surg 42B:840–843
86. Mann R (1978) Surgery of the foot, 4th edn. CV Mosby CO, St. Louis, pp 122–125
87. Biedert R (1993) Which investigations are required in stress fracture of the great toe sesamoids? J Orthop Trauma Surg 112(2):94–95
88. Burton EM, Amaker BH (1994) Stress fracture of the great toe sesamoid in a ballerina: MRI appearance. Pediatr Radiol 24:37–38
89. Orava S (2003) Uncommon stress fractures and their treatment principles. Instructional course on stress fractures, ICL no. 19, ISAKOS Congress March 2003, Auckland
90. McBryde AM, Anderson RB (1988) Sesamoid foot problems in the athlete. Clin Sports Med 7:51–60
91. Anderson RB, McBryde AM (1997) Autogenous bone grafting of hallux sesamoid nonunions. Foot Ankle 18:293–296
92. Hulkko A, Orava S, Pellinen P et al (1985) Stress fractures of the sesamoid bones of the first metatarsophalangeal joint in athletes. Arch Orthop Trauma Surg 104:113–117
93. Peterson L, Renstrom P (2001) Sports injuries. Martin Dunitz, London, p 421

94. Perez-Carro L, Echevarria-Llata JI, Martinez-Agueros JA (1999) Arthroscopic medial bipartite sesamoidectomy of the great toe. Arthroscopy 15(3):321–323
95. Hetsroni I, Mann G, Dolev E, Morgenstern D, Nyska M (2005) Base of fourth metatarsal stress fracture: tendency for prolonged healing. Clin J Sport Med 15(3):186–188
96. Saxena A, Krisdakumtorn T, Erickson S (2001) Proximal fourth metatarsal injuries in athletes: similarity to proximal fifth metatarsal injury. Foot Ankle Int 22(7):603–608
97. Rongstad KM, Tueting J, Rongstad M, Garrels K, Meis R (2013) Fourth metatarsal base stress fractures in athletes: a case series. Foot Ankle Int 34(7): 962–968
98. Black KP, Ehlert KJ (1994) A stress fracture of the lateral process of the talus in a runner. A case report. J Bone Joint Surg Am 76(3):441–443
99. Umans H, Pavlov H (1995) Insifficiency fracture of the talus: diagnosis with MR imaging. Radiology 197(2):439–442
100. Cline AD, Jansen GR, Melby CL (1998) Stress fractures in female army recruits – implications of bone density, calcium intake and exercise. J Am Coll Nutr 17:128
101. Okada K, Senma S, Abe E, Sato K, Minato S (1995) Stress fractures of the medial malleolus: a case report. Foot Ankle Int 16(1):49–52
102. Orava S, Karpakka J, Taimela S, Hulkko A, Permi J, Kujala U (1995) Stress fractures of the medial malleolis. J Bone Joint Surg Am 77(3):362–365
103. Shabat S, Mann G, Constantini N, Elyakim A, Shenkman Z, Nyska M (2002) Stress fractures of the medial malleolus in athletes. The 18th international Jerusalem symposium on sports medicine., March 2002. www.sportsmedicine.co.il
104. Lempainen L, Liimatainen E, Heikkila J, Alonso J, Sarimo J, Mattila K, Orava S (2012) Medial malleolar stress fracture in athletes: diagnosis and operative treatment. Scand J Surg 101(4):261–264
105. Shabat S, Sampson KB, Mann G, Gepstein R, Eliakim A, Shenkman Z, Nyska M (2002) Stress fractures of the medial Malleolus. Review of the literature and report of a 15-year-old elite gymnast. Foot Ankle Int 23(7):647–650
106. Kor A, Saltzman AT, Wempe PD (2003) Medial malleolar stress fractures. Literature review, diagnosis, and treatment. J Am Podiatr Med Assoc 93(4):292–297
107. Finestone & Lavon. Israel medical Corps. Command. Instruction no. 09:01, June 2006
108. Steckel H, Klinger HM, Baums MH, Schultz W (2005) Beidseitige Stressfraktur des Malleolus medialis [Bilateral stress fracture of the medial malleolus]. Sportverletz Sportschaden 19(1):41–45
109. Wilson ES Jr, Katz FN (1969) Stress fractures. An analysis of 250 consecutive cases. Radiology 92(3): 481–486
110. Mayer SW, Joyner PW, Almekinders LC, Parekh SG (2014) Stress fractures of the foot and ankle in athletes. Sports Health 6(6):481–491
111. Imerci A, Incesu M, Bozoglan M, Canbek U, Ursavas HT (2012) Bilateral calcaneal stress fractures: a case report. Ortop Traumatol Rehabil 14(5): 477–481
112. Pearce CJ, Zaw H, Calder JD (2011) Stress fracture of the anterior process of the calcaneus associated with a calcaneonavicular coalition: a case report. Foot Ankle Int 32(1):85–88
113. Miki T, Miki T, Nishiyama A (2014) Calcaneal stress fracture: an adverse event following total hip and total knee arthroplasty: a report of five cases. J Bone Joint Surg Am 96(2):e9
114. O'Malley MJ, Hamilton WG, Munyak J, DeFranco MJ (1996) Stress fractures at the base of the second metatarsal in ballet dancers. Foot Ankle Int 17(2): 89–94
115. Micheli LJ, Sohn RS, Solomon R (1985) Stress fractures of the second metatarsal involving Lisfranc's joint in ballet dancers. A new overuse injury of the foot. J Bone Joint Surg Am 67(9):1372–1375
116. Brunker P, Bennell K, Matheson G (1999) Stress fractures. Blackwell Science Asia, Carlton, pp 175–178
117. Harrington T, Crichton KJ, Anderson IF (1993) Overuse ballet injury of the base of the second metatarsal. A diagnostic problem. Am J Sports Med 21(4):591–598

New Trends in Rehabilitation

37

Stefano Della Villa, Francesco Della Villa,
Margherita Ricci, and Stefano Respizzi

37.1 Introduction

The evolution and the increasing interest in sport medicine have been powerful drives to improve the state of art in many aspects, from basic science through diagnosis, treatment, rehabilitation and return to sport.

The rehabilitation concept has widely evolved in the last decades, progressively embracing new concepts, focusing on the optimisation of the recovery process.

Orthopaedic and sports rehabilitation is now a new frontier of medicine in which clinical and organisational aspects have to coexist to optimise patient functional outcome.

The aim of this chapter is to describe the scientific background and the new trends in rehabilitation strategy.

S. Della Villa (✉) • F. Della Villa • M. Ricci
Isokinetic Medical Group,
FIFA Medical Centre of Excellence,
Via Casteldebole 8/4, 40132 Bologna, Italy
e-mail: s.dellavilla@isokinetic.com;
f.dellavilla@isokinetic.com;
m.ricci@isokinetic.com

S. Respizzi
Humanitas Research Hospital,
Via Manzoni 113, 20089 Rozzano, MI, Italy
e-mail: stefano.respizzi@humanitas.it

37.2 Scientific Background (From "Protection-Oriented" Rehabilitation to Functional Recovery)

The history of rehabilitation has been marked by several phases. We have to deeply analyse them to really understand where we are now.

The typical examples of this broad evolution are the anterior cruciate ligament (ACL) injury and postsurgical management.

In the early 1980s, a defensive strategy of rehabilitation predominated with long periods of immobilisation and no weight-bearing. This approach used to give rise to a series of very common complications, such as arthrofibrosis, permanent range of motion (ROM) deficit, delay in strength recovery and anterior knee pain [1].

In 1990, Shelbourne et al. [2] showed that *accelerated rehabilitation* with immediate recovery of knee extension, early weight-bearing and quadriceps strengthening led to faster recovery and better results. Even though the accelerated strategy after ACL reconstruction is still under debate, a new era of rehabilitation had begun.

In 1996, Dye [3] gave another significant contribution to the optimal recovery after knee surgery. His holistic approach is to consider the knee joint as an "envelope of function", in which different structures play a fundamental role in maintaining the joint homeostasis. The muscular and neuromuscular control assumed a decisive role to ensure system stability.

P. Volpi (ed.), *Football Traumatology: New Trends*, DOI 10.1007/978-3-319-18245-2_37

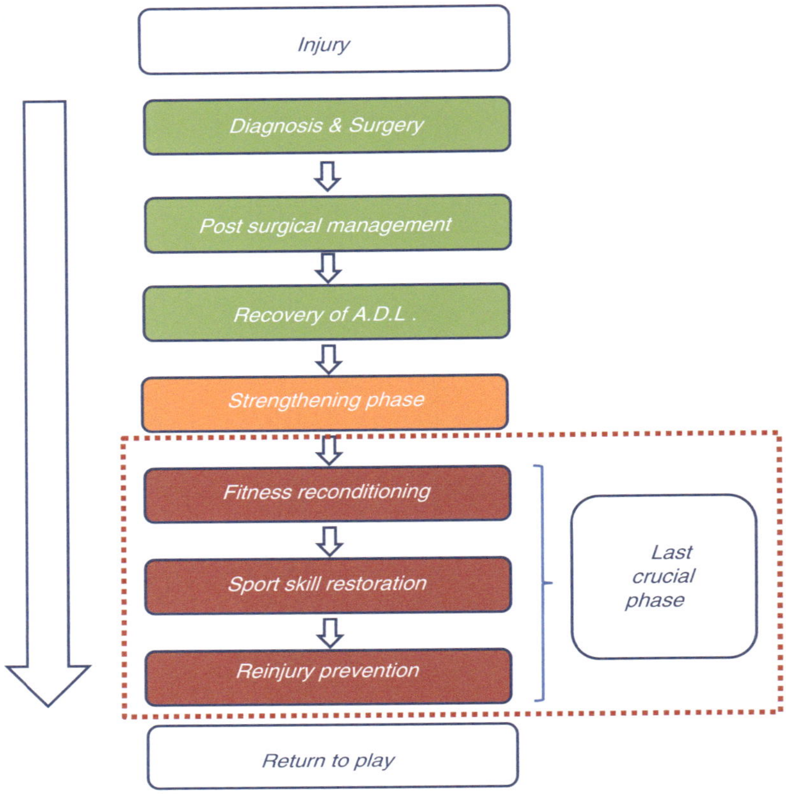

Fig. 37.1 From injury to return to play. The recovery pathway consists of three main phases. New trends may be addressed to the last one, which is the most challenging

This new perspective highlighted the fact that recovery time and loading progression were not strictly fixed by biological considerations but that timing depended on the stimuli given to the healing functional tissues.

According to this point of view, a rehabilitation strategy based on progression through *clinical and functional criteria*, instead of fixed time, started to gain popularity. In the early 2000s, Kvist et al. [4] formalised this approach and clarified the concept that certain criteria should be reached before allowing the patient to return to sport.

Nowadays, it is widely accepted that an accelerated rehabilitation protocol leads to important advantages without affecting knee stability [5]. Plus the scientific community is focusing on different aspects of human kinetics and on how certain *movement patterns*, involving the whole kinetic chain, may play a crucial role in functional recovery [6].

Through more than 30 years, there has been a progressive shift from "protection-oriented" to "functional-oriented" protocols.

37.3 Crucial Principles

We'd like to introduce our vision starting from the very beginning: the injured player. At the time of injury, our focus is on the lesion, trying to get the diagnosis and plan the treatment as soon as possible. The situation is different; in fact, we have to consider that making the correct diagnosis is only the first step of a long recovery process that goes from the injury to the return to play (Fig. 37.1).

Together with the Football Medicine Community, we assume to have a perfect control of the first phases and a pretty good control of the strengthening phase. Unfortunately, there is often an insufficient control of the last phases, when the goal is almost reached. We always have to remember that the last phases are important, both to really reach a complete recovery and for preventing re-injuries.

For this reason, we should change the classical medical paradigm, moving *from the lesion to the recovery*, embracing also fitness reconditioning, football skill restoration and re-injury prevention in the rehabilitation process.

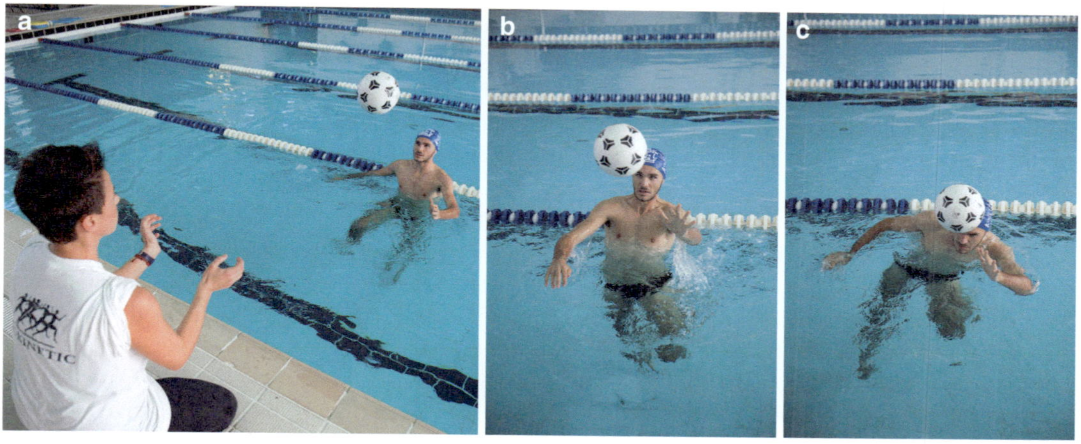

Fig. 37.2 Neuroplasticity exercises in the pool. (**a**, **b**, **c**) Different moments of football-specific heading exercises performed in the early phase of the rehabilitation

In other words, we should have the *complete control of the whole recovery process.*

In order to reach this challenging goal, we suggest the same sports medicine team to follow the player from the injury to the first official match.

37.4 Rehabilitation Strategy

As stated in the introduction, one of the main aspects of a successful rehabilitation is having a proper organisation. So we suggest a strategy based on three fundamental points including *the facility, the team and the method.*

In order to complete the rehab pathway of a football player, we surely need a proper facility consisting of *medical offices, rehabilitation gyms, rehabilitation pools and sport fields.* The use of these suitable areas at well-defined moments is critical for the best functional outcome.

Regarding the pool, the water environment allows the early introduction of sport-specific movement patterns, such as kicking or heading in football (Fig. 37.2). These exercises will be proposed again in the later phases, both in the gym and on the field, creating a sort of continuum. This approach is thought to favour the motor scheme reeducation. In fact, after the trauma, there may be a process of joint de-efferentation and central disorganisation. The early introduction of some complex stimuli is recommended to solve neuromuscular impairments.

The rehab gym is still considered the main rehabilitation area. Apart from the classical ROM and strength exercises, it is useful to introduce more neuromuscular exercises, considering not only the affected joint but also the whole kinetic chain and the biomechanical connection among different joints.

According to our philosophy, we have to progressively introduce sport-specific gestures on real sports field, to better restore player's self confidence in a supervised environment. The on-field rehabilitation (OFR) offers three main advantages: the complete recovery of specific movement patterns, metabolic reconditioning and a real education in prevention strategies.

Regarding the sports medicine team, we think it should be at least made by *a sport medicine physician, a physical therapist* and *a conditioning specialist.* They are supposed to follow together the player from the injury to the official return to play.

The last key point of a good strategy is having a working method shared by the team. According to our philosophy, the physician should act as the "case manager". He/she is in charge of controlling the process, from the beginning to the end, communicating regularly with the orthopaedic surgeon, coordinating the team around the patient and planning a customised protocol. Having a good and fluent communication model within the team is also mandatory to be successful. A frequent clinical update is important to constantly monitor patient's improvements and solve eventual complications. In fact, the strength of a sport medicine group has to be measured in the management of difficult cases, when logistical and clinical skills are required.

37.5 Criteria-Based Rehabilitation

The general feeling in the scientific community is that rehabilitation should be based on criteria progression, rather than on predefined times. Certain clinical and functional pitfalls have to be satisfied to safely progress in the recovery process.

According to literature, the goal of any criteria-based guideline is to maximise the patient response to exercise while minimising the risk of re-injury [7]. This approach is widely described about rehabilitation after ACL reconstruction [4, 5, 7–9]. Some authors individuated in *quadriceps strength*, *functional testing* and *patient-reported outcome scales (KOS-sport, IKDC2000)* [7] the best criteria to be fulfilled before returning to sport. Even if it is generally requested a limb symmetry of 90 %, we strongly suggest to aim to the 100 %. Only a few authors described a comprehensive protocol based on strict criteria to progress within the different phases, from the earliest to the latest [4]. A similar strategy is also applied in rehabilitation after articular cartilage repair [10]. Authors underline the importance of defined milestones to pass from one phase to the next. The criteria role is emerging also in other areas of sport traumatology. Heiderscheit et al. proposed a similar progression model in the hamstring injuries rehabilitation; objective criteria were individuated to progress through the three periods [11].

The described approach (without fixed times) is the only one that allows to build up a truly customised rehabilitation protocol. Basing on the literature and on our own philosophy, we advise to use this kind of mind setting in many different clinical situations. This can be done only if a perfect control of all the clinical and logistic factors is achieved. The real challenge still remains in identifying and respecting the stated criteria.

To better describe this new trend, we published papers showing our personal protocol following ACL reconstruction (ACL-R) and autologous chondrocytes implantation (ACI) in football players and other active patients [9, 12].

Our protocol is based on the so-called traffic lights concept. Predefined functional goals are allowed only if specific clinical and functional criteria are previously satisfied so that the time is a secondary issue. We individuated four functional goals (*(1) walk without crutches*, *(2) run on a treadmill*, *(3) start supervised OFR*, *(4) return to the team)* and their respective criteria (Fig. 37.3). This is the protocol we daily adopt for a wide variety of knee surgical patients, but the same model could be used for every kind of pathology.

For example, regarding recovery after ACL-R, we depicted and published data about timing. In a selected population of 50 footballers, patients were able to walk without crutches after 29 ± 8 days, run on the treadmill after 76 ± 26 days, start OFR after 90 ± 26 days and return to the team after 148 ± 36 days (4.9 months). The mean time to return to the first official match was 185 ± 52 days (6.2 months) [9].

Regardless from the clinical issue you are dealing with, we believe that the key of successful recovery is maintaining the balance between *biological healing* of the injured tissue and *functional recovery* of the patient. We know that biological maturation of tissues may take time, while functional recovery is faster and may help the tissue regeneration. A crucial example is the recovery of knee full extension (FE) after ACL-R. It is mandatory to reach the FE as quickly as possible, without affecting the graft healing [2].

37.6 Return to Sport Philosophy

According to what we previously described, we let the athlete to return to sport only if the criteria are completely satisfied and the light is "green". In order to allow a better comprehension of the issue, we will present you a case after ACL-R (Fig. 37.4). In the scheme, we present the same patient at different moments of his recovery process, focusing

Criteria based isokinetic rehabilitation protocol

1) Walk without crutches

- Knee full extension (as the controlateral)
- Absence of,or minimal (NRS<3) pain and intraarticular effusion
- Recovery of correct gait cycle

2) Run on a treadmill

- No pain during walking (NRS<3)
- Active knee flexion >120°
- Proper muscle tone of trunk, thigh and leg muscles

3) Start on field rehabilitation

- Strength: ≥80 % vs controlateral limb at the knee isokinetic test
- Being able to run on a treadmill at 8 km/h for at least 10'

4) Return to the team

- No giving way episodes
- Complete ROM
- Complete recovery of strength (100% at the isokinetic test)
- Complete metabolic recovery (reference values for sport level at the threshold test)
- Complete OFR
- Movement pattern restoration (≥ 90 pts at the movement analysis test)

Fig. 37.3 Traffic light concept. The four functional goals (walking, running, on-field rehab, return to the team) are permitted only when all the respected criteria are satisfied (*NRS* numeric rating scale, *ROM* range of motion, *OFR* on-field rehabilitation)

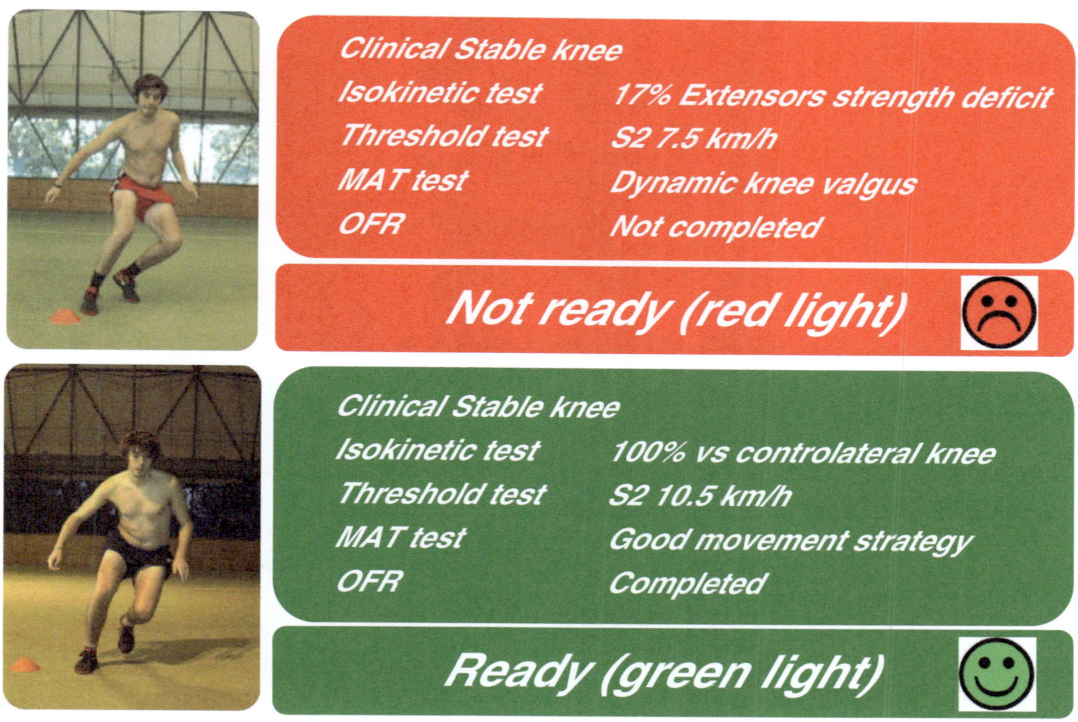

Fig. 37.4 To play or not to play. (**a**) The patient presents several impairments; certain criteria are not satisfied yet. So the patient is not allowed to return to sport. In the figure, we can observe a dynamic knee valgus in the cut manoeuvre. (**b**) The patient solved the impairments and he is now allowed to return to the team. In the figure, we can appreciate a better lower limb movement strategy

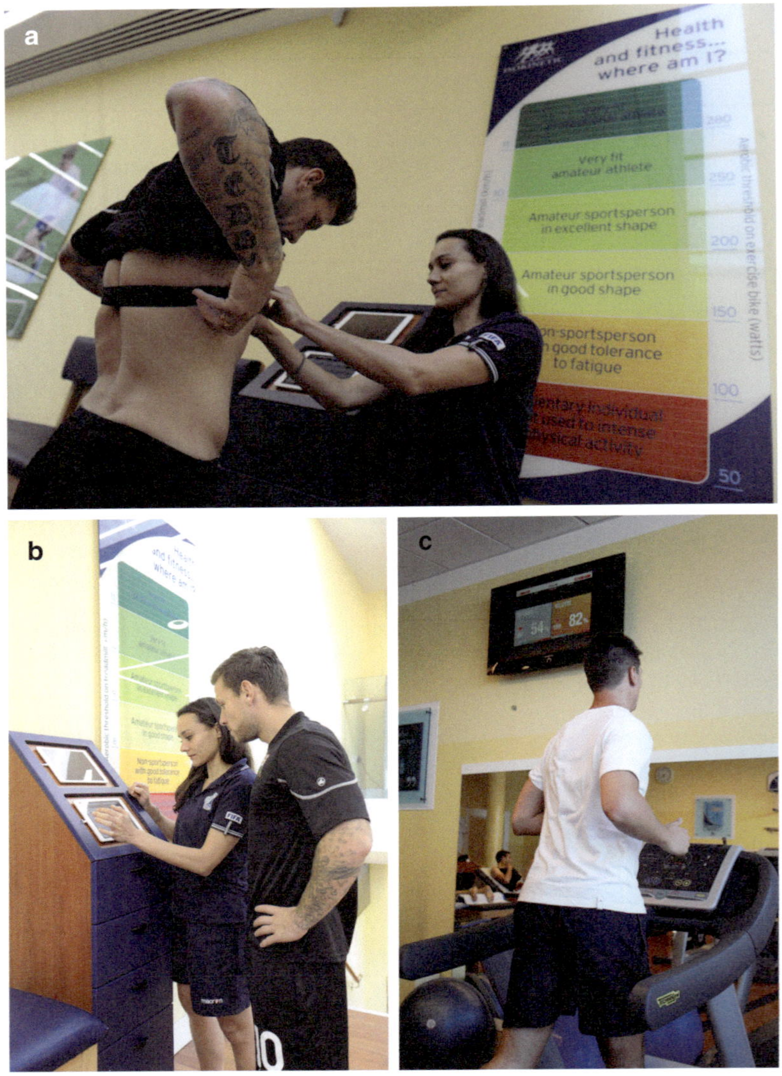

Fig. 37.5 Heart rate monitoring. (**a**) The patient wears the heart rate (HR) monitor. (**b**) The physiotherapist explains the system to the patient. (**c**) The visual feedback of the actual HR level is helpful in maintaining the desired threshold activity

on the ability to either pass or not the return to sport criteria. Considering only the knee stability is no more accepted. Many factors, evaluated through objective measurements, play a key role in ensuring a safe and effective return to sport.

Recovery of muscular strength is certainly a milestone in rehabilitation, both in the literature and in our experience. It is mandatory to reach the symmetry between the two limbs (for knee patients, we adopt 100 % both for extensor and flexor strength) evaluated with the isokinetic test. In case of strength deficit, the test must be repeated until the complete recovery.

Metabolic recovery also plays a role and has to be considered because fatigue leads to a potential risk of re-injury. We suggest checking aerobic and anaerobic lactate thresholds through specific tests. Customised threshold training is subsequently proposed to guarantee a proper metabolic reconditioning, and a continuous monitoring of the heart rate permits a tailored work on patient's thresholds (Fig. 37.5).

Movement pattern restoration, together with football-specific gestures, needs to be pursued. We know that specific movement patterns are frequently associated with a certain type of injury

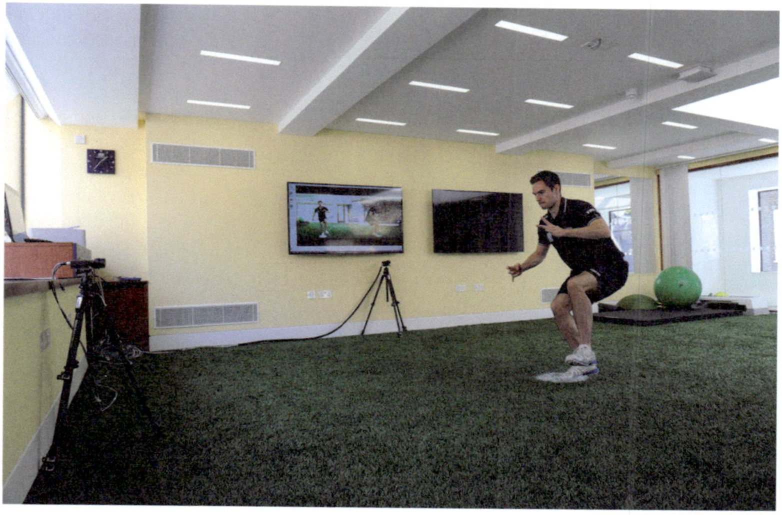

Fig. 37.6 Movement patterns evaluation. Example of a possible setting for biomechanics assessment and movement strategy biofeedback

(e.g. mild knee valgus and ACL injury [13]). These dangerous patterns have to be avoided in order to reduce the re-injury rate. Patients presenting with some kind of movement impairments need to be pro-habilitated to a more correct movement strategy. This is the main reason why we suggest to use a sport-specific movement analysis test (MAT). Plus the use of video technology during rehabilitation sessions allows a continued biofeedback helping the patient to restore proper biomechanics (Fig. 37.6). So, logistically, an *on-field rehabilitation programme* should be completed. The protocol needs to be progressive in terms of loading, complexity of the proposed exercises and velocity of the agility drills. Moreover, it should be focused on the whole athlete biomechanics. Regarding the duration of the OFR, it mainly depends on the clinical issue. We suggest 1 week OFR programme for partial meniscectomy, 5 weeks for ACL-R and 10 weeks for cartilage repair.

Prevention and psychological aspects are other "key topics" in the modern rehabilitation landscape. The prevention concept needs to be early introduced in the recovery process; there may be a continuum of interventions aimed to re-injury prevention (secondary prevention), from the first specific intervention in the pool to the more specific neuromuscular programmes (e.g. FIFA 11+) to be performed on the field. The programmes may be really effective in primary prevention, with a reduction up to 30 % of injuries, in case of maximal compliance to the programme [14]. Indeed a correct prevention education of the injured athlete is mandatory. Psychological factors have been already studied; it seems that both fear (fear of re-injury, kinesiophobia and other kinds of fear) and innate personality traits play a role in the return to sport decision [15]. We have to always remember that as Bruce Reider said one time: "sound mind, sound body" [16]. You cannot deal only with a joint, neither with a kinetic chain; you have to relate with the patient. With this assumption, it is easy to understand that a higher attention to this aspect may influence the final functional outcome.

The criteria philosophy is the natural evolution of sport rehabilitation, derived from the logical statement that objective parameters have to be measured to assess the readiness of the athlete.

Conclusions

Orthopaedic and sports rehabilitation is a unique branch of medicine. The progressive introduction of new technologies brought, is bringing and will bring great improvements in patient's outcome and perception of the proposed exercise. The bravery to use and implement new approaches, never forgetting the biological basis and timing of the tissue healing, will take the sports medicine community to the new era of rehabilitation.

References

1. DeHaven K, Cosgarea A, Sebastianelli W (2003) Arthrofibrosis of the knee following ligament surgery. Instr Course Lect 52:369–381
2. Shelbourne KD, Nitz P (1990) Accelerated rehabilitation after anterior cruciate ligament reconstruction. AJSM 18(3):292–299
3. Dye SF (1996) The knee as a biologic transmission with an envelope of function: a theory. Clin Orthop Relat Res 325:10–18
4. Kvist J (2004) Rehabilitation following anterior cruciate ligament injury: current recommendations for sports participation. Sports Med 34(4):269–280
5. van Grinsven S et al (2010) Evidence-based rehabilitation following anterior cruciate ligament reconstruction. Knee Surg Sports Traumatol Arthrosc 18(8):1128–1144
6. Hewett TE, Di Stasi SL, Myer GD (2013) Current concepts for injury prevention in athletes after anterior cruciate ligament reconstruction. AJSM 41(1):216–224
7. Adams D et al (2012) Current concepts for anterior cruciate ligament reconstruction: a criterion-based rehabilitation progression. JOSPT 42(7):601–614
8. Myer GD et al (2006) Rehabilitation after anterior cruciate ligament reconstruction: criteria-based progression through the return-to-sport phase. JOSPT 36(6):385–402
9. Della Villa S et al (2012) Clinical outcomes and return-to-sports participation of 50 soccer players after anterior cruciate ligament reconstruction through a sport-specific rehabilitation protocol. Sports Health 4(1):17–24
10. Mithoefer K et al (2012) Current concepts for rehabilitation and return to sport after knee articular cartilage repair in the athlete. JOSPT 42(3):254–273
11. Heiderscheit BC et al (2010) Hamstring strain injuries: recommendations for diagnosis, rehabilitation, and injury prevention. J Orthop Sports Phys Ther 40(2):67–81
12. Della Villa S et al (2010) Does intensive rehabilitation permit early return to sport without compromising the clinical outcome after arthroscopic autologous chondrocyte implantation in highly competitive athletes? AJSM 38(1):68–77
13. Alentorn-Geli E et al (2009) Prevention of non-contact anterior cruciate ligament injuries in soccer players. Part 1: mechanisms of injury and underlying risk factors. KSSTA 17(7):705–729
14. Soligard T (2008) Comprehensive warm-up programme to prevent injuries in young female footballers: cluster randomised controlled trial. BMJ 337:a2469
15. Tjong VK (2014) A qualitative investigation of the decision to return to sport after anterior cruciate ligament reconstruction: to play or not to play. AJSM 42(2):336–342
16. Reider B (2007) Sound mind, sound body. AJSM 35(12):1995–1996

Publisher's Erratum to: Injuries of the Lateral Collateral Ligament and Posterolateral Corner of the Knee

Andrea Campi and Stefano Campi

Erratum to:
Chapter 15 in P. Volpi (ed.), Football Traumatology: New Trends
DOI:10.1007/978-3-319-18245-2_15

The affiliation of the corresponding author, Andrea Campi and the co-author Stefano Campi was incorrect. It should read as follows:

Andrea Campi
Department of Orthopaedic Surgery
Azienda Ospedaliera San Giovanni - Addolorata
Rome, Italy
e-mail: and.campi@gmail.com

Stefano Campi
Università Campus Bio-Medico, Rome, Italy
e-mail: stefano.campi@gmail.com

The online version of the original book can be found under
DOI:10.1007/978-3-319-18245-2_15

P. Volpi (ed.), *Football Traumatology: New Trends*, DOI 10.1007/978-3-319-18245-2_38

MIX
Papier aus verantwortungsvollen Quellen
Paper from responsible sources
FSC® C105338

FSC
www.fsc.org

If you have any concerns about our products,
you can contact us on
ProductSafety@springernature.com

In case Publisher is established outside the EU,
the EU authorized representative is:
Springer Nature Customer Service Center GmbH
Europaplatz 3, 69115 Heidelberg, Germany

Printed by Libri Plureos GmbH
in Hamburg, Germany